HEALING

with the Herbs of Life

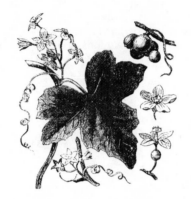

LESLEY TIERRA

L.Ac., Herbalist, AHG

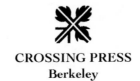

CROSSING PRESS

Berkeley

Copyright © 2003 by Tierra, L. Ac.
Illustrations by Akiko Shurtleff

All rights reserved. Published in the United States by Crossing Press, an imprint of the Crown Publishing Group, a division of Random House, Inc., New York.
www.crownpublishing.com
www.tenspeed.com

Crossing Press and the Crossing Press colophon are registered trademarks of Random House, Inc.

Library of Congress cataloging-in-Publication Data

Tierra, Lesley.
    Healing with the herbs of life / Lesley Tierra.
  cm.

    Includes bibliographic references and index
  Herbs – Theraputic use. 2. Medicine – Formulae, receipts and
    prescriptions. I. Title.

HD653.H632002
656.1'1'021 – dc21   2002165187

ISBN-13: 978-1-58091-147-4 (pbk.)

Printed in the United States

Cover design by Nancy Austin
Text design by Brad Greene

13 12 11 10 9 8

First Edition

IN THANKS...

Many people helped me bring this book into sharper clarity and purpose. I give my warmest thanks and appreciation:

All of my patients and students over the years, from whom I've learned much; Michael Tierra, for his constructive input; Ben Zappa, for his expertise, invaluable advice and technical input; Marjorie Wolfe, for her domestic and technical support; and all my apprentices for their teachings and constructive insights: Jen Holding, Dov Shoneman, Lauren Ruby Miller, Shala Pullvermacher, Rasa Amster and Susie Norris.

Many thanks to those who helped with the original version of this book, *The Herbs of Life*:

Michael Tierra, my first and greatest herb teacher, from whom I am always learning more; Shasta Tierra for her tremendous enthusiasm and wonderful insights; Holly Eagle, Christopher Hobbs and Roy Upton who gave so generously of their time and expertise; Steve Blake for his ideas and clarity; Mariah Wentworth and Candis Cantin for their encouragement and support; John Gill for his openness and belief in me for writing this book; Baba Hari Dass and the Sri Ram Foundation for their unending inspiration; Senta Tierra for her unflagging support with the household; Richard and Mary Jane Gunsaulus, for their warm hospitality that supported me while writing part of this book; Chetan Tierra for sharing his mom with the computer!

TABLE OF CONTENTS

INTRODUCTION

Healing with the Herbs of Life

After over 20 years of practice, I'm still continually amazed at the effectiveness of herbs and the wisdom of Traditional Chinese Medicine (TCM). More and more people seeking alternative medicine experience healing results with herbs when nothing else works. Consequently, the last decade has exploded with herbal information and new herbals, all essentially summarizing these two small words: *herbs work*.

Today, many people want to prove this scientifically. Studies regularly occur (particularly in Germany) to isolate a plant's components and investigate their effects. While providing much useful information, such studies essentially validate the traditional uses of those plants known for thousands of years. The resulting message is loud and clear: *it's time to trust nature again*.

For the last several years, I've seen a need to update my own book, *The Herbs of Life*. I wanted to enlarge the herbal section to encompass the greater range of herbs popularly known and used now. Further, because my own clinical work and herbal teaching center around educating and empowering people to care for themselves, I wanted to emphasize its self-healing focus. I feel it's important to not just help people heal, but to also teach them how their own body-mind-spirit complex works (from the viewpoint of energetic herbalism) so they can stay well and prevent disease.

The result is this herbal, *Healing with the Herbs of Life*. In it I've added a new and quite large chapter, *The Treatment of Specific Conditions*, increased the section on herbs (*Materia Medica*) and expanded several other chapters. Lastly, I've rearranged the sections, added a few more therapies, and addressed the contemporary issues of herbal safety and herb/drug interactions.

As I walk around my house and the neighboring roads, I see herbs everywhere—walnut trees shading the yard, dandelions covering the lawn, horsetail lining the creek, coltsfoot dotting the woods—the list is endless. If you'd take a look about your own home, you'd be amazed at how many surrounding plants are used as medicine. Purple coneflower decorating your garden, honeysuckle climbing your trellis, basil flavoring your pesto, chrysanthemum lining your window box, plantain cracking your sidewalk, jack-in-the-pulpit peeking through your woods, carnations scenting your bouquet, all are used as herbal medicines. Even cities are living concrete jungles harboring healing "weeds" such as plantain, comfrey, red clover, calendula, borage, rosemary, ginkgo, yarrow, chamomile and mint.

Take a look for yourself. Put on "nature eyes" and go for a walk. Search for plants wherever you live, work, drive, jog or eat. Soak in the vivid colors, inhale the fragrant odors, touch the rich textures. Then ask yourself, does this plant have any healing uses? More likely than not, it does, even if undiscovered yet. With all of nature's vast richness, there is still more to unfold and learn. Join in this treasure hunt and learn nature's secret for yourself: *herbs work and it's time to trust nature again*.

FOREWORD

By Michael Tierra, L. Ac., O.M.D.

The practice of herbalism can be defined as the systematic use and application of herbs and related materials for the purpose of healing. We find evidence of various systems and approaches to the use of herbs throughout ancient and native cultures of the world. *Healing with the Herbs of Life* shows how we in the West can benefit from the great herbal traditions of China and India which, as it turns out, are not unlike our own prior to the 18th century and the advent of so-called scientific rationalistic thought.

By offering a practical approach to the classification of the therapeutic properties of herbs and foods, this book integrates Eastern and Western approaches into a kind of Planetary Herbalism. Through a renewed appreciation of traditional "energetic" systems, especially Chinese herbal medicine, this allows us to go beyond the overly simplistic "this for that" approach so characteristic of many popular herbals.

It is at this point that one might ask what is meant by an energetic approach to healing and classifying herbs for medicine, and how or to what degree does it differ from the predominant Western medical model? To begin with, the Western medical model, which is often imitated by inexperienced herbal practitioners in a kind of "allopathic" herbalism, focuses almost exclusively on relieving the primary symptom of the patient. The traditional wholistic herbalist treats not only the primary symptom, but the underlying causes which precipitate it.

Healing with the Herbs of Life takes this second approach—recommending herbs and other foods which tend to strengthen underlying deficiencies as well as clear the body of toxic wastes. The reader will discover the true healing power of herbs and foods with absolutely no risk of the insidious long-term side effects of many, if not most, Western drugs.

Implied in this work is the belief that the essential principles and methods of traditional herbal medicine are capable of being understood and utilized not only by the professional health practitioner, but also by the lay public. Herbalism has been sometimes called "the simpler's art". This is to identify its common bond with folk practice based upon empirical evidence of "what works". This is in contrast to scientific medical knowledge which is primarily derived from research and laboratory experiments. With the present crisis in medicine and health care in the orthodox profession, its increasing exclusivity in terms of cost and availability, the side effects and risks of medical drugs and procedures, it is no wonder that natural medicine, especially herbal medicine, is on the rise.

Finally, this book invites the reader to share the experience of an herbalist, healer and teacher in the process of furthering the integration of the ancient healing wisdom of the East with the West as we evolve towards a more global awareness. Through this process, it is hoped that the reader will feel empowered to further continue to explore on his or her own the beautiful world of herbalism.

PART I
Herbal Fundamentals

CHAPTER 1
The Nature of Energetic Herbalism

❧

One night my husband and I visited a family party where we danced and enjoyed ourselves out on a deck full of people. I had my shoes off. As the night wore on, the dance floor became even more crowded and suddenly, my foot was impaled by a spike heel from a woman dancing a bit too close. The pain felt excruciating. Not only could I no longer dance, but also walking was out of the question. A perfect square indentation marked my foot and it instantly began bleeding, bruising and swelling.

Quickly looking around, my husband noted a tree overhanging the deck and climbed into its first branches where he picked several leaves. He chewed them into a pulp and spit them out, creating a poultice that he placed on my wound. Within ten minutes the pain decreased by 50% and in a half-hour I could walk by myself. We replaced the poultice with another, one or two more times that night, and by morning not only could I walk normally, but also hardly a sign of the wound remained. I was impressed!

This experience is one of many I've had proving over and over the powerful and practical healing ability of plants. In this case, leaves from an oak tree healed my wound. Oak leaves are high in tannins that relieve pain and promote wound healing. Yet, many other plants could have worked. The chlorophyll in plant leaves (creating their greenness) is extremely healing to wounds.

Combining the simple knowledge of making a poultice with the awareness of the healing abilities of green leaves, my wound was immediately treated, right there on the dance floor. There was no need to wait until getting home to locate something or someone to help me, or to suffer through several days of pain and debilitation before it slowly healed on its own, risking a possible infection.

Knowing basic herbal information like this helps many people tremendously. It is this useful practical wisdom which I desire to pass along and make available to more folks. Have you ever wondered what the plants and "weeds" growing around you are good for? Or has it ever occurred to you that the very thing you need for your sleep, cough or cold might be in your very own yard, or the local herb shop? There is a veritable pharmacy for most of our ailments right at our fingertips once we learn how to use them.

Applying herbs externally, like the poultice that healed my foot, is only one of many herbal uses. For thousands of years herbs have been employed all over the world and in a myriad of ways. They are still predominantly used for healing by several major cultures, such as the Chinese, East Indian and Tibetan. Herbal medicine prevailed in the West as well until the last hundred years or so when herbs became relegated to the status of spices, or quaint "folk medicines" with little or no healing value. There are two main reasons for this: 1) the loss of a systematic method for using herbs, and 2) the advent of science with technological industries and their resulting chemical medicines.

MECHANISTIC HEALING

Originally, herbs were used in the West according to a systematic approach, called the Humour system. Promoted by Hippocrates in Greece, this system categorized each person as one of several physiological types. It likewise classified herbs and applied them for healing in a corresponding fashion. In this system, like all traditional healing systems with a theoretical foundation, the individual was evaluated, taking into account any strengths and weaknesses causing the disease. Then the effect the herbal medicine had on the organs, the person and the disease was considered. It was next matched with the cause of the individual's condition.

With the advent of materialistic thinking in the 17th and 18th centuries, due largely to Newtonian physics, a mechanistic view of nature arose. This viewpoint proclaimed that only what can be substantiated materially is reality. Extending to the human body, this way of thought sees the body as a machine governed by mechanical laws and comprised of chemical constituents. As a result, modern medicine views and treats disease separately from the person who experiences it. The disease is identified and then the common treatment for it given. Thus, everyone who receives the same diagnosis gets the same cure.

Likewise, Western herbalism turned from applying herbs according to the Humour system to using them mechanistically. Herbs are applied to treat diseases solely according to their therapeutic properties and chemical constituents. The disease is separated from the individual and a plant's components are separated from the whole plant to treat the disease.

Such an approach is based on the fallacy of isolation. It sees that one aspect of a person can be isolated and treated separately regardless of all other aspects, or that an herb's part can be used in isolation irrespective

of the rest of its components. This results in the oversimplified approach, "What is in this herb and what is it good for?" and "What herb can I use for my headache?" This simplistic method of using herbs isolates the disease from the person and the chemical aspects of an herb from its overall individual therapeutic effects.

This view of modern medicine and western herbalism found footing when substantial financial support endowed only allopathic medical schools committed to scientific research and high technological needs in the early 20th century. This occurred after a survey of herbal and medical schools at the turn of the century to determine which ones were most interested in promoting "scientific medicine," or the newly developing drug and hospital industries.[1]

As a result, 80% of the then current schools, including naturopathy, homeopathy and herbalism, closed and became relegated to the status of interesting, but ineffective, folk medicine. Yet, these same schools were the ones that promoted a systematic way of viewing individuals, diseases and herbal medicine. This shift from traditional to modern medicine taught us to think that science knows more about us than we could ever understand about ourselves. Yet, as we gain further experience with chemical medicine, we are learning that perhaps nature knows more about healing people than we can ever assume with our modern approach.

We are finding that: chemical drugs often create worse problems than the ones they solve; chemical drugs frequently only maintain a person's condition without ever healing it; when a condition is cured, the person often develops other problems later; and, this method ignores other important and essential factors involved in true healing, such as a person's emotions, family life, work, lifestyle practices, dietary habits, personal needs and satisfaction. It is only when we take

---

[1] This survey resulted in the *Flexner Report*, which was subsidized by the Carnegie and Rockefeller foundations and issued by the American Medical Association in 1910.

these last factors into account that we are truly creating a holistic healing approach.

SYMPTOMATIC VERSUS ENERGETIC HERBOLOGY

Thus, a new model for healing is needed. As we search for this new healing model, we are experiencing a resurgence of interest in the West in herbs and their healing effects. In exploring this herbal renaissance, it's important to renew our use of herbs according to a holistic model, one that evaluates every element involved in an individual's condition, takes into account all aspects of an herb's energy and then matches the herbs to the condition accordingly.

Current Western herbalism is based on pathology, isolating the disease from the person. Then herbs are given to treat the disease symptoms, just like modern medicine. For example, if we get a headache, we take willow bark. Sometimes we combine several herbs into a formula for this ailment, yet our approach is always the same: willow bark is good for headaches, therefore, if we have a headache, we take willow bark. While this frequently works, it doesn't always, for not every headache is from the same cause and thus not relieved by the same herb. It's a "hit or miss" approach—something is missing.

Traditional cultures using herbs according to a theoretical system apply them energetically. Chinese, Ayurvedic, Tibetan, Middle Eastern Unani, Native American Cherokee and some traditional African medicines are all founded on an energetic basis, although each system is different. To use herbs energetically, we look beyond the symptoms of the disease to alleviating the underlying imbalance that caused the disease. This cause varies according to each individual because all aspects of a person are taken into account, not just the disease itself.

Likewise, each herb is evaluated energetically according to all of its aspects, such as its hot or cold effects, tastes, properties, colors, growing conditions and so on. The appropriate herbs are then selected that alleviate the underlying cause of the disease. The herb's energies are matched with that of the person, the disease and its cause. Thus, rather than making the headache the main treatment focus, we look at the *person* to see what is occurring in that body to cause the headache. The *cause* for it is then treated instead of just the headache itself. In eliminating the cause, the headache goes, too.

Some causes of a headache may be 1) liver congestion, 2) stomach upset, 3) tension, or 4) weakness in the body. The cause varies according to each person's body and whatever health imbalances exist. Dandelion and feverfew ease headaches due to liver congestion; catnip relieves headaches due to stomach upset; valerian alleviates tension headaches; and cinnamon eliminates headaches due to weakness. Each of these herbs is different, yet each relieves a headache due to a unique cause. This herbal treatment approach is quite different from simply giving willow bark for any type of headache, no matter the cause or origin.

What is missing in the symptomatic method of using herbs, therefore, is that only the headache is attended while the person having the headache is completely ignored. We assume that every headache is the same and forget that because every one of us is different, each of our headaches may be due to a different cause. The symptomatic way of using herbs treats *diseases*; the energetic method treats the *person* having the disease.

In the West we understand little about how to maintain health and prevent sickness. Instead, we focus on how to treat disease. The energetic concept of medicine is even more important, therefore, because it also provides a method for preventing as well as understanding and treating the cause of complex conditions. It also redefines disease so that when some of us think we have a particular ailment, like Candida or chronic fatigue syndrome, we find we don't when looking deeper at its cause. Further, many of us experience problems that can't be identified as a known disease and so told there's nothing wrong with us, or else to seek psychiatric help instead. That's why it's important to treat the person, not the condition: when treating the person, the imbalance can be discovered and corrected; when treating the condition, often a cure doesn't exist, or our condition doesn't exist!

Modern medicine definitely has strengths, including its ability to heal mechanical injuries, such as broken bones, perform surgery and probe the micro-universe. Interestingly, it is through this last means that science is now corroborating the energetics of herbs. Learning a plant's biochemical components actually validates its previously known energetic effects and traditional uses. This deepens our appreciation of traditional plant wisdom. For example, diaphoretic herbs that open the surface of the body (causing a sweat from their volatile oils) tend to be antibiotic and antiviral in action.

While many traditional cultures around the world now adopt modern medicine, they often do so by extracting its advantages and assimilating them into their traditional medicines. For example, many hospitals in China integrate both modern and traditional medicine by using modern medicine for surgery along with acupuncture for anesthesia and herbs for recovery. Such a synthesis could be extremely valuable for us in the West.

A NEW VIEW OF HEALING

This book, therefore, is not a typical Western herbal in which herbs are described symptomatically: this herb is good for that. Rather, it teaches how to treat the whole person and the underlying imbalance. It is geared both for those who know little, if anything, about herbs and their uses, and for those who already use herbs but want to move beyond using them symptomatically to applying them energetically.

Because we look at herbs and the process of healing differently in this book, it is important to put all your preconceptions about herbs, health and healing aside before reading further. Since the principles dis-

cussed here are quite new to Western thinking, they may not fit in with any preconceived notions of health. Instead, we'll build a concept of health based upon the ancient principles used by many other cultures around the world.

To learn an energetic herbal healing system, first identify the "correct" health imbalance pattern (type of headache, for example). Then learn an herb's energy, taking into account all its various aspects. Next, match the appropriate herbs to the determined condition. A further step is to look at any dietary, lifestyle or emotional factors involved, for it's not always enough to just give the right herbs in order to effect true healing. If someone eats foods that contribute to their health problem, then these counteract the herbal healing program. Therefore, disease-causing foods need be determined and eliminated along with health-promoting foods identified and substituted. Likewise, lifestyle habits contributing to the illness need to be recognized and changed.

How herbs are used is another important element. There are many different applications for the internal and external use of herbs, such as teas, fomentations, poultices, tinctures and pills. Each one has a different purpose and effect. Obtaining the herbs, making your own remedies, or knowing how to purchase them is also valuable to learn. Thus, a basic understanding of the extent and limitation of each herbal therapy is useful.

There are three different categories of herbs: mild, strong and toxic. Herbalists mainly use mild herbs because they are nutritive, energetic and therapeutic without causing reactions or toxic effects. This is one of the values of using herbs instead of chemical medicines. While mild herbs don't compete with the strong effects of drugs, their food-like natures with complex biochemical processes affect the entire body and mind. Likewise, they don't imbalance the body, or cause reactions or other diseases. Therefore, when you find the right herb, you can use less of it and affect more areas of the body than with chemical drugs.

Holistic herbal therapy is appropriate to use in most all conditions, either by itself or in adjunct to other methods. Because most mild herbs don't interfere with chemical drugs, they can be taken to assist modern medical procedures, from surgery and hospitalization to the intake of daily medicines. Herbal therapy can thus be used in complex, serious conditions as well as in more simple situations.

When using herbal therapy to heal illness, however, we must know when it's not working and other help is needed. For acute ailments, if no improvement is noted within three days, then it may be wise to consider other approaches. For chronic ailments, if no improvement is noted within a month, then another course of treatment might be considered. Quite often, treating ourselves is difficult since we can't always see our own conditions clearly. Going to an experienced professional, such as an herbalist, acupuncturist or naturopath, can be invaluable for obtaining evaluation and an herbal healing program.

Learning to use herbs can be simple. It can also be a joyous life-long pursuit when delving into all it's complex and various aspects. On whatever level you choose to encompass herbs into your life, I'm sure you'll feel enriched and rewarded. Reclaim the ancient knowledge of regaining and maintaining your health through holistic herbal healing and empower your own healing process.

CHAPTER 2
The Energy of Herbs

Traditional cultures throughout the world apply herbs according to their energetic effects on the body. The traditional Chinese, East Indian Ayurvedic, Unani and Tibetan healing systems, the ancient Greeks and Romans, herbalists throughout Europe until the 17th century and many African and Native American tribes, especially the Cherokee, all evolved energetic healing systems mostly still in use today.

In the West, we need to start using an energetic system of healing again. Doing so employs herbs efficiently and effectively and avoids their improper application, possibly either resulting in no effect or creating an opposite and undesired effect. Learning the components that comprise the energy of an herb enables us to apply these principles to herbs we aren't familiar with, in our own area or in other places we visit while traveling.

Traditional Oriental Medicine offers a useful system because it is practical, simple and has a tradition of 5,000 years experience and application. In this system, the energy of an herb has several different aspects that work together to give the herb a unique personality and use. They also determine the conditions for which the herb is effective or ineffective. These aspects are:

- heating or cooling energy
- the five tastes
- the four directions
- Organs and meridians entered
- other energies and special properties

The first and most important aspect of an herb's energy is it's heating or cooling quality. The effects of tastes, directions, Organs, meridians and other energies all contribute to this basic heating-cooling category. All together, these components comprise an overall energetic effect. This is then termed the energy of the herb. Each herb has a different effect on the body according to these various parts which comprise its energy.

HEATING-COOLING ENERGY

Imagine how you feel lying down in an open meadow on a bright summer day. Next imagine how you feel sitting by a bubbling stream in the woods. In the sun and meadow you feel warm, while by the stream in the shade of the woods you feel cool. Similarly, the energy of an herb has the capacity to warm or cool the body.

Every herb has a heating or cooling energy that is a natural part of that herb. When we use herbs their energies cause warmth or coolness in the body. Another way of looking at it is the effect an herb has on the body's metabolism. When it causes the body's metabolism to speed up, it is heating. When it causes the metabolism to slow down, it is cooling. In the first case, we feel warmer; in the second, cooler.

Overall, the heating energy of an herb warms the body, stimulates circulation and metabolism and gives energy. Herbs with a heating, or warming, energy are used when there are symptoms of Coldness and lowered metabolism. The cooling energy of an herb cools the body, slows metabolism and clears Heat. Herbs with a cooling energy are employed when there are symptoms of Heat and hyper-metabolism.

If there is already Heat in the body, then taking a warm-natured herb creates further Heat. However, taking an herb with a cool energy clears the Heat, creating balance. Likewise, if there is Coldness in the body, taking a cool-natured herb creates more Coldness. Taking a warm-natured herb warms that coldness and creates balance. This concept is simplified, but it demonstrates how the warming and cooling energies of herbs can affect the body and how we feel.

The energy of an herb is an inherent part of the herb. It can never be changed because it was created this way, just as a dog can't become a cat, nor a flower a rock because their inner natures are what they are. Yet, it can sometimes be slightly altered to be less cool or less warm through external applications, such as warming it up in the oven, or cooling it down in the refrigerator, although its inner nature still remains warm or cool.

Warming and cooling energies are on a continuum, as in the diagram below.

Some herbs are hot, some slightly warm, others cool, some very cold and others neutral. Each herb varies in energy, yet overall the herb is either hot, warm, neutral, cool or cold. There are very few hot or cold herbs, and so warming or cooling energies are the most commonly seen.

Let's use an example. **Peppermint** is an herb that has a cooling energy. It cools the body either by causing a sweat or slowing the metabolism. Drinking hot peppermint tea may make you feel warm at first since it is heated up, however, the peppermint eventually cools the body since its energy is cooling. Drinking cold peppermint tea cools you off since the peppermint is cooling and the tea is also cold from the refrigerator. Either way, if the outside temperature of peppermint is changed, it still doesn't alter its inner cooling energy.

Now let's try an experiment to test the warming or cooling energy of herbs. First, eat a few fresh mint leaves. Now, take a big breath in and out through your mouth. Does it feel cool or warm? Mint usually creates coolness in the mouth, and it has this same cooling effect inside the body. Next, sprinkle a little **cinnamon** powder on a finger and taste it. Notice how this makes your mouth feel after you eat it. Does it feel cool and numb, or tingly and warm? Cinnamon tastes spicy and warm and its warm energy stimulates metabolism.

It's easy to feel the energy of mint or cinnamon right away, but with most herbs it takes time to feel their warming or cooling energies in our bodies. Therefore, we want to learn what the energy of each herb is before we take it so we know which effect it will have and if this is the effect we want to happen.

There are some herbs that have a neutral inner nature. This means that they are neither warm nor cool, but balanced, and so don't change the energy of your body when you take them. **Licorice** is an example. If you chew on a slice of raw licorice root, it feels neither warm nor cool. This means it has a neutral energy and won't warm or cool the body.

The best key to learning the energy of an herb is how our bodies react from it. Usually herbs that give us more energy, strength and activate our blood circulation have a warm energy. Most herbs that make us go to the bathroom, sweat or feel calm, have a cool energy.

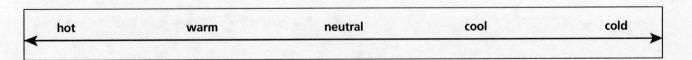

hot   warm   neutral   cool   cold

THE FIVE TASTES

The taste of an herb helps determine it's heating or cooling energy. It also gives the herb other qualities and effects that are helpful in learning more uses of the herb. In the West there are four tastes recognized, but in the Orient there are five: sweet, bitter, spicy, salty and sour. Sometimes astringent is placed in a sixth category, but essentially it belongs to the sour taste.

The various energies and tastes of herbs are assimilated into the body to nourish different Organs: the pungent taste is absorbed by the Lungs and Large Intestine; the salty taste by the Kidneys and Urinary Bladder; the sour taste by the Liver and Gallbladder; the bitter taste by the Heart and Small Intestine; and the sweet taste by the Spleen and Stomach.

The tastes may be used therapeutically. A small amount of a taste strengthens its corresponding Organs, whereas too much of the taste weakens them. For instance, a small amount of the sweet taste strengthens the Spleen and Stomach, or the digestive capacity in the body. However, too much sweet over time weakens digestion and assimilation.

Pungent

The pungent taste, also called acrid or spicy, is warm to hot in energy. It stimulates the circulation of Qi (energy), Blood, Fluids, saliva and nerve energy. The pungent taste counteracts poor digestion and circulation, feelings of coldness and mucus production. It moves energy from the inside to the outside of the body, opening the pores and promoting a sweat. Thus, it is especially useful for surface ailments such as colds, flu and mucus congestion. It also stimulates the circulation of fluid secretions and saliva. The spicy taste has a direct effect on the Lungs and Large Intestine.

Since spicy herbs are dispersing, in excess they can exhaust energy reserves, wither nails and tighten tendons, thus decreasing flexibility. Therefore, they should be used only as needed. Examples include **ginger**, **prickly ash** and **black pepper**.

Salty

The salty taste is cold in energy and stabilizes and regulates fluid balance. It also has a softening effect and so is good for hardened lymph nodes, tight muscles, constipation, hard lumps and cysts. The salty taste has a direct effect on the Kidneys, adrenals and Urinary Bladder. In fact, a craving for salt is often indicative of impending adrenal exhaustion.

In excess, the salty taste can cause water retention, high blood pressure and injure the Blood. Herbs high in mineral salts will not create the complications of excess salt in the body. All **seaweeds** are salty, and herbs such as **plantain** and **nettles**, while classified as bitter, are high in mineral salts.

Sour

The sour taste is cooling, drying, astringent and refreshing. It dries mucus and tightens tissues and muscles, thus toning them. The sour taste stops excessive perspiration, loss of fluids, diarrhea, seminal emission, spermatorrhea, frequent urination and mucus. It also stimulates digestion and metabolism and helps fat metabolism through its stimulation of bile, thus aiding their absorption. The sour taste has a direct effect on the Liver and Gallbladder, draining and expelling any Heat in those Organs.

In excess, however, the sour taste can actually harm digestion by coating the mucus linings of the stomach and intestines, thus causing poor digestion and absorption. It also toughens the flesh. Example sour herbs include **raspberries**, **blackberries**, **schisandra**, **orange peel** and lemons.

Bitter

The bitter taste is cooling, drying, detoxifying and anti-inflammatory. It stimulates the secretion of bile, which in turn sparks the digestive fires and stimulates normal bowel elimination. It also helps protect the body against parasites and clears the blood of cholesterol. As such, this taste strengthens the Heart and Small Intes-

pungent	full sweet		sour	bitter	salty
warm		neutral		cool	

tine and cleanses the Blood. Sweet cravings can be alleviated through ingestion of something bitter. It also dries Dampness and secretions, such as diarrhea, leucorrhea and skin abscesses.

In excess, the bitter taste can be too drying and eliminating, especially to the Blood and Yin, thus depleting them. It can also cause skin to wither and body hair to fall out. Example bitter herbs include **dandelion**, **gentian** and **goldenseal**.

Sweet

Perhaps the most well-known taste, sweet can actually be separated into two types: empty sweet and full sweet. Empty sweet includes simple sugars like honey, juices, sugar and sugary snacks. In small amounts honey, raw sugar and maltose can help strengthen the Spleen and Stomach, whereas in excess, they deplete energy even further, causing blood sugar to spike and dip sharply.

Full sweet includes complex carbohydrates and herbs that build, tonify, energize and nourish. The full sweet taste strengthens and builds those with weakness and lack of Qi (energy) and Blood (this is why people are so drawn to sweets when they are low in energy). Because they also satisfy the body's true craving for sweet, they directly tonify the Spleen and Stomach. However, in excess sweet produces congestion, lethargy and sedation of digestive fires. It can also cause the bones and joints to ache and hair to fall out. Example herbs with the sweet taste are **ginseng**, **red dates** and **cinnamon**.

Most herbs have two or more tastes in combination, which give them multiple uses, although usually one taste predominates. These tastes can also be used to alter the energy of an herb, or herbal combination, through their external application. For example, herbs stir-fried in vinegar have a greater effect on the Liver and are better absorbed. Stir-frying herbs in a little honey adds the sweet quality so that the herbs more strongly strengthen the digestive Organs (Spleen and Stomach). Adding salt to an herb tea helps take its energy to the Kidneys and Urinary Bladder. A small amount of a spicy herb added to a formula helps stimulate its circulation throughout the body, more quickly moving the herbs to their destination. Also, it takes the energy of the herbs to the Lungs and Large Intestine.

The diagram above gives a representation of herbal energies on a continuum from warm to cool energies.

THE FOUR DIRECTIONS

All herbs have a tendency to move in one of four directions in the body: rising or upward, sinking or downward, floating or outward, and descending or inward.

1. The *rising energy* moves toward the upper part of the body, removing obstructions and promoting circulation. Examples include **prickly ash** and **motherwort**.

2. The *floating energy* moves outward, toward the surface of the body. It disperses colds and flu, for example, and eliminates toxins through the pores of the skin. Herbs with volatile oils have this energy. Examples include **bupleurum**, **black cohosh** and **peppermint**.

3. The *sinking energy* moves downward and outward, causing elimination through the bowels or urine, activating menses and lowering fevers. Example herbs include **yellow dock**, **uva ursi** and **angelica**.

4. The *descending energy* moves inward, strengthening the inner Organs and treating the deep-level func-

tions of the body. Examples include **ginseng** and **rehmannia**.

Overall, lighter herbs, like leaves and flowers, tend to float and rise, making them effective for more acute and surface conditions like colds, flu and inflammations. Heavier herbs, such as roots, barks and seeds, tend to move inward, treating deep and chronic conditions.

The way herbs are prepared and taken also influence their directional energy. Herbs made into a tincture with wine or alcohol have a rising tendency, since alcohol itself has a rising energy. Herbs mixed with fresh ginger juice move outward to the extremities since ginger is spicy and has a floating energy. Herbs taken in vinegar sink downwards since vinegar is heavy in energy.

An herb's directional energy is used to move a formula to a particular Organ or part of the body. Further, the method of preparing herbs also has an effect upon where they are directed. For instance, adding herbs with a spicy rising energy to a formula causes it to ascend and treat the upper part of the body. Adding herbs with downward-moving energies to a formula makes it descend to treat the lower part of the body.

When treating ailments, herbs are used that have a similar movement tendency to that of the disease. For instance, if a disease is superficial and located in the outer part of the body, it is best to use rising and floating herbs that cause sweating and expectoration of mucus. For a disease in the intestinal or urinary tracts, sinking herbs with laxative or diuretic properties are appropriate. Inward-moving herbs with strengthening properties are used for internally weak Organs, such as a Deficient Spleen with poor digestion, lowered appetite, bloating and gas.

ORGANS AND MERIDIANS AFFECTED

Herbs are also defined according to the particular effects they have on one or more Organs and their associated channels and collaterals, called *meridians*

(refer to the Chapter, *Energy of Illness*, for more specifics). Herbs energetically enter specific Organs, affecting them with their unique qualities and functions. The Chinese determined these correspondences through thousands of years of observation, experimentation and knowledge of each herb's tastes, directions and functions. It is only over the last 25 years that the same assignments have been made to many (but not all) Western herbs.

HERBAL PROPERTIES

Each herb has a personality and this is its special properties. The property of an herb is its specific effect on one or more systems or general aspects of the body. For instance, herbs that clear mucus from the lungs are said to have an expectorant property, those that cause the urine to flow have a diuretic property and those that relax muscles have an antispasmodic property. Others, like **ginseng**, strengthen the energy of the entire body and so have a tonic property. Most herbs have several properties and all together they determine the unique personality of that herb. The physiological effects that the herb's biochemical constituents have on the body determine these properties.

For example, **peppermint**, **pueraria** and **ginger** are all diaphoretics. Yet, peppermint also lowers fevers, pueraria relaxes muscles and ginger aids digestion. If you want an herb to alleviate a cold, first determine what energy the diaphoretic should be, cool, warm or neutral. Then decide what additional effects are needed. If there is a cold with a fever, choose a diaphoretic herb that also lowers fevers **(peppermint)**. If there is tension, spasms or tight neck and shoulders choose an herb that is antispasmodic, too **(pueraria)**. If poor digestion, gas, bloatedness or stomachache accompanies the cold, select an herb that is carminative as well **(ginger)**. Fine tuning your herbal selection like this leads to more efficient and effective treatment, and also teaches a deeper knowledge of each herb's personality and abilities. This differentiation is part of the art of herbalism.

Since herbs have more than one effect on the body, they each have several properties. There are hundreds of terms to describe these properties, yet an understanding of the ones most frequently used is sufficient. These terms are defined as follows:

Alterative: improves or "alters" the body's ability to function, including enriching blood flow to the tissues and purifying or detoxifying blood; use for blood toxicity, infections, inflammations, arthritis, cancer and skin eruptions. Examples: **burdock root, dandelion, yellow dock, red clover, Oregon grape.**

Amphoteric: normalizes a process in the body. For example, garlic is amphoteric because it normalizes both high and low blood pressure. Examples: **garlic, vitex.**

Analgesic: relieves pain; use for any kind of pain, cramps, spasms and toothaches. Examples: **cloves, lobelia, valerian, willow bark, yarrow root, mints.**

Anodyne: powerfully relieves pain. These can be very strong and addicting. Examples: **valerian, skunk cabbage, wild lettuce.**

Anthelmintic: kills intestinal worms. Examples: **garlic, prickly ash, black walnut, wormwood, fennel, fenugreek.**

Antibiotic, antibacterial: stops the growth of, and destroys, germs, bacteria or amoebas (often working by stimulating the body's own immune response); use for infections and inflammations. Examples: **chaparral, echinacea, garlic, goldenseal.**

Antidiarrhetic: alleviates diarrhea. Examples: **blackberry root, oak bark, witch hazel, mullein.**

Anti-inflammatory: clears inflammations and inflammatory conditions. Examples: **aloe vera, eyebright, marshmallow, slippery elm.**

Antiphlogistic: counteracting inflammation; use for infections and inflammation. Examples: **echinacea, goldenseal, garlic.**

Antipyretic: lowers fever; use for fevers, infections and inflammations. Examples: **boneset, chrysanthemum, yarrow, elder, catnip.**

Antirheumatic: alleviates rheumatic conditions; use for painful conditions of the joints and muscles with inflammation and stiffness. Examples: **motherwort, prickly ash, black cohosh, boneset.**

Antiseptic: kills or prevents growth of bacteria and counters sepsis; use for wounds, cuts, sores, bites, stings and skin infections. Examples: **calendula, goldenseal, garlic oil.**

Antispasmodic: prevents or relaxes muscle spasms. Include in most herbal formulas to relax the body and allow for more rapid healing. Examples: **black cohosh, dang gui, lobelia, skullcap.**

Antitumor: prevents, or helps alleviate, tumors. Examples: **chaparral, red clover, astragalus, reishi, fu ling.**

Antitussive: helps stop coughs and coughing spasms. Examples: **coltsfoot, mullein.**

Antiviral: prevents, or helps eliminate, viral conditions. Examples: **echinacea, garlic, St. John's wort.**

Aperient: mildly causes bowel movements; use for constipation, mildly sluggish bowels. Examples: **yellow dock, Oregon grape,** bitter herbs in general.

Aromatic: having a sweet, spicy or fragrant aroma. Examples: **peppermint, fennel, cardamom, cloves, ginger, angelica.**

Astringent: dries up secretions and has a constricting or binding effect to the tissues and thus, tones tissues and muscles; use for any undesired secretions, swollen tonsils and hemorrhoids. Examples: **bayberry bark, partridgeberry, schisandra.**

Carminative: relieves gas and cramping in bowels; use for stomach pains, gas, indigestion and lack of appetite. Examples: **cumin, fennel, ginger, peppermint.**

Cholagogue: stimulates flow of bile; use for indigestion

and constipation. Examples: **goldenseal, Oregon grape root, yellow dock, gentian, dandelion root.**

Demulcent: soothes and moistens, usually with mucilage; use for Kidney and Urinary Bladder irritations, mucus membranes and inflammations. Examples: **comfrey, licorice, marshmallow, slippery elm.**

Diaphoretic: induces sweating, either by relaxing the pores, or stimulating Blood circulation to surface of body; use for colds, flu and fevers. Drink the herb teas hot for this. Examples: **basil, chrysanthemum, ginger, lemon balm, peppermint.**

Digestant: helps process of digestion; use for indigestion, feelings of stuck or congested food, overeating, gas, bloatedness. Examples: **hawthorn, pueraria, gentian, chamomile.**

Diuretic: causes and increases flow of urine; use for water retention, obesity, lymphatic swellings, edema (tissue swelling), kidney stones and bladder infections. Drink the herb tea cool for this. Examples: **parsley root, uva ursi, corn silk.**

Emetic: induces vomiting, usually when taken in larger quantities; use for food poisoning, and stomach congestion. Examples: **lobelia, licorice, peppermint, mustard, Ipecac.**

Emmenagogue: promotes, and sometimes regulates, menstruation, usually causing it to come earlier and often with increased flow; use for any menstrual and related problems; normally not used when there is excessive bleeding. Examples: **angelica, black cohosh, dang gui, mugwort.**

Emollient: softens, soothes and protects skin; use for dry and chapped skin, cuts and sores. Examples: **chickweed, comfrey, slippery elm.**

Expectorant: expels mucus from Lungs and throat; use for cough, Lung congestion, asthma and bronchitis. Examples: **coltsfoot, elecampane, mullein.**

Febrifuge: reduces fevers; an antipyretic. Examples: **honeysuckle, yarrow, boneset.**

Galactogogue: increases flow of mother's milk; use to improve nursing. Examples: **dandelion, fennel, fenugreek.**

Hemostatic: stops bleeding and hemorrhaging; use for bleeding from any body opening and for internal bleeding and hemorrhage. Examples: **cayenne, tienchi ginseng, fresh shepherd's purse.**

Hepatic: cleanses and regulates Liver function; use for Liver congestion and toxicity, side and rib pain, bitter taste in the mouth, hepatitis, jaundice, enlargement of the liver. Examples: **barberry, dandelion** root, **Oregon grape, gentian.**

Hypotensive: alleviates high blood pressure. Examples: **garlic, motherwort.**

Laxative: promotes bowel movements; use for constipation, irregularity and poor digestion. Examples: **cascara sagrada, dandelion root, psyllium seed.**

Lithotriptic: dissolves and eliminates urinary and gall bladder stones. Examples: **dandelion, parsley root, Oregon grape root, turmeric.**

Nervine: calms, quiets, nourishes and strengthens nervous system; use for nervousness, stress, restlessness, insomnia, crying and nervous tension. Examples: **lobelia, scullcap, valerian.**

Oxytocic: stimulates uterine contraction; use to assist and induce labor. Examples: **angelica, black cohosh, partridgeberry.**

Parasiticide: destroys parasites and worms in the digestive tract or on skin. Examples: **chaparral, garlic, rue, wormwood, mugwort, black walnut.**

Parturient: helps prepare uterus for childbirth during pregnancy. Examples: **raspberry, partridgeberry, black cohosh.**

Purgative: a strong laxative that causes increased intestinal peristalsis. Example: **rhubarb.**

Rejuvenative: renews body and mind, increasing quality of life and possibly counteracts effects of aging; use for premature wrinkles and gray hair, loss of body strength and endurance, senility, general debility and dryness. Examples: **American ginseng**, **aloe vera**, **he shou wu**, **reishi**.

Rubefacient: increases flow of blood at surface of the skin and produces redness where applied; use for inflammations, congestion in deeper areas, arthritis, rheumatism and sprains. Examples: **black pepper**, **cayenne**, **mustard**.

Sedative: strongly quiets nervous system; use as you would nervines and antispasmodics. Examples: **skullcap**, **valerian**, **hops**.

Sialagogue: increases flow of saliva. Example: **echinacea**.

Stimulant: stimulates Blood circulation, breaks up obstructions, increases energy and warms the body; use for coldness, menstrual cramping, painful obstructions, colds, flu, and lack of energy or vitality. Examples: **cayenne**, **black pepper**, **bayberry bark**, **cinnamon**, **ginger**, **prickly ash**.

Stomachic: promotes digestive ability; use for poor digestion, gas and lack of appetite: Examples: **codonopsis**, **elecampane**, **gentian**.

Tonic: strengthens and promotes the overall body processes, or particular Organs, to function better; use to improve any Organ or system function and to strengthen and build Qi, Blood, Yin or Yang. Examples:
> *bile tonics:* **goldenseal, Oregon grape root**
> *bitter tonics:* **gentian, citrus peel**
> *Blood tonics:* **dang gui, lycii berries, rehmannia**
> *Heart tonics:* **hawthorn, motherwort**
> *Qi (energy) tonics:* **astragalus, ginseng, jujube dates, licorice**
> *immune tonics:* **reishi, astragalus, schisandra**
> *Liver tonics:* **dandelion, fennel**
> *nerve tonics:* **skullcap, valerian**
> *nutritive tonics:* **marshmallow, slippery elm**
> *sexual function tonics:* **ginseng, damiana, epimidium**

> *Stomach tonics:* **codonopsis, elecampane**
> *urinary tonics:* **parsley, rehmannia**
> *Yin tonics:* **American Ginseng, ophiopogon, Chinese asparagus root**
> *Yang tonics:* **dipsicus, cuscuta, walnuts**

Vermifuge: expels intestinal worms. Examples: **garlic**, **wormwood**.

ALTERING ENERGIES

The energy of an herb can be altered somewhat by where it grows and how and when it is picked. These do not change the herb's inherent warm or cool energy, but can alter it slightly so that it becomes warmer or less warm, cooler or less cool than normal. For instance, herbs that grow in cold, northern climates, such as long roots or the barks of trees, tend to be more warming and building in energy. Herbs that grow in warm, southern climates, such as many fruits and flowers, tend to be more cooling and eliminating in energy.

This makes sense, as people tend to use what grows locally. People living in colder climates need herbs and foods that are heartier and warmer. Thus, the herbs that grow there tend to have a warmer energy to help warm the body in cold weather. Likewise, those living in hotter climates need herbs and foods that are more cooling and eliminating in nature. Herbs growing in hot climates tend to have a cooler energy to help cool the body in hot weather.

Herbs that grow in higher and more mountainous regions also tend to be warmer while those growing in flat lowlands near water are more cooling. These locations can make some difference in the energy of an herb, also. For instance, **dandelion** has a slightly less cold energy when grown in northern climates than when grown in southern climates.

Herbs picked in late morning after the sun rises, at noon or middle afternoon become more warming in energy. When herbs are dried in the sun (this is done quickly and with much turning of the herbs to prevent them from burning) their warming energy is also enhanced. Similarly, herbs picked in the early evening, at night or before dawn are more cooling. Herbs exposed to the cooling rays of the moon also have their cooling energies increased.

The energy of an herb can also be altered somewhat by external applications. To make an herb warmer in energy (or less cool): 1) add heat or cook; 2) cook a long time; 3) use pressure (pressure cook or use weights, as for making pickles); 4) roast; or 5) use dry. To make an herb cooler in energy (or less warm): 1) add liquid or make soupy; 2) prepare with vinegar; 3) add simple sweets such as sugar, fruit or fruit juice; 4) cook quickly; 5) use cool; or 6) use raw.

OVERALL

Putting it together, we can look at the overall qualities that give an herb its warming or cooling energy and other effects. In general, warming herbs tend to have a spicy or complex sweet taste (made up of complex carbohydrates), with more minerals. Examples include **fennel**, **elecampane**, **angelica**, **prickly ash**, **cinnamon**, **ginseng** and **astragalus**. Overall, cooling herbs have a sour, bitter or salty taste. They are more eliminating in effect. Examples include **dandelion**, **goldenseal**, **red clover** and **peppermint**.

As with everything in nature, there are exceptions to the rule. Although the pungent taste is warm in energy, there are some herbs that are pungent with a cool energy, such as peppermint and lemon balm. Similarly, though the bitter taste is cooling in energy, there are some bitter herbs with a warm energy, like **angelica** and **ginseng**. It's necessary to not be dogmatic with herbal energies. The most definite aspect of an herb that determines its energy is the final effect it has on the body. The two most important criteria for this are tastes and actions (properties), and each only serves as one determining factor.

CHAPTER 3

Herbal Fundamentals

There are many aspects to learn about herbs. Other chapters cover herbal energetics and materia medica. Here we cover plant parts and chemistry, herbal families, safety, herb/drug interactions and herbal forms, administration, formulary, processing, harvesting, preparing and storing.

PLANT PARTS

Any part of an herb may potentially be used as medicine: **root**—grows into the ground; **rhizome**—grows horizontally under the ground; **root bark**—a root's outer bark; **above ground parts**—entire herb growing above the ground—leaves, stems, seed, flowers; **bark**—bark of a tree or shrub; **twigs**—the small branches of a shrub or tree; **leaf, stem, seed, flower, fruit, vine**—these are exactly as named.

HERBAL FAMILIES

Taxonomy, the science of plant classification, groups plants according to their botanical classification, usually based upon the comparative study of their flower, fruit and leaf structures (botany is the study of plants). These groupings are ordered according to kingdom, division, class, subclass, order, family, genus, species and common name. Plants are generally identified by their genus and species (the two Latin words botanically naming a plant), much like the last (genus) and first (species) names of people. An example classification of **lemon balm** (*Melissa officinalis*) follows:

Kingdom: Plantae (plant kingdom)

Division: Magnoliophyta (the angiosperms, including flowering plants)

Class: Magnoliopsida (the dicots)

Subclass: Asteridae (gentian-aster subclass)

Order: Lamiales (mint order)

Family: Laminaceae (mint family)

Genus: Melissa

Species: officinalis

Common Name: lemon balm

Knowing these details enables herbalists to not only peg one exact herb, but also to identify commonalties between herbs sharing the same family and genus, giving hints at what possible uses other herbs in that family might have. For example, most herbs in the Rose Family (*Rosaceae*), such as **blackberry** and **agrimony**, have an effect on the intestinal tract, while many of those in the *Umbelliferae* family have a zesty flavor.

On the other hand, because Chinese **ginseng** and North American **spikenard** are both members of the *Araliaceae* family and both plants have saponins as major constituents, **spikenard** may have similar tonifying effects to **ginseng**. Further exploration in these areas could be very valuable for learning the uses of lesser known herbs of North America.

PLANT CHEMISTRY

The science and study of plant chemistry, called pharmacognosy, covers all aspects of a plant's structure, growth, reproduction, active ingredients and nutrients. The primary compounds of a plant are the elements it needs to live: vitamins, minerals, sugars, starches and so forth. Yet, plants also produce secondary compounds in small quantities that have various biological effects. These are the **chemical constituents** (or active parts) of a plant studied for therapeutic use.

When scientists began separating individual constituents and looking at them closely, they found out why plants affect the body. Further, they learned that these effects correspond to the way the whole plant is traditionally used. For instance, Digitoxin was created from a cardiac glycoside found in **foxglove**, an herb (though a poisonous one) known to regulate the heart.

Likewise, salicylic acid was extracted from **meadowsweet** to form aspirin, having the same analgesic effect as the herb does (salicylic acid is also found in **willow bark** and **poplar bark** and buds). Thus, active ingredients were separately extracted, then concentrated, to treat specific conditions. Later, these laboratories synthetically produced the drugs without using the herbs, usually changing one molecule to make the product stronger or "better" (and, of course, patentable and more expensive).

While learning chemical constituents can be very useful to scientifically determine how and why herbs work, it is not a holistic method for using herbs themselves. Keep the big picture in mind, for the territory is not the map: the isolated components are not responsible for the healing action of a plant—the whole plant is.

Herbs are a complex synergistic whole in which each of its chemical parts contributes to, or buffers, the other parts. In separating out and concentrating one active principle from the rest, this important balance is lost. Since an herb can actually be separated into hundreds, even thousands, of isolated constituents, it ultimately teaches us *less* about a plant, not more. Further, each individual constituent may have different uses on its own than when combined within the whole plant.

Therefore, only learning about herbs through their chemical constituents limits the use of an herb to the effects of that constituent rather than using its traditional broad functions. The result is possible toxic side effects and, eventually, a drug rather than a useful herb. Further, it perpetuates the symptomatic approach to treating illness rather than treating the person and his/her unique condition. Several valuable herbs are being lost to this way of thinking, which doesn't represent herbalism as a healing system.

Interestingly, those who do experience difficulty with certain plant chemicals (like pyrrolizidine alkaloids) are generally the folks with Liver imbalances, since this Organ is responsible for processing anything foreign in the body. If the Liver is imbalanced in any way, then it can't properly process chemicals and symptoms arise.

Thus, those who have Liver congestion (stagnation), Heat, or Damp-Heat (see the *Glossary* or *The Energy of Illness* for descriptions of these terms), liver diseases, or who are taking medications with liver side effects, are more susceptible to any potential issues around certain plant chemicals. Liver imbalances generally arise from long-term or excessive consumption of alcohol (including those who don't drink but are children of alcoholics), caffeine, fats, fried foods, nuts and nut butters, avocados, cheese and/or turkey, as well as taking drugs (including recreational), or having a history of hepatitis or mononucleosis.

As there are thousands of chemical constituents in plants, only the main ones are listed here. This is a brief reference and not intended to fully describe the details of plant constituents or plant chemistry (consult the *Bibliography* for further informational sources).

Carbohydrates: A carbohydrate is any form of sugar; it provides basic nutrition and energy. It appears as starch, monosaccharide, disaccharide, polysaccharide, inulin, pectin, gum and mucilage (a slippery stringy exudate that serves as a soothing and healing gel on damaged mucus membrane linings in the lungs, digestive and urinary tracts, the tissues and nerves). Gums are commonly used as stabilizers in cosmetics and foods. Examples: **marshmallow**, **comfrey**, **plantain**, **slippery elm**, **aloe vera**.

Glycosides: A glycoside is a sugar combined with a non-sugar (a-glycone) compound. Found in many combinations, they are soluble in water and alcohol. There are many types of glycosides

> *Cardiac glycosides:* These have a marked effect on the heart and increase its efficiency by increasing the force and power of the heartbeat without increasing the amount of oxygen needed by the heart muscle. These are very dangerous plants and shouldn't be used internally. Examples: **foxglove** (from which the drug, Digitoxin, is made) and **lily of the valley**.

> *Anthraquinone glycosides:* These irritate the large intestine, creating a laxative or purgative effect. They should always be combined with a carminative, like **ginger** or **fennel**, to relieve any gripping pain they can cause. Examples: **rhubarb** and **senna**.

> *Flavonoids and Flavonone glycosides:* These compounds are safe for people and animals, but toxic to microorganisms. Many are antiviral, antispasmodic, anti-inflammatory, antifungal, antibacterial, diuretic, heart and circulatory stimulants and antioxidants; Vitamins C, E and P are flavonoids. Examples: **hawthorn berries**, **raspberry**, **ginkgo**.

> *Phenols and Phenolic Glycosides:* Phenols, always carbon-based, are basic building blocks of many plant constituents and other glycosides. Some have antiseptic, febrifuge, analgesic and anti-inflammatory activities and externally, antiseptic and rubefacient properties. Examples: **clove**, **thyme**.

> *Coumarins:* There are more than 100 kinds of coumarins and they have a sweet smell (best known for their aromatic components used in perfumery) and anti-inflammatory and antibacterial properties. They are also anticoagulants, thus thinning the blood and reducing blood clots (and therefore, shouldn't be taken by those on blood-thinning medication and vice versa). Examples: **black haw**, **red clover**, **angelica**, **licorice**

> *Saponins:* These glycosides dissolve in water (water-soluble) and form lather when shaken. Saponins have a structure similar to human sex and stress hormones and so have been used in synthesizing these types of drugs. Examples: **fenugreek**, **licorice**, **sarsaparilla**, **wild yam**.

> *Other glycosides:* Others include sulfur glycosides, cyanide glycosides and furanocoumarin glycosides.

Acids: Weak acids are found throughout the plant kingdom in many forms. Acids cleanse and detoxify, astringe tissues and stimulate pancreatic and bile secretions. *Citric* and *tartaric acids*, for example, are most concentrated in unripe fruit. They stimulate saliva flow and are mildly laxative, diuretic and antibacterial. Citric acid provides vitamin C to the body whereas *oxalic acid*, found in spinach, chard and sorrel, binds with calcium, making it unavailable and ultimately causing kidney stone formation. *Salicylic acid*, found in **meadowsweet**, **willow bark**, **white poplar** and **wintergreen**, has recognized analgesic effects that were synthesized into the drug, aspirin. **Formic acid**, found in animals and plants to protect themselves, causes a temporary inflammation but easily breaks down with cooking.

Tannic acid, as its name suggests, tans leather. In small amounts, tannins are astringent, acting on protein to form protective skin on wounds and inflamed mucus membranes, thus promoting their rapid healing. Tannins are used externally for minor burns, cuts, inflammations and infections, swellings, hemorrhoids and varicose ulcers. Internally they treat diarrhea, peptic ulcers, colitis secretions and bleeding. Tannins are soluble in water, glycerine and alcohol.

Example herbs with acids: **red clover**, **yarrow**, **willow bark**, **black haw**, **blackberry**.

Alkaloids: When nitrogen isn't fully utilized by plants for protein production, it accumulates in the form of alkaloids. There are around 5,000 known alkaloids that produce diverse and profound effects. Alkaloids act on particular parts of the body, such as the liver, nerves, lungs, digestive system and especially, the central nervous system.

Usually alkalinizing and having a bitter taste, some alkaloids are anti-inflammatory and antibacterial while others are irritating stimulants, narcotics or toxic. Some are in poisonous and hallucinogenic plants, including nicotine, caffeine, morphine, opium poppy and codeine (all characterized by their -ine ending). Plants normally contain several alkaloids in combination. Alkaloids have limited solubility in alcohol and are comparatively insoluble in water. Some better known alkaloids include **indole**, **quinoline**, **isoquinoline**, **purine**, **tropane**, **pyridine**, **piperidine**, **quinolizidine** and **terpenoid alkaloids**.

One alkaloid group, **pyrrolizidine alkaloid**, causes liver blockage in humans and cancer in mice. Usually this occurs when the plant is taken in very high doses over a long period of time since this alkaloid slowly accumulates in the body. If you are uncertain how to use a plant containing PAs, then consider taking it only for short periods of time, and avoiding it altogether if pregnant, nursing, a young child, having liver disease or Liver stagnation, Heat or Damp Heat (**comfrey** and **coltsfoot** have PAs).

Example herbs with alkaloids: **Oregon grape root**, **goldenseal**, **barberry**.

Essential or Volatile Oils: As the name implies, volatile oils are unstable and easily separate from the plant to vaporize into air, especially when the plant is crushed or exposed to the sun. In various combinations these oils provide plants' rich smells, and because they permeate and travel through the body quickly and easily, they have a wide range of use. Essential oils are antiseptic, carminative, antispasmodic, anti-fungal, analgesic, febrifuge, vermifuge, sedative, diaphoretic, anti-inflammatory and/or rubefacient in action and stimulate the production and activity of white blood cells. They are also used in perfumes, aromatherapy and insect repellents. Most are soluble in alcohol and slightly soluble in water. Examples: **rosemary, thyme, mint**.

Bitter Principles: Because these substances have a very strong bitter taste, they stimulate the secretion of digestive juices and bile, thus activating digestion, bowel elimination and bile flow and increasing appetite. Bitters, as some herbal combinations have traditionally been called, are often taken before meals for just these reasons, although they are valuable after meals for indigestion. They are also antibiotic and antifungal in action. Bitter compounds are soluble in water and alcohol. Examples: **gentian, wormwood, goldenseal**.

Resins: These transparent or translucent plant secretions or excretions are usually yellowish to brown in color and sticky or gummy. Formed from oxidized volatile oils, they are expectorant, stimulating, diaphoretic and diuretic in action, and are soluble in alcohol, fixed oils and volatile oils, and insoluble in water. Examples: **myrrh, frankincense**.

Plants have other components, such as vegetable oils, vitamins, trace elements, chlorophyll, oleoresins, alcohols, acrids, latex, gelatins, lipids, enzymes and other proteins, balsams and coloring matter. The myriad aspects that comprise a plant's chemistry truly give it a unique character which, when combined with the plant's energy, properties and special qualities, yield the unique healing ability of that plant.

HERBAL SAFETY

Most herbs are mild and act like special foods in the body. With some exceptions, they lack the concentration of active biochemical ingredients that cause side effects, as do Western drugs. They also possess hundreds to thousands of constituents that counterbalance each other, making most herbs quite safe. Generally, herbs *regulate* chemical physiological imbalances, not cause adverse reactions, and when taken together in formula, they buffer any of the strong effects of one individual herb while synergistically enhancing each other's functions and purposes.

People rarely consider foods as toxic, yet when exposed to sunlight the green tuber of potatoes creates a poisonous alkaloid. Wheat, rye, barley and oats contain protein gluten that can irritate the intestines. Similarly, there are toxic herbs most people know to avoid, such as **oleander**, **hemlock** and **poison oak**, **ivy** and **sumac**. The point is that just because a few plants are poisonous doesn't mean all herbs are dangerous or unsafe. Rather, it's wise to familiarize yourself with and avoid the few toxic plants (**aconite**, **belladonna**, **foxglove**, **mandrake**, **may apple**, and **arnica** are some, though they are not commonly available, except perhaps in homeopathic remedies). Most herbs are safe to use if you heed their dosage and precaution guidelines.

Periodically, public warnings against herbs occur. These often arise either when the herb is used inappropriately, such as for the wrong intention or in excessive doses, or when the whole herb is ignored and instead only the actions of one particular constituent is investigated and condemned (and it's usually given in much higher doses than can ever be taken when consuming the whole plant). Such information can be misleading because some specimens of an herb may contain a constituent that others do not, or occur in higher amounts in one plant part versus another.

Sometimes warnings are issued before all the evidence is in, or is checked for true accuracy. For example, women with estrogen-sensitive tumors and fibroids were warned against using **dang gui** for several years because people believed it contained phytoestrogenic substances, while later studies demonstrated it doesn't after all. Another time a study pointed to the false presence of colchicine in **ginkgo**, yet it later was learned that the paper itself was flawed, as the herb doesn't contain this substance (this is actually herbal slander).

HERB STANDARDIZATION: PROS AND CONS

Many warnings actually arise from using standardized herbal extracts. This is because some of these extracts take one constituent and concentrate it to a much higher percentage than is naturally found in the plant (for instance, a **turmeric** extract containing 95% curcumin), thus displacing the herb's ratio of other naturally occurring constituents. These extracts create something different than the herb itself and thus they often have drug-like actions.

Further, when one constituent is pumped up at the expense of the others, it can create actions that aren't present in the whole herb itself (for instance, **ginkgo** taken in its whole herb form doesn't cause bleeding, but in its 24% flavoglycoside extract form it does). On the other hand, all of ginkgo's circulatory and memory-enhancing properties are based on this standardized extract, and so this is the form that should be used to treat those issues.

Thus, not only are all of an herb's uses lost, but now a different product is created that has no precedent in traditional herbal practice. While a ginkgo standardized extract is valuable in certain circumstances, this general approach can be dangerous to herbalism as a whole. Not only do such products create herbal warnings, but eventually the herb may be taken away from public use, and the more drug-like standardized product eventually be exclusively used by doctors (and become patentable). While this may seem far-fetched, it's exactly what's occurring in Europe today.

Interestingly, and perhaps most importantly, standardizing herbs doesn't always increase their effectiveness. In fact, according to herbalist and researcher, Roy Upton, tests of various herbs, like **St. John's wort** and **echinacea**, determine that the whole plant extracts containing all the herbs' compounds are more effective than their standardized extracts. To avoid these problems, some standardized products use a chemical component only as a marker, presuming that if the herb meets a certain content level of that component, the other chemical constituents will meet it as well (for instance, a **feverfew** extract that contains 2.6% parthenolides, or a **goldenseal** extract that contains 5% hydrastine). Others use standard markers in their extracts and then add it back into the whole herb (called "full spectrum"), thus buffering some of the boosted constituent's side effects and making a very potent, but safe product.

Currently, the whistle is blowing about heavy metals in herbs, particularly Chinese patent medicines. Virtually all animal products and plants (including vegetables) contain minute amounts of naturally occurring heavy metals, such as lead, mercury, cadmium, arsenic, nickel and aluminum (lead alone is in food/plant sources from petroleum by-products in the air). These don't pose a health threat unless safe levels are exceeded.

Some Chinese patents and Ayurvedic medicines do contain heavy metals usually either because minute amounts are added in *purified* form for their medicinal effects, or the herbal products are prepared in aluminum pots or with water from iron pipes. When in doubt, only purchase those products produced in the United States, or those manufactured by companies that follow GMP standards (good manufacturing practice—some of these are listed in the *Resources*).

Other Chinese patents contain small amounts of pharmaceuticals or artificial colors and flavors. Again, these can be avoided if patents are chosen from GMP manufacturers. As well, imported herbs are usually sprayed with sulfur to kill microorganisms. While a few people are highly allergic to sulfur, I have many times treated people with severe allergies who were still able to consume Chinese and other foreign herbs to their great benefit and improvement. Other patents contain endangered animal parts, and these I definitely recommend be avoided.

Overall, the majority of most readily available herbs are extremely safe for general use, particularly

Herbal Safety Guidelines

- ➴ Mild herbs are specific foods, as safe as practically any vegetable.

- ➴ Examine all the evidence on an herb rather than swallowing a little carte blanche.

- ➴ Know your sources—only purchase herbs from quality sources, companies with GMP. If an herbal product company withholds information about, or won't tell you who's in charge of quality control, search for another source.

- ➴ Be cautious when purchasing herbs that are commonly adulterated, such as **chickweed**, **plantain** and **skullcap** and make sure you obtain the correct one. Also beware of herbs that are sometimes substituted by others, such as **true unicorn** for **false unicorn**, **barberry**, **Oregon grape** or some other berberine-containing herb for **goldenseal**, or Russian **comfrey** for *Symphytum officinale* (it's more concentrated in PA's and so less desirable).

- ➴ Don't exceed given doses and heed the few herb/drug interactions.

- ➴ Read labels and doses carefully.

- ➴ Use common sense.

- ➴ Choose commonly available herbs and if you don't experience results within several weeks, stop and rethink your approach.

- ➴ Don't believe sensational claims about miraculous cures.

- ➴ Monitor yourself for reactions and discontinue use if you notice any adverse effects.

- ➴ Don't use herbs just for specific vitamin and mineral supplementation, as they have many other effects you may be unaware of.

- ➴ Only use herbs as necessary during pregnancy or lactation, or to promote those functions (such as **raspberry** for pregnancy and **fennel** for lactation).

- ➴ If you have any questions, consult a professional herbalist for guidance.

when consumed in their whole, rather than standardized, forms. When an herb has been used for thousands of years and we "suddenly" believe it's toxic, perhaps the investigation should turn to our stressful and toxin-laden lives and how this disables our bodies to handle such herbs, rather than labeling the herb itself as dangerous. In other cases, herbs cause problems because they are used improperly.

For instance, in most of the **kava kava** cases reported in Europe, the users also heavily drank alcohol, had hepatitis or a history of drug abuse, or took medications with known liver disease-causing side effects. Yet, kava kava was reported to be the cause for hepatotoxicity rather than the other factors, all of which are known to cause liver damage. In other cases, the herb is used inappropriately, such as **ephedra** (*ma huang*), a major Chinese herb for treating asthma, taken as a power pill to reduce weight and stimulate energy. This is inappropriate lifestyle usage and herbal substance abuse.

The real issue then isn't if an herb is safe or not, but the data given and how it's reviewed. It's important such information be discriminately checked for inaccuracies and true issues needing attention. Thus, don't throw the baby out with the bath water, assuming the current hype on an herb tells the whole story. This type of sensationalism is generally inaccurate and overemphasized, especially in relation to the acceptable daily consumption of known dangerous substances such as alcohol and tobacco. Further, people generally turn to herbs in the first place because they're safer than drugs. You do not have to be a professional herbalist to use herbs safely. Look at the whole picture, be informed and critically review all the data.

HERB/DRUG INTERACTIONS

As the spotlight turns on herbs more, how they affect medications (and vice versa) is now coming into focus. In general, it's safe to take most herbs while taking medications. According to herbalist Christopher Hobbs, 20 million people take herbs and drugs together with only a handful of adverse reactions reported. Many people like to study the theoretical adverse interactions between herbs and drugs and get others excited about potential problems, but most of their study results are just that: hypothetical and not actual.

In fact, I frequently see people who are on 5–10 medications (I am not exaggerating) and, with the use of herbs and diet, I am able to help these folks eliminate most, if not all, of them. To me, this is the ideal goal, and rather than looking at which herbs you should not take while on medications, you might consider which medications you won't take while on herbs.

As some herbs do have interactions with certain medications, it's wise to know about them. There are two main **red flag categories** of drugs to watch when taking herbs: **blood thinners** and **tranquilizers/antidepressants**:

Blood thinners: If you are undergoing surgery or taking any blood-thinning medications (including anti-coagulants, Warfarin, etc.), then any herb with *coumarin* should be avoided: **angelica** (*Angelica archangelica*), **prickly ash**, **red clover** and western **licorice**. Further, herbs that thin blood should be avoided, too (**garlic** and standardized **ginkgo**). However, seriously consider that if your blood needs thinning, perhaps taking a blood-thinning herb, such as red clover, might do the job without needing to use medication. If on blood thinners and you take herbs with coumarins, then have your doctor monitor your clotting time and adjust your medication appropriately.

Tranquilizers/antidepressants: Certain herbs can interact with tranquilizers and antidepressants, increasing their actions, such as **St. John's wort** or **kava**. On the other hand, these herbs can be extremely useful alternatives after eliminating these medications. Any herb with MAO inhibitors can also interfere with certain antidepressants (and anesthesia—St. John's wort has MAOs). As well, **ephedra** (*ma huang*) should never be taken while on MAO inhibitors, or it can skyrocket blood pressure.

Other: Other possible herb/drug interactions to be aware of include taking herbs that alter thyroid function (**bugleweed**, **lemon balm**, **myrrh**) if on hypothyroid medication, or herbs that interfere with interferon, such as **bupleurum**. Further, because spices, like **cayenne**, **black pepper** and **kava** speed absorption of various chemicals, including phytochemicals (since they influence how the liver processes and eliminates these substances), taking them in frequent or high doses while on medications can make drugs more potent. As well, it is wise to avoid combining herbs and drugs that have opposite effects, such as taking **astragalus** while on an immuno-suppressive medication (and vice versa).

DOSAGE OF HERBS

The proper dosage of herbs is very important. First, it's necessary to take a sufficient quantity of herbs for them to be effective. Quite often people take the right herbs or formulas but don't realize results simply because they didn't take enough of them. Most traditional herbalists give herbs in fairly high doses, while Western herbalists tend to give lower ones. On the other hand,

---

Guidelines for Taking Herbs and Medications

↳ Check the "red flag" categories of herb/drug interactions.

↳ Take herbs in formulas rather than singly.

↳ Begin herbs at low doses, then gradually increase.

↳ Take herbs and medications separately, about 3-4 hours apart.

↳ Monitor your body's response for any adverse reactions after taking herbs.

↳ Have you doctor monitor your body's response and reduce medication doses as appropriate.

↳ If you have any questions, consult a professional herbalist for guidance.

---

it's possible to take too many herbs (and supplements), for over a long period of time excessive quantities can injure digestion, eventually impairing the body's ability to metabolize food. At other times, a low dose of a formula over time can give results without any aggravating effects, especially if it contains strong-acting herbs.

How do you know which dose to use? Once you've chosen an herbal treatment plan, take the herbs for three days. If after this time you experience a positive reaction, continue your plan until your symptoms are relieved. If you don't experience any changes, increase the dose and continue for another week, then re-evaluate your condition. Sometimes subtle changes occur slowly which take time to feel. Other times you have the right herbs but need to take a higher dose for better results.

If you experience a mild negative reaction, cut down to a minimal dose (1 tablet or 10 drops tincture, 2 times/day) and continue for another 3 days. If the reaction continues, or if you experience a marked negative reaction, stop the herbs until the reactions disappear, then restart at a lower dose. If reactions recur again, you definitely know that it's the wrong herbal approach and needs re-evaluation. Don't be discouraged if this occurs. Herbal medicine is a matter of strategy and herbalists often give a test formula or treatment to see if they have the right diagnosis. If an adverse reaction occurs, this may be used diagnostically to help reveal the correct treatment plan.

The most effective form to take herbs is as teas since they assimilate easily. Yet, some herbs are too bitter to drink as teas while others are more potent in alcoholic extract form. Thus, other forms are useful, such as liquid extracts, powdered extracts, pills and tablets. Generally, most herbs are better absorbed when taken warm, either by drinking the warm teas, or by swallowing the pills, powders, capsules, tablets or extracts with warm water. This is because warm water assists their assimilation and protects digestion.

General dosages are calculated for a person weighing about 150 pounds. However, even if weighing this, each body responds differently to herbs and therefore, a particular dosage may be too high or too low for your own needs and sensitivities. As a guideline, start with the given dosage, then increase or decrease according to your body's response and size.

For **children**, a convenient rule of thumb helps determine herb dosages by calculating according to the child's body weight as compared to the adult dosage:

$$\frac{\text{Child's weight in pounds}}{150 \text{ pounds}} = \frac{\text{the fraction of the adult}}{\text{dose to use}}$$

For example, if a child weighs 50 pounds:

$$\frac{50}{150} = .33 = \frac{1}{3} \text{ of the adult dose is used for this child}$$

DOSAGE GUIDELINES

Age	Fractional Adult Dosage
0 to 1 year	$\frac{1}{10}$ to $\frac{1}{75}$ of adult dosage
2 to 6 years	$\frac{1}{8}$ to $\frac{1}{10}$ of adult dosage
6 to 12 years	$\frac{1}{4}$ to $\frac{2}{3}$ of adult dosage
15 to 70 years	Full adult dosage
Over 70 years	$\frac{1}{2}$ adult dosage

For **babies**, the same dosage rule may be used. However, the best way to treat nursing babies with herbs is to treat the mother. Any herbs mom takes go directly into her milk and then to the baby (the same is true of

GENERAL DOSAGE FOR DIFFERENT HERBAL FORMS

For those who are sensitive to herbs, start with the lower dosage and increase or decrease as appropriate. Of course, dose changes according to each herb (refer to each herb in the *Materia Medica*, for its specific dose). Dosage can be varied according to body weight, age and severity of condition (for instance, heavier bodies need a higher dosage while lighter bodies need a smaller dosage; the more severe the condition, the more herbs need to be taken).

Bulk herbs in formulas	3-9 gm ($\frac{1}{9}$-$\frac{1}{3}$ oz.)
Teas	1 oz. herbs/1 pint water; drink 1 cup, 3 times/day
Tinctures *	20-60 drops, 3-4 times/day (traditional herbalists tend to give 1 tsp., 3 times/day—depending on the herb)
Capsules	2-4 capsules, 3-4 times/day
Dry Concentrated and Freeze-dried extracts	3-5 gms., 3 times/day
Tablets/Caplets	2-6 tablets, 3-4 times/day
Patents	4-8 pills, 3 times/day (depending on patent)
Powdered Herbs	1 tsp, 3-4 times/day
Standardized Extract	Follow directions on bottle
Syrups	1 Tbsp., 3-4 times/day (every 2 hr. for acute conditions)
Compress/fomentations	1-2 times/day leaving on for 20-60 minutes
Poultices	Replenish 2-3 times/day and continue generally for 3 days
Essential Oils	Add 1-2 drops to an oil and apply locally
Liniments, salves, cremes, oils, sprays and other external ointments	As needed

*To evaporate the undesirable alcohol, boil tincture in water uncovered for 20 minutes.

any foods or substances). Use the same herbs given for baby's ailment and drink as a tea. Start with teaspoon doses at first to make sure the baby doesn't have a reaction, then increase to a cup, twice a day, if needed.

For those who cannot nurse, there are several other effective ways to give herbs to babies. A plastic eyedropper is useful for administering mild herbal teas. Squeeze a dropperful of tea into baby's mouth several times throughout the day. Keep fresh tea in dropper bottle for convenient traveling and administration throughout the day. (This is especially a good method for treating colic—try a combination of equal parts **chamomile, fennel** and **lemon balm** for this.)

Herbal baths are also very effective for treating babies and quite safe. Baby quickly absorbs the herbs' healing properties through the skin and from there into the bloodstream. This can be done 2-3 times/day until the problem is alleviated. (Fevers respond especially well to **poplar bark** bath.)

ADMINISTERING HERBS

How herbs are taken also affects their efficiency:

- Take herbs that treat the lower part of the body (Bladder, Kidneys, Intestines, genital area, lower body conditions and sometimes the Liver and Gallbladder) between and up to $1/2$ hour before meals.

- Take herbs that treat the middle of the body (Stomach, Spleen, Liver, Gallbladder and digestive disorders) with meals.

- Take herbs that treat the upper part of the body (Heart, Lungs and upper body ailments) $1/2$ to several hours after eating.

- If a diaphoretic or tonic effect is desired, take the herbal tea warm.

- When a diuretic effect is wanted, take the herbal tea cool.

- Take herbs on an empty stomach for detoxification (creates a stronger effect).

- Taking herbs before meals most effectively treats intestinal issues, tonifies and reduces fat.

- Herbs taken after meals treat gas, indigestion, lung conditions, sinus ailments and prevents mucus.

- Herbs mixed with food, or taken with a meal, are best for weak individuals, or those with poor digestion or having digestive disturbances.

- Taking herbs between meals is best for urinary and nervous disorders.

- Infants and young children respond well to herbal baths and fomentations, or to teas (add **licorice** or **slippery elm** to improve taste) when put into dropper bottle and given several dropperfuls throughout the day. Children over two may be given herbs powdered and mixed with honey to form a paste.

- Herbs with strong therapeutic actions, such as strong diaphoretics, and purgatives, should be used with great care in those with severe weakness.

- Blood-moving herbs, emmenagogues and purgatives with a strong downward action should not be used by pregnant women or during menses.

- Excessively cooling and bitter herbs should not be taken too frequently, or over a prolonged period, since they can damage digestion and injure Blood and Yin.

- Excessively Heating herbs should rarely be used in summer, while Cold herbs with strong eliminative properties should rarely be used in winter.

- For a more rapid recovery from skin diseases and disorders of the throat, vagina, rectum, lungs, eyes, ears and nose, use external applications along with internal ones, such as fomentations, gargles, douches, boluses, herbal enemas, suppositories, eye and ear drops, syrups, fomentations, poultices and herbal vapor inhalations.

- If there is an acute disease occurring at the same time as a chronic one, the acute disease should be treated first by using fewer herbs in a formula.

Small frequent doses should be taken every 1-2 hours, tapering off frequency as symptoms subside. If too many herbs are combined for acute conditions, their individual effects are weakened and effectiveness diluted. Acute diseases should show improvement within 1-3 days at most. If they don't, herbs should be re-evaluated and possibly changed.

- Chronic diseases are treated more slowly and gently with a balanced formulation given over a prolonged period of time. If treated too quickly or strongly, the body's reserves may diminish, or the body itself weaken. Combine several herbs together in a formula to temper any strong effects of one individual herb. Take larger amounts of the herbs regularly, 2-3 times/day, and last the equivalent of one month to each year since the symptoms began. Chronic diseases should show benefit within two weeks or so. If they don't, re-evaluate and possibly change your treatment approach.

- When treating illness naturally, it is important to take plenty of herbs and use several natural therapies to heal the condition. For example, if you have pneumonia, then it isn't effective to only drink three cups of herb tea a day. Instead, you also need to rest, use onion poultices on the chest twice a day, do a ginger foot bath, take an herbal syrup and herbal formula every 2-4 hours as well as drink 4-6 cups of strong herb tea per day. This may be why some people who try herbs don't feel they are effective: they didn't take enough herbs nor do enough therapies to overcome the disease.

- In general, Excess diseases are easier to cure while Deficiency conditions take longer and can be more difficult to heal (refer to *The Energy of Illness*, to understand Excess and Deficiency). This is because it is easier to eliminate too much of something than it is to build from a depleted physical state. Deficient conditions often involve more complex issues, such as healing emotional needs, work or relationship issues, or poor dietary habits. On the

other hand, prolonged Excess conditions ultimately cause Deficiency in the body because over time they deplete the body's resources and reserves. As with Deficiencies, healing then becomes harder, taking more attention, time and patience.

HERBAL FORMULARY

Herbs are very potent when taken singly, yet when combined carefully with several other herbs, they act synergistically, enhancing each other's actions, covering a broader range of application and effects and having less potential for causing side effects (since the other herbs in the formula tend to balance and soften each other's effects). For example, while taking **ginseng** alone increases energy, it can also over-stimulate and cause chest pains. Thus, it is usually combined with **licorice**, **fu ling** and **citrus** to prevent these reactions.

Creating an herbal formula is an art. To do so, first decide the formula's major thrust and desired effects. Are you clearing mucus from the lungs, nose and sinuses from a cold, improving digestion, or strengthening a weak and lethargic system with low resistance? Each of these requires different herbs and a different herbal approach.

Next, determine the energy involved in these conditions *and* in the person experiencing them. Is there Heat, Coldness, Dampness, Deficiency, Excess or stagnation, for instance? (Be sure to review *The Energy of Illness*). Then choose herbs according to the desired herbal properties, such as warming or cooling expectorants and diaphoretics in the first condition, Qi regulating carminatives in the second and Qi tonics in the third (review *The Energy of Herbs*). Now you know which herbs to choose with the specific properties indicated for that illness and the appropriate cooling or warming energies.

For instance, if a person has a cold with thick yellow mucus and a fever, then you want to clear mucus from the lungs and nose with cool expectorating and febrifuge herbs. If the person's indigestion is characterized by gas and bloating after eating with a feeling of food getting stuck or not moving well, then warming carminatives, with a few cool cholagogue herbs are chosen. Lastly, if you desire to strengthen a weak system with low energy and immunity, then combine warm energy tonics with warm, immunity-enhancing herbs.

After this is determined, deciding which herbs to combine together and their ratios and proportions is the next step. Standard guidelines exist for this and include combining herbs with main, supporting, assisting and conducting functions. Their ratios and proportions, or parts, are then decided by the function each herb has in the formula.

A part is defined as the proportion each herb has to the entire formula in either weight or volume. Main herbs generally comprise one or more parts of the formula, assisting herbs may include 1/2 to 1 part, supporting herbs usually make up 1/2 part and conduction herbs 1/4 part. The part you choose relates to the total amount that you want to make of the formula, be it weight or volume. Thus, the part can be any measurement, such as 1 ounce or one handful.

Main Herb: This category provides the major therapeutic effect desired and encompasses the bulk of the formula. Most herbs in a formula are main ones, having similar functions and treating the same area.

Supporting Herbs: These herbs support the action of the main herbs and develop their functions. They are fewer in number than the main ones and provide subsidiary effects.

Assisting Herbs: These herbs are added to treat associated symptoms and bring out the effects of the main and supporting herbs.

Conducting Herbs: A few herbs direct the other herbs to the desired location in the body, called envoys. These transport the entire herbal formula quickly so its actions aren't dissipated in the process of assimilation. Only one or two herbs in this category are included.

As an example, let's create a formula to treat a cold with thick yellow mucus in the lungs, coughing, restlessness, severe sore throat and high fever with slight chills. Such a cold is caused by Heat (from the signs of thick yellow mucus, restlessness, severe sore throat and high fever). The thrust of the formula, therefore, is to clear Heated mucus, lower fever, soothe coughing and the throat and open the surface to expel the cold.

FORMULA TO CLEAR A COLD WITH MUCUS FROM HEAT

Herb	Function	Parts	Energy
Coltsfoot	Main herb	1 part	Neutral
Mullein	Main herb	1 part	Cool
Loquat	Main herb	1 part	Cool
Yarrow	Assisting herb	1/2 part	Neutral
Honeysuckle	Assisting herb	1/2 part	Cool
Licorice	Supporting herb	1/2 part	Neutral
Lobelia	Supporting herb	1/2 part	Neutral
Raw ginger	Conducting herb	1/2 part	Warm

The main herbs, **coltsfoot**, **mullein** and **loquat**, are all expectorants, well known for their usefulness in clearing Heated mucus, alleviating cough and soothing inflamed conditions. The assisting herb **yarrow** opens the surface, causing a sweat through its diaphoretic action. In addition its anti-spasmodic effect allays cough. **Honeysuckle** is assisting because it opens the surface, lowers fevers and clears Heat toxins.

The supporting herbs, **licorice** and **lobelia**, aid expectoration of mucus, but have additional antispasmodic properties that soothe and heal inflammations. Licorice also adds a pleasant taste to the formula and harmonizes so all the herbs work better together. Lastly, raw **ginger** is included as the conducting herb because its stimulating and circulating energy opens the surface to cause a sweat and its upward energy moves the other herbs to the upper part of the body. Because only 1/4 part is included, ginger's warm energy won't aggravate the Heat condition. Further, a little warm energy helps soften the predominantly cool formula.

In general, formulas for acute conditions contain fewer herbs and most of them are main and supporting in function. This is so the formula quickly and strongly affects the acute ailment and isn't diluted by other functions. The formula is generally taken frequently, such as a cup every 2 hours or so, up to 6 cups of tea per day.

Chronic conditions are better treated with a variety of herbs that support and complement one another. Here it's important to gradually change the body's condition because energy is weak. As the chronic condition improves and the body gets stronger, it may eventually have the power to manifest the ailment as an acute disease. At this point the formula should be changed to target any acute condition that may arise (see "Healing Crisis" in *The Process of Healing)*. Formulas for chronic conditions are taken less frequently, for example, 2 to 3 cups of tea per day.

When choosing herbs, pick those that complement the formula. For instance, when a demulcent is needed in a diuretic formula, **marshmallow** is a good choice since it's also diuretic; yet in a tonic formula **licorice** is the preferred demulcent since it's not only tonic, but also harmonizes the many herbs in that formula. Likewise, when choosing an antispasmodic, **lobelia** is used for acute ailments because of its strong direct action; **valerian** is better for treating superficial chronic ailments; whereas **skullcap** is best in treating deeper and more debilitating chronic ailments affecting the nerves.

As well, balance herbs with each other in formulas. For example, if making a Blood-moving formula, then include an herb that also moves Qi, such as **citrus**, and vice versa. If making a formula that tonifies Yang, then include an herb that tonifies Yin and vice versa. This is because Qi and Blood, and Yin and Yang, are so inter-related, they enhance each other's functions. If creating a formula comprised of moistening or cloying herbs, include an herb that metabolizes Dampness, such as **fu ling** (most Qi, Blood and Yin tonics are moistening).

Balancing herbs with each other to soften, enhance or counteract their actions is another art of creating formulas. It's fine to combine heating and cooling herbs together, and some of the most power-ful formulas do this. Yet, their functions should be mutually supportive, or their energies could dilute each other. Thus, a formula should predominantly contain either warming or cooling herbs. On the other hand, if a formula's heating or cooling energy is too strong for the patient or disease, it could possibly cause a reaction. In this case add a small amount of herbs with opposing energies and actions. For example, warming **ginger** or **cinnamon** may be added to a cold formula, or cooling and soothing **marshmallow** may be added to a hot formula.

General Guidelines in Creating Formulas

- ↬ Cold purgatives, such as **rhubarb**, can cause abdominal cramping and so need a small amount of a warming carminative, such as **ginger** or **fennel**, added to counterbalance possible griping, relax the stomach and better assimilate the herbal properties.

- ↬ A formula containing many bitter herbs is balanced by adding sweet herbs, such as **licorice**, **jujube dates** and/or honey, to protect the stomach from the over-secretion of hydrochloric acid stimulated by the bitter taste.

- ↬ When using a majority of diuretic herbs, such as **uva ursi**, it's important to include some demulcents, such as **marshmallow**, to soften any irritating diuretics and ease the release of possible kidney stones.

- ↬ Add demulcent herbs to a strongly spicy or laxative herbal formula, such as **slippery elm** or **licorice**, to buffer any irritating effects.

- ↬ Adding an antispasmodic herb to formulas relieves spasms and nervous tension, enhances assimilation and helps prevent reactions to any strong effects of the formula, for instance bitter herbs possibly causing stomach upset. **Lobelia**, **valerian** and **scullcap** are commonly used this way.

PROCESSING HERBS

Many traditional medicines, such as Chinese, Ayurvedic and Tibetan, have developed methods of processing herbs to reduce toxicity, increase therapeutic effectiveness, alter energies or properties and remove any offending odors. For example, when **astragalus** is uncooked it is diaphoretic and diuretic, but when stir-fried with honey, it more directly tonifies the Spleen and Stomach and raises Qi, lifting prolapsed organs. Uncooked **dang gui** lubricates the intestines, acting as a laxative, while dang gui in wine form more strongly tonifies Blood. You may process your own herbs, or purchase them prepared from herb suppliers. Following are a few of the processing methods and their effects:

Steamed and Dried: When herbs are steamed with wine and then dried, the herb's energy becomes warmer. Example: cooked **rehmannia** (*Rehmannia glutinosa*).

Dry-Roasted: Herbs dry-roasted in a dry pan (in the oven or on the stove, while stirring constantly until slightly brown) creates a warmer energy and enhances flavor. Examples: roasted **dandelion** and **chicory** roots.

Stir-Fried: Stir-frying herbs in a wok or skillet with honey enhances moistening properties and tonification (particularly of the Spleen and Stomach). Examples: **licorice** and **astragalus**.

Spirits or Wine: Herbs soaked in grain spirits or wine increases Blood-moving, warming and ascending energies. Generally the herbs are left in the alcohol and taken in teaspoon doses 3-4 times/day as a tonic, or for rheumatic or circulatory complaints. Examples: **deer antler** and **dang gui**.

Processing with Salt: Salt added to an herbal formula enhances its descending and Kidney-tonifying energies (although omit if cleansing the urinary system).

Processing with Vinegar: Processing herbs with sour substances, such as vinegar, increases their descending and contracting energies and actions on the Liver, and helps extract alkaloids found in herbs.

Charring/Carbonizing: Charring (calcining, carbonizing) herbs is cooking them until burnt. This increases their astringency so they more effectively stop bleeding, diarrhea, dysentery and other undesirable discharges. Examples: charred **agrimony**.

HARVESTING HERBS

Harvesting, preparing and storing your own herbs is an enriching and satisfying experience. Directly working with herbs teaches invaluable information that can't be substituted by reading books. Pick herbs from your own garden as well as in fields, woods or mountains. Harvesting your own herbs is called *wildcrafting* and provides the purest and best source for making herbal medicines.

When wildcrafting, harvest plants in a manner that increases their number and perpetuates healthy plant populations. Indiscriminate harvesting practices in the past have endangered several herbs native to America, such as **goldenseal**, wild **American ginseng** and **lady's slipper**. Thus, it's important to follow ethical harvesting practices to protect the plants and their environment. Following are several guidelines for picking and processing your own herbs, whether they are wildcrafted or grown yourself:

1. **Bring along** gloves, cutting knives, shears, string and large bags to carry your harvest home. Avoid wearing hard-soled shoes that damage delicate hillside ecosystems.

2. **Choose your harvesting locations wisely.** Pick herbs far from common highways to avoid pollution and car exhaust. Harvest in areas not used by other herbalists. Don't pick herbs growing near high-tension electric wires (this may cause mutation), on lawns or in public parks that are chemically fertilized, or located downstream from mining or agribusiness, around parking lots and areas sprayed with chemicals, herbicides or pesticides. Avoid picking herbs in fragile locations and ecosystems, as one irresponsible wildcrafter can easily destroy an herbal environment.

3. **Pick herbs during their prime therapeutic state** as follows:

Roots and rhizomes: in early spring before sap rises, after seeding, in the early morning before sunshine, or in late autumn when sap returns to ground and aerial parts have died back.

Barks and root-barks: in spring or fall when they easily peel from wood.

Seeds, fruits and berries: when fully ripened and mature.

Leaves and stems: when fully matured, usually before full development of flower.

Flowers: when fully developed, scent is strong, oil content is evident and before fruiting and seeding stages.

Saps and Pitches: in late winter or early spring.

Buds: when sticky.

All plant parts: in early morning after dew dries and before noon when life force is strongest. Avoid wilted or withered plants, as they have weaker energy.

4. **Harvest herbs in such a way as to not deplete or inhibit their future growth and development.** Take only what you immediately need. Pick where there's an abundance of herbs and only take about one-third. Don't harvest the same stand year after year. You may need to tend the area by thinning, cleaning and preserving a selection of grandparent plants to seed and guard young plants. Spread any seeds to help propagation, especially when taking roots. Fill any holes you dig and cover with leaves. When harvesting leaves, don't pull the roots. Flower pruning of certain plants increases root yields as well as foliage. Keep your picking places secret so others don't crudely plunder them.

5. **Taste, but don't swallow, a plant you don't know.** Have positive identification of the plant before harvesting. Use identification keys or a specimen when necessary.

6. **When getting barks from trees**, only take longitudinal strips—never strip a complete circumference around the tree, as this kills the tree. Only pick from smaller branches.

7. **Never gather endangered or threatened plant species,** such as **goldenseal**, **American ginseng** and **lady's slipper**. Harvest no more than 10% of the native and 30% of the naturalized plant species from an area. Gather only from abundant stands. The over-harvesting of certain wild herbs has caused many to become endangered. Rather than harvesting any endangered or at-risk herbs, purchase cultivated ones. To learn more about this as well as to help protect endangered plants and locate seeds and cultivated plants, contact the organization, *United Plant Savers* (listed in the *Resources*). The following herbs are now endangered or at risk:

Endangered Herbs

American ginseng (*Panax quinquefolius*)

Black Cohosh (*Cimicifuga racemosa*)

Bloodroot (*Sanguinaria canadensis*)

Blue Cohosh (*Caulophyllum thalictroides*)

Echinacea (*Echinacea spp.*)

Eyebright (*Euphrasia spp.*)

Goldenseal (*Hydrastis canadensis*)

Helonias Root (*Chamaelirium luteum*)

Lady's Slipper (*Cypripedium spp.*)

Lomatium (*Lomatium dissectum*)

Osha (*Ligusticum porteri, L. spp*)

Slippery Elm (*Ulmus rubra*)

Sundew (*Drosera spp.*)

Trillium, Beth Root (*Trillium spp.*)

True Unicorn (*Aletris farinosa*)

Venus' Fly Trap (*Dionaea muscipula*)

Virginia Snakeroot (*Aristolochia serpentaria*)

Wild Yam (*Dioscorea villosa, D. spp.*)

Endangered in Hawaii: **Kava Kava** (*Piper methysticum*)

At-Risk (To Watch) Herbs

Arnica (*Arnica spp.*), **Butterfly Weed** (*Asclepias tuberosa*), **Cascara Sagrada** (*Rhamnus purshiana*), **Chaparro** (*Casatela emoryi*), **Elephant Tree** (*Bursera microphylla*),

Gentian (*Gentiana spp.*), Goldthread (*Coptis spp.*), Lobelia (*Lobelia spp.*), Maidenhair Fern (*Adiantum pendatum*), Mayapple (*Podophyllum peltatum*), Oregon Grape (*Mahonia spp.*), Partridgeberry (*Mitchella repens*), Pink Root (*Spigelia marilaandica*), Pipsissewa (*Chimaphilla umbellata*), Spikenard (*Aralia racemosa, A. californica*), Stillingia (*Stillingia sylvatica*), Stone Root (*Collinsonia canadensis*), Stream Orchid (*Epipactis gigantea*), Turkey Corn (*Dicentra canadensis*), White Sage (*Salvia apiana*), Wild Indigo (*Baptisia tinctoria*), Yerba Mansa (*Anemopsis californica*), Yerba Santa (*Eriodictyon californica*)

PREPARING HERBS

1. First, wash herbs gently, scrubbing roots well and rinsing barks (usually flowers, leaves and seeds don't need to be washed—instead, shake to remove bugs and dust). After washing, immediately slice roots into small pieces (they are too hard to cut when dry).

2. Dry herbs in a shaded and well-ventilated area, spreading on screens or sheets (avoid wire screens and newspaper print). It's important to keep most herbs out of sunlight or else they'll scorch and lose medicinal properties (although some barks, like **wild cherry**, may be dried in the sun to activate their medicinal properties). If plants are too close to each other, they'll mold or turn brown, losing much healing value. Don't dry too quickly. If plants contain natural oils, dry slowly to retain.

3. Herbs may also be gathered together and tied in a bundle (with a diameter no bigger than 1^1/2") near the end of the stems. Suspend upside down from a ceiling beam or wall. This allows the plant's sap to run from the stems into the leaves and flowers while drying, making those parts more potent. Hang in a well-aired, dry and shady place for several weeks, or until completely dry. All plant parts are dry when they feel brittle. You can pinch the lowest part of hanging plants to check this, or cut a sample root in half to see if the center is dry.

4. Crush and "garble" harvested herbs for easy storage (clean by removing stems and other unwanted items). Strip leaves from stems by running your hand along the stem from the top towards its bottom.

STORING HERBS

Herb potency is destroyed by heat, bright light, exposure to air and bacteria. Therefore, store herbs in well-sealed or tightly capped and dark-colored jars and containers. Place in a cool, dry place away from windows, direct sunlight, the stove or other places of high heat. Be sure to label herbs and herbal preparations with date, name of herb(s), name of preparation, if wildcrafted, organically grown or store bought, location, and any other relevant information you think necessary.

The shelf life of dried loose herbs is 1-2 years, and some parts, like barks, last much longer and even improve with age, such as **cascara bark**. Broken or crushed herbs lose potency more rapidly than whole, uncut herbs. If herbs begin to lose smell, taste and/or color, they are best used in an herbal bath rather than as medicine. Herbs bought at the store, especially if whole, should last about one year in a well-sealed jar. Herbs you harvest and dry can last 1-2 years. Herbs with strong plant oils lose potency first, while roots and barks keep medicinal energies longer.

An herbal tea keeps about three days when tightly bottled and refrigerated (when reheating, do not boil the tea). Tinctures and wines last 7-10 years. Vinegar extracts last 3 years or more if stored in a cool, dark place. Oils last up to seven years if a small amount of vitamin E or benzoin tincture is added as preservative and they're stored in tightly covered jars in a cool, dark place. Likewise, salves last for 5 years or more when properly preserved and stored in the same way. Powders last from 3 months to a year or two at most, depending on how well they are stored. Powders particularly need to be well sealed to prevent exposure to air and kept in a cool, dark place. Herbal poultices, fomentations, washes, plasters, milks, gargles, gruels and potherbs are not stored, but made as needed.

CHAPTER 4

Materia Medica

Most herbalists use a group of herbs with which they are very familiar. It may be 10, 50 or 100 herbs, but usually no more, if even that. To begin knowing herbs, it is best to choose 10-30 herbs and get to know them very well, then you can branch out and learn more. Because each herb has several uses, one can cover a wide range of conditions and situations. With time you'll find favorites and use them over and over again. To begin, first learn one herb's energy, tastes, actions, properties and indications. Then experiment with it, trying several remedies and preparations. Next, try to identify it in the wild, or plant it. If possible, observe the herb's growth patterns throughout the seasons.

Each herb has a unique personality. It has a primary property, such as causing a sweat (diaphoretic), and a secondary one, such as relaxing or calming (antispasmodic, calmative or sedative). Most herbs have several properties that together determine its unique personality. For example, **peppermint, pueraria** and **ginger** are all diaphoretics. Yet, **peppermint** also lowers fevers, pueraria relaxes muscles and ginger aids digestion. If you're looking for a diaphoretic herb to treat a cold, first determine the herbal energy needed: cool, warm or neutral. Then decide what additional actions are desired.

If a fever accompanies the cold, for instance, choose a diaphoretic that also lowers fevers (**yarrow** or **elder**). If tight neck and shoulders arise with the cold, choose a diaphoretic that is antispasmodic, too (**pueraria**). If there's poor digestion, gas, bloatedness or stomachache with the cold, select a diaphoretic that is carminative as well (**ginger** or **mint**). Fine tuning your herbal selection this way leads to more efficient treatment and deeper knowledge of each herb's personality and abilities. Such differentiation is part of the art of herbalism.

The herbs included in this materia medica are commonly used in Western, Chinese and Ayurvedic herbology. They represent a range of energies and variety of properties. Since so many Western herbs are great cleansers and eliminators (laxatives, diuretics, diaphoretics, etc.), the Chinese herbs I have included are mostly tonics because they are rarely found in Western herbalism. Effective in treating several conditions, the included herbs are basically mild and safe for general use. Most are well known and easily obtained. In fact, several can probably be found along the roads or in vacant lots near your own home, if not in your own back yard. You may also be surprised to learn that varieties of Chinese herbs grow as ornamentals in your gardens, such as "pinks" (**dianthis**), quince (**chaneomales**) and **clematis**. As well, many Chinese herbs may be purchased in stores or through the mail.

In choosing which herb to use from this materia medica, be sure to first review *The Energy of Illness*. The broad indications given for each herb need to be modified according to the illness and energy of the person you are treating. An herb that treats headaches, for instance, is not useful for every person's headache. Be sure to first identify the correct pattern (type of headache) along with its energy and then discriminate among the headache-relieving herbs to choose the appropriate one. This comes more easily with experience. As well, refer to *The Treatment of Specific Conditions*, for determining the appropriate pattern needing treatment.

Rather than listing the Western, Chinese and Ayurvedic herbs separately in this materia medica, I have integrated them. First of all, many of these herbs are used in common by all three systems and secondly, I wanted to make locating them in this book as easy as possible. Further, each herb is listed in alphabetical order according to its most frequently used name, be it common, Latin, Pin Yin or Sanskrit. While most garden enthusiasts are familiar with purple coneflower, they'd be surprised to learn it's a commonly found herb in stores, but under its Latin name, **echinacea**. Many beginning herbalists are familiar with using **coltsfoot** for coughs, but they'd rarely recognize it by the Latin name professional herbalists normally use, *Tussilago*.

Lastly, you'll notice that the term "herb" is used loosely in this materia medica, for along with plants and weeds, some foods, minerals and animal parts are included. Cultures throughout the world recognize an "herb" to be anything that heals. Iron filings, ashes, amber and scorpians are all part of the Chinese pharmacopoeia, while Ayurvedic medicine commonly employs silver, gold and honey.

A particular format is followed in describing each herb:

Most commonly used name of herb: This is the common, Latin, Ayurvedic or Pin Yin name of the herb most commonly used.

A, C, W: A means this herb is used by Ayurvedic herbalists; **C** by Chinese herbalists; and **W** by Western herbalists.

Botanical, or Latin, name: The Latin name of the herb is given; if it says "spp." after the name, it means any member of the species.

Family: This is the plant family the herb belongs to; I have used the most recent family names.

Pin Yin: If Chinese herbalists use the herb, the Mandarin (pin yin) name of the herb is given here.

Sanskrit: if Ayurvedic herbalists use the herb, the Sanskrit name of the herb is given here.

Part used: This covers what parts of the herbs are used, such as the whole herb, root, flowers or above ground part.

Energy, taste and Organs affected: The herb's energies, tastes and Organ's affected are listed here (refer to *The Energy of Illness*, for further details).

Actions: This describes how the herb affects the fundamental properties and Organs in the body (refer to *The Energy of Illness*, for more details).

Properties: These are the ways in which the herb acts on the body, such as diaphoretic (causes sweating) or antispasmodic (stops spasms); (refer to *The Energy of Herbs*, for a description of these).

Biochemical constituents: This outlines most of the herb's biochemical constituents. These are not meant to be all-inclusive or detailed, but give a general idea and further understanding of the herb (refer to *Herbal Fundamentals*, for descriptions of plant constituents and their effects).

Dose: The common dosage is given here (refer to *Herbal Fundamentals*, for information on proper herb dosages.

Precautions: These are the conditions in which you should not take the herb, along with possible warnings or side effects. Sometimes a caution is included about not using the herb with certain other herbs. This comes from the Chinese 5,000-year-old system of empirical herbalism, and is not traditional to Western herbalism.

Other: Any other important or interesting details about the herb are included here.

Indications: This summarizes the most common ailments for which the herb is used. It is not exhaustive by any means, but a quick reference and guideline.

Uses: This section provides more detailed information gleaned from the author's and other herbalists' experiences and training along with the common uses that herbal literature describes.

MATERIA MEDICA CATEGORIES

In Chinese medicine, herbs are categorized according to their shared common properties. For instance, all herbs that drain Dampness are grouped together, and the herbs that tonify Qi are classified collectively. Although each herb displays several different properties, such as **dandelion** clearing Heat and toxins and acting as a laxative and diuretic, the herb is classified according to its primary strength and use, in this case, clearing Heat and toxins. Grouping herbs this way can be very useful. First of all, it's a great way to learn the shared, but unique properties of each herb. Further, If you don't have a needed herb, you can refer to its category and quickly find the most closely matching substitute.

Because TCM and Western properties are termed differently, I have grouped them together. This enables you to learn their similarities through the different terminology, and learn further uses for the Western properties because of their TCM terms. The following TCM/Western categories include a short description of their functions, purposes and herbs from this materia medica (although some common foods are included for interest).

EXTERIOR-RELEASING HERBS release disorders lodged in the superficial layers of the body. Most are **diaphoretics** that promote sweating and peripheral circulation, while others release the muscles, or vent measles and other rashes. When releasing the Exterior, the pores of the skin open, helping push pathogens and toxins out to the surface of the body. These herbs are used for colds, flu, fevers, skin diseases, arthritis, rheumatic pains, muscular tension, edema and swelling in the upper part of the body (drain Dampness herbs are used for these in the lower body). Those who are very weak, have Deficient Blood or Yin, or have signs of physical wasting should avoid excess sweating. This category is divided into two more specific groupings:

■ **WARMS AND RELEASES THE EXTERIOR** herbs are warming, stimulating and dispersing in nature. They are used for surface Wind Cold conditions with symptoms of stronger chills and mild fever, no sweating or thirst, mild sore throat, mild headache, body aches, stiff neck, floating and tense pulse, thin white tongue coating and copious, runny white phlegm.

HERBS:

fresh ginger	ephedra
angelica spp.	magnolia flowers
cinnamon twig	sassafras

■ **COOLS AND RELEASES THE EXTERIOR** herbs are cooling and dispersing in nature. They are used for surface Wind Heat conditions with symptoms of mild chills and high fever, sweating and thirst, severe sore throat, intense headache, floating and rapid pulse, thin yellow tongue coating and thick, yellow phlegm.

HERBS:

bupleurum	pueraria
mint	lemon balm
elder	chrysanthemum
yarrow	boneset
mulberry leaves	feverfew
Chinese black cohosh	horse chestnut bark

HEAT-CLEARING HERBS treat both Exterior and Interior Excess Heat, such as inflammations, infections, high fevers, restlessness and toxins, and Deficient Heat (from Deficient Yin), like night sweats, low-grade afternoon fever, sensation of heat in palms, soles and chest, malar flush and dry mouth at night. There are five categories of Heat-clearing herbs:

■ **CLEAR HEAT AND DRAIN FIRE** herbs are **antipyretic** (anti-Fire), **anti-inflammatory** and **antimicrobial**, treating acute high fever, severe thirst, sweating and eye problems due to Wind Heat. Moistening and cold in energy, they protect against burning up body Fluids.

HERBS:

gardenia	bugleweed

■ **CLEAR HEAT AND COOL BLOOD** herbs are **demulcent** and Blood-nourishing **febrifuges** that treat more advanced stages of fevers where the fever has already burnt up the vital Fluids (Yin) and Blood, causing acute Internal Deficiency, dehydration, bleeding or hemorrhage. Thus, they treat both Excess Heat with symptoms of high fever, thirst, delirium, rapid thready pulse and dark red or purple tongue with no coating, along with Deficient Heat symptoms of low-grade afternoon fever, malar flush, night sweats, sensation of heat in palms, soles and chest and dry mouth at night.

HERBS:

raw rehmannia	marshmallow root
tree peony (moutan)	

■ **CLEAR HEAT, DRY DAMPNESS** herbs treat Damp Heat conditions with symptoms of diarrhea, dysentery and leukorrhea with burning, itching, yellowish discharge with odor, urinary tract infections, jaundice, hepatitis, boils, septicemia, eczema, herpes, ulcers, gastrointestinal tract inflammations and some fevers, like malaria. They are typically cold and bitter in energy and are strongly **antibacterial**, **antimicrobial**, **antipyretic** and **anti-inflammatory**. Taken alone, they are inappropriate for those with Coldness, Deficient Yin or Blood, emaciation and weak digestion.

HERBS:

gentian	goldenseal
barberry	Oregon grape
scute	coptis

■ **CLEAR HEAT AND TOXINS** herbs have a broad **antibiotic**, **antibacterial** and **antiviral** action, **detoxifying** and treating infectious and contagious diseases, including hot, swollen, painful swellings or sores with a fever, mastitis, pulmonary and breast abscesses, appendicitis, mumps, encephalitis and similar conditions. These are the most commonly used blood-cleansing Western herbs.

HERBS:

echinacea	red clover
burdock root	dandelion root
yellow dock	sarsaparilla
isatis	baptisia
honeysuckle	forsythia
neem	gotu kola
olive leaf	milk thistle
andrographis	chaparral
usnea	pau d'arco
chickweed	St. John's wort

■ **CLEAR SUMMER HEAT:** Summer heat is a particular acute condition arising from over-exposure to heated conditions, very similar to heat exhaustion, with symptoms of profuse sweating, fever, irritability, diarrhea, dysentery, sunburn, sunstroke, exhaustion and extreme thirst. Diuretic and antipyretic, none of these herbs are included in this materia medica, but examples include watermelon, mung beans, black soybeans and cucumber.

DOWNWARD DRAINING HERBS (LAXATIVES) increase elimination and regulate colon function by stimulating or lubricating the gastrointestinal tract and facilitating the expulsion of stools. There are three main categories:

■ **PURGATIVES** are also called "attaching" herbs because they strongly attack and dispel toxins and pathogens in the body. They treat acute or severe constipation, often accompanied by fevers, with symptoms of abdominal fullness, distention and pain on palpation, infrequent hard or dry stool, strong pulse and yellow-coated tongue. The bitter taste of these herbs stimulates the release of bile and then peristalsis.

Those herbs with a cold energy treat accumulation of Heat, and should be taken with a small amount of warming carminative herb, like **ginger** or **fennel**, to prevent griping pains. Those with a warm energy treat accumulation of Cold, and should be taken with herbs that warm the Interior. Generally, these herbs shouldn't be used during lactation, pregnancy, at the onset of menstruation, or in the weak, very young, elderly, or convalescent. Excessive or inappropriate use of these laxatives can injure the Qi. Thus, curb their use to limited periods of time.

HERBS:

rhubarb	cascara sagrada
aloe	walnut bark

■ **MOIST LAXATIVES** herbs are mild, oily, lubricating, bulk and demulcent laxatives, specific for constipation due to lack of bulk in the diet, or to Deficient Yin. They are used to counteract Dryness and lubricate the colon, allowing for easier bowel movements. Initially combine with a purgative as needed. Suitable for chronic constipation, including that of the elderly and convalescent, do not use if there is stagnant or Excess Dampness. They are safer to use during pregnancy, but caution is still advised. Of the following, only castor oil and triphala are included in this materia medica.

HERBS:

flaxseed	psyllium
marijuana seeds	castor oil
triphala	

■ **CATHARTIC LAXATIVES** are very powerful laxatives and diuretics used to treat constipation due to stagnation of Fluids in the thoracic or abdominal cavities, or to poor water metabolism. Thus, they not only purge feces, but also water, and treat pleurisy and ascites. Harsh herbs, they are generally toxic and dangerous to use (the "drastics" in Western herbalism). There are no cathartics in this materia medica, but examples include mandrake, euphorbiae, poke root and croton.

■ **DRAIN DAMPNESS HERBS** eliminate excessive fluid by draining it downward through the urinary system (kidneys and bladder) and/or helping proper fluid metabolism. Similar to **diuretics**, they treat difficult, painful or burning urination, urinary tract infections or stones, dribbling or turbid urine, lymphatic conges-

tion, clear mucus discharges, skin diseases, venereal diseases, arthritic and pneumatic complaints, edema and swelling in the lower part of the body (**diaphoretics** are used for this in the upper body). Some also purify the blood, while others lower fevers and relieve infections, including jaundice and hepatitis. Use with caution in those with Deficient Yin or Blood.

HERBS:

fu ling	nettle
dandelion leaf	parsley
plantain	gravel root
uva ursi	alisma
kava kava	coix

■ **DISPEL WIND AND DAMPNESS HERBS**, either cool **antiinflammatories**, or warm **stimulants**, dispel Wind and transform Dampness. Spasmodic pains and derangement of movement (associated with the nervous system) characterize Wind. Dampness is congestion of Fluids, primarily lymphatic fluid. Together, both cause blockage and pain in the channels and muscles resulting in arthritis, rheumatism and joint pains with accompanying swelling, pain, limitation of movement and inflammation. These herbs combine varying degrees of **diuretic, antiinflammatory, antispasmodic, diaphoretic** and **stimulant** properties. Some strengthen the tendons, ligaments and bones. Use with caution in those with Deficient Blood or Yin.

HERBS:

Western black cohosh	kava kava
mulberry branch	

■ **HERBS THAT DISSOLVE PHLEGM AND RELIEVE COUGH** are **expectorants** and **antitussives** that dissolve Phlegm in various parts of the body—the respiratory and digestive tracts, muscles and other body tissues. Symptoms include coughing, wheezing, asthma, bronchitis and other lung ailments as well as epilepsy, convulsions, scrofula, goiter, wheezing, stifling sensation in the chest, pain in the ribs, nausea, vomiting, loss of appetite, epigastric distention, wind-stroke, coma, lockjaw and contracted limbs. There are two categories:

■ **COOL AND DISSOLVE PHLEGM AND STOP COUGH** herbs cool and clear Phlegm Heat, treating cough with difficult-to-expectorate mucus, yellow, sticky phlegm, swollen lymph glands, lung or breast abscesses, scrofula, goiter and convulsions. Do not use if there's Coldness, weak digestion or watery white mucus

HERBS:

comfrey	mullein
platycodon (treats Hot or Cold Phlegm)	
seaweeds (kelp, kombu, sargassum and so on)	

■ **WARM AND DISSOLVE PHLEGM AND STOP COUGH** herbs warm and dissolve Phlegm Cold or Phlegm Dampness, treating cough with clear to white mucus and copious, watery, runny phlegm, coldness and pale complexion. They should not be used for dry cough or inflammatory conditions.

HERBS:

elecampane	thyme
platycodon	

■ **HERBS THAT RELIEVE COUGH AND ASTHMA** are cough-sedating herbs with **antitussive**, **expectorant**, **anti-asthmatic**, **bronchodilating**, antibiotic, diuretic and laxative properties and symptomatically treat coughs and wheezing. They should always be combined with herbs that treat the root cause of these symptoms.

HERBS:

wild cherrry bark	apricot seed
coltsfoot flower	loquat
mulberry root bark	

■ **HERBS THAT EXPEL PHLEGM BY INDUCING VOMITING (emetics)** induce vomiting for the express purpose of expelling Phlegm, similar to the Ayurvedic treatment of clearing excess *Kapha* from the body. These should only be used under the guidance of a trained practitioner and by those with robust constitution. Thus, no examples are included in this materia medica (although **lobelia** and **ipecac** may be used this way).

■ **AROMATIC STOMACHICS** are fragrant herbs that strengthen and "revive" the Spleen in its transforming (metabolizing) function, treating digestive disturbances due to Dampness (mucus) in the Spleen/Stomach. Symptoms include abdominal distension and fullness, bloating, fluid retention, nausea, vomiting, loss of appetite, possible acid regurgitation, diarrhea, mucus, cough or the need to clear the throat after eating, excessive drooling, snoring, runny nose and post-nasal drip. Because Dampness is blocking the digestive functions, there may be no thirst, or a desire to only sip in small amounts. As well, these herbs assist lymphatic metabolism, reducing lymphatic congestion, edema and swelling. Because these herbs are generally warm and drying in action, they should be used with caution in those with Deficient Blood and Yin.

HERBS:

cardamom	agastache
magnolia bark	asafoetida
black atractylodes	

■ **HERBS THAT RELIEVE FOOD STAGNATION** are **digestants** that break up food stagnation, help metabolize, assimilate and move food through the gastrointestinal tract and increase gastric secretions, enzymatic functions and peristalsis. They treat symptoms of bloatedness, fullness, distension and pain in the abdomen, no appetite, nausea, vomiting, foul breath, sour regurgitation and abdominal masses. Some specifically aid in digestion of starches, while others assist meat digestion.

HERBS:

hawthorn berry	shen qu
radish seeds	sprouted wheat

■ **HERBS THAT REGULATE QI** normalize the smooth flow of Qi, move blocked energy and promote digestion and regularity of body functions (like **carminatives**). They especially treat stagnant Qi in the Spleen, Stomach, Liver or Lungs with symptoms of gas, epigastric pains, abdominal distension, belching, acid regurgitation, nausea, vomiting, alternating constipation and diarrhea, mood swings, depression, PMS, breast distention before menses, pain in the chest, ribs, flank or abdomen, general dull pains that come and go or change in severity, chest tightness and some types of shortness of breath and wheezing. Many are drying to Blood and Yin and shouldn't be taken long during pregnancy. These herbs are rarely taken alone, but combined with others based on the disorders.

HERBS:

citrus peels	cyperus
fennel	vitex

HERBS THAT REGULATE BLOOD includes two groupings of herbs: those that stop bleeding and those that invigorate (move stagnant) Blood:

■ **HERBS THAT STOP BLEEDING** are **hemostatic** herbs that stop many types of bleeding: hemorrhage, nosebleeds, coughing or vomiting of blood, blood in the urine or stool, excessive menstrual bleeding and bleeding from trauma. Many herbs in this category are astringent and are usually combined with Heat-clearing herbs, or herbs to treat the underlying condition (stagnant Blood, Deficient Yin and so on). Their stop-bleeding action is enhanced by burning (charring) the herbs to ash and taking in water internally, or applying externally.

HERBS:

agrimony	shepherd's purse
tienchi ginseng	mugwort

■ **HERBS THAT INVIGORATE BLOOD** are similar to **emmenagogues** with vasodilatory, antihypertensive and analgesic properties. They break up Blood stagnation, treating delayed menses, painful menstruation, amenorrhea, blood clots, tumors and cancer, abdominal masses, injuries and trauma, abscesses, ulcers, appendicitis, angina, heart disease and intense fixed pain with a boring, sharp or stabbing quality. They may also be used with other herbs to treat sciatica, arthritis and muscle and joint pains. These herbs are contraindicated during pregnancy, excessive menstrual bleeding and in those who bleed easily.

HERBS:

corydalis	angelica
motherwort	ligusticum
turmeric	blue cohosh
calendula	frankincense
myrrh	red peony
horse chestnut seed	salvia
safflower	arjuna

■ **WARMS THE INTERIOR AND DISPELS COLD** are herbal **stimulants** that raise the body's vitality, increase circulation and generate warmth in the Interior by warming, or reviving, the Yang, including that of the heart and pulse. They stimulate circulation, ignite digestive fires and counteract shock and collapse, treating symptoms of coldness, pallor, cold hands and feet, no thirst or sweating, loose stools, poor circulation, frequent and copious urination, poor digestion, lack of appetite, copious white discharges, low libido and infertility. Their heating and drying energies contraindicate them for those with Deficient Blood and Yin, or during pregnancy.

HERBS:

cayenne	black pepper
prickly ash	cinnamon bark
bayberry	dried ginger

■ **HERBAL TONICS** are herbs that strengthen or supplement an area, Organ or process of the body. There are no equivalents to this property in Western medicine ("bitter tonics" are really herbs that support digestion and elimination through stimulating the secretion of bile, and "blood tonics" such as yellow dock, are really high in iron and must be combined with blood nurturing (tonifying) herbs, such as molasses or **mulberries**, to effectively tonify the Blood). Tonics are used for Deficient Qi, Blood, Yang or Yin, and to strengthen immunity. They are contraindicated in stagnation, Excess Heat, high fever, Exterior disorders and most inflammatory and acute conditions.

Tonics are generally combined to enhance their effectiveness. Thus, when tonifying Qi, add a small amount of a Blood tonic and vice versa. The same is true when tonifying Yin and Yang. Further, it is generally important to move any stagnation present before using tonification therapy, otherwise you may be adding more cars to a bad traffic jam (with a worsening of symptoms such as gastrointestinal fullness and chest pains or tightness). Combining tonics with herbs that regulate Qi and/or Blood best alleviates this. Since food is considered the best tonic, many tonifying herbs are cooked with food, or taken in soup form.

■ **TONIFY QI** herbs increase energy, stamina, improve Organ functions and boost immunity, treating weakness, tiredness, poor digestion, shortness of breath on exertion, shallow breathing, lowered immunity, frequent colds and flu, palpitations, spontaneous sweating, chronic diarrhea, sluggishness, lack of motivation, frequent urination, weak voice, lack of appetite and prolapsed organs. Many are adaptogenic, fostering a sense of well-being and vitality. In excess, their sweet dampening nature can cause fullness in the chest and diaphragm, or sensations of Heat.

HERBS:

ginseng (panax)	codonopsis
astragalus	jujube date
reishi	white atractylodes
Chinese wild yam	eleuthro
honey-fried licorice	

■ **TONIFY BLOOD** herbs nourish the Blood, strengthen the body and improve its nutrition. They treat anemia, pale face, lips, nails and tongue, dizziness, vertigo, blurry vision, lethargy, palpitations, dry skin, poor memory, delayed and scanty menses and insomnia (hard to fall asleep). Blood tonics tend to foster compassion, patience, tolerance and devotion. Overuse can cause indigestion; thus, combine with herbs that tonify and regulate Qi and Blood.

HERBS:

dang gui	white peony
prepared rehmannia	lycii berries
longan berries	mulberries
he shou wu	

■ **TONIFY YANG** herbs generate warmth and stimulate metabolism. Having a direct effect on the endocrine sys-

tem, energy metabolism, sexual function and growth, they strengthen the mind, stamina and immunity. Symptoms include coldness, exhaustion, no appetite, timidity, lack of will power, fear of cold, withdrawal, low back and joint pains, impotence, frigidity, infertility, pallor, spermatorrhea, clear chronic leukorrhea, frequent and copious urination, wheezing, asthma and morning diarrhea. Like Qi tonics, these herbs generate well-being, vitality and charisma. They should generally not be used in Excess Heat or Deficient Yin conditions unless combined with Heat-clearing herbs, or Yin tonics.

HERBS:

walnuts	fenugreek
false unicorn	damiana
cuscuta	dipsacus
epimidium	ashwagandha
deer antler	cordyceps
eucommia	saw palmetto

■ **TONIFY YIN** herbs nourish, lubricate and moisten various aspects of the body, including blood, lymph, muscles, connective tissues, reproductive and hormonal secretions and various Organs. They treat Deficient Heat conditions with symptoms of malar flush, night sweats, burning sensation in the palms, soles and chest, dry throat at night, low-grade afternoon fever, wasting diseases (diabetes, TB, AIDS), dizziness, ringing in the ears, many peri/menopausal symptoms and Dryness, such as dry cough, stools, skin, mouth and nails. Like Blood tonics, these herbs also generate compassion, tolerance, patience and devotion. Because they are dampening in nature, do not use if there is Spleen or Stomach Deficiency, Dampness or Phlegm, abdominal distention, or diarrhea unless combined with herbs to treat those conditions.

HERBS:

American ginseng	asparagus root
marshmallow	slippery elm
comfrey	ophiopogon
black sesame seeds	

■ **STABILIZE AND BIND HERBS** are **astringent**, contracting, drying and tightening tissues. Helping stop excessive discharges from Deficiency, they treat diarrhea, excessive sweating or urination, mucus discharges, chronic diarrhea or cough, leukorrhea and bleeding. As well, they treat prolapsed uterus and rectum, and externally function as **vulneraries** to promote the healing of tissues in wounds or sores. Many herbs become astringent when charred or toasted. Combine with herbs to treat the root cause of the problem, generally Deficiency. Do not use astringents if there's Dryness, Exterior disorders, Dampness or severe nerve disorders.

HERBS:

horse chestnut seeds	blackberry
huckleberry	raspberry
eyebright	schisandra
cornus	partridgeberry
bilberry	ginkgo

NOURISH THE HEART AND CALM THE SPIRIT HERBS include both strong and mild sedatives and treat disturbances of the Spirit. There are two categories

■ **ANCHOR, SETTLE AND CALM THE SPIRIT (STRONG SEDATIVES)** herbs are minerals that weigh down and calm the mind. A category unique to Chinese medicine, they treat palpitations, insomnia, anxiety, nervousness, irritability, fright and hysteria. As well, they alleviate coughing, belching, hiccoughs and wheezing. In excess, minerals are very difficult to digest causing poor appetite, indigestion, and bloatedness. Thus, they are largely given for only acute conditions. Of the following only oyster shell is discussed.

HERBS:

oyster shell	magnetite
pearl	flourite
amber	hematitie

■ **CALM THE SPIRIT** herbs are mild **sedatives**, **calmatives** and **nervines** that calm and nourish the heart. More suited for chronic conditions, they treat nervousness, anxiety, insomnia, emotional instability, pain, cramps, spasms, tremors and epilepsy. Some also relieve stress and muscle tension. They are contraindi-

cated in Deficiency conditions unless combined with Blood or Yin tonics.

HERBS:

valerian	skullcap
hops	passionflower
California poppy	chamomile
polygala	zizyphus (jujube seeds)
Cactus grandiflorus	albizzia

■ **FRAGRANT HERBS THAT OPEN THE ORIFICES** are strongly fragrant herbs used to help restore consciousness in coma or fainting, and for stroke, coma, delirium, convulsion, lockjaw, clenched fists and/or rigid limbs. None are included in this materia medica, however examples include **camphor, musk** and **bay**.

■ **HERBS THAT EXTINGUISH INTERNAL WIND** are similar to **antispasmodics** and treat symptoms of Internal Wind, including neurological disorders, nervous depression, muscle spasms and twitches, pains and itching, emotional disturbances, palpitations with anxiety, Parkinson's disease, facial paralysis, lockjaw, rigidity, paralysis, epilepsy, hemiplegia, aphasia, tremors, convulsions, tinnitus, headaches, hypertension, dizziness and blurred vision. Because Internal Wind generally arises from Excess Heat, high fever or Deficient Blood or Yin, they are combined with herbs that treat these.

HERBS:

American/Mexican wild yam	gambir
black haw	lobelia

■ **EXPEL PARASITES HERBS** kill external and internal parasites (**vermifuges**). For them to be effective, it's essential to also eliminate those foods that feed parasites: sugar, sweets, juices, fruit, rich, greasy foods and flour products.

HERBS:

garlic	wormwood
black walnut hulls, leaves and bark	raw rice

■ **SUBSTANCES FOR EXTERNAL APPLICATIONS:** Certain herbs that are toxic and too strong to be used internally are applied externally to treat parasites, swelling, pain, injuries, bleeding, inflammation and skin lesions. None are included in this materia medica, but examples include **alum, borax** and **sulfur**.

MATERIA MEDICA

🐾 AGASTACHE

Agastache rugosa; Pogostemon cablin; Laminaceae   **C, W**
huo xiang

Part used: leaf

Energy, taste and Organs affected: slightly warm; acrid; Lungs, Spleen, Stomach

Actions: aromatic stomachic

Properties: stomachic, antiemetic, antifungal, diaphoretic

Biochemical constituents: methylchavicol, anethole, anisaldehyde, *d*-limonene, *p*-methoxycinnamaldehyde, *3*-octanone, 3-octanol, *p*-cymene, locten-3-ol, linalool, beta-humulene, alpha-ylangene, alpha-pinene

Dose: 4.5-9 gms; decoct 2 tsp./cup water for no more than 15 minutes, drink 1-3 cup/day

Precautions: Stomach Heat, Deficient Yin with Heat signs

Other: This herb is not the **anise hyssop** (Agastache foeniculum); patchouli (Pogostemon cablin) may be used instead.

Indications: *nausea, vomiting, bloatedness, edema, mucus in the lungs or throat after eating, a feeling of heaviness, poor appetite, lack of a desire to drink fluids, edema in thighs, legs and buttocks, indigestion, abdominal distention and fullness, nausea, vomiting, reduced appetite, bad breath, diarrhea, morning sickness, summer colds and flu*

Uses: A very common digestive problem occurs from eating excessive amounts of iced drinks, raw foods and cold foods/drinks directly out of the refrigerator, freezer, or eating/drinking any of these along with fats, such as chips, fries, greasy foods and flour products that cause mucus. The result is Dampness that obstructs the Spleen transformative function. This fancy term means those cold and damp drinks and foods cause poor and sluggish metabolism so that food and Fluids are not fully digested, but collect as Dampness and undigested food in the body. Further, the cold food/fluids encapsulate the fat, making it unable to properly assimilate, resulting in *ama* (to Ayurvedic practitioners), or cholesterol, toxic fat and cellulite (to Western practitioners).

Agastache is one of the very best herbs for reviving the Spleen transforming process, helping it better metabolize food and fluids. Thus, it effectively treats symptoms of nausea, vomiting, bloatedness, indigestion, abdominal distention and fullness, edema, mucus in the lungs or throat after eating, a feeling of heaviness, poor appetite, diarrhea and lack of a desire to drink fluids, and is commonly included in Chinese pill formulas for these. This herb may be used for morning sickness, especially with **cardamom** seeds and fresh **ginger**, and is very useful for prolonged or chronic diarrhea. It is also one of the best herbs to take for summer colds and flu when the body's heat is dispersed to the Exterior (its surface), leaving Coldness in the Interior with resulting chills/fever, diarrhea, stomachache and vomiting.

This herb is so effective in eliminating Dampness that I have seen it drain edema on heavy thighs, legs and buttocks, clearing out much of what is called cellulite. Now, before you rush right out to purchase this herb and start madly dosing yourself with it, know that it also drains fluid from the breasts (reducing their size) but even more importantly, its drying nature aggravates, or eventually causes, Deficient Blood or Yin with many undesirable symptoms like blurry vision, dizziness, dry skin, nails and hair, numbness in the limbs, or night sweats to name a few. Thus, like all herbs, it should be used with respect and in the right conditions.

🐾 AGRIMONY

Agrimonia pilosa, A. eupatoria; Rosaceae   **C, W**
xian he cao

Part used: whole plant

Energy, taste and Organs affected: neutral; bitter, acrid; Lungs, Liver, Spleen

Actions: stops bleeding

Properties: hemostatic, astringent, antiparasitic, anti-inflammatory, antifungal

Biochemical constituents: tannins, bitter glycosides, nicotinic acid amide, silicic acid, vitamins B and K, iron and essential oil

Dose: 9-15 gms; 15-30 gms fresh; 1 Tbsp./cup water; drink 1-3 cups/day; also used as an external wash or suppository

Precautions: in excess may cause nausea and vomiting

Other: Western herbalists use agrimony (*A. eupatoria*) to stop bleeding and diarrhea as well as to restore tone to flaccid muscles of the stomach and intestines.

Indications: *nosebleeds, vomiting blood, coughing blood, bleeding gums, blood in urine or stools, colitis, uterine bleeding, hemorrhoids, diarrhea, dysentery, parasites, trichomonas vaginitis, tapeworm*

Uses: Agrimony (*A. pilosa*) is widely used by the Chinese for various types of bleeding such as nosebleeds, vomiting blood, coughing blood, bleeding gums, blood in the urine or stools, or uterine bleeding. Because of its neutral energy, it can be combined with other herbs to treat bleeding due to Cold, Deficiency, Heat or Excess. Agrimony is even more effective at stopping bleeding if the burnt herb is used (put ash in water and drink). The Chinese frequently use ashes—from the fireplace, herbs, even human hair—to stop bleeding as this increases the astringent effects.

Agrimony's astringent nature also stops diarrhea and dysentery, including chronic problems of this nature. For this it may be used as a suppository as well as taken internally. It is frequently combined with **sophora flowers** for bloody stools. As a suppository it also treats hemorrhoids. Since it is astringent and stops bleeding, it is a great herb for colitis. Agrimony also kills parasites, such as trichomonas vaginitis and tapeworm, either as an external wash, or taken internally. For best results, decoct 30–60 gms (1-2 oz.) agrimony flowers (*he cao ye*) and drink first thing in the morning before breakfast. Reportedly the tapeworm should be dislodged in 5 to 6 hours.

🦎 ALIBIZZIA

Albizzia julibrissin; Fabaceae   C
he huan pi (bark); *he huan hua* (flower)

Part used: bark, flowerheads

Energy, taste and Organs affected: neutral; sweet; Heart, Liver

Actions: calm the Spirit

Properties: sedative, analgesic

Active constituents: tannin, saponin, albizzin, albitocin

Dose: bark: 9-15 gms.; flowerheads: 3-9 gms.

Precautions: none noted

Other: This is the **mimosa tree**; some Chinese herbalists call it "herbal Prozac" while its literal Chinese name is "happiness bark".

Indications: bark: *depression, bad temper, insomnia and palpitations due to anger and anxiety, irritability and poor memory due to stagnant Liver Qi, pain and swelling due to trauma, abscesses, carbuncles, furuncles and similar swellings;* flowerheads: *insomnia and palpitations due to anger and anxiety, fullness of the chest, poor memory, irritability due to stagnant Liver Qi*

🦎 ALISMA

Alisma orientale; A. plantago-aquatica, Alismataceae   C
ze xie

Part used: rhizome, tuber

Energy, taste and Organs affected: cold; sweet, bland; Kidneys, Bladder

Actions: drains Dampness

Properties: diuretic, antihypertensive, antibacterial

Active constituents: alisol A, alisol B, alisol A monacetate, alisol B monacetate, epialisol A, asparagine

Dose: 6-15 gms; decoct

Precautions: spermatorrhea, vaginal discharge, and presence of Deficient Kidney Yang or Damp Cold

Other: Although this is a diuretic, it is less harmful to the Yin than other diuretics.

Indications: *edema, urinary difficulty, painful urination, scanty urine with abdominal distention, dizziness, tinnitus, vertigo, heat in the bones, kidney infections, lumbago, diarrhea, high blood pressure, low back pain*

✿ ALOE (Aloe Vera)

Aloe vera; A. chinensis; A. barbadensis-officinalis; A. ferox; Liliaceae   **A, C, W**
lu hui (except *A. barbadensis-officinalis*); Sanskrit: *Kumari* (*Aloe spps.*)

Part used: gel (inner mucilaginous part of leaf); dried concentrate of the leaf gel

Energy, taste and Organs affected: cold; bitter; Large Intestine, Liver, Stomach, female reproductive organs

Actions: purgative

Properties: fresh gel: vulnerary, demulcent, emollient, rejuvenative, antiparasitic, Yin tonic; dried concentrated gel: purgative, cholagogue, emmenagogue, antiinflammatory, alterative, bitter liver tonic

Biochemical constituents: Two aloins, barbaloin and isobarbaloin, polysaccharides including glucomannans, anthraquinones, glycoproteins, sterols, saponins and organic acids, aloctin A., emodin

Dose: topically as needed; gel: 0.3-1.5 gms; 2 tsp. mixed in water 3 times a day; $1/2$-1 tsp. of powdered gel; 2 "00" caps 3 times/day; whole leaf: small pieces about size of little fingernail for laxative effect

Precautions: internal use: pregnancy, lactation and during menstruation (because in large doses aloe strongly stimulates blood circulation and has a downward energy); hemorrhoids, uterine or rectal bleeding, Coldness from Spleen or Stomach Deficiency (ex: indigestion with gas and bloatedness) chronic internal use of whole leaf causes potassium depletion and Kidney inflammation and ulcerative colitis, Crohn's disease and inflamed hemorrhoids; it is completely safe for external use

Other: The outer leaf is the part that is a laxative; the bottled gel has the bitter yellow latex beneath the outer skin removed. There are 325 species of aloe native to Africa, Arabia and the Cape Verde Islands.

Indications: gel: *burns, inflammatory skin problems (rashes, sores, insect bites and stings, poison oak and ivy, acne, herpes and wounds, eczema) PMS, gynecological and peri/menopausal conditions*; concentrated powder of gel: *constipation, parasites—especially roundworm and ringworm, fungus, red eyes, dizziness, headache, tinnitus, irritability, childhood nutritional impairment*

Uses: Aloe vera gel, the inner mucilaginous part of the leaf, is best known for its use in treating burns. I always have an aloe plant at my home and office, so that if anyone gets burned, I immediately clip a piece of aloe leaf, slit it open and smear its gel onto the burn (alternatively, the bottled gel may be used this way). Relief is almost instantaneous and the burn quickly clears without forming blisters or scars. I can think of many a bad burn healed this way and have heard many stories where aloe miraculously healed burns. Everyone should keep an aloe plant near his or her kitchen!

Aloe has many other uses than treating burns, though. Its soothing, cooling and healing nature rapidly heals the discomfort of skin rashes and itch, injuries, sores, insect bites and stings, poison oak and ivy, acne, herpes and wounds when applied topically. I have seen it heal eczema sores, but of course the internal cause must be addressed, too, or the eczema will return (this is true of any skin condition). As well, the gel treats gastric ulcers, diabetes, and diabetic wounds and lowers cholesterol.

In Ayurvedic medicine aloe gel is one of the most important tonics for the female reproductive system, the liver and for cooling excess fire in the body. Termed *kumari*, or "goddess", in Sanskrit, it is considered to impart beauty and youthful energy, rejuvenate the uterus, ease PMS and prevent wrinkles from forming (this makes one wonder if aloe contains phytoestrogens). The Chinese use the concentrated powder of aloe gel as a purgative. It is considered relatively mild and used for chronic constipation. It also clears Heat, especially that of the Liver, and so is used for red eyes, dizziness, headache, tinnitus and irritability. If that's not enough, aloe also kills fungus and parasites, especially roundworm and ringworm.

🜨 AMERICAN GINSENG

Panax quinquefolium; Araliaceae　　　　　　**C, W**
xi yang shen

Part used: root

Energy, taste and Organs affected cold; sweet, slightly bitter; Heart, Kidneys, Lungs

Actions: tonifies Yin (and Qi)

Properties: tonic, demulcent, rejuvenative, adaptogen

Biochemical constituents: triterpenic saponosides, (known as ginsenosides), traces of essential oils, traces of germanium (which may be partially responsible for its remarkable action)

Dose: 3-9 gms; use plants that are 3–6 years old; decoct 1 tsp./cup water; 20-60 drops, 1-4 times/day

Precautions: avoid when there is Damp Cold of the Spleen or Stomach, such as poor digestion with watery diarrhea

Other—Important Note: American ginseng has been widely over-harvested, both for sale in China and lately, in the States, and so is now endangered. Thus, *purchase only the cultivated plant instead.* American Ginseng has a very different energy from **Chinese** or **Korean ginsengs.** The latter tonify Qi and Yang (stimulating metabolism) while American ginseng mainly tonifies Yin (quieting metabolism).

Indications: *low-grade fevers (especially in the afternoon), thirst, spontaneous sweating, night sweats, irritability, wheezing, coughing up blood—all with weakness and Deficiency; AIDS, TB*

Uses: Many Native American tribes, especially the Cherokee, considered American ginseng the herb of choice. They used the root for colic, nausea, vomiting, asthma and chronic coughs. The Jesuits were primarily responsible for beginning the booming American-Chinese ginseng trade that has eventually led to it being overharvested and now an endangered plant in the wild (thus, only purchase if cultivated). The Chinese widely use American ginseng because its cooling demulcent energy tonifies Yin at the same time it strengthens Qi (this is quite different than Panax ginseng, which is a warming Qi tonic).

Thus, American ginseng is used for chronic, afternoon or low-grade fevers and irritability and thirst after a fever, since Yin (fluids) becomes depleted from fevers (heat evaporating moisture). It also treats irritability, thirst and night sweats due to general Yin Deficiency, all accompanied by weakness, deficiency and debility. American ginseng is also great for nourishing the Lungs to treat loss of voice, wheezing and coughing up of blood. As such, it is valuable for wasting conditions such as AIDS and pulmonary tuberculosis. Western herbalists use American ginseng as an adaptogen to counteract the effects of stress and to increase endurance.

🜨 ANDROGRAPHIS

Andrographis paniculata; Acanthaceae　　　**C, W**
chuan xin lian

Part used: aerial parts of herb

Energy, taste and Organs affected: cold; bitter; Lung, Stomach, Large and Small Intestines

Actions: clears Heat and toxins

Properties: antiviral, antiinflammatory (antiphlogistic), febrifuge, antipyretic, antibacterial, analgesic, cholagogue, bitter tonic

Biochemical constituents: deoxyandrographolide, andrographolide, neoandrographolide, homoandrographolide, Beta-sitosterol

Dose: 9-15 gms; this herb is extremely bitter and so best taken powdered in capsules or tablets: use 1-1.5 gms in powdered form; take every 2 hours during acute conditions, then taper down dosage as condition clears. Take with a pinch of powdered ginger for those with Coldness or Deficient Spleen symptoms.

Precautions: long-term use can injure Stomach Qi, causing digestive problems

Indications: *colds, flu, acute infections of the gastrointestinal tract, staph, asthma, lung abscesses, sore throat infections, strep throat, hepatitis, dysentery, heated diarrhea (yellowish with odor), urinary tract infections, weeping eczema, sores, carbuncles, snakebites, poor appetite, gas, hyperacidity*

Uses: Andrographis is a fantastic antiviral herb that is little known in the West, although it is available. I have seen it quickly eliminate in a few days (especially along with **isatis** and **dandelion** in the Chinese patent, *Chuan Xin Lian*—Formula #142), bacterial, and particularly viral, colds and flu that would normally linger for three to four weeks in most people. The Chinese specifically use it for a wide variety of Heat disorders, such as acute infections of the gastrointestinal tract, staph and other bacterial infections, asthma, lung abscesses, strep and other severe sore throat conditions, hepatitis, dysentery, diarrhea from Heat (yellowish with odor) and urinary tract infections. It is also applied topically to treat weeping eczema, sores, carbuncles and snakebites.

❦ ANGELICA spp.

Angelica archangelica (Western); A. dahurica, A. pubescens (Chinese), **C, W**
Apiaceae; bai zhi (A. dahurica); du huo (A. pubescens)

Part used: root

Energy, taste and Organs affected:
A. dahurica: warm; acrid; Lungs, Stomach
A. pubescens: warm; bitter, acrid; Kidneys, Bladder
A. archangelica: warm; acrid, bitter; Lungs, Stomach, Intestines

Action:
A. dahurica and *A. pubescens:* warms and releases the Exterior
A. archangelica: warms and releases the Exterior, invigorates Blood

Properties:
A. dahurica: diaphoretic, analgesic, antibacterial
A. pubescens: antirheumatic, antiarthritic, analgesic, diaphoretic

A. archangelica: diaphoretic, expectorant, carminative, stimulant, emmenagogue, antiseptic, diuretic

Biochemical constituents:
A. dahurica: byak-angelicin, byak-angelicol, oxypeucedanin, imperatorin, isoimperatorin, angelic acid, angelicotoxin, xanthotoxin, marmesin, scopoletin, isobyak-angelicol, neobyakangelicol, alloisoimperatorin
A. pubescens: angelol, angelicone, glabralactone, bergapten, osthol, umbelliferone, scopoletin, angelic acid, tiglic acid, palmitic acid, sterols, stearic acid, linolenic acid, oleic acid, glucose, essential oils
A. archangelica: essential oil with phellandrene, pinene, angelica acid, coumarin compounds, bitter principle and tannins

Dose: 3-9 gms; decoct 1 tsp./cup, drink 1-3 cups/day; 25-50 drops as needed, or 1-4 times/day

Precautions: do not use *A. dahurica* and *A. pubescens* if there is anemia, Deficient Blood or Yin because they are very drying; do not use *A. dahurica* with **elecampane** flowers; excessive amounts may cause convulsions and paralysis; do not use *A. archangelica* in pregnancy, diabetes, bleeding

Indications:
A. dahurica: common cold, flu, allergies, headaches, migraines, nasal congestion, pain above the eyes, stuffy nose, sinus congestion, allergies, sores and carbuncles, vaginal discharge
A. pubescens: sciatica, arthritis, rheumatism, colds, flu, headache, toothache
A. archangelica: colds, flu, pleurisy and other lung diseases, rheumatism, menstrual disorders from coldness, indigestion, spasms, ulcers and gas from coldness, arthritis, rheumatism

Uses: Different angelica species are used quite similarly: for colds, flu and lung conditions, headache and arthritis. Its warm energy stimulates blood circulation to warm the body and alleviate rheumatic pains. As well, Western angelica (*A. archangelica*) treats gas, colic, eructations, indigestion due to coldness, spasms of the stomach and intestines, stomach ulcers, anorexia and poor appetite. Daily doses can help cold folks stay warm all winter. Being a strong emmenagogue, it also promotes menstruation and eases menstrual disorders due to Coldness.

It is said that regular use of Western angelica creates a distaste for alcohol (but because it can increase sugar in the blood, diabetics should avoid it). In fact, frequently used as a flavoring and bitter digestive, angelica oil is included in various liqueurs such as Benedictine and Chartreuse, the leaves as a garnish or in salads and the stems in candies. Externally Western angelica may be applied as an oil, poultice or liniment to treat rheumatism, arthritis and skin disorders. The root oil prevents bacterial and fungal growth.

❧ APRICOT

Prunus armeniaca; Rosaceae　　　　　　　　　　**C**
xing ren

Part used: seed

Energy, taste and Organs affected: slightly warm; bitter; slightly toxic; Large Intestine, Lung

Actions: relieves coughing and wheezing

Properties: antitussive, antiasthmatic, demulcent

Biochemical constituents: amygdalin, amygdalase, prunase and oils

Dose: 3-9 gms, decoction; chop before decocting, add near end of cooking other herbs.

Note: because this herb is slightly toxic, do not eat more than 20 seeds in one day—overdose can cause dizziness, nausea, vomiting, headache, dyspnea, spasms, dilated pupils, arrhythmias and coma. Excess dosage in adults is around 50-60 kernels and in children at 10 kernels. Cooking, removal of the outer coating and mixing with sugar reduces its toxicity. In cases of overdose, take activated charcoal and syrup of **ipecac**, or drink a strong decoction from the bark of the apricot tree.

Precautions: diarrhea, infants; do not use with **astragalus**, **pueraria** or **skullcap**.

Indications: *coughs due to either Heat or Cold, especially dry coughs, wheezing, bronchitis, asthma, constipation due to dryness*

Uses: Laetrile, used in cancer therapy, is extracted from its seeds. Apricot seed is one of the very best remedies for coughs, bronchitis and asthma, especially since it can be used for either Hot or Cold conditions depending on the herbs with which it is combined, although it's best for dry coughs. It moistens the intestines as well, treating dry constipation, especially when combined with **dang gui** and **cannabis seeds**. One of the best formulas I've seen for treating prolonged colds and flu with cough is *Apricot and Gypsum Combination* (see Appendix, *Formula #134*). It is seemingly miraculous in these conditions when nothing else works.

❧ ARJUNA

Terminalia arjuna; Combretaceae　　　　　　　　**A**
Sanskrit: *arjuna*

Part Used: bark

Energy, taste and Organs affected: cool; spicy, astringent; Heart, Kidneys, Uterus

Actions: invigorates Blood

Properties: cardiac stimulant and tonic, hemostatic

Biochemical constituents: triterpenoid saponins, calcium carbonate and other calcium salts, tannin

Dose: 2 gms, 2-3 times/day dried powder; 20-40 drops, 2-3 times/day tincture; it is usually prepared in milk or ghee and taken daily for up to a year

Precautions: none noted

Uses: This tree is a myrobalan, in the same family as two other fruits in Triphala. It is the herb of choice for cardiac debility, as it's a heart tonic and stimulant, strengthens and improves cardiac function and regulates heart rhythm, treating angina and arrhythmias. It also prevents accumulation of fluid and thus, reduces edema and lowers blood lipids.

Indications: *heart tonic, angina, arrhythmia, edema, malpresentation of the fetus, frequent urination, spitting up of blood, wounds*

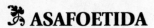 ASAFOETIDA

Ferula asafoetida; Apiaceae **C, A, W**
ai wei; Sanskrit: *hingu*

Part used: gum resin

Energy, taste and Organs affected: hot; acrid, bitter; Liver, Spleen, Stomach

Actions: aromatic stomachic

Properties: stimulant, digestive, carminative, expectorant, antispasmodic, analgesic, anthelmintic, antiparasitic, antimycobacterial

Biochemical constituents: essential oil, resin, ferulic acid, glue, sec-butyl-propenyl disulfide, farnesiferol

Dose: 100 mg–1 gm powder; 2-4 caps or tablets, 2-3 times/day

Precautions: Excess or Deficient Heat, high fever, hyperacidity, rash, urticaria, pregnancy

Other: Sometimes referred to as *Hing.*

Indications: *gas, bloatedness, indigestion, abdominal distention, colic pain, constipation, fungus, Candida albicans, arthritis, rheumatism, whooping cough, asthma, convulsions, epilepsy, hysteria, worms*

Uses: This hot spicy herb is a major component in the famous Ayurvedic herbal formula *Hingashtak,* used to alleviate gas, bloatedness, cramping, abdominal pain and indigestion, especially due to Coldness. It also moves food stagnation, impacted fecal matter and destroys worms, especially round worms and threadworms. A pinch may be added to food (especially beans) at the end of their cooking to prevent these symptoms. As it also dries Cold-Dampness and cleanses intestinal flora, it eliminates clear to white-colored mucus and such fungal conditions as Candida albicans overgrowth. Externally it is applied as a paste for arthritis and painful joints. The Chinese use it similarly to treat parasites and dysentery due to Coldness.

Asafoetida is used as a cooking spice in the West, especially in the southern states. Because it has an extremely strong odor, it is a good idea to keep the tin of powder stored in a glass jar. My southern grandmother used to pin a tiny muslin bag of asafoetida (pronounced ass-a-FOE-ti-da in the south) on my mother's undershirt to keep her from catching colds and flu. My mother reports that she did, indeed, stay healthy, but it sure wreaked havoc on her social life.

ASHWAGANDHA

Withania somnifera; Solanaceae **A**
Sanskrit: *ashwagandha*

Part used: root (of Winter Cherry)

Energy, taste and Organs affected: warm; bitter, sweet; Kidneys, Lungs

Actions: tonifies Yang (and possibly Yin and Qi)

Properties: aphrodisiac, sedative, astringent, nervine, rejuvenative, adaptogen

Biochemical constituents: bitter alkaloid somniferin, withaferin A, sitoindoside IX, carbon-27-glycowithanolides, acylsteryl glucosides, tropine, pseudotropine, isopelletierine, anaferine

Dose: 3-12 gms; 3 gms in powder, 2 times/day in boiled warm milk; decoct 1 Tbsp. dry root/cup water; 10-60 drops, 3-4 times/day

Precautions: severe congestion or stagnation; acute conditions; pregnancy; do not use with barbituates because it could potentiate the drug's effects

Other: Ashwagandha means "that which has the smell of a horse," as it gives the vitality and sexual energy of a horse.

Indications: *general debility, sexual debility, nerve exhaustion, problems of old age, emaciation of children, memory loss, loss of muscular energy, spermatorrhea, insomnia, paralysis, multiple sclerosis, rheumatism, cough, difficulty breathing, fatigue, infertility*

Uses: The ginseng of Ayurvedic medicine, ashwagandha is one of the best rejuvenative herbs because it tonifies without being overly stimulating and, in fact, calms and strengthens the nervous system. Thus, it can be widely used in all conditions of weakness, chronic debilitation due to overwork, stress, insomnia, or nervous exhaustion, in other words, for all of you "burned-out" Type A folks. It is especially good for the elderly, including signs of premature aging and senile dementia, and for children who aren't growing properly. For any of these conditions take as a mild decoction with sugar, honey, **pipply long pepper** and rice added. Traditionally it is mixed in a 50/50 ratio with ghee and taken in teaspoon doses, 2–3 times daily.

Ashwagandha is also one of the best herbs for calming the mind, improving memory and promoting deep, dreamless sleep (as indicated by part of its name, *somnifera*) and calming nervousness and an over-worked nervous system. As well, it treats lumbago and sciatica. In general, ashwaganda regenerates the hormonal system, is good for weak pregnant women as it helps stabilize the fetus and traditionally used to promote conception. Externally it is used on wounds and sores, and the leaves are applied to cancerous growths. Another species of ashwagandha, *W. convolvulus*, is used similarly but has a much stronger aphrodisiac effect.

ASPARAGUS

Asparagus cochinchinensis; Liliaceae	**C, A**
tian men dong; Sanskrit: *shatavari*	

Part used: tuber

Energy, taste and Organs affected: very cold; sweet, bitter; Kidneys, Lungs

Actions: tonifies Yin

Properties: Yin tonic, nutritive, diuretic, expectorant, demulcent, adaptogen

Biochemical constituents: asparagine, citrulline, serine, threonine, proline, clyccine, smilagenin, B-sitosterol, 5-methoxymethylfurfural, rhamnose

Dose: 6-15 gms, decoction

Precautions: coldness, loss of appetite, diarrhea, Wind-Cold cough with clear to white phlegm, Damp stagnation

Other: A similar species of this herb, *A. springerii*, is a common ornamental sold in nurseries. The asparagus vegetable is a wonderful diuretic.

Indications: *dry mouth, thick blood-streaked mucus, dry cough, tuberculosis, mouth sores, low-grade afternoon fever, constipation due to Dryness, thirst*

Uses: Chinese asparagus tuber is a wonderful Yin tonic for nourishing Kidney and Lung Yin while clearing Lung Heat. It generates Fluids in both Organs, treating dry cough, dry mouth, thirst and thick, or blood-streaked, sputum that is difficult to expectorate. It is a stronger and more effective herb than **ophiopogon** but more cloying and dampening in nature. It also treats wasting and thirsting disorder, tuberculosis, and consumption with low-grade afternoon fever and constipation due to Dryness. The Chinese believe that this herb engenders love and compassion and so Chinese pharmacists routinely set aside some of the sweetest roots for their personal use. Ayurvedic medicine uses *A. racemosus*, called *shatavari*, to strengthen female hormones, promote fertility, increase breast milk, relieve menstrual pain, nourish the female reproductive system and as an aphrodisiac.

ASTRAGALUS

Astragalus membranaceus; Fabaceae	**C**
huang qi	

Part used: root

Energy, taste and Organs affected: slightly warm; sweet; Lungs, Spleen

Actions: tonify Qi

Properties: adaptogen, diuretic, anhydrotic (stops sweating), antitumor, antiviral, cardiotonic, antioxidant, hepatoprotective

Biochemical constituents: asparagine, 2'4'-dihydroxy-5, 6-dimethoxyisoflavane, calycosin, formononetin, cycloastragenol, astragalosides, choline, betaine, kumatakenin, sucrose, glucoronic acid, B-sitosterol

Dose: 9-30 gms; decoct 2-3 long sticks/1 cup water; 10-60 drops, 1-4 times/day

Precautions: Qi stagnation, Damp stagnation, food stagnation, Excess Heat, skin lesions, Yin Deficiency with Heat signs

Other: This is yellow vetch. There are many grades of astragalus. Choose roots with the sweetest flavor. The seeds of *A. complanati* (*sha yuan ji li*) are used as a Yang tonic for low back pain, tinnitus, impotence, frequent urination and incontinence, or vaginal discharge.

Indications: *lowered immunity with frequent colds and flu, exhaustion, poor digestion and metabolism, low appetite, weakness, shortness of breath, prolapsed organs, excessive or spontaneous sweating, fatigue, diarrhea, uterine bleeding from Deficiency, postpartum fever due to Deficiency, night sweats, recovery from severe loss of blood, edema, chronic sores and wounds*

Uses: One of the best known Chinese herbs in the West, astragalus is a major herb that boosts immunity, building resistance to colds, flu and other externally contracted diseases. It does this by tonifying the *Wei Qi*, the part of Yang that circulates just below the skin surface, imparting radiance and suppleness as well as properly contracting the pores, (which causes goosebumps or sweating as appropriate). I frequently combine astragalus with **reishi** mushroom to improve immunity and instruct patients who easily get sick to drink a daily dose of the two throughout fall and winter. Similarly, it may be included in soups or cooked with grains and eaten on a weekly basis to help the whole family get through the winter without a single cold (people are always impressed with how well they feel and avoid colds and flu).

Astragalus also strengthens chronically weak Lungs, treating shortness of breath, excessive or spontaneous sweating and low energy. It regulates fluid metabolism, promotes urination and reduces deficiency edema, chronic nephritis with edema and swellings due to Deficiency and weakness, including a puffy face. I have seen it successfully treat kidney and bladder infections that do not respond to diuretics and dribbling of urine from coughing or sneezing. Since the Lungs act like a finger over one end of a straw that holds the Fluids in, weak Lungs result in lifting the finger off the straw, allowing Fluids to leak out. Similarly, astragalus's function of raising the Yang is effective for lifting prolapsed organs, collapsed energy and exhaustion.

As if this were not enough, astragalus also tonifies Spleen Qi, strengthening digestion, improving metabolism, increasing appetite and treating malnutrition and diarrhea. Every sort of wasting disease is benefited by it. The raw root helps heal chronic sores and ulcerations that have formed pus but have not drained or healed well and speeds the healing of all sorts of wounds.

In cancer patients undergoing chemotherapy, astragalus protects adrenal cortical function, decreasing bone marrow suppression, increasing white blood cell count, lessening chemotherapy and radiation side effects and inhibiting spreading of tumors. I have seen cancer patients taking this herb quickly raise their white blood cell count to the amazement of their doctors. Since it also tonifies Blood, it is used for uterine bleeding and when given with Blood tonics, for postpartum fever due to Deficient Qi and Blood and in the recovery stage from severe loss of blood.

🜨 ATRACTYLODES, Black

Atractylodes lancea; Asteraceae   **C**
cang zhu

Part used: rhizome

Energy, taste and Organs affected: warm; acrid, bitter, aromatic; Spleen, Stomach

Actions: aromatic stomachic

Properties: digestant, aromatic, carminative, diaphoretic, antirheumatic

Biochemical constituents: atractylodin, atractylol, atractylin, hinesol, Beta-eudesmol, vitamins A and B1

Dose: 4.5–9 gms, decoction; note that this is a very drying herb and so it is best to eat rice gruel after taking it to counteract this effect

Precautions: excessive sweating due to Qi Deficiency, Yin Deficiency with Heat signs

Other: Black atractylodes is very similar to **agastache** in action.

Indications: *reduced appetite, diarrhea, epigastric distention and pressure, fatigue, nausea, vomiting. swollen hips,* *thighs and legs, vaginal discharge, swollen, sore joints, headache and body aches with lack of sweating and oozing sores, all due to Wind-Damp Cold influences, night blindness, diminished vision with a rough sensation in the eyes.*

❦ ATRACTYLODES, White

Atractylodes macrocephala; Asteraceae   **C**
bai zhu

Part used: rhizome

Energy, taste and Organs affected: warm; bitter, sweet; Spleen, Stomach

Actions: tonify Qi

Properties: diuretic, carminative, digestive

Biochemical constituents: atractylol, atractylon, butenolide A, butenolide B, acetoxyatractylon, hydroxy-atractylon, vitamin A

Dose: 4.5–9 gms, decoction; use raw to dry Dampness and promote urination; dry-fry to strengthen the Spleen, tonify Qi and stop diarrhea

Precautions: Yin Deficiency with extreme thirst

Indications: *lowered appetite, fatigue, lack of strength, vomiting, loose stools or diarrhea, fluid retention, edema, stagnant water in the stomach, spontaneous sweating caused by low energy, fever and chills without sweating, chronic wheezing or cough with thin watery sputum, spermatorrhea, frequent urination, vaginal discharge, diabetes*

Uses: One of the most revered tonic herbs of Chinese medicine, white atractylodes tonifies the Qi of the Spleen and Stomach at the same time it dispels Dampness. The Stomach is responsible for physically breaking down the food we eat while the Spleen is responsible for extracting Qi (or vital energy) from it. If we lack Qi, then symptoms such as lowered appetite, fatigue, lack of strength, vomiting, loose stools or diarrhea and heaviness in the arms and legs result.

These are exactly the symptoms that white atractylodes alleviates along with eliminating fluid retention, edema and stagnant water in the stomach. As well, it tonifies Lung Qi, helping stop spontaneous sweating

caused by low energy, fever and chills without sweating and chronic wheezing or cough with thin watery sputum. It helps calm a restless fetus from Spleen Deficiency. It is generally combined with **ginseng**, **fu ling**, **licorice** and sometimes **tangerine peel** and **pinellia** to enhance its digestive and assimilation abilities.

❦ BAPTISIA

Baptisia tinctoria; Fabaceae   **W**

Part used: leaves, root

Energy, taste and Organs affected: extremely cold; bitter; toxic; Liver

Actions: clears Heat and toxins

Properties: alterative, antibiotic, antibacterial, anti-inflammatory, antiseptic, emmenagogue, emetic

Biochemical constituents: babtitoxine (baptisine), two glucosides, baptin, a cathartic, yellowish resin

Dose: 3-9 gms; infuse 1-2 tsp./cup water, take $^1/_2$ cup tea every 2-3 hours

Precautions: Deficient Yang, coldness; this herb is very strong and toxic in high doses; reduce dosage if feeling nauseous

Other: Also known as **wild indigo**, this herb is at risk of becoming endangered, thus *only use the cultivated plant*.

Indications: *inflammations, septicemia, disintegration of tissues, putrid ulcerations, malignant ulcers, mouth sores, scrofula, malignant sore throat, diphtheria, tonsillitis, typhoid dysentery, typhoid pneumonia, meningitis, fetid leukorrhea, ulceration of cervix, foul discharges with dark-purplish discoloration, cancer, tumors, boils, ulcers, genital herpes*

❦ BAYBERRY

Myrica cerifera; Myricaceae   **A, W**
Sanskrit: *katphala*

Part used: bark of the root

Energy, taste and Organs affected: warm; spicy, astringent; Spleen, Lungs, Liver

Actions: warms the Interior and expels Cold

Properties: stimulant, astringent, expectorant, diaphoretic

Biochemical constituents: volatile oil, starch, lignin, albumen, gum, tannic and gallic acids, acrid and astringent resins, an acid resembling saponin

Dose: 1–4 gms; decoct 1 tsp./cup water, drink $1/2$ cup 2-3 times/day; powder—1 tsp. per cup boiling water, or 2 "00" capsules 3 times/day; 10–30 drops tincture, 1-3 times/day

Precautions: avoid in pregnancy; in large doses it is emetic; use cautiously in Blood or Yin Deficiency

Other: Wax from the berries was used for making candles.

Indications: *colds, flu, sore throat, sinus and lung congestion, diarrhea, excessive menstrual bleeding, uterine prolapse, vaginal discharge, sores, ulcers*

Uses: Bayberry is a powerful stimulant that disperses Coldness in the body and raises vitality and resistance to disease (especially in the initial stages) in those who have Coldness or Cold signs. Use for fear of cold, chills with lowered fever, clear to white mucus, lack of thirst, body aches and moderate sore throats or headaches. It also treats colds, flu and coughs with white to clear mucus and sinus congestion with clear to white discharge. I've fended off many a sore throat or cold by sipping a tea of bayberry mixed with **cayenne, ginger** and **cinnamon**. While quite stimulating to the palate, as you can imagine, it quickly warms the body and brings on a sweat. As well, bayberry cleanses the lymphatics and, in general, eliminates all Cold mucus conditions in the body, treating ulceration of the mucous membranes and digestive tract. For any of these situations take in capsule or tea form, gargle for sore throats, smoke to clear the lungs and snuff to clear the sinuses.

Bayberry also treats Coldness-caused persistent diarrhea, bowel inflammation, excessive menstrual bleeding, uterine prolapse and uterine and vaginal white discharges with little odor (use as a douche for the latter). Its stimulant action warms and circulates Qi and Blood, thus promoting the healing and toning of tissues after checking the undesired discharge.

Externally, the powdered bark may be made into a paste, poultice or wash to help old wounds, ulcers and sores that do not heal. It makes an excellent toothpowder and mouthwash, astringing and cleansing receding and bleeding gums (combine with powders of **cinnamon, myrrh, echinacea** and salt). A bayberry fomentation can be applied nightly to relieve, cure and prevent varicose veins.

✿ BILBERRY (also Blueberry and Huckleberry)

Vaccinium Spp.; Ericaceae   **W**

Part used: leaf and berry

Energy, taste and Organs affected: leaves: cool, astringent; Liver; berries: cool; sweet; Liver and Kidneys

Actions: tonify Blood

Properties: leaves: astringent, diuretic; berries: also nutritive, antioxidant

Biochemical constituents: berries: anthocyanosides, arbutin, ericolin, beta-anyrin; leaves also have tannins

Dose: leaves: decoct 1 Tbsp./cup water, drink 2–3 cups daily; 20–40 drops tincture 1-4 times daily; eat the berries freely

Precautions: large doses of the leaves may cause gastric irritation

Other: Blueberry and **huckleberry** may be used similarly to bilberry. Frozen blueberries are the best antioxidant known, stronger than any antioxidant supplements. A little known cure that works well for certain types of chronic bladder infections is to eat 1 cup cooked blueberries in the morning and another in the evening for two weeks in a row. Then reduce to 1 cup per day for two weeks and reduce again to 1 cup every other day. I have seen this work in a number of cases, particularly in people who tend to have Dampness. Interestingly, blueberries, like **raspberries** and **blackber-**

ries, contain less sugar than most other fruits. **Cranberries**, also a *Vaccinium* species, are well known to treat bladder infections due to hyperacidity.

Indications: *impaired night vision and eyesight, diabetic retinopathy, macular degeneration, cataracts, glaucoma, eyestrain, varicose veins, hemorrhoids, easy bruising, chronic bladder infections, diarrhea, dysentery, mild adult-onset diabetes*

Uses: Bilberry is best known for its ability to restore night vision and eyesight. This action was first discovered in World War II when British Royal Air Force pilots reported improved visual acuity on nighttime raids after consuming bilberries. Since then, the berry's colorful anthocyanodise compounds have been found to strengthen capillary walls, reduce capillary leakage and neutralize free radicals. This enhances microcirculation, particularly to the eyes, improving night vision and visual acuity, treating (or preventing) night blindness, diabetic retinopathy, macular degeneration, cataracts, glaucoma, eyestrain, myopia and more generally, varicose veins, hemorrhoids and easy bruising. (Interestingly, the Chinese also use **green raspberries** for poor vision.) Use bilberry's astringent leaves along with the fruit to treat diarrhea and dysentery and help regulate blood sugar in mild adult-onset diabetes.

🐾 BLACKBERRY

Rubus fruticosus and other species; Rosaceae **W**

Part used: leaves, root bark, fruit

Energy, taste and Organs affected: cool; Liver, Kidneys; leaves and root bark: astringent; fruit: sweet, sour

Actions: leaves, root bark: stabilize and bind; fruit: tonify Blood and Yin

Properties: leaves, root bark: antipyretic, astringent, hemostatic; fruit: nutritive

Biochemical constituents: leaves, root bark: both are high in tannins; fruit: isocitric and malic acids, sugars, pectin, momoglycoside of cyanidin and vitamins A and C

Dose: leaves: infuse 2 tsp./cup water; root bark: decoct 1

tsp./cup water; both: drink 3 cups a day or use 3-9 gms in formulas; fruit: 9-15 gms, decoction; eat as desired

Precautions: Deficient Yin with Heat signs

Indications: root bark: *diarrhea, dysentery*; root bark and leaves: *uterine tonic, excessive menstrual bleeding*; leaves: *fever, colds, sore throat, vaginal discharge*; berries: *anemia*

Uses: Blackberry root bark is perhaps one of the best remedies for diarrhea and dysentery, even in infants. For this, simmer 1 Tblsp. with 1 tsp. **cinnamon** powder in 1 cup milk for 5 minutes on low heat, or take powdered in capsule form (2-4 capsules as needed). The leaves also work for this, but are less astringent. They are better as a uterine tonic and, along with the root, help inhibit excessive menstrual bleeding. The leaves are also used for fever, colds, sore throat and vaginal discharge. The berries and juice build Blood, alleviating anemia. In excess, however, they cause loose stools, (which is interesting since the leaves and root firm loose stools).

🐾 BLACK COHOSH

Cimicifuga racemosa (Western), *C. foetida* (Chinese); *Ranunculaceae*   **C, W**
sheng ma

Part used: rhizome

Energy, taste and Organs affected: cool; sweet, spicy, slightly bitter; Liver, Spleen, Stomach, Large Intestine

Actions: *C. racemosa*: clears Wind and Damp; *C. foetida*: cools and releases Exterior

Properties: antispasmodic, expectorant, emmenagogue, diaphoretic, alterative, parturient, uterine tonic, antirheumatic

Biochemical constituents: various glycosides such as triterpine and actein, salicylic acid, ferulic acid, woferulic acid, cimicifugoside, formononetin, bitter principles, racemosin, triterpenes, isoferulic acid, salicylic acid, tannin

Dose: decoct 1 tsp. dried root/1 cup water, take 2-3 cups/day; 2 "00" caps 3 times/day; tincture, 10-40 drops, 1-4 times/day; 3-9 gms in formulas; prepare *C. foetida*

with wine or stir-fry to increase its ascending action; stir-fry with honey to nourish the lungs and relieve cough

Precaution: too large a dose causes nausea, dizziness, vomiting, light headedness, low blood pressure, dilated pupils and dimness of vision; Heat due to Yin Deficiency, fully erupted measles, in those with breathing difficulty and in those with Excess above and Deficiency below

Other: Its other names of **black snakeroot** and **rattle snake root** refer to its past use in North America to treat snakebites, including that of the rattlesnake. Also known as **bugbane** (in Latin *cimicifuga* means "to chase insects away"), this herb is currently under heavy demand and is now endangered, thus, ***only use the cultivated plant***.

Indications: *hot flashes, menstrual irregularity, headaches right before the period (due to low-estrogen levels), menstrual cramps, excessive menstrual bleeding, delayed and painful menses, ovarian pain, post-hysterectomy symptoms, endometriosis, late menstruation, childbirth and afterbirth pains, menstrual pain, all nervous conditions, hysteria, neuralgia, cramps, whooping cough, asthma, bronchitis, rheumatism, arthritis, neuralgia, sciatica, amenorrhea, PMS, colds, flu, fever, headache, sore throat, swollen or painful gums, ulcerated lips or gums, canker sores, skin rashes, measles, prolapsed organs, epilepsy*

Uses: Although black cohosh has been used for centuries in the West, it has recently hit the popular market after German tests showed its beneficial use in the treatment of menopausal and ovarian insufficiency symptoms. Some studies also claim it to be a phytoestrogen, meaning it has estrogenic compounds that bind to estrogen receptor sites, causing the body to act as if it has been given estrogen. However, it only seems to do this in the brain and bone, not the uterus, while other studies don't show it to have any estrogenic activity at all. Regardless, realize that phyto-hormonal herbs don't contain hormones, but mimic their functions by latching onto a cell's hormonal receptor sites. Thus,

black cohosh may bring benefits of estrogen to the body but without stimulating the growth of estrogen-sensitive tumors.

Black cohosh tones the uterine muscles, countering prolapse of the uterus, and alleviates hot flashes, poor vaginal tone, vaginal dryness, fatigue, mood swings, menstrual irregularity, headaches right before the period (due to low estrogen levels), menstrual cramps and spasms, excessive menstrual bleeding, delayed and painful menses, ovarian pain, post-hysterectomy symptoms, endometriosis and late menstruation. Native American women also used it to relieve childbirth (it stimulates uterine contractions during labor), afterbirth pains and menstrual pain. To facilitate childbirth, combine with **raspberry leaves** and **blue cohosh,** and take daily for the last two weeks of pregnancy. If needed, it may be used throughout pregnancy to relax spasmodic uterine activity (use with **black haw** and **wild yam**).

Western herbalists use black cohosh as an antispasmodic useful for all nervous conditions, hysteria, neuralgia, cramps and nerve pains. When combined with lung and cough herbs it eases whooping cough, asthma and bronchitis since it helps dilate the bronchioles. It is also used in Europe for rheumatism, arthritis, neuralgia, sciatica, amenorrhea, PMS and respiratory disorders. I have successfully used black cohosh with white peony to treat epilepsy, lessening the frequency and severity of seizures.

Chinese herbalists use *C. foetida* and related species as a cooling diaphoretic for colds, flu, fever, headache, sore throat, swollen or painful gums, ulcerated lips or gums, canker sores, and to ripen and bring out skin rashes in the early stages, such as measles. Like **bupleurum**, it raises the Yang and lifts the sunken, treating Deficient Qi with symptoms of shortness of breath, fatigue and prolapsed stomach, intestines, bladder, uterus, rectum or veins. Because of its rising energy, this herb may be combined with other herbs to direct their energy upward in the body. It also means it should be avoided in hypertension.

❧ BLACK HAW

Viburnum prunifolium; Caprifoliaceae W

Part used: stem and root bark

Energy, taste and Organs affected: cool; bitter; Liver, nervous system

Actions: extinguish Internal Wind

Properties: antispasmodic, uterine tonic, sedative, nervine

Biochemical constituents: amentoflavone, coumarins (including scopoletin), scopoletine, aesculetine, arbutin, oleanolic and ursolic acids, sterol, salicin, 1-methyl-2,3-dibutyl hemimillitate, viburnin, plant acids, volatile oils, tannin

Dose: 3-9 gms; decoct 1 tsp./cup water, drink 3 cups/day; tincture, 10–20 drops

Other: *V. opulis* (**cramp bark**) is very similar to black haw, though weaker in action.

Indications: *PMS, dysmenorrhea, irregular menstruation, menstrual cramps, spasms, pain, morning sickness, habitual miscarriage, pain and bleeding after childbirth, nervous conditions, convulsions, hysteria*

Uses: A powerful antispasmodic, black haw treats PMS, dysmenorrhea, irregular menstruation, menstrual cramps, spasms and all painful conditions. It helps to control morning sickness and can change the mental attitude of an expectant mother from depression to cheerfulness. As a uterine tonic, it is used for habitual miscarriage anytime during pregnancy, although it should be taken preventatively several weeks before the miscarriage usually occurs. Combined with **false unicorn** (and sometimes **cramp bark**), it has worked brilliantly for several women I know to prevent threatened miscarriage, even in the last trimester. It is also used after childbirth to check pain and bleeding. Black haw treats all nervous conditions, including convulsions and hysteria as well.

❧ BLACK PEPPER

Piper nigrum; Piperaceae A, C, W
hu jiao; Sanskrit: *marich*

Part used: fruit

Energy, taste and Organs affected: hot; spicy; Large Intestine, Stomach

Actions: warms the Interior and expels Cold

Properties: stimulant, expectorant, carminative, stomachic

Biochemical constituents: essential oil that contains phellandrene, two acrid resins, hot tasting amides, 5-9% piperdine, piperdine and aromatic acids

Dose: 2-5 gms; $1/4$ to $1/2$ teaspoon powder as needed

Precautions: Excess or Deficient Heat; inflammatory conditions; prolonged daily use of black pepper can cause the tendons to contract, thus injuring flexibility

Other: Black pepper is the immature fruit; **white pepper** is the dried mature fruit after processing.

Indications: *weak digestion, gas, stagnant food in the stomach, bloatedness, nausea, vomiting, diarrhea, belching, abdominal pain, mucus in the colon, colds, coughs, mucus conditions, toothache*

Uses: While predominantly used as a spice, black pepper is an important metabolic stimulant and expectorant for weak digestion, gas, stagnant food in the stomach, bloatedness, nausea, vomiting, diarrhea, belching, abdominal pain and mucus in the colon. It also dries Cold mucus in the Lungs, throat and sinuses, clearing out colds, coughs and other mucus conditions. Once when our young son was coming down with a mucousy cough, my husband and I sprinkled some black pepper on his hand while we ate at a restaurant, which he delightedly licked off. His cough immediately disappeared and didn't return. Black pepper may also be used as a powder for toothache.

One of the best ways of taking black pepper is in its traditional Ayurvedic combination, *Trikatu*, where it is ground in equal parts together with **pippli long pep-**

per, ginger root and enough honey to form a paste, and taken in $1/2$-1 tsp. doses with a little hot water 3 times/day. If the pippli long pepper cannot be located (try Indian food stores) use 2 parts anise seed instead. At the first signs of a cold, mucus congestion or sinus infections from Cold, I give this paste with great results, even to children in small doses.

BLUE COHOSH

Caulophyllum thalictroides; Berberidaceae   **W**

Part used: rhizome

Energy, taste and Organs affected: warm; acrid, bitter; mildly toxic; Liver

Actions: invigorates the Blood

Properties: emmenagogue, antispasmodic, diuretic, diaphoretic, parturient, uterine tonic

Biochemical constituents: the alkaloid methylcytisine, the glycosides caulophyllosaponin and caulosaponin, gum, starch, salts, phosphoric acid, soluble resin

Dose: 3–9 gms; decoct 1 tsp./cup water; 10–30 drops tincture, 1-4 times/day

Precautions: avoid during first eight months of pregnancy, heavy menstruation; angina or cardiac insufficiency; overdose may cause nausea, vomiting, headache, thirst, dilated pupils, muscle weakness, incoordination, constriction of coronary blood vessels, cardiovascular collapse, convulsions, enlarged heart in newborns, elevated temperature and blood pressure, sweating

Other: It is also known as **papoose root**, referring to its ability to bring on labor and ease childbirth pains; this herb is now endangered, thus *only use the cultivated plant.*

Indications: *menstrual irregularities, amenorrhea, dysmenorrhea, delayed menses, menstrual cramps that are heavy, achy and spasmodic in nature, childbirth and afterbirth pains, spasmodic muscular pain, rheumatic pain, arthritis, epilepsy, chronic inflammation, edema, swelling*

Uses: A strong blood-moving herb, blue cohosh is used for menstrual irregularities, amenorrhea, dysmenor-

rhea, delayed menses, menstrual cramps that are heavy, achy and spasmodic and to ease childbirth and afterbirth pains. It tonifies uterine tissue while relaxing spastic uterine muscles. It is also used for spasmodic muscular pain, rheumatic pain, arthritis, epilepsy, chronic inflammation, edema and swelling.

BONESET

Eupatorium perfoliatum; Asteraceae   **W**

Part used: aerial portions

Energy, taste and Organs affected: cool; bitter; toxic; Liver, Lungs

Actions: cools and releases the Exterior

Properties: febrifuge, diaphoretic, expectorant, laxative, diuretic, antispasmodic

Biochemical constituents: sesquiterpene lactones, eupafolin, euperfolitin, eufoliatin, eufoliatorin, euperfolide and others; immunostimulatory polysaccharides; flavonoids, quercetin, kaempferol, hyperoside, astragalin, rutin, eupatorin, diterpenes including dendroidinic acid, hebenolide, vitamin C, volatie oil and sterols

Dose: acute: infuse 1 Tbsp./cup water, drink $1/2$ to 1 cup every 2-3 hours; tincture: 10-40 drops 1-4 times daily; reduce its toxicity by drying the herb.

Precautions: chronic use or overdose can result in nausea, vomiting, weakness, loss of appetite, thirst, constipation

Other: This herb has a nasty bitter taste, but is very effective and so worth the effort. It was considered a miracle herb in 1918-1919 when it successfully treated the influenza epidemic.

Indications: *fevers, dengue fever, colds, flu, pulmonary inflammations, pleurisy, all due to Heat*

Uses: Simply put, boneset is a fabulous herb for fevers, including dengue fever, intermittent fever, colds and flu, pleurisy and rheumatism, all due to Heat. Once when my young son came down with the flu at an herbal conference, several herbalists determined boneset was the herb of choice and so gave him the tea. It was so nasty, not much got down, but what did reach him effectively cleared the flu very quickly. To this day my son remembers his boneset cure. According to the herbalist Sharon Tilgnar this herb contains tremerol, which can cause fatty degeneration of the liver and kidneys and so should only be taken for acute conditions and for a limited time. Given this, it is still far safer than Acetomenophen, which is known to cause death from stomach bleeding.

❧ BUGLEWEED

Lycopus virginicus (Western); L. lucidus (Chinese);
Laminaceae   C, W
ze lan

Part used: herb

Energy, taste and Organs affected: *L. virginicus*: slightly cool; bitter; thyroid, Liver, Heart, Lungs; *L. lucidus*: slightly warm; bitter; Liver, Spleen

Actions: clear Heat, drain Fire

Properties: *L. virginicus*: anti-inflammatory, astringent, antitussive, sedative; *L. lucidus*: emmenagogue, diuretic

Biochemical constituents: *L. virginicus*: various phenolic acid compounds: caffeic, rosmarinic, chlorogenic and ellagic acids; *L. lucidus*: glycosides, flavones, saponins, lycopose, raffinose

Dose: infuse 1 tsp./cup water, drink 1, cup 3 times/ day; 10-20 drops tincture, 1-3 times/day

Precautions: pregnancy, nursing mothers, hypothyroidism

Other: Both the Western and Chinese varieties of this herb grow in marshy areas.

Indications: *L. virginicus: hyperactive thyroid; L. lucidus: painful menses, traumatic injuries, abscess, systemic or facial edema, postpartum edema, abdominal pain or painful urinary dysfunction*

Uses: Bugleweed is a specific for hyperactive thyroid: it blocks the conversion of thyroxin to T3 in the liver and inhibits TSH by interfering with iodine metabolism in the thyroid.[1] For Grave's disease, combine with **lemon balm**, **motherwort** and **reishi**. Additionally, it is beneficial for tachycardia and arrhythmia in conjunction with insomnia. Interestingly, in Chinese medicine the thyroid is associated with the Heart. Thus, any Heart imbalance can affect thyroid function as well (as shown in Heart imbalance symptoms, such as tachycardia, arrhythmia and insomnia). The Chinese use *L. lucidus* as an emmenagogue for painful menses, pain and swelling from traumatic injury or abscess, systemic or facial edema and postpartum edema, abdominal pain or painful urinary dysfunction.

❧ BUPLEURUM

Bupleurum Chinensis; Apiaceae   C
chai hu

Part used: root

Energy, taste and Organs affected: cool; acrid, bitter; Liver, Pericardium, Gallbladder, Triple Warmer

Actions: cools and releases the Exterior

Properties: antipyretic, diaphoretic, carminative, alterative, antihypertensive, antibacterial, antiviral, antimalarial, analgesic, antiinflammatory

Biochemical constituents: bupleurumol, saponin, phytosterol, adonitol, angelicin, oleic acid, linolenic acid, palmitic acid, stearic acid, lignoceric acid

Dose: 3-15 gms in decoction; use raw for Exterior disorders; with honey for cough; with vinegar to invigorate Blood in the Liver

Precautions: Deficient Yin with Heat; signs of Liver Fire rising: splitting headache, red eyes and face, bitter taste in the mouth and hypertension; may occasionally cause nausea or vomiting; this herb is very drying—do not use long term; if there is anemia or Deficient Heat, always combine with **dang gui** or **lycii berries**; long-term use can cause dizziness; **DO NOT USE WHILE ON INTERFERON**, as their adverse interaction is toxic to the body, as discovered by the Japanese (of course, interferon has well-known toxic side effects by itself—further, the combination of both is redundant and unwarranted).

---

[1] Tilgnar, *Herbal Medicine from the Heart of the Earth*, Wise Acres Press, Inc. 1999.

Other: Due to its rising energy, some people have anger and irritability after taking bupleurum. If this occurs, stop for several days and then restart with a lower dose.

Indications: *alternating chills and fever along with a bitter taste in the mouth, colds, flu, irritability, vomiting, dizziness, vertigo, menstrual difficulties and irregularity, mood swings, emotional instability, PMS, depression, uterine prolapse, hemorrhoids, epigastric and flank pain, a stifling sensation in the chest, abdominal bloating, nausea, indigestion, alternating diarrhea and constipation*

Uses: Bupleurum is one of the most commonly used Chinese herbs. As a cooling diaphoretic, it is used raw to relieve alternating chills and fever along with a bitter taste in the mouth, colds, flu, flank pain, irritability, vomiting and a sensation of constriction in the chest. Because it harmonizes both External and Internal problems, it is especially beneficial when an acute condition lingers and becomes chronic. Quite often colds and flu move deeper into the body to a place that is part Exterior and part Interior, but neither exclusively (this is when the acute symptoms have passed, but you still don't feel well yet).

At this point normal diaphoretics no longer work, yet the body is still under the pathogenic influence of the cold or flu, with symptoms of low energy, lowered appetite and impaired function in general. In fact, the body can easily have a relapse of the cold or flu because it is still stuck in the body, inaccessible from the surface. This is where bupleurum is useful because it pulls the pathogen out of the partially Interior position in the body and then releases it on the surface. There are dozens of formulas based on bupleurum alone because of this function.

Bupleurum is also one of the best harmonizing Liver herbs since it "spreads", or regulates, Liver Qi (and further improves Liver function when stir-fried in vinegar). This means that bupleurum unblocks the flow of stuck energy not only in the Liver, but also throughout the whole body, relieving chest and flank pain and congestion, dizziness, vertigo and menstrual difficulties. It also stabilizes emotions, regulates mood swings and depression and eases PMS symptoms. Any time I treat de-pression, mood swings, PMS or menopausal symptoms, I always use a formula based on bupleurum, as it effectively alleviates all these symptoms. Many a woman has been able to sidestep or eliminate antidepressants because of this.

If this were not enough, bupleurum has a strong ascending energy that picks up the body's energy, lifting vitality, anal or uterine prolapse, hemorrhoids, and sagging spirits (although for some, this strong rising energy causes feelings of unwarranted anger—if this occurs, lower dosage until anger disperses). As well, it is used for disharmonies between the Liver and Spleen, treating epigastric and flank pain, a stifling sensation in the chest, abdominal bloating, nausea, indigestion and alternating diarrhea and constipation.

☘ BURDOCK

Arctium lappa; Asteraceae C, W
niu bang zi (seeds)

Part used: root and seeds

Energy, taste and Organs affected: root: cool; bitter, slightly sweet; Kidneys, Spleen, Stomach, Liver, skin; seeds: cold; acrid, bitter; Lungs, Stomach

Actions: root: clears Heat and toxins; seeds: cools and releases the Exterior

Properties: alterative, diuretic, diaphoretic, nutritive, antibacterial, antiinflammatory

Biochemical constituents: root: essential oil, nearly 45% inulin; seeds: arctiin, l-arctigenin, isoarctigenin, arachidonic acid, steric acid, oleic acid, linolenic acid, palmitic acid, gobosterin, vitamins A and B2, essential and fatty oils, calcium, phosphorus, sodium, iron

Dose: root: 3-10 gms; decoct 1 Tbsp./1 cup water, drink 3 cups/day; 20-60 drops tincture, 1-4 times/day; seeds: 3-9 gms; crush first before decocting

Precautions: root: diarrhea; seeds: Deficient Qi, diarrhea, open sores, carbuncles, later stages of measles

Indications: root: *skin diseases, rashes, boils, eczema, styes, carbuncles, acne, psoriasis, canker sores, anger, irritability,* *restlessness, low back pain, fluid retention, sciatica; seeds: sore, red, swollen throat, fever, cough, toxic red swellings, carbuncles, erythemas, mumps, skin conditions, acute febrile rashes, skin lesions, boils, early stages of measles, chicken pox and smallpox, psoriasis, alopecia*

Uses: A good blood, liver and lymphatic cleanser, burdock root is an excellent remedy for all skin diseases. It clears rashes, boils, eczema, styes, carbuncles, acne, psoriasis and canker sores. For skin diseases it may be combined for further effectiveness with **yellow dock** and **sarsaparilla**. Because burdock provides an abundance of iron, it strengthens as well as cleanses the blood. Burdock also detoxifies the liver, clearing Heat, anger, irritability and restlessness with beneficial effects on arthritis, rheumatism, cancer, tumors, gout, infections, inflammations and mastitis. It further has a diuretic action on the kidneys which clears the blood of harmful acids, alleviating low back pain, fluid retention, urinary calculi and sciatica. As a bitter herb, it stimulates digestion by increasing bile secretion.

The raw root may be used as a food. Called *Gobo*, the Japanese first thinly slice and soak it for 15 minutes in vinegar water, then boil in salted water. This is a cleansing and strengthening food and eaten in this way in the morning lessens sweet cravings and aids digestion (a good way to incorporate the bitter taste into our diets, which is notably lacking in most Western meals). The roots may be roasted and added to roasted **dandelion** for a useful coffee substitute that cleanses Damp Heat from the Liver and supports the Kidneys, the opposite of what coffee does!

The Chinese use burdock seeds to treat sore, red, swollen throats fever and cough. They also clear Heat and relieve toxic red swellings, carbuncles, erythemas, mumps and skin conditions such as acute febrile rashes, lesions, boils, and the incomplete expression of rashes, such as the early stages of measles, chicken pox and smallpox. They may be used externally as a wash, tincture, or oil to treat psoriasis and alopecia.

🦎 CACTUS (Night-blooming Cereus)

Cactus grandiflorus; Selenicereus grandiflorus, Cereus grandiflorus, Cactaceae **W**

Part used: fluid extract made from the flowers and green stems

Energy, taste and Organs affected: cool, sweet; Heart, Lungs

Actions: calm the Spirit

Properties: sedative, diuretic, cardiac tonic

Biochemical constituents: unavailable

Dose: 1-15 drops tincture, 1-3 times/day

Precautions: pregnancy; overdose may cause rapid and erratic heartbeat, cardiospasm or feeling of constriction in the chest, carditis, pericarditis, mental confusion, headaches, vertigo, gastrointestinal upset and noise sensitivity.

Indications: *heart problems, heart weakness, palpitations, anxiety, tachycardia, angina, carditis, pericarditis, arrhythmia, valvular disease, mitral insufficiency, irregular, feeble pulse accompanied by shortness of breath and a sensation of tightness and constriction around the chest*

Uses: A specific for heart problems, *Cactus grandiflorus* is especially indicated for irregular, feeble pulse accompanied by shortness of breath and a sensation of tightness and constriction around the chest. It works especially well when combined with **hawthorn**, **salvia**, **motherwort** and **tienchi** ginseng.

Note: Cactus can potentiate cardiac drubs like Digitoxin and Digoxin, so be sure to have your doctor monitor you while taking cactus along with these or any cardiac glycosides.

🦎 CALENDULA

Calendula officinalis; Asteraceae **W**

Part used: flowers

Energy, taste and Organs affected: neutral to warm; spicy, bitter; Liver, Heart, Lungs

Actions: invigorate Blood

Properties: vulnerary, emmenagogue, astringent, diaphoretic, antispasmodic, stimulant, antifungal, antiviral, antiseptic, demulcent, antiinflammatory, cholagogue

Biochemical constituents: essential oil containing carotenoids (carotene, calenduline and lycopene), flavonol glycosides, saponins, triterpene alcohols, sterols, carotenes, xanthophylls, polysaccharides, tannins, resin and bitter principle

Dose: 3-6 gms; infuse 2-3 Tbsp./cup water; acute—drink 1 cup tea every hour until symptoms lessen, then drink 1 cup 2-4 times/day until problem is gone, other—drink 3 cups/day; 20-50 drops tincture, 1-4 times/day

Precautions: pregnancy

Other: This herb is similar in action, but weaker than, **safflower**; the common garden **marigold** is a distinctly different plant.

Indications: *fevers, skin eruptions, measles, rashes, chicken pox, skin fungus, diaper rash, wounds that will not heal, ulcers, burns, bruises, boils, injuries, varicose veins, sore, red and irritated eyes*

Uses: Calendula is a very old herb, employed since the 12th century in Europe and even earlier in Egypt, where it originated. It is often used as a dye; in fact, cheese was originally dyed yellow by its flower. The larger flowers are more medicinal and make beautiful garden plants. The volatile oils of calendula stimulate blood circulation and cause sweating, thus lowering fevers and assisting skin eruptions to come out faster. For this reason it is specific for the beginning stages of measles, rashes and other eruptive diseases. When my son had the chicken pox, I only had to apply calendula tincture once to each pox for the itching and eruption to stop. Within the day he was feeling much better and the chicken pox rapidly cleared. Calendula oil or wash works well for this, too.

In general, calendula is a wonderful herb for cleansing the liver, and as it is neutral to warm in energy, it may safely be used for any type of liver condition without overheating it. As well, it is a great lymphatic cleanser, moving lymphatic congestion in the chest, under the armpit and in the groin area. It is hands-down one of the best herbs for any skin problems, and I have seen it useful for fungal conditions (take internally and apply topically). Many mothers find it wonderful for diaper rash. Used as a salve, oil or poultice it promotes the rapid healing of slow-healing wounds and eases persistent ulcers, burns, bruises, boils, rashes, injuries, varicose veins and bleeding, including bleeding hemorrhoids. Like **mullein**, calendula flowers can be made into oil and used for earaches and other infections. As a natural antiseptic it prevents the growth of harmful bacteria. Cooled calendula tea can be used as an eyewash for sore, red and irritated eyes.

🦎 CALIFORNIA POPPY

Eschscholzia californica; Papaveraceae   W

Part used: whole plant

Energy, taste and Organs affected: cool; bitter; Liver, Heart

Actions: calm the Spirit

Properties: sedative, analgesic, antidiarrheal, antitussive, diaphoretic, antispasmodic

Biochemical constituents: californidine, eschscholzin, protopine, N-methyllaurotanin, allocryptopine, chelerythrine, sanguinarine

Dose: infuse 1-2 tsp./cup water, drink 1–3 times daily; tincture: 20-60 drops 1-4 times daily

Precautions: pregnancy (due to the uterine-stimulating effects from the alkaloid cryptopine)

Other: This herb is completely free of any toxicity, unlike some other poppies. This is the State flower of California.

Indications: *anxiety, nervous tension, agitation, neuralgia, pain relief (including acute), nervousness, sciatica, herpes, shingles, heart palpitations, insomnia*

Uses: California poppy wonderfully sedates, calms and relaxes the nervous system, treating symptoms of anxiety, nervous tension and agitation. As well, it repairs nerves and alleviates nerve pain, especially from sciatica, herpes and shingles. It is also used for heart palpitations and insomnia due to nervousness.

⚘ CARDAMOM

Elettaria cardamomum; Amomum villosum; A. tsao-ko;
Zingiberaceae   **A, C, W**
sha ren (A. villosum); cao guo (A. tsao-ko) Sanskrit: *ela*

Part used: seed

Energy, taste and Organs affected: warm; spicy; Spleen, Stomach, Lungs, Kidney

Actions: aromatic stomachic

Properties: stomachic, carminative, expectorant, tonic

Biochemical constituents: essential oil including *d*-borneol, bornylacetate, *d*-camphor, nerolidol, linalool

Dose: 1.5-6 gms; decoct 1 tsp. seeds/cup water for 5 minutes; $1/4$ to $1/2$ tsp. powder as needed

Precautions: Deficient Yin with Heat signs

Other: Note that there are several different species of this herb, but they are all used similarly.

Indications: *Elettaria cardamomum: indigestion, gas, bloatedness, diarrhea, colic, nervous digestive upset, belching, vomiting, acid regurgitation, abdominal distention, stagnant food, headaches due to indigestion, mucus congestion in the lungs and sinuses, colds, cough, bronchitis, asthma, hoarse voice; Amomum villosum: vomiting, nausea, abdominal pain, loss of appetite, indigestion, diarrhea, morning sickness, threatened abortion, restless fetus; A. tsao-ko: malaria disorders*

Uses: A delicious spice, cardamom is one of the best digestive stimulants used by Ayurvedic, Chinese and Western herbalists, alleviating indigestion, gas, bloatedness, diarrhea, colic, nervous digestive upset, belching, vomiting, acid regurgitation, abdominal distention, stagnant food in the stomach and headaches due to indigestion.

It also counteracts mucus congestion in the lungs and sinuses, clearing colds, cough, bronchitis, asthma, and hoarse voice. When added to milk or fruit it neutralizes their mucus-forming properties. For a Lung tonic recipe core a hard winter pear, stuff it with honey and $1/2$ to 1 teaspoon cardamom powder and bake.

The Chinese actually use two types of cardamom: the seeds, *Amomum villosum*, and the fruit cluster containing the seeds (*A. tsao-ko*). *A. villosum* transforms phlegm, stops vomiting and moves stagnant Qi in the middle and upper parts of the body with symptoms of vomiting, nausea, abdominal pain, loss of appetite, indigestion, diarrhea, morning sickness, threatened abortion and a restless fetus. It is added to herbal formulas with tonifying herbs to prevent them from causing stagnation. *A. tsao-ko* not only treats digestive disorders but also malarial disorders, especially with Dampness. Ayurvedic medicine uses *Elettaria cardamomum* similarly to the Chinese use of cardamom, and adds it to milk to neutralize its mucus-forming properties.

⚘ CASCARA SAGRADA

Rhamnus purshiana; Rhamnaceae   **W**

Part used: bark of tree, dried and aged at least a year

Energy, taste and Organs affected: cold; bitter; Spleen, Stomach, Liver, Gallbladder, Large Intestine

Actions: purgative

Properties: laxative, bitter tonic, nervine, emetic

Biochemical constituents: anthraquinone glycosides of rhamnoemodine, rhamnicoside and shesterine, emodin, cascarosides, chrysaloin, chrysophanol, aloe-emodin, bitter principle, tannins, ferment and resin

Dose: 3-9 gms; infuse 1-2 tsp./cup water, drink 1 cup at bedtime (though it's usually taken in capsule or tincture form since it's too bitter for most people); 20-70 drops tincture, 1-4 times/day, or $1/2$-$3/4$ tsp. for faster action

Precautions: while some herbalists believe cascara shouldn't be used for extended periods since it may deplete potassium levels and cause muscle weakening, promoting laxative dependent constipation, others, like Dr. Christopher and Michael Tierra, have found it to be a lower bowel tonic that doesn't' create laxative dependency.

Other: Only the dried bark which is a year or older should be used, as fresh bark is too irritating; this is NOT the same herb as *Cascara amarga*, which is an entirely different herb used for diarrhea and dysentery, this herb is at risk of becoming endangered, thus **only use cultivated plant.**

Indications: *constipation, anal fissures, colitis, hemorrhoids due to poor bowel function, liver congestion or sluggishness, cirrhosis, jaundice, indigestion*

Uses: The cold bitter properties of cascara stimulate secretions of the entire digestive system, including the liver, gallbladder, stomach and pancreas, and stimulate peristalsis in the large intestine. Such secretions cause a laxative action and aid digestion. Thus, cascara is good for chronic constipation, anal fissures, colitis, hemorrhoids due to poor bowel function, liver congestion or sluggishness, cirrhosis, jaundice, indigestion and to help move bowels after rectal operations. It tones the entire intestinal tract. For those with sensitive bowels, it should be combined with a little **ginger**, **anise** or **fennel** seed to prevent griping or cramping.

🦎 CASTOR

Ricinus communis; Euphorbiaceae　　　　　　**A, C, W**
bi ma zi; Sanskrit: *eranda*

Part used: expressed oil from the seed

Energy, taste and Organs affected: neutral; sweet; bitter; toxic; Liver, Large Intestine

Actions: moist laxative

Properties: demulcent, laxative, antirheumatic, analgesic

Biochemical constituents: fixed oil consisting of glycerides of ricinoleic, isoricinoleic acid, stearic acid, linoleic acid, dihydroxystearic acid

Dose: 1-2 Tbsp. before bed

Precautions: avoid during pregnancy; *WARNING:* **do not ingest seeds—they are poisonous.**

Other: Although the castor bean is poisonous, this toxicity is left in the meal after the oil is pressed out.

Indications: *constipation, food poisoning, chronic or acute skin eruptions, worms, hard swellings, boils, abscesses, enlarged lymph nodes, bunions, corns, warts, adhesions, cysts, fibroids*

Uses: Castor oil has been used for a very long time and, in fact, is known as *Palma Christi*, meaning the Palm of Christ, so named because of its many incredible healing powers. What child does not know the "delight" of taking castor oil to move those stubborn bowels? One patient told me her parents used to give it periodically just on general health principles!

Most known as a reliable laxative to Ayurvedic, Chinese and Western herbalists, castor oil is also used for food poisoning, to expel worms when combined with anthelmintics and for chronic or acute skin eruptions. Rapidly absorbed by the body's cells, castor oil quickly heals tissues and breaks down fibrous tissue, dissolving adhesions, scars, cysts and fibroids. Topically it is applied to heal boils, abscesses, enlarged lymph nodes, hard swellings and other abnormal growths, to soften bunions and corns on the feet and to dissolve warts. The Chinese use it this way and to heal gunshot wounds.

One woman I know used it as a fomentation over her bladder for two years to effectively resolve a chronic weak bladder with recurring bladder infections. Perhaps best known as one of Edgar Cayce's favorite remedies, he frequently prescribed castor oil fomentations for toxic conditions in the body, even effective for such stubborn skin ailments as psoriasis. He recommended applying the fomentation for four days in a row, then taking three days off, repeating this process for months at a time. I frequently recommend patients do this to detoxify an area, dissolve cysts or fibroids, or to strengthen specific Organs such as the Kidneys.

Castor oil has many other wonderful uses. One of my Native American teachers uses castor oil topically for any pain conditions. She has found it to be effective even on the terrible Agent Orange pain. The Chinese also use castor oil to relieve pain by applying the leaves to swollen, painful joints. Several people I know take 5 drops of castor oil daily to prevent allergies, and have even been able to stop their long-term allergy shots by doing this. In India the leaves are steamed, softened and directly applied to arthritic joints and other painful areas for speedy, lasting relief.

❧ CAYENNE

Capsicum anuum; Solanaceae   **A, W**
Sanskrit: *marichi-phalam*

Part used: the ripe fruit (peppers)

Energy, taste and Organs affected: hot; acrid; Kidneys, Lungs, Spleen, Stomach, Heart

Actions: warms the Interior and expels Cold

Properties: stimulant, astringent, carminative, hemostatic, antispasmodic

Biochemical constituents: a pungent alkaloid (capsaicin), a red carotenoid pigment, capsanthine, high in vitamins A and C

Dose: 2 "00" capsules, 2-3 times daily; 1-5 drops tincture, 1-4 times daily; 1/4-1 tsp. powder/cup water, 2-3 times/day. Since it is quite hot and spicy to taste, cayenne powder takes getting used to: begin with a small amount and slowly increase. At first one may feel nauseous, but the feeling soon passes and a wonderful sense of well-being follows. In general, cayenne may be taken in larger doses for a beneficial short-term effect in acute conditions, but in small doses as a long-term tonic.

Precaution: pregnancy, Deficient Yin, Excess Heat; large doses cause vomiting, duodenal ulcers

Other: Cayenne and fresh **ginger** both cause sweating, which ultimately can cool the body; dried ginger warms the body Internally.

Indications: *headaches, cramping or pains of the stomach and bowels, indigestion, poor appetite, gas, arthritis, diabetic neuropathy, artherosclerosis, stomach ulcers, low vitality, first sign of colds and flu, external bleeding, acute hemorrhaging, high or low blood pressure, toothaches, cramps, sprains, muscle pain and stiffness, swellings, sore joints, laryngitis, sore throat, eye problems, trigeminal and post-hepatic neuralgia (shingles)*

Uses: Since cayenne is so hot, the idea that it's harmless is sometimes hard to believe, yet it is not irritating when uncooked. Its hot, stimulating properties make it perfect for breaking up congestion in the body, clearing mucus, moving blood and dispelling Internal and External Cold and Cold Dampness. It treats headaches, cramping or pains of the stomach and bowels, indigestion, poor appetite, gas, arthritis, diabetic neuropathy and artherosclerosis. If used carefully (starting with small doses and gradually increasing tolerance), it can heal stomach ulcers and inhibit the growth of *Helicobacter pylori* pathogen. It also stimulates energy and vitality and counteracts depression.

Considered a superior crisis herb, cayenne is a useful first-aid remedy for the first sign of colds, flu, indigestion, bleeding, or that "low" feeling (in Africa, where it is known as African Bird Pepper, it is taken daily to prevent colds, flu and other common ailments). For any type of external bleeding, sprinkling cayenne powder on the wound stops the bleeding without burning the skin or causing pain. It also arrests acute hemorrhaging internally and externally because it normalizes circulation. For the same reason, it is well suited for those who have either high or low blood pressure.

Cayenne is a terrific stimulant for the heart, circulation and for preventing heart attacks and strokes and may be taken as a daily tonic for these. It also inhibits platelet aggregation, therefore treating atherosclerosis and blood clotting. Western herbalists regularly add small amounts of cayenne in formulas as a stimulant to carry the herbs quickly and effectively throughout the body, potentizing the other herbs in the formula (this is similar to how the Chinese use **ginger**), since the spicy taste bypasses the liver detoxification process.

Externally, cayenne tincture or oil rubbed on toothaches, cramps, sprains, muscle pain and stiffness, swellings and sore joints heals and stops pain. For arthritis, apply to painful areas, then wrap in flannel cloth and keep in place throughout the night. As well, cayenne oil is used topically to alleviate the pain of trigeminal and post-hepatic neuralgia (shingles). Cayenne powder may be used as a gargle for laryngitis and sore throat and a pinch diluted in water as an eye wash to improve circulation and vision (be careful, it stings).

❧ CHAMOMILE

Matricaria recutita (German chamomile); Asteraceae **W**
Anthemis nobiles (Roman chamomile)

Part used: flowers

Energy, taste and Organs affected: neutral; bitter, spicy; Liver, Stomach, Lungs

Actions: calms the Spirit

Properties: nervine, carminative, diaphoretic, mild sedative, antispasmodic, vulnerary, antiseptic, emmenagogue, antiinflammatory, analgesic

Biochemical constituents: essential oil comprised of a blue-colored azulene; a coumarin, flavonic heterosides, tannic acid

Dose: infuse 1 heaping Tbsp./cup water, drink 1-4 cups tea a day or more as needed; 20-75 drops tincture, 1-4 times daily

Precautions: some say that large doses are emetic

Indications: *nervousness, irritability, restlessness, hypertension, insomnia, pains, cramps, spasms, indigestion, gas, fevers, colds, flu, headaches due to indigestion, constipation, menstrual cramps, children's crying, whining, restlessness, teething, colic, gas, ulcers, constipation and difficulty sleeping; externally for burns, cuts, sore muscles, painful joints, ulcers, wounds, diaper rash and earaches*

Uses: Traditionally the stronger, bitter German chamomile is preferred over the sweeter Roman chamomile because it has a stronger anti-inflammatory action. German chamomile has a high concentration of easily assimilable calcium, making it particularly useful for soothing nerves and treating nervousness, irritability, restlessness, insomnia (difficulty falling asleep), night-

mares, hypertension, pains, cramps and spasms. A common European beverage, it calms the gastric system, soothing nervous stomachs and alleviating indigestion, gas, pain, ulcers and other stomach disorders. It also treats fevers, colds, flu and headaches (especially when due to indigestion). Further, it is a gentle laxative, brings on the menses and eases menstrual cramps, especially when combined with **ginger**. Externally, a chamomile poultice, bath or herbal wash heals burns, cuts, sore muscles, painful joints, ulcers and rashes. It also makes a good hair rinse for blond hair.

Because it is a safe, calming herb, chamomile is one of the best herbs to use for crying, whining and restless children. It's also invaluable in teething, both for aiding the teeth to come in as well as calming any irritation, restlessness or fever this process causes. Used in baby's bath water or as a wash, it clears diaper rash and heals burns, wounds, cuts and abrasions. The tea eases children's colic, gas and constipation and the oil can be combined with **mullein** or **calendula** for earaches.

❧ CHAPARRAL

Larrea tridentata; L. mexicana; Zygophyllaceae **W**

Part used: leaves

Energy, taste and Organs affected: cold; bitter, spicy, slightly salty; Lungs, Liver, Kidneys

Actions: clears Heat and toxins

Properties: alterative, antiseptic, antibiotic, parasiticide; alterative, expectorant, diuretic, antitumor, laxative

Biochemical constituents: NDGA (nordihydroguaiaretic acid) is a powerful antioxidant that is vasodepressant and increases ascorbic acid levels in the adrenals

Dose: 3-6 gms; infuse 1 tsp.-1 Tbsp./cup water for 25 minutes, drink 1/2-1 cup tea 2-3 times/day; 2 "00" capsules 2-4 times/day; 10-60 drops tincture, 1-4 times/day

Precautions: pregnancy

Other: This herb is not to be confused with chaparral, a type of ecological region.

Indications: *bacteria, viruses, parasites, wounds, itching*

eczema, scabies, dandruff, warts, dental caries, infections, inflammations

Uses: Often known by the name greasewood, chaparral grows bountifully as a tall, yellow flowering bush in ring formation in desert areas. One of the oldest living plants on earth, some rings are 7,500 years old! Eating the leaf straight off the bush is a great way to acclimate one's self to the desert and cool your body (although it is usually taken in capsule or tincture form because the leaves are quite bitter).

Chaparral is antiinflammatory, or clears Heat and toxins from the respiratory, intestinal and urinary tracts, and detoxifies and decongests the liver. It is also valuable for treating bacteria, viruses and parasites. Chaparral is often combined with **goldenseal** and **echinacea** for an antibiotic effect in infections and inflammations. Externally, it is applied to heal wounds, itching eczema, scabies and dandruff, and a concentrated extract can be applied to reduce warts. A mouthwash used on a daily basis helps prevent dental caries.

☙ CHICKWEED

Stellaria media; Caryophyllaceae   **W**

Part used: above ground portion

Energy, taste and Organs affected: cool; bitter, sweet; Lungs, Stomach

Actions: clears Heat, cleans toxins

Properties: expectorant, demulcent, emollient, antitussive, antipyretic, alterative, vulnerary

Biochemical constituents: saponins, coumarins and hydroxycoumarins, flavonoids, carboxylic acids, triterpenoids, vitamin C

Dose: 6-15 gms; decoct 1 Tbsp./cup water, drink 3 cups or more as needed/day; 20-75 drops tincture, 1-4 times/day; this herb may be eaten abundantly as a food

Indications: *any itching conditions, skin eruptions, cuts, wounds, bruises, hemorrhoids, rheumatism, boils, ulcers, abscesses, sore throat, ulcers, fevers, excess fat*

Uses: This very commonly found "weed" is one of the best herbs to stop itching, alleviating mosquito bites, eczema, scaly scalp, dandruff, hives, seborea, hemorrhoids and other itchy skin conditions. Further, it can be used as a drawing poultice for boils, ulcers and abscesses. For these, it is applied externally as an oil or salve (especially with olive oil), juice, ointment or poultice. As well, it treats skin eruptions, cuts, wounds, bruises and hemorrhoids. The juice directly expressed from the leaves is especially effective for healing scalp problems. A demulcent, it also relieves sore throats, soothes stomach and duodenal ulcers, expectorates mucus from the lungs and lower fevers. It treats blood toxicity, inflammation and other "hot" type diseases. Chickweed may also be used to reduce excess fat, being both mildly diuretic and laxative.

☙ CHRYSANTHEMUM

Chrysanthemum morifolium; Asteraceae   **C**
ju hua

Part used: flowers

Energy and taste: slightly cold; pungent, sweet, bitter; Lungs, Liver

Actions: cools and releases the Exterior

Properties: antipyretic, antiinflammatory, antihypertensive, diaphoretic

Biochemical constituents: essential oil, adenine, choline and stachydrine

Dose: 5-15 gms, infusion

Precautions: Deficient Qi with poor appetite and/or diarrhea

Other: The yellow-flowered chrysanthemums are preferred; **wild chrysanthemum** flowers (*ye ju hua*) are white, colder in energy and seem more similar to **feverfew** (*C. parthenium*). They are a stronger detoxifyer for hypertension, skin ailments, eczema, scrofula, boils and inflammation of the throat, eyes and cervix.

Indications: *fevers, headache, colds, flu, pneumonia, red, painful, dry eyes, excessive tearing, blurry vision, dizziness,* *spots in front of the eyes, anger, irritability, headaches, hypertension, deafness due to ascendant Liver Yang*

Uses: Yellow chrysanthemum flowers are included in many cold and flu formulas, including the well-known *Yin Chiao (Qiao) Chieh Tu Pien*, to treat fevers, headache, colds, flu and pneumonia. Chrysanthemum also clears Heat from the Liver and soothes red, painful, dry eyes, or excessive tearing. It also treats Yin Deficient Heat of the Kidneys and Liver causing blurry vision, dizziness or spots in front of the eyes. As well, it calms the Liver and extinguishes Wind, treating anger, irritability, dizziness, headaches, hypertension and deafness due to ascendant Liver Yang. The Chinese drink chrysanthemum as a summer beverage for its refreshing taste and cooling properties.

🦎 CINNAMON

Cinnamomum cassia; Lauraceae   **A, C, W**
rou gui (bark); *gui zhi* (twigs); Sanskrit: *twak* (bark)

Part used: inner bark of tree; twigs

Energy, taste and Organs affected: bark: hot; sweet, acrid; Heart, Kidneys, Liver, Spleen; twigs: warm; sweet, acrid; Heart, Lungs, Bladder

Actions: bark: warms Interior and dispels Cold; twigs: warms and releases the Exterior

Properties: bark: stimulant, analgesic, astringent, carminative; twigs: diaphoretic, aromatic, stimulant, astringent, stomachic

Biochemical constituents: bark: cinnamic oil (cinnamic aldehyde, cinnamyl acetate, phenylpropl acetate); twigs: cinnamic aldehyde, cinnamic acid, cinnamyl acetate

Dose: bark: 1.5-4.5 gms; decoct last 5 min, or infuse 1 tsp./cup water for 25 min; crush into small pieces before using; 10-60 drops tincture; twigs: 10 min. decoction, covered, 3-9 gms for sweating, 9-15 gms for pain or to stop bleeding

Precautions: bark: Deficient Yin with Heat signs, Interior Excess Heat, bleeding from Heat, pregnancy; twigs: colds, flu and fever due to Heat (high fever, sweating, little chills), Deficient Yin with Heat signs, Heat in Blood with vomiting, pregnancy or excessive menstruation

Other: Cassia is Chinese cinnamon; it is stronger in effects than the common cinnamon used as a spice; Ayurvedic medicine uses cinnamon similarly as well as combines it with **cardamom** and **bay** to promote digestion and help absorption of medicines.

Indications: bark: *fear of the cold and being cold, cold limbs, weak back, impotence, frequent urination, cold abdominal pain, gas, spasms, reduced appetite, diarrhea, pain, amenorrhea, dysmenorrhea, arthritis, rheumatism and abscesses or sores that do not heal, all due to coldness; flushed face, wheezing, severe sweating, weak and cold, lower extremities;* twigs: *fevers, colds, flu, absence of sweating and more chills, cough, wheezing, palpitations, joint pain, chest pain, arthralgia, lumbago, arthritis, dysmenorrhea, amenorrhea, anemia or abdominal masses, bleeding*

Uses: One of the world's oldest spices, cinnamon is considered one of the seasonings in "Five Spice Powder" (the other four being **anise**, **star anise**, **cloves** and **fennel** seeds). Medicinally, the inner **bark** of the cinnamon tree (cassia) strongly warms, raising vitality, stimulating circulation and clearing congestion. It treats a variety of problems due to Coldness, such as the Deficient Kidney Yang symptoms of cold limbs, weak back, impotence, frequent urination and fear of cold, and Deficient Spleen Yang symptoms of poor digestion, cold abdominal pain, gas, spasms, reduced appetite and diarrhea. As well, it warms and unblocks the channels, alleviating Coldness that stagnates Qi or Blood, causing pain, amenorrhea, dysmenorrhea, arthritis, rheumatism and abscesses or sores that don't heal.

Cinnamon bark also "leads the body's metabolic fires back to their source", alleviating symptoms of a hot upper body and cold lower body, such as a flushed face, wheezing, severe sweating, weak and cold, lower extremities and diarrhea. Common kitchen cinnamon is also warming. Mixed with milk, it alleviates diarrhea in the elderly, and with honey, it forms a delicious paste that keeps one warm in winter and improves digestion, eliminates gas and clears mucus in the chest. Cinnamon powder may be effectively added to fruits, milk and deserts to aid their digestions.

Cinnamon **twigs** have a slightly different use. Releasing Exterior Wind Cold, they treat strong chills, lower fever, colds, flu and absence of sweating (eat a bowel of rice afterwards to replenish strength lost during the sweating process). They also treat cough and wheezing due to Wind and Cold, and spread the Yang of the Heart throughout the chest and arms, treating palpitations, warming cold hands and clearing pain in the chest and joints (especially shoulders, arthralgia, lumbago and arthritis). As well, they are widely used for gynecological problems from Coldness stagnating Blood, such as dysmenorrhea, amenorrhea, anemia, or abdominal masses. In high doses, cinnamon twigs stop bleeding as well.

🦎 CITRUS

Citrus reticulata; Rutaceae   **C**
Chen pi (aged peel)

Part used: aged dried peel of the ripe tangerine (the strongest acting) or of the orange or mandarin orange (fresh peel may be used for a weaker action

Energy, taste and Organs affected: warm; spicy, bitter; Lung, Spleen, Stomach

Actions: regulates Qi

Properties: carminative, stimulant, expectorant, antitussive, antiemetic, stomachic, antiasthmatic

Biochemical constituents: limolene, linalool, perpineol, hesperidin, carotene, cryptosanthin, vitamins B1 and C

Dose: 3-9 gms, decoct only 10 minutes

Precautions: dry cough due to Deficient Yin or Qi, Hot phlegm, spitting of blood

Other: For *chen pi*, the longer the peel is aged, the better. The green peel of immature tangerine (**green citrus**, or *qing pi*) is specifically used to regulate Liver Qi with symptoms of distention and pain in the chest, breasts or hypochondriac regions, or hernia pain. The immature (unripened) fruit of the bitter orange (*zhi shi* or *chih-shih*) has a cool energy and is used like *chen pi*, but also unblocks the bowels, treating abdominal pain, constipation and dysenteric diarrhea that is difficult. The mature ripened fruit of the bitter orange (*zhi ke*) is milder in action than *zhi shi* and is used when the patient is deficient or weak. Tangerine seed (*ju he*) is used for hernia, lumbago, mastitis, and pain and swelling of ascites.

Indications: *indigestion, gas, watery diarrhea or loose stools, nausea, vomiting, cough with profuse phlegm, abdominal swelling or fullness, bloating, belching, lack of appetite, cough with copious sputum, stifling sensation in the chest*

Uses: Citrus peels are widely used in Chinese medicine to alleviate indigestion (interestingly, the Italians use lemon peel tea for the same purpose). Both the mature and green tangerine peels are most commonly used along with the unripe and ripened fruits of the bitter orange. Aged tangerine peel moves stagnant energy in the abdomen and strengthens the digestive functions, alleviating indigestion, gas, watery diarrhea, nausea, vomiting, abdominal swelling or fullness, bloating, belching, lack of appetite and cough with profuse phlegm.

Whereas the inner fruit is cold and creates mucus, the peel warms and eliminates mucus from the Lungs and the digestive system, treating cough with copious sputum, loss of appetite, fatigue, loose stools and a stifling sensation in the chest. Thus, it is always good to eat a bit of the peel whenever eating citrus (in fact, Ayurvedic medicine says eating a bit of the peel from any fruit counteracts its potentially imbalancing properties). Finally, include citrus peel in tonifying formulas to prevent an herb's cloying nature from causing stagnation. **Grapefruit peels** also dry mucus.

🦎 CODONOPSIS

Codonopsis pilosula; Campanulaceae   **C**
dang shen

Part used: root

Energy, taste and Organs affected: neutral; sweet; Lungs, Spleen

Actions: tonifies Qi

Properties: energy tonic, demulcent, expectorant

Biochemical constituents: saponin, starch, sugar, inulin, alkaloids, sucrose, glucose

Dose: 9-30 gms, decoct for 20-30 minutes; eat root after cooking

Precautions: do not use with **veratri** (*li lu*)

Other: Codonopsis is frequently substituted for Chinese **ginseng** particularly in the summer

Indications: *lack of appetite, fatigue, tiredness, weakness, poor digestion, gas, weak arms and legs, bloatedness, diarrhea, vomiting, prolapse of uterus, stomach or rectum, chronic cough, shortness of breath, copious white to clear mucus*

Uses: Codonopsis is a primary herb used to tonify Qi, particularly of digestion (the Spleen) and immunity (the Lungs). It is similar to Chinese **ginseng**, but milder in energy and actions (and cheaper, too!) and so is safe for long-term treatment, in all climates (it is typically given in summer rather than ginseng) and by both sexes. Codonopsis increases vital energy, strengthens digestion and assimilation and treats diabetes and hyperacidity. It is given in all diseases associated with weakness, debility after illness, tiredness, lack of strength, poor appetite and anemia. It also alleviates diarrhea, vomiting, gas, bloatedness, chronic cough and shortness of breath. When combined with **astragalus**, it builds immunity. It may be given along with Exterior-releasing herbs (diaphoretics) for colds and flu in those who are weak. Include codonopsis in a weekly tonic soup or morning cereal as a general tonic. It's useful for teething babies, as its hard, sweet tasting root can be held like a stick.

❧ COIX

Coix lachryma jobi; Poaceae　　　　　　　　　**C**
yi yi ren

Part used: seeds

Energy, taste and Organs affected: slightly cold; sweet, bland; Spleen, Lungs, Kidneys

Actions: drain Dampness

Properties: diuretic, antirheumatic, antispasmodic, antiinflammatory, antidiarrheal, antitumor

Biochemical constituents: coixol, coixenolide, vitamin B1, leucine, lysine, arginine

Dose: 9–30 gms; this herb is a food and can be taken long term

Precautions: use with caution during pregnancy because it's diuretic

Other: Also known as coix; pearled barley has very similar, but milder, properties; this is **Job's Tears** (the inner kernel of the plant is used medicinally).

Indications: *edema, urinary difficulty, fluid retention in the legs, hips and thighs, moistens the skin, diarrhea, carbuncles, lung or intestinal abscesses, arthritis, rheumatism, plantar warts, fatty tumors, cancer*

Uses: Coix is quite an amazing herb as it tonifies Spleen Qi, eliminates Dampness and kills cancer cells all at the same time. Further, it is a delicious therapeutic food—make into congee porridge (dry-fry until light brown, then grind into flour and cook in water), or cook with equal parts rice and eat as a grain. Medicinally, coix drains Dampness, treating edema, urinary difficulty and fluid retention in the legs, hips and thighs, at the same time it moistens, clears and softens the skin (it does this by strengthening the Spleen to properly metabolize Fluids—taking them from where they don't belong to where they do).

Coix also stops diarrhea, clears Heat, expels pus from carbuncles and lung or intestinal abscesses, alleviates joint pain in arthritis and rheumatism from Wind-Damp and increases joint mobility while reducing spasms. It may also be used externally to treat plantar warts and fatty tumors. Research has shown coix to be an effective anticancer and antitumor herb.

❧ COLTSFOOT

Tussilago farfara; Asteraceae　　　　　　　**C, W**
kuan dong hua

Part used: leaves, flowers (the Chinese only use the flowers)

Energy, taste and Organs affected: leaves: neutral; bitter, sweet; Lungs; flowers: warm; spicy; Lungs

Actions: relieve coughing and wheezing

Properties: antitussive, expectorant, demulcent, anti-inflammatory, astringent, sedative

Biochemical constituents: leaves: mucin, abundant tannin, sitosterol, saltpeter, inulin, a glycosidal bitter principle, pyrrolizidine alkaloids in very small amounts; flowers: tannin, triterpenoid saponins, taraxanthin, mucin, two flavonoids (rutin and hyperin), phytoserols arnidiol and faradio, essential oil

Dose: 3-9 gms; infuse 1 Tbsp./cup water, drink 3 cups/day; 2 "00" caps 3 times/day; 10-50 drops tincture, 1-4 times/day; use with honey to relieve cough and moisten the Lungs

Precautions: since coltsfoot contains pyrrolizidine alkaloids, it should be avoided in pregnancy, nursing, liver disease and for prolonged use in infants and children (although it's nontoxic in low doses); use with caution for any cough due to Heat or Deficient Yin; do not use with **fritillaria**, **magnolia flowers**, **ephedra**, **scute**, **coptis** or **astragalus**

Other: The Chinese use the flowers that bloom just before winter, while Western herbalists use the leaves.

Indications: *cough, wheezing, asthma, bronchitis, whooping cough, emphysema, laryngitis, hoarseness, flu, colds, sore throat, difficulty in breathing, shortness of breath*

Uses: Meaning "cough dispeller" in Latin, coltsfoot is one of the best cough remedies available. It relieves dry, irritating or persistent coughs, wheezing, asthma, bronchitis, emphysema, whooping cough and difficulty breathing. It is especially useful in chronic respiratory conditions and for persistent or acute episodes of spasmodic cough (one mother I know found this herb amazingly effective for her child's whooping cough). It also helps the bronchioles recover after damage from smoking. Additionally, coltsfoot's demulcent and anti-inflammatory actions effectively soothe sore throats, laryngitis, hoarseness, flu and colds. For these, take as a tea, cough syrup, or smoke (as the Native Americans used it). A cup of hot coltsfoot tea first thing in the morning is especially valuable for clearing the air passages in chronic cases.

🐾 COMFREY

Symphytum officinale; Boraginaceae   **W**

Part used: leaves and root

Energy, taste and Organs affected: cool; bitter, sweet; Lungs, Stomach, bones, muscles

Actions: tonify Yin

Properties: demulcent, vulnerary, expectorant, nutritive tonic, alterative, astringent, antitussive

Biochemical constituents: leaves: allantoin, pyrrolizidine alkaloids, tannins, mucilage, starch, inulin; root: allantoin, mucilage, tannins, starch, inulin and traces of oil

Dose: root: 6-15 gms; decoct 1 tsp./cup water; leaves: 3-9 gms; infuse 2 tsp./cup water, acute—drink $1/2$ to 1 cup tea every hour until condition lessens, then drink 2 cups a day until problem is gone; 10-30 drops tincture, 1-3 times/day

Precautions: Because of its pyrrolizidine alkaloids (PAs), it should be avoided internally in pregnancy, children, nursing and liver disease. Mainly use the leaf from *S. officinalis*, as both are lower in PAs than other species or plant parts.

Indications: *fractures, skin wounds and tears, bites, stings, boils, sores, ulcers, hemorrhage, bleeding from stomach, lungs, bowels, kidneys, ulcers and piles, broken bones, diarrhea, bronchitis, tonsillitis, pharyngitis, pleurisy, pneumonia and consumption, coughs, including whooping cough, expels phlegm, sore throat, fever, poor digestion rejuvenates the lungs and mucous membranes*

Uses: Comfrey's nickname, knitbone, is highly appropriate as one of its constituents (allantoin) actually causes cell proliferation, quickly healing broken bones, fractures, torn skin (try it on torn perineums after childbirth, using the fresh herb poultice daily), and strengthening tendons, bones and ligaments (take internally and apply externally). The root can be used as well as the leaf, and is stronger in tonic properties for healing lungs and mucous membranes, especially in cases of Dryness, Heat, Deficient Yin and inflammation. The leaves are more astringent and antiinflammatory.

Because comfrey has the highest mucilage content of any herb, it is very moistening and lubricating. As a poultice or salve it soothes burns, wounds, psoriasis, eczema, inflammations, ulcers, varicose veins and draws out poisons from boils and insect bites or stings. I have found comfrey, along with perhaps **plantain** and **echinacea**, to be incomparable in drawing out the poison from spider bites, healing them quickly and painlessly. It is the fastest wound healer around. A wonderful herb for the Lungs (tonifies Lung Yin), comfrey's cooling moistening effect heals bronchitis, tonsillitis, pharyngitis, pleurisy, pneumonia, pulmonary TB, coughs (including whooping cough), expels phlegm, soothes the throat, lowers fevers and overall, rejuvenates the Lungs and mucous membranes. It helps the pancreas regulate blood sugar levels and promotes the secretion of pepsin, thus aiding digestion. Comfrey also stops bleeding from the stomach, lungs, intestines, kidneys, ulcers and piles.

While comfrey is a powerful nourishing tonic that rapidly promotes tissue growth, it is now a controversial plant because of its pyrrolizidine alkaloids causing liver disease in humans. Many herbalists feel the plant causes no threat to humans if consumed only as needed and avoided in prolonged high doses, while others have stopped using it altogether. It is important to realize that a constituent with a negative effect may be neutralized, or greatly diminished, when combined with other herbs in formulas. To help make your own choice, those with a personal and/or parental history of alcoholism, hepatitis or mononucleosis, a history of drug use (recreational or otherwise) and caffeine users should all probably avoid using this herb internally. However, it may safely be used externally by everyone. Further, certain herb companies offer PAs-free comfrey products.

✤ COPTIS

Coptis chinensis; Ranunculaceae   C
huang lian

Part used: rhizome

Energy, taste and Organs affected: cold; bitter; Heart, Large Intestine, Liver, Stomach

Actions: clears Heat, dries Dampness

Properties: antiinflammatory, antibiotic, antipyretic, cholagogue, vasodilator

Biochemical constituents: berberine, coptisine, worenine, palmatine, columbamine, obacunone, obaculactone, palmatine, jatrorrhizine, magnoflorine, ferulic acid

Dose: 1.5-9 gms; 1 tsp./cup water; 10-60 drops tincture, 1-4 times/day; take with wine for upper body symptoms, with ginger for stomach symptoms, with salt for lower body symptoms, with vinegar to clear Liver and Gallbladder Heat

Precautions: Deficient Yin and Essence with Heat signs, nausea or vomiting due to Stomach Cold and Deficiency, diarrhea due to Deficient Spleen or Kidneys; pregnancy; long-term use can injure the Spleen and Stomach; do not use with **chrysanthemum**, **scrophularia**, **coltsfoot** or **achyranthis**

Other: Also known as "goldthread", coptis is very similar to **goldenseal** in its effects (both are high in berberine) and so is a good substitute for the overused goldenseal. As a Chinese *huang*, or one of the "four yellows" (**coptis**, **scutellaria**, **phellodendron** and **rhubarb**), it is specific for treating inflammations and infections in the lower, middle and upper parts of the body; as this herb is now endangered in the States, *only used the cultivated plant*.

Indications: *high fever, irritability, meningitis, disorientation, delirium, painful, red eyes, sore throat, boils, carbuncles, abscesses, vomiting and/or acid regurgitation due to*

Stomach Heat, insomnia due to Heart Fire, hepatitis, gallstones, cirrhosis, jaundice, herpes, conjunctivitis, nosebleed, hemorrhage, blood in urine, stool or vomit, bad breath—all due to Heat; topically, for red, painful eyes, ulcerations of tongue and mouth, canker sores and scabies, dysentery, gastric pain (clears pylori bacteria)

❀ CORDYCEPS

Cordyceps sinensis; Clavicipitaceae　　　　　C
dong chong xia cao

Part used: fungus growing on caterpillar larvae (sometimes called a mushroom)

Energy, taste and Organs affected: warm; sweet; Lungs, Kidneys

Actions: tonify Yang (and Yin)

Properties: tonic, hemostatic

Biochemical constituents: cordyceptic acid, cordycepin, glutamic acid, phenylalanine, proline, histidine, valine, oxyvaline, arginine, alanine, d-mannitol, vitamin B12

Dose: 4.5-12 gms, decoction, 1-3 cups/day

Precautions: acute Exterior conditions (colds, flu, etc.)

Other: Because it tonifies both Yang and Yin, it is safe and can be taken over a long time; this herb is at risk of becoming endangered, ***thus only use the cultivated plant***.

Indications: *impotence, sore and weak lower back, legs and knees, cough, coughing up blood, chest pain, wheezing from Deficient Yin, emphysema, pulmonary TB, lowered immunity, spontaneous sweating, weakness, dizziness; increases stamina*

Uses: This unique "herb" tonifies Kidney Yang and Lung Yin, clears Phlegm and stops bleeding, thus making it very safe and useful for a variety of deficiency complaints. Use for dry cough with difficult to expectorate mucus, blood in mucus, when it's more difficult to inhale, wheezing, emphysema, frequent urination, urinating on sneezing, weakness, low back pain and/or lowered immunity. Chinese Olympic athletes used it to increase their effectiveness and endurance. To double its effectiveness, cook with duck, chicken, pork or fish (use whole herb or tablets). As this herb is very gentle, it should be taken for several months for lasting results.

❀ CORNUS

Cornus officinalis; Cornaceae　　　　　C
shan zhu yu

Part used: Chinese dogwood berries

Energy, taste and Organs affected: slightly warm; sour; Kidneys, Liver

Actions: stabilize and bind

Properties: astringent

Biochemical constituents: verbenalin, saponins, morroniside, loganin, cornusiin A & B, ursolic acid, tannin, vitamin A

Dose: 3-12 gms, 30-60 gms in shock, decoction

Precautions: painful or difficult urination, Damp Heat; do not use with **platycodon** or **sileris**

Other: The astringency of cornus berries retains Essence in a weak body (or holds "Fluids that leak out"). This means it helps those who deplete their Kidney Qi through stress and overworking physically, mentally or emotionally. North American and European dogwood berries are edible and some very delicious. They are a much under-utilized botanical resource.

Indications: *excessive urination, incontinence, spermatorrhea, excessive sweating, especially from shock, lightheadedness, dizziness, sore and weak lower back and knees, impotence, excessive uterine bleeding, excessive and prolonged menstruation, night sweats, loss of hearing, tinnitus*

❀ CORYDALIS

Corydalis yanhusuo; Papaveraceae　　　　　C
yan hu suo

Part used: rhizome

Energy, taste and Organs affected: warm; spicy, bitter; Heart, Liver, Lungs, Stomach;

Actions: invigorates Blood

Properties: analgesic, anodyne, circulatory stimulant, emmenagogue, antispasmodic

Biochemical constituents: corydaline, dl-tetrahydropalmatine, corydalis L. protopine, corybulbine, coptisine, dehydrocorydaline, corydalmine

Dose: 4.5-12 gms, decoction

Precautions: do not use during pregnancy

Indications: *menstrual, chest and abdominal pain, traumatic injury, hernia pain, migraines, headaches, arthritis, rheumatism*

Uses: As a member of the poppy family, corydalis is the most valued herb for pain in Chinese medicine. As well, it stimulates Blood and Qi circulation and breaks up stagnant Blood. I always give it for painful conditions due to stagnant Blood. It is commonly available in tablet patent form, called *Yan Hu Suo* (Formula #157).

❦ CUSCUTA

Cuscuta chinensis; Convolvulaceae   C
tu si zi

Part used: Chinese dodder seeds

Energy, taste and Organs affected: neutral; pungent, sweet; Kidneys, Liver

Actions: tonify Yang

Properties: demulcent, aperient, diuretic, aphrodisiac, ophthalmic, antifungal

Biochemical constituents: glycosides, cholesterol, campesterol, Beta-sitosterol, vitamin A

Dose: 9-15 gms, decoction

Precautions: Deficient Yin with Heat signs, constipation, scanty and dark urine

Other: Cuscuta not only tonifies Yang, but also supports Yin and Essence. As well, it is antifungal and supports digestive functions. It is also used to increase male sperm count.

Indications: *impotence, nocturnal emission, premature ejaculation, tinnitus, frequent urination, sore painful back, vaginal discharge, dizziness, blurred vision, spots in front of the eyes, diarrhea or loose stools, lack of appetite, restless fetus, threatened miscarriage; strengthens tendons and bones*

❦ CYPERUS

Cyperus rotundus; Cyperaceae   C, W
xiang fu

Part used: rhizome

Energy, taste and Organs affected: neutral; spicy, slightly bitter, slightly sweet; Liver

Actions: regulate Qi

Properties: carminative, antispasmodic, emmenagogue

Biochemical constituents: 0.5% essential oil comprised of cyperol, cyperene, cyperone, pinene and sesquiterpenes

Dose: 4.5-12 gms, decoction

Precautions: Deficient Qi (weakness, fatigue) without stagnation, Deficient Yin, Heat in the Blood (bleeding with Heat signs); this herb is very drying, use with caution in Deficient Blood

Other: Also known as **sedge**, this herb is similar to **bupleurum**, though it doesn't have the Exterior-releasing properties to treat colds and flu; the Native Americans of Northern California roasted the rhizomes and ate them as food, thus its popular name, "**nutgrass**". Natives of the Peruvian Amazon use cyperus for gynecological problems and birth control.

Indications: *painful or irregular menstruation, menstrual disorders, pain in the ribs and chest, upper abdominal distention, depression, moodiness, menstrual cramps, indigestion, gas, nausea—all due to stagnant Qi*

❦ DAMIANA

Turnera diffusa: Turneraceae   W

Part used: leaves

Energy, taste and Organs affected: warm; spicy; Kidney

Actions: tonify Yang

Properties: aphrodisiac, diuretic, nervine, aperient, expectorant

Biochemical constituents: volatile oil, hydrocyanic glycoside, bitter principle, tannin, resin

Dose: infuse 1 tsp./cup water 1 cup, 3 times daily; 10-30 drops tincture, 1-4 times/day

Precautions: Deficient Yin, pregnancy

Indications: *impotence, frigidity, poor digestion, cough, depression*

❧ DANDELION

Taraxacum mongolicum; Asteracea   **A, C, W**
pu gong ying; Sanskrit: *atirasa*

Part used: leaves and root

Energy, taste and Organs affected: cold; bitter, sweet; Liver, Stomach, Kidneys, Gallbladder, Bladder, Spleen, Pancreas

Actions: clears Heat and toxins

Properties: lithotriptic, astringent, cholagogue, galactagogue, mild laxative, diuretic (especially leaves), antibacterial, bitter stomachic

Biochemical constituents: eudesmanolides, germacranolides, triterpenes, sterols, carotenoids, flavonoids, carbohydrates (root), fructose, mucilage, potassium (leaves), inulin, aesculin (leaves), a bitter principle, tannin, vitamin A

Dose: 9-30 gms; decoct 1 tsp./cup water; drink 1 cup tea 3 times/day; 2 "00" caps, 3 times/day; 10-60 drops tincture, 1-4 times/day

Precautions: overdose can cause mild diarrhea

Indications: *red, swollen and painful eyes, firm and hard abscesses and sores, breast abscesses, sores, tumors and cysts, mastitis, gout, arthritis, skin problems, painful urination; promotes lactation; indigestion, liver congestion, hepatitis,* *jaundice, cirrhosis, constipation, skin eruptions, urinary bladder and kidney infections, gallbladder and kidney stones, diabetes, hypoglycemia*

Uses: This notable "weed" is often needed most by those who love to pull it—excitable, fiery and angry folks—because it clears the Liver Heat and congestion that causes this energy. One of the best liver and blood-cleansing herbs, **dandelion root** treats hepatitis, jaundice and cirrhosis (I have seen it effectively heal hepatitis in doses of 6 cups tea of raw root daily for 1-2 weeks) and skin conditions such as skin rashes, measles, chicken pox, eczema, poison oak and ivy and other skin eruptions (especially when combined with burdock seeds and calendula).

I always include dandelion in my liver formulas, often combining it with **isatis** and **andrographis** for a premier antibacterial, antiviral and Heat-clearing formula to treat inflammations anywhere in the body and for flu, sore throats, bladder infections and constipation (Formula #142). Dandelion root acts on the digestive system by stimulating secretion of bile, assisting digestion and elimination, dissolving gallbladder and kidney stones and regulating blood sugar in diabetes and hypoglycemia. As well, it helps detoxification and stagnation from overeating meat, fatty and fried foods, treating gout and arthritis.

The root can be roasted and made into a strong tea that Europeans call Dandelion Coffee, an excellent coffee substitute since its full-bodied bitter flavor is satisfying and counteracts the effects of previous caffeine by cleansing the injured liver. It combines well with **chicory root** for a closer coffee flavor (use roasted roots if there's Coldness and raw roots if there's Heat). I frequently recommend it to help people eliminate their daily coffee by slowly decreasing the caffeine and commensurately increasing the dandelion/chicory tea. Grind the roots and place in a filter, just like your coffee ritual.

The Chinese use dandelion root's Cold properties to treat Hot (and painful) toxic swellings, infections, inflammations, boils, abscesses, dental caries, red, swollen and painful eyes or throat, fever and mumps. Having a special affect on the breasts, the Chinese also use it to reduce breast sores, tumors, mastitis, swollen lymph nodes and cysts. As such, it is a breast cancer preventative. It also stimulates the production of mother's milk. Externally, the Native Americans applied its juice to snake bites. Ayurvedic practitioners use it for dysentery, fevers, vomiting and as an antipoison.

Dandelion leaves are very high in iron, vitamins and minerals, especially vitamin A and potassium. Grown as a vegetable in Europe, they are eaten when young in the spring (they are less bitter then—add olive oil and lemon juice) to help clear winter's excesses and prevent spring's colds and flu. Taken cool, dandelion leaf tea is one of the most effective diuretics, as effective as Lasix, and because it is rich in potassium, it isn't as harsh, thus cleansing the kidneys, eliminating water retention and lowering blood pressure.

❀ DANG GUI

Angelica sinensis; Apiaceae   **C**
dang gui

Part used: Chinese angelica root

Energy, taste and Organs affected: warm; sweet, spicy, bitter; Heart, Liver, Spleen

Actions: tonify Blood

Properties: emmenagogue, analgesic, mild laxative, sedative

Biochemical constituents: butylidene phthalide, ligustlide, sequiterpenes, carvacrol, dihydrophthalic anhydride, sucrose, vitamins B12 and E, carotene, folic acid, folinic acid

Dose: 3-15 gms; 10-60 drops tincture, 1-4 times daily; char to stop bleeding, take with wine to invigorate blood

Precautions: diarrhea, abdominal distention due to Dampness, Deficient Yin with Heat; pregnancy, excessive menstrual flow; nosebleeds, sore throat, blood clotting difficulty, if taking blood thinning medication

Other: This is also known as **dang gui** or **tang kuei**; usually the entire root is prescribed, as the tail, body and head have slightly varying functions (the head is more tonic, the tail more Blood invigorating while the body does both equally).

Indications: *builds blood, regulates menses; anemia, for all gynecological problems: irregular menstruation, amenorrhea, dysmenorrhea; tinnitus, blurred vision, palpitations, numbness in the limbs, abdominal pain, traumatic injury, arthritis, rheumatism, sores, abscesses, constipation due to anemia, dry skin and skin eruptions*

Uses: Dang gui is the supreme woman's herb for tonifying Blood and regulating menses. It is used for most gynecological complaints, promoting blood circulation, stimulating the uterus and stopping pain. As such, it is also used for abdominal and menstrual pain, traumatic injuries, arthritis, rheumatism, sores and abscesses. Because dang gui actually causes red blood cell proliferation, it is invaluable for anemia (including pernicious), pale face, blurred vision, dizziness, numbness in the limbs, palpitations, weakness (particularly during menses), thrombosis and headaches due to Deficient Blood (although usually given to women, men can take it for this, too). As well, it normalizes heart contractions and dilates coronary blood vessels, increasing peripheral blood flow.

Dang gui smoothes menopausal complaints and promotes feelings of compassion. Studies are mixed, with some showing estrogen activity while others don't. Regardless, the Chinese successfully use it to reduce fibroids in those with Deficient Blood and so it doesn't seem to aggravate estrogen-sensitive tumors or growths. In fact, dang gui exemplifies one of the mysterious ways that many herbs work: despite it having or not having phyto-estrogens, it promotes healthy pelvic blood circulation, which thus normalizes gynecological or hormonal imbalances.

Dang gui moistens the intestines, alleviating constipation due to Deficient Blood (dryness in intestines). While normally not taken during menses (it increases blood flow), women with scanty menses or those in peri/menopause may take it during the end of their cycles to help complete sloughing of the uterine lining.

🦎 DEER ANTLER

Cornu cervi parvum; Cervidae   C
lu rong

Part used: velvet of young deer antler

Energy, taste and Organs affected: warm; salty, sweet; Kidney, Liver

Actions: tonify Yang

Properties: tonic, stimulant

Biochemical constituents: calcium, magnesium, phosphorus, estrone (small amounts)

Dose: 3-4.5 gms, decocted; 1-3 gms powder divided into 2-3 doses. **NOTE:** It is very important to start off with low doses and gradually work up; otherwise symptoms of dizziness or red eyes can occur.

Precautions: Deficient Yin with Heat signs, Heat in the Blood, Damp Heat in Lungs, Stomach Heat, fevers

Other: When deer antler is cooked a long time, a residue collects. This is powdered into the herb, **antler glue** (*lu jiao shuang*), used to nourish Blood, stop bleeding and tonify Kidney Yang. This powerful Yang tonic also supports Yin and Essence and tonifies Qi and Blood, thus making it very beneficial herb for many conditions.

Indications: *fatigue, infertility, low sex drive, impotence, frigidity, cold extremities, lightheadedness, ringing in the ears, sore and weak lower back and knees; frequent, copious, clear urination; children's physical and/or mental developmental disorders, failure to thrive, mental retardation, learning disabilities, insufficient growth or skeletal deformities; vaginal discharge, uterine bleeding, chronic ulcerations or boils, peri/menopause*

🦎 DIPSACUS

Dipsacus asper; Dipsacaceae   C
xu duan

Part used: root

Energy, taste and Organs affected: slightly warm; bitter, pungent; Kidney, Liver

Actions: tonify Yang

Properties: tonic, hemostatic, antirheumatic, bone-healing, analgesic, promotes growth of flesh

Biochemical constituents: alkaloid, essential oil, vitamin E

Dose: 6-21 gms, decoction; fry in vinegar to enhance its blood invigoration and pain-alleviating properties; roast in salt to enhance its Kidney-tonifying properties; dry-fry or char for excessive uterine bleeding; powder to apply topically

Precautions: Deficient Yin with Heat signs

Other: Also known as **teasel**, the literal translation of the pinyin name is "restore what is broken" or "heal fracture", referring to its ability to strengthen weak bones, knees and tendons.

Indications: *sore and painful lower back and knees, stiffness in the joints, weak legs, uterine bleeding, white vaginal discharge, bleeding during pregnancy, restless fetus, threatened miscarriage, pain, traumatic injuries, healing of bones, skin sores, arthritis, rheumatism*

Uses: Teasel, a beautiful herb with a tall bristly head, grows many places. I once saw multitudes of dried teasel heads in a wool combing machine in Scotland, as it is still used today. In fact, it is widely available throughout the world and, except for the Chinese, is underutilized.

Medicinally, dipsacus tonifies Kidney Yang, treating sore and painful lower back and knees, stiffness in the joints, weak legs and arthritis and rheumatism from Wind-Cold-Damp. As it stops white vaginal discharge and bleeding, especially uterine, it's used to stop bleeding during pregnancy, calm a restless fetus and treat threatened miscarriage, all due to Coldness and Deficiency with lower back pain. Because it moves Blood, alleviates pain and promotes growth of flesh, dipsacus is also used for traumatic injuries, healing of bones (as it's name implies) and skin sores. For these, it may be applied externally and taken internally.

ECHINACEA

Echinacea spp.; Asteraceae   **W**

Part used: root

Energy, taste and Organs affected: cool; spicy, bitter; Lungs, Stomach, Liver

Actions: clears Heat and toxins

Properties: alterative, antibiotic, vulnerary, stimulant, antiseptic, antibacterial, antiviral

Biochemical constituents: echinacoside, unsaturated isobutyl amides, polysaccharides, a heteroxylan and an arabinorhamnogalactan, polyacetylenes, essential oil

Dose: 3-9 gms; decoct 1 tsp./cup water; 2 "00" caps, 3 times/day; 10-75 drops tincture, 1-4 times/day; acute conditions—take 1 dropperful of tincture, or 2 "00" capsules, every 1/2 hour. As symptoms lessen, take same dosage every two hours and taper off until problem is gone.

Precautions: Coldness; Deficient Yang

Other: Also known as **purple coneflower**; often grown as a garden ornamental; this herb is now endangered, thus *only use the cultivated plant.*

Indications: *all infections and inflammations, swollen glands, offensive discharges, bites, wounds, immune enhancing, colds, blood poisoning, fevers, poison oak and ivy, boils and other skin infections, cancer*

Uses: Echinacea, nature's incredible natural antibiotic, activates leukocytes (white blood cell infection fighters) and T-cell formation, which assist the healing process, raise the body's immune level and encourage wounds to heal. It also inhibits the hyaluronidase enzyme that causes the spread of bacteria. Thus, it is one of the most powerful and effective remedies against all kinds of bacterial infections and inflammations. Large doses can be taken because it is not toxic, and its effects are potentiated if you exercise within 10 minutes after taking it.

Echinacea is a wonderful blood cleanser, effective for blood poisoning and toxicity, cancer and other poisonous conditions. It further decongests the lymph, treating swollen glands and offensive discharges, alleviates the negative effects of vaccinations, lowers fevers (including typhoid fever) and prevents and cures colds, flu and sore throats. Note that while echinacea treats these conditions, according to herbalists Christopher Hobbs and Michael Tierra, if used preventatively for more than ten days, it looses effectiveness. This points to its main use as an herb for acute inflammations and infections rather than as a "tonic" herb. For those with Internal Heat, echinacea is fine alone, but for those with Coldness or any Deficiencies, it works best when combined with **eleuthro** or **astragalus**.

Externally, echinacea is excellent for all venomous bites, such as snake, insect and spider, poison oak and ivy, boils, cuts, wounds and other skin infections, and for teething. It is even more effective when taken both externally and internally, the more frequently the better, or when combined with other remedies, such as salves, washes, baths and poultices. It is such a valuable herb, I always have echinacea tincture nearby for first aid and emergencies.

☙ ELDER

Sambucus nigra; S. canadensis; Caprifoliaceae   **W**

Part used: flowers (also berries and leaves)

Energy, taste and Organs affected: cool; bitter, spicy; Lungs, Liver

Actions: cools and releases Exterior

Properties: antiviral, diaphoretic, alterative, stimulant, expectorant, diuretic, mild laxative

Biochemical constituents: essential oil, terpenes, glycosides, rutin, quercitin, mucilage, tannin; berries high in vitamin C, aribino A, alpha and beta-amyrin, palmitate

Dose: infuse 1 Tbsp./cup water, 3 cups/day; 10-60 drops tincture, 1-4 times/day; 1 Tbsp. syrup as needed

Precautions: Only black elder is safe to use internally; red elder (*S. racemosa*) is toxic; unripe fruit and excessive use of leaves, root and bark can cause nausea, vomiting, diarrhea, dizziness, tachycardia and convulsions.

Other: The aged bark is used as a laxative and the berries as an antirheumatic; elder berries are frequently made into jams, wine and eaten as fruit; often called the Tree of Music, the hollowed branches are made into flute pipes and whistles (as well as pea shooters and play arrows!).

Indications: flowers: *colds, flu, fever, coughs, rashes, burns, wrinkles*; berries: *chronic sinusitis, night sweats, rheumatism, neuralgia*; leaves: *rashes, burns, skin ailments, wrinkles*

Uses: An herb revered around the world for its effectiveness, folklore invests elder with magical powers of protection and long life. Indeed, the delicious elder berries are a fantastic antiviral herb that effectively dispel colds, flu, fever, cough, spasmodic croup, chronic sinusitis and night sweats, and the berry juice treats rheumatism and neuralgia. The leaves treat these as well and soothe rashes, burns and other skin ailments and diminish wrinkles. Elder flowers soften and soothe the skin, healing burns, cuts, scratches, sores and abrasions (combine with **chamomile** and **calendula** flowers).

✿ ELECAMPANE

Inula helenium (Western); *I. Japonica, I. chinensis* (Chinese); *Asteraceae*   **A, C, W**
xuan fu hua; Sanskrit: *pushkaramula*

Part used: root, flowers

Energy, taste and Organs affected: warm; sweet, spicy, bitter; Liver, Lungs, Spleen, Stomach

Actions: warms and dissolves Phlegm and stops cough

Properties: carminative, expectorant, diuretic, antiseptic, astringent, stimulant

Biochemical constituents: flower: britanin, inulicin, inulin, quercetin, isoquercetin, caffeic acid, chlorogenic acid, taraxasterol, sterols; root: essential oil, bitter principles, resin, inulin

Dose: flower: 3-12 gms; infuse 1 Tbsp./cup water; root: 3-9 gms; decoct 1 tsp./cup water; drink 3 cups/day; 1 "00" cap, 3 times/day; $^1/_2$ tsp. or 10-40 drops tincture, 1-4 times/day; take with honey to moisten Lungs and relieve cough

Precautions: cough due to Wind and Heat; large doses of the root can cause vomiting, diarrhea or gastric spasms

Other: Western herbalists use the root while the Chinese mainly use the flowers; the Chinese use the leaves (*jin fei cao*) for similar uses as the flowers, but for more superficial problems.

Indications: *colds, cough, wheezing, asthma, bronchitis, vomiting, hiccoughs, poor or weak digestion, nervous debility*

Uses: Elecampane root and flowers eliminate Cold Dampness from Lungs and Spleen, clearing and inhibiting the formation of mucus due to poor digestion and assimilation. The flowers particularly redirect Qi downwards, alleviating cough and wheezing with copious phlegm, treating bronchitis, asthma, sinusitis and stopping irritable or chronic cough, vomiting and hiccoughs from Dampness, Coldness or weakness in Spleen and Stomach. It is particularly useful for the elderly or convalescent. For chronic lung ailments combine with **wild cherry** bark, **comfrey** root and **licorice**, or extract one ounce of the bruised root in a pint of red wine and take 1 tablespoon every several hours. To increase its tonic properties, roast the roots in a dry pan with honey.

The root contains a starch-type carbohydrate called inulin, which has a sweetish taste and is used as a sugar substitute for diabetics (this is NOT insulin, however). The flowers contain quercetin, very useful for upper respiratory allergies and hayfever. Ayurvedic medicine uses elecampane not only to clear the lungs, but as a lung rejuvenative tonic since it promotes the longevity of lung tissue.

✿ ELEUTHRO (see SIBERIAN GINSENG on page 120)

Eleutherococcus senticosus; Araliaceae   **W**

✿ EPHEDRA

Ephedra spp.; Ephedraceae   **C**
ma huang

Part used: twigs or stems

Energy, taste and Organs affected: warm; spicy, slightly bitter; Lungs, Bladder

Actions: warms and releases the Exterior

Properties: diaphoretic, stimulant, diuretic, expectorant, astringent, antiasthmatic, antitussive

Biochemical constituents: ephedrine alkaloids, pseudoephedrine, norephedrine

Dose: 3-9 gms, decoction

Precautions: Deficiency (any type) with sweating or wheezing; high blood pressure, glaucoma, hyperthyroidism, heart palpitations, if on MAO inhibitors[2]; excessive use can cause heavy sweating and weaken the body. Symptoms of ephedra overdose include palpitations, rapid heartbeat, elevated blood pressure, restlessness, tremors, insomnia, nervousness and sweating.

Other: Western ephedra is often called **Mormon Tea**, **Brigham Tea**, or joint fur. It has similar effects but is far less stimulating and so milder acting. As a diuretic it is more useful for treating water retention. Ephedra root (*ma huang gen*) is used to stop spontaneous sweating and night sweats, opposite effects to the stems/twigs.

Important note: There are Ma huang products on the market used to stimulate energy or weight loss. This is a dangerous and inappropriate use of a valuable herb. That said, the well-known pharmaceutical stimulant *dexedrine*, is widely sold as a weight-loss stimulant and is at least equally, or more, dangerous as concentrated ma huang in such formulas. Both should be used cautiously by those with a tendency to cardiovascular disease.

Indications: *colds with chills, slight fever, colds, flu, headache, lack of sweating, cough, asthma, bronchitis, wheezing, edema*

Uses: Chinese ephedra is a strong stimulant with an action like adrenaline. Included in most formulas to treat asthma (and quite effective for this, especially when honey-roasted), ephedra is a powerful bronchodilator valuable for treating bronchitis, wheezing, cough and difficulty in breathing. As ephedra causes sweating, it is helpful in relieving colds, flu and fever without sweating in those with strong constitutions. It also has a diuretic effect, reducing acute edema. Ephedra is a useful

and powerful herb, but should definitely be avoided by those with high blood pressure and/or heart problems.

🦁 EPIMEDIUM

Epimedium grandiflorum; Berberidaceae C
yin yang huo

Part used: aerial parts

Energy, taste and Organs affected: warm; acrid, sweet; Kidneys, Liver

Actions: tonify Yang

Properties: yang tonic, aphrodisiac, antirheumatic, antitussive, expectorant, antiasthmatic

Biochemical constituents: flavonol glycoside (icariin), olivil, icariresinol, epimidine, tannin, palmitic acid, linolenic acid, oleic acid, vitamin E

Dose: 6-15 gms, infusion; steep in wine to enhance its properties

Precautions: Deficient Yin with Heat signs, hypersexuality and wet dreams; do not take for prolonged periods as it can damage the Yin, causing dizziness, vomiting, dry mouth, thirst and nosebleed

Other: This genus is composed of about 25 species and is often grown as an ornamental ground cover for shady borders. Also known as "licentious (or **horny**) **goat wort (weed)**", it is commonly available from nurseries. Grow in a shaded, moist environment.

Indications: *impotence, frigidity, spermatorrhea, involuntary and premature ejaculation, frequent urination, forgetfulness, withdrawal, painful cold lower back and knees, lower back pain, dizziness, headache, hypertension, menstrual irregularity, arthritis, rheumatism, spasms or cramps in the hands and feet, joint pain, numbness in the extremities, high blood pressure, chronic bronchitis*

Uses: Although epimedium has been used by the Chinese for quite a long time, it is hitting the Western market now as a sexual tonic and aphrodisiac, just as its name, horny goat weed, implies. Indeed, epimedium is used in China to stimulate sexual activity

---

[2] Tillotson, *The One Earth Herbal Sourcebook*, Kensington Publishing Group, 2001.

and sperm production, treating symptoms of impotence, frigidity, spermatorrhea, involuntary and premature ejaculation, frequent urination, forgetfulness, withdrawal and painful cold lower back and knees. Now, as with most Kidney Yang tonics (and tonics in general) results take awhile to appear, so don't expect any immediate miracles like some medications. At the same time, be sure to eliminate all cold/cooling foods and drinks, such as iced drinks, ice cream, raw foods, fruit juices and soy milk, as well as sugar, caffeine and alcohol, as these foods cause all the symptoms for which you want to take epimedium in the first place (sounding harder now?).

Epimedium also tonifies Yin along with Yang and harnesses ascendant Liver Yang due to underlying Kidney and Liver Deficiency. All this means that it's useful for lower back pain, dizziness, menstrual irregularity, peri/menopausal symptoms, headaches and hypertension. As well, this versatile herb expels Wind-Damp-Cold, treating arthritis, rheumatism, spasms or cramps in the hands and feet, joint pain and numbness in the extremities. Epimedium further strengthens the bones (the Kidneys rule the bones), lowers blood pressure and treats chronic bronchitis, especially when there is Coldness (white phlegm) and difficulty on inhalation. I always include it in any peri/menopausal formula along with Yin tonics.

❧ EUCOMMIA

Eucommia ulmoides; Eucommiaceae **C**
du zhong

Part used: bark

Energy, taste and Organs affected: warm; sweet, slightly spicy; Kidneys, Liver

Actions: tonify Yang

Properties: antihypertensive, diuretic, sedative

Biochemical constituents: gutta-percha, aucubin, alkaloids, glycosides, potassium, vitamin C

Dose: 6-15 gms, decoction; salt-water fry to increase its Kidney-tonification glycosides properties

Precautions: Deficient Yin with Heat signs; do not use with **scrophularia**

Other: commonly given with Chinese **scutellaria** to effectively lower high blood pressure

Indications: *weakness and pain in lower back and knees, fatigue, frequent urination, calms fetus, bleeding during pregnancy, prevents miscarriage, hypertension, premature aging, impotence; strengthens tendons and bones*

❧ EYEBRIGHT

Euphrasia officinalis; Scrophulariaceae **W**

Part used: above ground portion

Energy, taste and Organs affected: cool; bitter, mildly astringent; Liver, Lungs

Actions: stabilize and bind

Properties: astringent, antiinflammatory, expectorant, alterative

Biochemical constituents: tannins, iridoid glycosides including aucubin, ancuboside, phenolic acids, caffeic and ferulic acids, sterols, choline, volatile oil

Dose: 2-5 gms; infuse 1-2 tsp./cup water, drink 3 cups a day; 2 "00" caps, 3 times/day; 10-60 drops tincture, 1-4 times/day

Precautions: none noted

Other: This herb is now endangered, thus *only use the cultivated plant.*

Indications: *conjunctivitis, blepharitis, scrofulous eye conditions, eye infections, eye weakness, ophthalmia, sinus infections, congestion and inflammations of nose, throat and lungs*

Uses: As eyebright clears Heat in the Liver and toxins from the Blood, helping promote clarity of vision, it treats many eye problems such as blepharitis, scrofulous eye conditions in children, eye infections, eye weakness and ophthalmia. It also treats conjunctivitis with thick, yellow discharge and swollen red eyes that are encrusted in the morning. Also use externally as eyewash, especially combined with **raspberry**, **bayberry** and **goldenseal**. It may also be used as a compress to give rapid relief of redness, swelling and visual disturbances in acute inflammations and eye injuries. As well, eyebright decongests the upper sinuses, useful for inflammations of the nose, throat and bronchioles and nasal and sinus congestion, especially if the discharge is thin and watery. A specific for "snuffles," even in infants, place 5-10 drops tincture in $1/2$ glass water and administer 1 tsp. every 15-30 minutes.

❧ FENNEL

Foeniculum vulgare; Apiaceae   **A, C, W**
xiao hui xiang; Sanskrit: *mahdurika*

Part used: seeds

Energy, taste and Organs affected: warm; spicy, sweet; Liver, Kidneys, Spleen, Stomach

Actions: regulate Qi

Properties: stimulant, carminative, antispasmodic, diuretic, expectorant, galactagogue

Biochemical constituents: volatile oil (up to 8%) consisting mainly of anethole, 10-30% fenchone, flavonoids, alpha-phellandrine, limonene, methylchavicol, amesaldehyde, alpha-pinene, protein, fixed oil, organic acids

Dose: 3-9 gms; eat directly or decoct 1 tsp.-1 Tbsp./cup water for 5 minutes, drink 3-4 cups/day; 2 "00" caps, 3 times/day; 10-60 drops tincture, 1-4 times/day

Precautions: Deficient Yin with Heat signs, pregnancy (relaxes uterus)

Other: Fennel stalks may be eaten raw like celery and are a delicious and beneficial addition to any meal.

Indications: *indigestion, gas, bloatedness, spasms of gastrointestinal tract, abdominal pain due to cold, cough, reduced appetite, vomiting, abdominal pain, spasms, cramps, colic, hernia pain, cough; promotes lactation*

Uses: In medieval times the fennel plant, along with **St. John's wort** and **rosemary**, were hung over doors on Midsummer's Eve to ward off evil spirits. Today the delicious taste of fennel makes it a wonderful after-meal tea to ease gas, indigestion, abdominal pain and spasms of

the gastrointestinal tract (the roasted and sweetened seeds are eaten this way in India). Fennel is also excellent for digestive weakness and colic in children or the elderly, as its warm energy isn't over-stimulating.

Fennel regulates Liver Qi, smoothing energy flow, calming nerves, easing cramps and spasms, aiding bowel movements and treating hernia pain. It is often combined with purgatives to prevent any attendant griping. It helps clear mucus from the Lungs, treating cough and promoting lactation. According to herbalist Sharon Tilgnar, this herb has phytoestrogen effects. Chinese herbalists use fennel to treat lower abdominal pain, indigestion, decreased appetite, vomiting, gas and intestinal spasms due to Coldness.

❧ FENUGREEK

Trigonella foenum-graecum; Fabaceae   **A, C, W**
hu lu ba; Sanskrit: *methi*

Part used: seeds

Energy, taste and Organs affected: warm; bitter; Kidneys, Liver

Actions: tonify Yang

Properties: nutritive, carminative, stimulant, demulcent, alterative, expectorant, antipyretic, rejuvenative, diuretic

Biochemical constituents: gentianine, carpaine, choline, trigonelline, disogenin, yarnogenin, gitogenin, tigogenin, vitexin, orientin, quercetin, triptophan, vitamin B, protein

Dose: 3-9 gms; decoct 1 Tbsp./cup water, drink 3 cups/day; 10-50 drops tincture, 1-4 times/day; as a tonic: 1 tsp. powder/cup heated milk, once/day

Precautions: Dampness, Deficient Yin with Heat signs; pregnancy (stimulates uterus)

Other: Fenugreek seeds are included in curry powders and used as a flavoring.

Indications: *indigestion, mucus, tuberculosis, anemia, convalescence, promotes lactation and hair growth, regulates blood sugar balance, low back pain, hernia pain*

Uses: One of the oldest known herbs, the ancient Egyptians, Romans and Greeks used fenugreek seeds for both medicinal and culinary purposes. Greatly benefiting the nervous, digestive and respiratory systems, it clears mucus, easing cough, preventing fever and alleviating stomach and digestive disorders, including colic. It is very nourishing for wasting diseases such as tuberculosis, anemia, debility, neurasthenia and convalescence (especially when combined with milk) and diarrhea in infants. Made into gruel, the seeds stimulate mother's milk and promote hair growth. In Chinese medicine fenugreek is used as a Yang tonic for coldness, pain in the lower back, abdomen, sides, ribs and/or extremities, hernia, gastric problems and morning sickness. The seeds may be sprouted and eaten to aid digestion and seminal debility. A poultice treats sores, ulcers and boils, and the eyewash sooths inflamed eyes.

❀ FEVERFEW

Tanacetum parthenium; Asteraceae　　　　**A, W**
Sanskrit: *atasi*

Part used: leaves, flowers

Energy, taste and Organs affected: cool; bitter; Stomach, Liver

Actions: cools and releases the Exterior

Properties: antipyretic, carminative, purgative, bitter tonic, diaphoretic, antiinflammatory

Biochemical constituents: volatile oils (camphor, terpene, borneol), various esters, bitter principle

Dose: 3-9 gms; infuse 1 tsp./cup water, drink 2-3 cups/day; 10-40 drops tincture, 1-4 times/day

Precautions: do not use for migraines resulting from weakness or Deficiency; pregnancy (emmenagogue effects)

Indications: *headaches and migraines due to Liver Heat (use long-term for best results), colds, flu, fever, digestive problems, arthritis*

❀ FORSYTHIA

Forsythia suspensa: Oleaceae　　　　**C**
lian qiao

Part used: fruit (seed)

Energy, taste and Organs affected: cool; bitter, slightly spicy; Heart, Liver, Gallbladder

Actions: clear Heat and toxins

Properties: antibacterial, antimicrobial, antiemetic, parasiticide, antipyretic, antiinflammatory

Biochemical constituents: forsythin, matairesinoside, betulinic acid, phyillygenin, pinoresinol

Dose: 6-15 gms, infusion

Precautions: Spleen and Stomach Deficiency with diarrhea; carbuncles that have already ulcerated, concave ulcers oozing clear fluid (called Yin ulcers)

Indications: *skin ailments, acne, toxic and hot sores, boils, carbuncles, neck lumps, colds, flu, fever, slight chills, sore throat, headache, urinary tract infections, scrofula, abscesses*

Uses: Forsythia is a wonderful Heat-clearing herb that treats many skin ailments, such as acne, toxic and hot sores, boils, carbuncles and neck lumps. I always combine it with my skin-clearing remedies as it also opens the surface to release toxins. This same action makes it useful in alleviating colds and flu with high fever, slight chills, sore throat, thirst, sweating and headache. It is an ingredient (along with its "cousin" **honeysuckle**) in the well-known Chinese cold and flu patent, *Yin Chiao (Qiao) Chieh Tu Pien* (Formulas #109 and 110). As well, it treats urinary tract infections, scrofula and abscesses.

❀ FRANKINCENSE

Boswellia carterii, B. serrata; Burseraceae　　**A, C**
ru xiang (B. carterii), Sanskrit: *shallaki (B. carterii)*;
Hindi: *salai guggul (B. serrata)*

Part used: gum (resin)

Energy, taste and Organs affected: warm; spicy, bitter; Heart, Liver, Spleen

Actions: invigorates Blood

Properties: circulatory stimulant, emmenagogue, analgesic, vulnerary

Biochemical constituents: boswellic acids, olibanoresene, arabic acid, bassorin, pinene, dipentene

Dose: 3-9 gms; fry with vinegar to enhance its Blood-invigorating properties

Precautions: avoid in pregnancy; caution in Deficient Spleen conditions

Other: The pharmaceutical name for *B. carterii* is *Gummi olibanum.*

Indications: *traumatic injuries, sprains, aches, osteoarthritis, rheumatoid arthritis, arthritic aches and pains, joint pains, chest, epigastric or abdominal pain, sores, carbuncles; redness and swelling of gums, mouth and throat; bronchial asthma, ulcerative colitis, psoriasis, Crohn's disease, edema, boils, arthritis*

Uses: Frankincense is a powerful pain reliever, treating traumatic injuries, sprains, aches, osteoarthritis, rheumatoid arthritis, arthritic aches and pains, joint pains and chest, epigastric or abdominal pain due to stagnant Blood (boring, stabbing pain). I almost always include it in formulas for the above, combining it with **myrrh** and **corydalis**. As well, frankincense may be applied topically to reduce swelling and generate flesh, promoting healing of sores, carbuncles, traumatic injuries and pain, redness and swelling of gums, mouth and throat. Ayurvedic medicine uses a purified form of frankincense, referred to as **Boswellia**, as an anti-inflammatory to treat bronchial asthma, ulcerative colitis, psoriasis, Crohn's disease, edema and boils. It is also one of the most effective herbs for relieving arthritic pains.

🐾 FU LING

Poria cocos; Polyporaceae   C
fu ling

Part used: whole fungus (mushroom, usually found adhering to the roots of pine trees)

Energy, taste and Organs affected: neutral; sweet; Heart, Lungs, Spleen

Actions: drains Dampness

Properties: diuretic, sedative, lowers blood sugar

Biochemical constituents: tetracyclic triterpenic acid (eburicolic acid, pachymic acid), polysaccharide (pachyman), ergosterol, tumulosic acid, chitin, protein, glucose, sterols, histamines, lecithin, gum, lipase, choline, adenine

Dose: 9-15 gms, decoction; up to 60 gms for acute facial edema

Precautions: frequent, copious urination due to Cold (Deficient Yang), or prolapse of urogenital organs; do not use with **sanguisorbae**, **gentian** or **tortoise shell**

Other: Also known as **Hoelen**; a species was used by Native Americans found adhering to the roots of pine trees, known as **Tuckahoe**, or **Indian Bread**; the central part of the sclerotium with the root of *Pinus densiflora* or *P. massoniana* still in the center is specifically used by the Chinese (as *fu shen*) to calm the mind and sedate nerves.

Indications: *difficult urination, excessive Dampness, edema, loss of appetite, diarrhea, abdominal distention, insomnia, forgetfulness, anxiety, palpitations, moodiness, tachycardia from Dampness*

Uses: In Chinese medicine, an herb that drains Dampness acts not only as a diuretic, but also aids proper cellular fluid metabolism. Interestingly, Western science has found fu ling to be high in potassium salts that free interstitial fluid for excretion and regulate intercellular fluid metabolism while not causing thirst or potassium depletion. In general, medicinal mushrooms aid in this process, which helps alleviate toxic Dampness causing tumors and cancer. Thus, they are also used to treat tumors and cancer. Fu ling specifically promotes urination, treating urinary difficulty, diarrhea, edema and scanty urine due to Damp Heat. As well, it alleviates poor appetite, epigastric distention, headache and dizziness due to Phlegm and calms the spirit, alleviating palpitations, insomnia and forgetfulness.

❧ GAMBIR

Uncaria rhynchophylla; Rubiaceae   C
gou teng

Part used: stems with hooks (thorns) of vine

Energy, taste and Organs affected: cool; sweet; Heart, Liver

Actions: extinguish Internal Wind

Properties: sedative, anticonvulsant, antipyretic, lowers blood pressure

Biochemical constituents: rhynchophylline, isorhynchophylline, corynoxeine, isocorynoxeine, corynantheine, nicotinic acid, hirsutine, hirsuteine

Dose: 6-15 gms; decoct no more than 10 minutes

Precautions: none noted

Other: Gastrodia (*Gastrodia elata; tian ma*) has very similar uses except it supports the Yin, costs more and is becoming endangered.

Indications: *tremors, spasms, seizures, headache (including migraine), irritability, red eyes, dizziness, hypertension, fever, convulsions*

Uses: Gambir is a fantastic herb for extinguishing Wind and clearing Liver Heat, treating tremors, seizures, jerks and spasms. It also pulls down ascendant Liver Yang, alleviating headaches, irritability, red eyes, dizziness and hypertension. I frequently give it along with gastrodia for migraines and vertex headaches, particularly for hypertension of peri/menopausal women.

❧ GARDENIA

Gardenia jasminoides; Rubiaceae   C
zhi zi

Part used: fruit

Energy, taste and Organs affected: cold; bitter; Heart, Liver, Lungs, Stomach

Actions: clear Heat and drain Fire

Properties: cholagogue, antiinflammatory, antipyretic, promotes blood circulation

Biochemical constituents: gardenin, crocin, crocetin, sitosterol, gardenoside, geniposide, shanzhiside, genipin-1-glucoside

Dose: 3-12 gms; crush herb before decocting; use charred herb to stop bleeding

Precautions: loose stools, loss of appetite

Other: Gardenia is an important herb for clearing Heat, Dampness and toxins in all parts of the body.

Indications: *irritability, high fever with restlessness and insomnia, painful urination, jaundice, hepatitis, hypertension, depression, ulcers, red eyes, nosebleeds, blood in vomit, stool or urine*

❧ GARLIC

Allium sativum; Liliaceae   A, C, W
da suan; Sanskrit: *lasunam*

Part used: bulb

Energy, taste and Organs affected: hot; spicy; Lungs, Spleen, Large Intestine, Stomach

Actions: expels parasites

Properties: stimulant, diuretic, diaphoretic, hypotensive, alterative, digestant, carminative, expectorant, antiseptic, antispasmodic, parasiticide, antibiotic, antibacterial, antifungal, anticoagulant, lowers cholesterol

Biochemical constituents: volatile oil (about 0.2%) including allicin and aliin, B vitamins, minerals

Dose: 6-15 gms; since the volatile oils hold its active ingredients, garlic must be taken fresh for acute ailments rather than deodorized in capsules; acute conditions: 1 tsp. every hour of syrup, oil or juice; 3-5 raw cloves/day; 30-60 drops tincture, 1-4 times/day

Precautions: avoid in high doses during pregnancy; do not use with Excess Heat or Yin Deficiency with Heat signs, acute inflammations, or take with problems of the mouth, tongue or throat; prolonged direct contact of fresh garlic to the skin can cause irritation; excessive use can irritate the stomach

Other: Purple-skinned garlic has a stronger effect against parasites; eat with food as a preventative.

Indications: *respiratory conditions, colds, flu, sore throats, infections, earaches, cough, high and low blood pressure, high cholesterol and triglyceride levels, atherosclerosis, weak digestion, poor circulation, arthritis, rheumatism, lower back and joint pains, genitourinary diseases, nervous disorders, cramps, spasms, heart weakness, parasites, intestinal worms (particularly hookworms), pinworms, ringworm of the scalp, amoebic dysentery, staphylococcus, streptococcus, vaginitis, leukorrhea, Candida, yeast infections*

Uses: Garlic is said to be a cure for every ailment but the one it causes: bad breath! Its delightful fragrance comes from the presence of sulfur compounds, nature's own antibiotic, yet if you eat parsley after the garlic much of its undesirable odor is eliminated. Garlic is a rejuvenating herb because it both stimulates metabolism and detoxifies. In fact, the body absorbs it so quickly that when you rub a clove on your feet you can taste it within seconds.

Specifically, garlic treats respiratory conditions, colds, flu, sore throats, infections and earaches. Because it so powerfully heals Lung ailments, I recommend it to most all patients with coughs or mucus (especially white or clear mucus). I have found two methods to be particularly effective for Lung ailments: garlic juice or garlic appetizer.

Once when visit my parents, I developed walking pneumonia (and didn't know it). I tried a variety of different herbs but had no results. Finally, I purchased a bottle of garlic juice at a chain grocery store and drank one teaspoonful every 2–3 hours. Within the first day I was well on the road to recovery and by the end of the third day, completely healed.

Another time I had a terrible debilitating cough on Mother's Day. My son and husband wanted to take me out to lunch to celebrate and since I didn't want to disappoint them, I went along thinking I would keep them company but not eat. Luckily we found an Italian restaurant where, as we waited to order, a large appetizer of bread with raw garlic in olive oil sat on our table. Knowing garlic would help me, I coated several pieces of the bread with masses of the raw garlic dipped in olive oil and ate them with relish. By the time our meals had arrived, my cough was nearly gone and the next day I had fully recovered. I have seen many a patient experience similar results using garlic juice or appetizer.

Also a specific for regulating blood pressure, garlic is beneficial for both high and low blood pressure and lowers blood cholesterol and triglyceride levels and plaque in vessels, thus treating atherosclerosis. The deodorized garlic capsules work well in this case, which is a blessing for it is quite convenient and of course, odorless (in fact, the aged garlic may be superior for these actions). As well, raw garlic effectively improves weak digestion, stimulates circulation and treats arthritis, rheumatism, lower back and joint pains, genitourinary diseases, nervous disorders, cramps and spasms and heart weakness. For any of these eat the raw cloves, or drink the juice or syrup. It may also be used in food poisoning due to shellfish.

The Chinese use garlic as a preventative and treatment for parasites and intestinal worms, particularly hookworms, pinworms and ringworm of the scalp. Either insert an oiled garlic clove in the rectum, use garlic enemas (made from garlic tea), eat 3-5 raw cloves of garlic, 3-6 times daily, apply the paste (mashed garlic in sesame or olive oil) topically for ringworm, and in general, heavily dose oneself with it.

Garlic is also good for amoebic dysentery and an effective antibiotic for staphylococcus, streptococcus and bacteria resistant to standard antibiotic drugs. It is effective for vaginitis and leukorrhea (coat cloves in oil, wrap in muslin, saturate in olive oil and directly insert into vagina) and antifungal for the treatment of Candida albicans and yeast infections.

🦎 GENTIAN

Gentiana spp.; Gentianaceae **A, C, W**
long dan cao; Sanskrit: *kirata, katuki, trayamana*

Part used: Chinese gentian root

Energy, taste and Organs affected: cold; bitter; Gallbladder, Liver, Stomach

Actions: clears Heat, dries Dampness

Properties: cholagogue, antibacterial, antihypertensive, anti-inflammatory, bitter tonic

Biochemical constituents: gentianine, gentiopicrin, gentianose, gentisin, gentropicroside

Dose: 3-9 gms; decoct 1/4 tsp./cup water; drink 1/2 cup, 3 times/day; 2 "00" caps, 3 times/day; 10-30 drops tincture, 1-4 times/day; take 1 tsp. 20 minutes before meals as a bitter tonic

Precautions: Deficient Spleen and Stomach (poor digestion) with diarrhea; gastric inflammation and irritation

Other: This herb is at risk of becoming endangered, thus *only use the cultivated plant.*

Indications: *red, swollen sore throat and eyes, swollen and painful ears, sudden deafness, jaundice, pain or swelling in genital area, foul-smelling vaginal discharge and itching, infantile convulsion, headache, fever, spasms, pain in sides, hepatitis, herpes, anal itch, gas pains, urinary tract infections, hypertension with dizziness and ringing in the ears, insufficient acid for digestion*

🦎 GINGER

Zingiberis officinalis; Zingiberaceae **A, C, W**
fresh ginger: *sheng jiang*, Sanskrit: *ardraka*; dried ginger: *gan jiang*; Sanskrit: *sunthi*

Part used: rhizome

Energy, taste and Organs affected: fresh: warm; spicy; Lungs, Spleen, Stomach; dried: hot; spicy; Heart, Lung, Spleen, Stomach

Actions: fresh: warm, surface relieving; dried: warms Interior, expels Cold

Properties: stimulant, diaphoretic, carminative, emmenagogue, expectorant, antiemetic, analgesic, antispasmodic, stomachic, antipyretic, antimicrobial

Biochemical constituents: zingiberene, phellandrene, camphene, shogaol, gingerol, zingiberone, borneol, zingiberol, citral

Dose: fresh: 1-3 gms; decoct 2-6 thin slices or 1" root grated/cup covered no more than 5-10 minutes, drink 2-4 cups tea a day; acute—drink 1/2 cup every 2-3 hours until symptoms lessen, then decrease frequency until problem is gone; dried: 3-12 gms; infuse 1 tsp./cup water for 10 minutes; 10-60 drops tincture, 1-4 times/day

Precautions: fresh: Deficient Qi with profuse sweating; headache due to Deficient Blood; cough due to Deficient Yin; dried: Deficient Yin with Heat signs; Heat in Blood causing bleeding; caution during pregnancy (avoid large doses)

Other: The Chinese use fresh ginger to reduce toxicity of fish, crabs and some herbs.

Indications: fresh: *colds, flu, lung complaints, sore throat, diarrhea, pains, cramps, spasms, indigestion, nausea, gas, mucus conditions, poor circulation, earache, dandruff, diarrhea, menstrual difficulties due to cold;* dried: *Coldness, cold hands and feet, poor digestion, watery, thin phlegm, hemorrhage and uterine bleeding due to Cold (chronic bleeding with pale blood)*

Uses: Most people associate ginger as a spice cooked in gingerbread, pumpkin pie, or candied ginger (which the Chinese especially like). In addition, some know that when ginger is cooked with meat it helps the body better digest and assimilate the meat, thus detoxifying it. More recently it has garnered fame for its value in easing motion sickness. For this, it's best to take 3-4 ginger capsules before boarding a plane or boat, or traveling by car. Yet, ginger has many more multi-healing applications; in fact, it is so highly regarded in the Orient that it's included in about 50% of all formulas (its stimulating action quickly moves other herbs through the blood, increasing their effectiveness and absorption rate).

Internally, **fresh ginger's** warming and stimulating energy alleviate digestive upset, nausea (use tincture for chemotherapy-induced nausea), motion sickness, poor digestion and circulation, gas, colic, burping and excessive mucus. It also treats colds, flu, lung congestion with white to clear, runny mucus, cramps, pains, spasms, sore throat, diarrhea, fevers and general Coldness. It combines well with **chamomile** for menstrual cramps. Add ginger to milk to aid its assimilation and increase its tonifying properties. **Dried ginger** root is also used and has a slightly different purpose. Hotter and drier, it warms the body, dispels cold hands and feet, treats poor digestion, clears watery, thin phlegm and stops hemorrhage and uterine bleeding due to Coldness (chronic bleeding with pale blood).

Externally, ginger juice rubbed into the skin relieves muscle pain; ginger oil applied to the scalp clears dandruff and in the ear treats earaches; ginger foot or body baths can stop the onset of colds and flu, warm cold feet and ease body pains; and ginger tea or tincture can be gargled for sore throats.

A ginger fomentation placed on sore joints or muscles eases pain, arthritis, rheumatism, or on a sore throat, relieves pain (I successfully treated a patient with chronic low-grade lingering sore throats with this therapy along with improving her diet and rest). Over the lungs, it breaks up congestion and expels mucus. Over the lower abdomen and perineum during childbirth, it speeds delivery and eases tearing. Over the kidneys (located on either side of the spine at waist level of the back), it supports Kidney function and immunity. It's useful to employ both external applications along with internal ones, so that when treating a cold, flu or sore throat, drink a cup of ginger tea, place a ginger fomentation over the throat or lungs, sit in a hot ginger bath, and/or soak feet in ginger tea.

🦋 GINKGO

Ginkgo biloba; Ginkgoaceae   **C, W**
nut: *bai guo*; leaf: *yin guo ye*

Part used: nut and leaf

Energy, taste and Organs affected: both: neutral; sweet, bitter, astringent; nut: Lungs, Kidneys; leaf: Lung

Actions: both: stabilize and bind

Properties: nut: expectorant, antitussive, antiasthmatic, sedative, mildly astringent, antibacterial, antifungal; leaf 50:1 extract: improves circulation to brain, antihypertensive, lowers cholesterol, antioxidant

Biochemical constituents: nut: gibberellin, ginkgolic acid, hydroginkgolinic acid, bilobol, ginnol, aspartine, calcium, phosphorus, iron; leaf: terpene lactones, ginkgolides A, B, C, bilobalide, quercetine, isohamnetin, kaempferol

Dose: nut: 4.5-9 gms in formula, less if fresh; leaf: 3-6 gm; decoct 1 Tbsp./cup water for 5 min.; 20-60 drops tincture 1-3 times/day; 40 milligrams of the 24% standardized extract 3 times/day for a minimum of three months

Precautions: as nuts are mildly toxic, do not taken in large doses for prolonged periods—toxic symptoms include headache, fever, tremors, irritability and dyspnea (60 gms raw licorice boiled may be used as an antidote); caution in Excess conditions; leaf 50:1 extract: avoid standardized extract if on blood thinners, as this concentrated form can cause excessive bleeding, or if having low blood pressure, Deficient Blood, excessive menses, or hemophilia

Other: The ginkgo tree, one of the world's oldest living plants, can live over 1,000 years; it even survived the Hiroshima atomic blast at the end of World War II.

Indications: nut: *wheezing, cough, asthma, frequent urination, incontinence, vaginal discharge, leukorrhea, spermatorrhea;* leaf 50:1 extract: *wheezing, asthma, cough, Raynaud's, varicose veins, erectile dysfunction, headache, vertigo, arthritis, rheumatism, hearing loss, ringing in the ears, poor circulation, high cholesterol, hypertension, angina pectoris, anxiety tension, visual problems, prevents macular degeneration, poor memory and concentration, mental confusion, senility*

Uses: Ginkgo **nut** expels mucus from the lungs, stops wheezing and cough, treats frequent urination or incontinence, alleviates asthma and stops leukorrhea, vaginal discharge and spermatorrhea. Ginkgo **leaf 50:1 extract,** a powerful antioxidant that tones blood vessels and stimulates peripheral blood circulation, especially to the brain, eyes and limbs, calms wheezing, stops pain and treats Raynaud's disease, varicose veins, erectile dysfunction and helps prevent organ transplant rejection.

As well, the leaf 50:1 extract improves memory, mental efficiency and concentration, treating mental confusion and senility. It also lowers cholesterol and hypertension, eases angina pectoris, decreases anxiety tension, headaches, vertigo, visual problems, ringing in the ears, arthritis, rheumatism, diabetic retinopathy and hearing loss and prevents macular degeneration. It is especially good for the elderly. Note that ginkgo leaf tea or extracts less than 50:1 are not effective for the above uses.

❦ GINSENG

Panax ginseng; Araliaceae　　　　　　　　**C**
ren shen

Part used: aged Chinese ginseng root

Energy, taste and Organs affected: slightly warm; sweet, slightly bitter; Lungs, Spleen

Actions: tonify Qi

Properties: stomachic, stimulant, nutritive, rejuvenative, demulcent, adaptogen

Biochemical constituents: panaxadiols, panoquilon, panaxin, ginsenin, panacene, panaxynol, panaenic acid, panose, dammarane, glucose, fructose, maltose, sucrose, nicotinic acid, riboflavin, thiamine

Dose: 1-9 gms, up to 30 gms for hemorrhage shock; decoct 1 tsp./cup water; 20-60 drops tincture, 1-4 times/day; freeze-drying may increase potency

Precautions: Deficient Yin with Heat signs, Excess Heat, hypertension with ascendant Liver Yang, high blood pressure; according to Tilgnar in *Herbal Medicine*, concurrent use with the drug phenezine has resulted in manic-like symptoms

Other: The many types of ginseng can seem confusing as they all share the ability to strengthen the body and its energy, yet otherwise they have different specific uses. **American ginseng** tonifies Yin, **Tienqi ginseng** moves Blood circulation. **Eleuthro** is not a true ginseng, but does act as an adaptogen, increasing energy, vitality and endurance. (see each of these separately for more details). Chinese white ginseng, usually found as a white powder, is less potent (avoid unless from a reputable source or company as it is easily adulterated). The more potent Korean ginseng is red from steaming Chinese ginseng. Ginseng is also known as "man root" because its shape looks like a person.

Indications: *all Deficiency diseases, chronic fatigue, shortness of breath, profuse sweating, lethargy, lack of appetite, chest and abdominal distention, chronic diarrhea, prolapse of stomach, uterus or rectum, palpitations with anxiety, insomnia, forgetfulness, restlessness, excellent for convalescence, debility and weakness in old age, tiredness, poor appetite and digestion, emaciation, shortness of breath, profuse sweating, palpitations, shock*

Uses: As a primary herb for Deficiencies, ginseng revitalizes the body and mind, strengthening weakness, low energy and vitality, shock, collapse due to loss of blood, chronic fevers, heart weakness, debility, convalescence and weakness in old age. It promotes weight and tissue growth and increases longevity and resistance to disease.

Ginseng particularly benefits digestion and Lung function, treating lethargy, lack of appetite, abdominal and chest distention, chronic diarrhea, prolapse of stomach, uterus or rectum, shortness of breath, profuse sweating, wheezing, tuberculosis and restlessness. As a cardiac tonic, ginseng relieves palpitations with anxiety, insomnia and forgetfulness. It also increases adrenal cortex function and stimulates the pituitary gland to produce more sex hormones. Traditionally, it is taken regularly by men age 40 and over, although women may take it, too.

Ginseng may be used when the root is four years old, but it's best to harvest when at least seven years as the older the root, the more valuable (and unfortunately, more expensive). I remember a Chinese pharmacist once showing me a selection of very old and large ginseng roots, valued from $1,000 to $10,000 each (all truly looking like a man!) According to Michael Tierra, who studied with him, this Taoist herb teacher claimed certain wealthy Chinese and American celebrities visited him annually for his rejuvenation technique: a week of avoiding all greasy and fried foods along with drinking the Yin tonic formula, *Liu Wei Di Huang Wan* (Formula #74) 2-3 times/day. Afterwards, they'd purchase an expensive ginseng root, cook and eat it, along with drinking the tea, to rejuvenate their physical and sexual energy.

GOLDENSEAL

Hydrastis canadensis; Ranunculaceae   **W**

Part used: root

Energy, taste and Organs affected: cold; bitter; Stomach, Intestines, Heart, Liver

Actions: clears Heat, dries Dampness

Properties: bitter tonic, alterative, antiinflammatory, aperient, astringent

Biochemical constituents: hydrastine, berberine, resin, traces of essential oil, chologenic acid, fatty oil, albumin, sugar

Dose: 3-6 gms in formula; infuse 1 tsp./cup boiling water; tincture, 10-60 drops tincture, 1-4 times/day; 2 "00" capsules, 1-3 times a day or more for short-term use in acute conditions

Precautions: pregnancy; Deficient Blood and Yin, dizziness; long-term use can weaken intestinal flora and diminish vitamin B absorption

Other: This herb is now endangered, thus *only use the cultivated plant.*

Indications: *infections, inflammations, ulcers, colds, flu, severe sore throat, fever, hemorrhoids, leukorrhea, bladder infections, chronic middle ear infections, conjunctivitis, vaginitis, dysentery, constipation, colitis, heartburn, indigestion, liver congestion, cancer*

Uses: Goldenseal treats infections and inflammations caused by Heat. It cleanses mucous membranes and lymph glands, dries yellow discharges, treats leukorrhea and vaginal yeast and clears bladder infections. It specifically clears Heat from the Liver and Blood, treating liver diseases, tumors, cancer, hepatitis, jaundice and cirrhosis. Because it stimulates bile secretion, it is also useful for indigestion, hemorrhoids, heartburn, colitis, constipation and ulcers.

As well, it has a laxative action, stimulates uterine muscles, contracts blood vessels and inhibits excessive bleeding. It is effective against colds, flu, severe sore throats, fevers, chronic middle ear infections, conjunctivitis and treats amoebic dysentery (giardia) when used continuously for 10 days. Include a pinch of goldenseal in eyewashes for inflamed eyes (be warned—it stings), or in salves, powders and tinctures for eczema, inflammation of the ear and other infections. I successfully used the powder on my baby's umbilicus after birth to prevent infection until the cord fell off.

GOTU KOLA

Centella asiatica; Hydrocotyle asiatica; Apiaceae   **A, C, W**
(Centella asiatica): luo de da; Sanskrit: *brahmi*
(Hydrocotyle asiatica): ji xue cao; Sanskrit: *mandukaparni*

Part used: leaves

Energy, taste and Organs affected: cool; bitter, astringent; Liver, Bladder

Actions: clears Heat and toxins

Properties: antiinflammatory, antibiotic, diuretic, circulatory stimulant

Biochemical constituents: essential oil, tannin, asiaticoside

Dose: 15-30 gms; 1 tsp./cup water; 20-60 drops tincture, 1-4 times/day

Precautions: pregnancy (emmenagogic effect)

Other: Bacopa (*Bacopa monniera*), named **brahmi**, is found more in the south of India and was added to the pharmacopeia later than gotu kola. It has a warming and stimulating energy, but is also used to improve memory and concentration and is perhaps even stronger than ginkgo in doing so. As well, it is commonly sold as a fish aquarium plant!

Indications: *poor memory, mental confusion, poor concentration, ADD, high blood pressure, varicose veins, nervousness, mental chatter, boils, toxic fevers, stress-induced ulcers, burns, wounds, scar tissue buildup after injuries (take internally)*

✿ GRAVEL ROOT

Eupatorium purpureum; Asteraceae   **W**

Part used: root

Energy, taste and Organs affected: neutral; bitter, spicy; Kidneys, Bladder, Stomach, Liver

Actions: drains Dampness

Properties: diuretic, lithotriptic, nervine, antirheumatic, carminative

Biochemical constituents: volatile oil, flavonoids, euparin, pyrrolizidine alkaloids

Dose: 3-9 gms; 2 tsp./cup water; 0-40 drops tincture, 1-4 times/day

Precautions: don't use long term, and only in small amounts, because of its pyrrolizidine alkaloids; pregnancy, blood in urine

Indications: *urinary tract infections, kidney stones, frequent and nighttime urination (causes bladder to fully empty so you go less frequently), inability to urinate*

✿ HAWTHORN

Crataegus oxyacantha, C. pinnatifida (Chinese), *C. spp.; Rosaceae*   **C, W**
shan zha (C. pinnatifida)

Part used: berry

Energy, taste and Organs affected: slightly warm; sour, sweet; Liver, Spleen, Stomach, Heart

Actions: relieves food stagnation

Properties: cardiac tonic, digestant, antispasmodic, astringent, sedative, regulates blood pressure, lowers cholesterol, diuretic, antioxidant, cardioprotective

Biochemical constituents: crategolic acid, citric acid, tartaric acid, procyanidins, proanthocyanins, sugars, glycosides, flavonoids including hyperoside, vitexin 2"rhamnoside, rutin, oligomeric procyanidins; vitamin C

Dose: 5-9 gms, up to 30 gms when used alone; infuse 1 Tblsp. berries or flowers/cup water, drink 3 cups a day; 10-30 drops tincture or wine, 3 times/day; use raw for stagnant Blood, dry-fried for food stagnation; take long term for best results

Precautions: may potentiate the effects of cardiac glycosides, such as digitalis; caution in Spleen/Stomach Deficiency without food stagnation; acid regurgitation

Other: Western herbalists also use the leaves and flowers to treat heart conditions.

Indications: *tachycardia, heart weakness, aging heart problems, palpitations, angina, valvular insufficiency, coronary artery disease. high and low blood pressure, ADD, arrhythmia, arteriosclerosis, high cholesterol; food stagnation, particularly of meats or greasy foods; abdominal distention, pain, diarrhea, dysentery, hypertension,*

Uses: Hawthorn is highly recognized in the West as a strong cardiac tonic, treating both emotionally and physically induced heart issues including high and low blood pressure, rapid or arrhythmic heartbeat, tachycardia, inflammation of the heart muscle, angina pectoris, arteriosclerosis, enlarged heart, heart strain and valvular heart diseases. Hawthorn increases the uptake of oxygen to the heart, enzyme metabolism in the heart muscle and mildly dilates both coronary and peripheral vessels bringing more blood to the heart.

This incredible herb stimulates circulation and moves stagnant Blood, regulates blood flow, blood pressure and heart rate, dilates coronary vessels, brings more blood to the heart, reduces cholesterol and blood lipids, strengthens the heart muscle and helps maintain a healthy heart, arteries and veins. I have seen it stabilize irregular heartbeats and eliminate palpitations many times. Therefore, hawthorn is a specific for all cardiovascular diseases, particularly good for heart problems of old age, high cholesterol and nervous palpitations, or other heart conditions. It is considered to be gentle and safe with long-lasting effects.

Although the Chinese are aware of its Blood-moving and heart-protective properties, they primarily use the berries to move food congestion, particularly due to meats or greasy foods. Hawthorn also stimulates appetite and eases abdominal distention, gas, bloating and pain. The green fruit treats diarrhea while the roasted and charred fruit relieves both diarrhea and chronic dysentery. As the berries have an affinity for alcohol, they are often made into herbal wine.

✿ HE SHOU WU

Polygonum multiflorum; Polygonaceae   **C**
he shou wu

Part used: root

Energy, taste and Organs affected: slightly warm; bitter, sweet, astringent; Liver, Kidneys

Actions: tonify Blood

Properties: blood tonic, laxative, antibacterial, anticholesterol

Biochemical constituents: chrysophanic acid, emodin, rhein, anthrone, lecithin, emodin methyl ester, rhophantin

Dose: 9-30 gms; decoct 1-2 tsp./cup water (but not in a steel container); 20-60 drops tincture, 1-4 times/day; generally the treated root is used

Precautions: Spleen Deficiency (weak digestion), phlegm, diarrhea; do not take with onion, chives or garlic; this safe, non-toxic herb may be taken over a long time

Other: Also known as **fleeceflower, Ho Shou Wu** and **Fo Ti**; he shou wu is treated by being cooked with black bean juice

Indications: treated: *anemia, dizziness, blurred vision, premature gray hair, premature aging, weak and sore lower back and knees, insomnia, nocturnal emission, spermatorrhea, in-fertility, impotence, persistent vaginal discharge (leukorrhea), Wind rash from Deficient Blood, chronic malaria with Deficient Qi and Blood;* raw: *carbuncles, sores, boils, abscesses, scrofula, goiter, neck lumps, constipation from Deficient Blood*

Uses: He shou wu is said to have mysterious properties: when taken for a year, the 50-year-old root preserves the black color of hair, the 150-year-old root causes new teeth to grow in the elderly whereas the 300-year-old root gives earthly immortality. This herb obviously has restorative and reviving powers to the body!

As a Blood, Liver and Kidney tonic, **treated he shou wu** alleviates dizziness, blurred vision, prematurely gray hair, weak lower back and knees, insomnia, infertility, impotence, premature senility, withered skin, wrinkles, nocturnal emission, spermatorrhea and leukorrhea. It builds Blood and sperm, strengthens muscles, tendons, ligaments and bones and counters the effects of aging. I have seen it restore gray hair to black, although it needs be taken continuously for a long time for it to work. Like **dang gui**, it moistens the intestines and helps relieve constipation from Dryness. It also reduces the heart rate, slightly increases blood circulation through the heart and moves cholesterol from the liver plasma, preventing its deposit as plaque along the inner arterial walls.

Raw he shou wu clears Heat and treats boils, carbuncles, sores, scrofula, goiter, neck lumps and constipation from Deficient Blood. **He shou wu vine** (or stem *ye jiao teng*) is used to treat insomnia, irritability, dream-disturbed sleep, general weakness, soreness, pain and numbness due to Deficient Blood. This vine grows rapidly and can easily take over your garden if you're not careful!

✿ HONEYSUCKLE

Lonicera japonica; Caprifoliaceae   **C**
jin yin hua

Part used: flower

Energy, taste and Organs affected: cold; sweet; Large Intestine, Lungs, Stomach

Actions: clear Heat and toxins

Properties: alterative, febrifuge, antibiotic, diuretic, refrigerant, diaphoretic, antibacterial, antimicrobial

Biochemical constituents: luteolin, inositol, tannin

Dose: 9-15 gms, infusion

Precautions: diarrhea due to Deficient Spleen and Stomach Yang; sores and ulcers due to Deficient Qi (those with clear fluid)

Other: Honeysuckle stem (*jin yin teng*) is used similarly and for dysentery, infectious hepatitis and rheumatic arthritis; this herb is another example of a commonly available plant that is underutilized.

Indications: *inflammations, infections, fever, viruses, headache, sore throat, colds, flu, conjunctivitis, swellings, acute feverish conditions, headache, dysentery, painful urination; hot, painful sores and swellings of breast, throat or eyes; intestinal abscess*

Uses: These beautiful flowers with the sweet nectar children so love to suck are quite valuable for treating infections, inflammations, fevers, viruses, staph and strep infections and other conditions needing antibiotics. They are also useful in colds and flu, sore throat, headache, conjunctivitis, hot painful eyes, boils and dysentery. Honeysuckle reduces swellings of various types and in any stage, especially of the breast, throat or eyes and intestinal abscess. I always include it in my skin formulas along with **forsythia**, as it opens the surface to release Heat toxins. As well, honeysuckle clears inflammations of the intestines, urinary tract and reproductive organs.

🦋 HORSE CHESTNUT

Aesculus hippocastanum; Hippocasanaceae **W**

Part used: bark, seeds

Energy, taste and Organs affected: neutral; bitter; Intestines

Actions: bark: cools and releases Exterior; seeds: stabilizes and binds

Properties: bark: febrifuge: seeds: astringent, antispasmodic

Biochemical constituents: bark: aesculin, ash, tannin; seeds: phytosterol, starch, sugar, linoleic, palmitic and stearic acids, aescin

Dose: bark: decoct 1 tsp./cup water; take only 1 Tbsp., 3-4 times daily; seeds: 1-5 drops tincture, 1-4 times/day

Precautions: bark can be narcotic; do not exceed dosage, or nausea, vomiting, diarrhea, dizziness, weakness, incoordination and coma may result; seeds: **DO NOT EAT!** Pregnancy; in children under 4; acute kidney inflammation, gastrointestinal ulcers, bleeding disorders

Indications: bark: *intermittent fevers; externally on ulcers and sores;* seeds: *varicose veins, hemorrhoids, rectal diseases, rheumatism, neuralgia, ureter spasms (especially left-sided), bronchial spasms*

🦋 ISATIS

Isatis tinctoria; Brassicaceae **C**
ban lan gen

Part used: root

Energy, taste and Organs affected: cold; bitter; Heart, Lungs, Stomach

Actions: clear Heat and toxins

Properties: antiviral, antibacterial, parasiticide, anticancer

Biochemical constituents: isatin, arginine, glutamine, proline, tyrosine, glucosides

Dose: 15-30 gms, decoction

Precautions: weakness, absence of Heat toxins

Other: Also known as **woad**, the Chinese use the leaf (*da quing ye*) similarly and often combine it with the root; this commonly found antiviral herb is widely underutilized.

Indications: *viral infections, colds and flu from Heat, fever, encephalitis B, meningitis, extreme sore throat, acute laryngitis, mumps, salmonella, strep, mouth and gum sores, infections and inflammations, hepatitis, jaundice, scabies*

Uses: Isatis is one of the best antiviral and broad-spectrum antibiotic herbs for viral infections, colds and flu from Heat and fever, even preventing epidemics. I always include it in my cold and flu formulas, as it prevents them from occurring long-term or quickly rids the body of prolonged ones. As well, it treats encephalitis B, meningitis, extreme sore throat, acute laryngitis, mumps, salmonella, strep, mouth and gum sores, infections and inflammations, hepatitis, jaundice and externally, scabies.

🦎 JUJUBE

Ziziphus jujuba (fruit); *Z. spinosa* (seeds); *Rhamnaceae* **C**
da zao (fruit); *suan zao ren* (seeds)

Part used: fruit, seeds

Energy, taste and Organs affected: fruit: neutral; sweet; Spleen, Stomach; seeds: neutral; sweet, sour; Gallbladder, Heart, Liver, Spleen

Actions: fruit: tonify Qi and Blood; seeds: seeds: calms the Spirit

Properties: fruit: energy tonic, expectorant, nutritive, mild sedative; seeds: sedative, nutritive, tonic, analgesic

Biochemical constituents: fruit: vitamins A, B2, and C, calcium, phosphorus, iron; seeds: betulin, betulic acid, jujuboside, jujubogenin, ebelin lactone, other saponins, vitamin C

Dose: fruit: 10-30 gms (3-12 pieces); seeds: decoction of 9-18 gms (crushed first) or 1.5-3 gms powder

Precautions: fruit: excess Dampness, food congestion, intestinal parasites, bloating; seeds: severe diarrhea, Excess Heat

Other: The red dates are more medicinal than the black ones; both dates and seeds are moistening, nurturing, strengthening and safe for children and the weak or elderly.

Indications: fruit: *weakness, shortness of breath, lack of appetite, loose stools, emotional instability, low energy, insomnia; poor digestion, appetite and memory; diarrhea, moodiness;* seeds: *insomnia, palpitations with anxiety, irritability, spontaneous sweating, night sweats, forgetfulness, nervous exhaustion, poor memory*

Uses: The delicious large red **jujube dates** tonify both Qi and Blood, treating poor digestion, weakness, low energy, nervous exhaustion, insomnia, diarrhea from Coldness and poor appetite, digestion and memory. Nourishing to the Spirit, they calm and stabilize emotions when feeling irritable, sad or crying for no reason. They are added like licorice to sweeten and harmonize other herbs in a formula. After cooking the dates in a tea or soup, eat them for their full medicinal value (remove pits first). They increase weight gain and help malnourished children thrive.

Because **zizyphus seeds** clear Liver and Heart Heat, they help calm the mind and emotions, treating insomnia, irritability, palpitations, anxiety, nervous exhaustion, amnesia and poor memory. They also reduce spontaneous sweating or night sweats.

🦎 KAVA KAVA

Piper methysticum; Piperaceae   **W**

Part used: root

Energy, taste and Organs affected: warm; bitter, spicy; Liver, Kidneys

Actions: drain Dampness

Properties: calmative, antispasmodic, diuretic, analgesic, muscle relaxant, anesthetic, anti-anxiety, sedative

Biochemical constituents: kavapyrones, other alkaloids, resin, lactones, kawain, yangonin, methysticin, glycosides, starch

Dose: 2-4 gms; 1-2 tsp./cup water; 10-60 drops tincture, 1-4 times/day; 100-250 mg of standardized extract, 3 times daily (100 mg of 70%, 140 mg of 50%, 220 mg of 30%); **DO NOT exceed recommended doses**

Precautions: avoid in pregnancy, lactation, with alcohol or anticoagulant medications; do not use if taking antidepressants, such as Xanax; as Kava potentiates the effects of barbiturates and benzodiazepines[3]; excessively large doses can cause dry skin, scaly rash, yellow

---

[3] Tillotson, *The One Earth Herbal Sourcebook*, Kensington Publishing Group, 2001.

discoloration of skin, hair and nails and bloodshot eyes; avoid if you have Excess Liver Heat, stagnant Liver Qi, regularly use alcohol or other recreational drugs, have liver disease or a history of hepatitis, jaundice, mononucleosis or drug use, or take medications with known adverse liver side effects. **Note:** While in Europe there were reports of kava causing hepatotoxicity, when looked at closely most all cases were due to other causes, such as alcohol and drug abuse, a history of hepatitis, taking medications with known liver disease-causing side effects, or driving with an illegal level of alcohol in the blood but having a bottle of kava in the car (so the accident was attributed to kava). However, because the spiciness of kava potentiates drugs and has a direct action on the liver, avoid use as given in the above precautions.

Other: As Kava is now endangered in Hawaii, *only use the cultivated plant*.

Indications: *anxiety, nervousness, insomnia, stress, restlessness, muscle spasms, asthma, fibromyalgia, ureter spasms, interstitial cystitis pain and spasms, irritable bladder, hyperactivity, ADD, tension headaches*

Uses: Long used by the Polynesians as a group ritual and recreational beverage (or intoxicant), kava is a mild tranquilizer that relaxes the mind, clarifies thoughts and induces mild euphoria. Very effective for anxiety, it also treats nervousness, insomnia, stress, restlessness, muscle spasms, asthma, fibromyalgia, hyperactivity, ADD and tension headaches. As kava relaxes muscles and numbs pain, it's useful for irritable bladder, ureter spasms and interstitial cystitis pain and spasms. Kava is frequently combined with **St. John's wort** to treat anxiety and depression together (note that kava only treats anxiety and anxiousness with possible palpitations, while St. John's wort just treats depression—can't get out of bed in the morning with lack of interest in life).

🦎 LEMON BALM

Melissa officinalis; Lamiaceae   **W**

Part used: leaves

Energy, taste and Organs affected: cool; sour, spicy; Lungs, Liver

Actions: cools and releases Exterior

Properties: carminative, diaphoretic, calmative, antipyretic, antispasmodic

Biochemical constituents: essential oil with citral, citronellal, geraniol and linalool, bitter principle, acids and tannin

Dose: 1-6 gms; infuse 1 Tblsp./cup water, drink 1 cup every 2 hours until fever or cold breaks, 1 cup 2-3 times daily otherwise; 10-60 drops tincture, 1-4 times/day

Precautions: Exterior Deficiency, Deficient Yin with Heat signs, hypothyroidism

Other: Sometimes known as **balm** and **sweet balm**.

Indications: *colds, flu, melancholia, depression, nervousness, hysteria, anxiety, restlessness, irritability, insomnia, whining, crying, colicky or teething children, herpes simplex, hyperthyroidism*

Uses: As an antiviral, lemon balm is very effective for breaking fevers and treating colds and flu, especially in children since it has a delicious lemony taste and smell they love. For these conditions, drink several cups tea, take a hot bath and follow by sweating therapy (see *Home Therapies*). Repeat several times for high fevers. Lemon balm also calms, relaxes and tranquilizes the nervous system, excellent for melancholia, depression, nervousness, hysteria, anxiety, restlessness, irritability and digestive problems due to nervousness. It may be combined with **chamomile** for nervous states and insomnia, or for whining, crying, colicky or teething children. A refreshing summer drink, people in England drank it daily during the 16th and 17th centuries.

Today Europeans use **lemon balm tea extract** in salve form to treat herpes simplex. As well, it interferes with TSH binding to thyroid cell membranes and prevents iodine synthesis, conversion of T4 to T3 and binding of auto-antibodies found in Grave's disease[4]. Thus, it is also useful in hyperthyroidism, especially when combined with **bugleweed**.

---

[4] Tilgnar, *Herbal Medicine from the Heart of the Earth*, Wise Acres Press, Inc. 1999.

✴ LICORICE

Glycyrrhiza glabra (Western); *G. uralensis* (Chinese);
Fabaceae   **A, C, W**
Raw: *gan cao*, Sanskrit: *madhukam*
Honey-fried: *zhi gan cao*; Sanskrit *yashti madhu*

Part used: root

Energy, taste and Organs affected: neutral; sweet; enters all meridians, especially Heart, Lungs, Spleen and Stomach

Actions: honey-fried: tonify Qi; raw: clears Heat and toxins

Properties: antiinflammatory, cholagogue, antitussive, antihistamine, detoxicant, nutritive, expectorant, demulcent

Biochemical constituents: *G. glabra:* glycyrrhizin, flavonoids, isoflavonoids, chalcones, triterpenoid saponins, sterols, starch, sugars, amino acids, asparagine, betaine, choline, gums, wax, volatile oil; *G. uralensis:* glycyrrhizic, glycyrrhizinic and glycyrrhetinic acids, glycyrrhizin, uralenic acid, liquiritigenin, isoliquiritigenin, liquiritin, neoliquiritin, neoisoliquiritin, licurazid, formononetin, sitosterol, coumarins (in Western licorice, not the Chinese species

Dose: 2-12 gms; decoct 1 tsp. Western or 2-3 slices Chinese/cup water, drink 2-3 cups/day; 20-60 drops tincture, 1-4 times/day; use raw to clear Heat and relieve toxicity; stir-fry with honey to tonify Qi

Precautions: Excess Dampness, nausea, vomiting, edema with high blood pressure, tendency towards fluid retention; do not use with **polygala**, **euphorbiae** or **sargasum** (seaweeds); causes vomiting in high doses; according to Tilgnar in *Herbal Medicine*, licorice potentiates activity of anthraquinone drugs and toxicity of cardiac glycosides (like digitalis)

Other: Also known as **liquorice**.

Indications: Western licorice: *sore throats, gastric and duodenal ulcers, other stomach problems; soothes mucous membranes, urinary, respiratory and intestinal passages; tuberculosis, coughing, wheezing, throat and bronchial irrita-tions, mild laxative, stress, muscle spasms of abdomen or legs;* deglycyrrhizinated licorice: *intestinal and stomach pains and spasms;* Chinese raw licorice: *detoxifies poisons, carbuncles, sores; when added to other herbs it harmonizes their characteristics and sweetens a formula;* Chinese honey-fried licorice: *can be used for either Heat or Cold in the Lungs; shortness of breath, bronchitis, low energy, laryngitis, weakness, general debility, poor digestion, loose stools, Qi or Blood Deficiency, palpitations, coughing, wheezing, sore throat, painful spasms of abdomen or legs, stomach and duodenal ulcers*

Uses: One of the most widely used herbs in the world, licorice is restoring and rejuvenative. Children especially like licorice (remember sucking on licorice ropes at a show or fair?), and they can suck on a root or several slices when hiking or traveling to help quench thirst. As well, it can be safely given to teething babies to stimulate and relieve gum pain. The demulcent property of **Western licorice** eases sore throats, remedies gastric and duodenal ulcers and other stomach problems (especially when combined with **chamomile**), soothes mucous membranes, urinary, respiratory and intestinal passages and treats tuberculosis, coughing, wheezing and throat and bronchial irritations. It also has mild laxative properties and can safely be taken by children and debilitated people. Licorice's calming properties alleviate stress and relax muscle spasm of abdomen or legs. **Deglycyrrhizinated licorice**, or DGL, doesn't contain the substances that cause edema, headache and other symptoms of overdose. It is particularly healing to intestinal membranes and stomach pains and spasm.

Licorice is the most used herb in Chinese medicine for several reasons: it harmonizes all the herbs in a formula so they work together better, it alleviates the harsh stimulating effects of bitter herbs without interfering with their use, its neutral energy makes it effective with both warming and cooling herbs, and it adds a wonderful sweet taste. **Raw Chinese licorice** is used for carbuncles, sores, sore throat due to Heat, or to treat any toxicity or poisoning in the body, externally or internally, including lessening the toxicity of many toxic substances. When Chinese **licorice is honey-fried**, it's a general tonic for the whole body, strengthening digestion, improving energy and treating poor digestion and assimilation from Coldness and weakness. It also tonifies Qi and Blood in those with palpitations, irregular pulse, shortness of breath, lassitude and loose stools.

ꙮ LIGUSTICUM

Ligusticum wallichii; Apiaceae   **C**
chuan xiong

Part used: root of Szechwan lovage

Energy, taste and Organs affected: warm; spicy; Liver, Gallbladder

Actions: invigorates Blood

Properties: emmenagogue, antibacterial, antihypertensive, sedative, anticonvulsive

Biochemical constituents: tetramethylpyrazine, perlolyrine, ferulic acid, chrysophanol, sedanoic acid

Dose: 3-6 gms, decoction; up to 9 gms for irregular menses

Precautions: pregnancy, excessive menstrual bleeding, Deficient Yin with Heat signs, Deficient Qi, headaches due to Deficient Yin with rising Liver Yang; vomiting and dizziness may occur from over-dosage; do not use with **cornus**, **astragalus** or **coptis**

Other: *L. porteri*, or **Osha**, is used similarly for colds, flu, viral conditions, sore throat, stomach upset, cuts, sores, snake bite, gas, arthritis, rheumatism, bruised muscles, body aches and seizures. As this herb is now endangered, *only use cultivated osha*.

Indications: *menstrual disorders and pain such as dysmenorrhea, amenorrhea, endometriosis, difficult labor, pain and soreness of chest, sides and ribs, headache, dizziness, skin problems*

Uses: One of the primary herbs used to move Blood and Qi, it is specific for gynecological issues including painful menses (stabbing pain), amenorrhea and difficult labor. As well, it alleviates pain and soreness in the chest, sides and ribs, and treats dizziness and skin problems due to Wind. It is also one of the finest herbs for many types of headaches due to Wind, Heat, Cold or Deficient Blood.

ꙮ LOBELIA

Lobelia inflata (Western); *L. chinensis* (Chinese);
Campanulaceae   **C, W**
ban bian lian

Part used: above ground portion

Energy, taste and Organs affected: neutral; bitter; Liver, Lungs, Heart, Small Intestine

Actions: extinguish Internal Wind

Properties: antispasmodic, expectorant, stimulant, emetic, sialagogue

Biochemical constituents: alkaloids (lobeline is the most important one), pyridine and other alkaloids, resin, gum, chelidonic acid and a pungent volatile oil

Dose: acute conditions: infuse 1 tsp./cup water, drink 1 cup 3 times/day; 1 "00" capsule, 1-2 times/day; 4-5 drops tincture, 1-6 times/day; 6-15 gms in formula

Precautions: overdose can cause nausea and vomiting; while some caution lobelia's use in certain conditions, no single case of lobelia toxicity has been reported and in fact, one would vomit before any toxicity could occur. Lobelia is actually a very active, safe and important herb.

Other: The Chinese use *L. chinensis* to remove water retention and edema, and as a detoxicant, particularly as a primary herb to treat tumors and cancer.

Indications: *spasms and twitches, muscles tension, asthma, bronchitis, pleurisy, pneumonia, hiccough, whooping cough, relaxing respiratory passages, stop smoking, emetic, cough*

Uses: Lobelia is a wonderful antispasmodic, relaxing muscles and nerves and treating asthma, bronchial spasms, whooping and other spasmodic coughs, muscle spasms and twitches, lockjaw and any pains, including lessening the strength of contractions during natural childbirth (it's most frequently combined with other herbs). For muscle spasms, boils and ulcers, apply lobelia externally in baths, fomentations, poultices and liniments.

Add to enemas for fevers and infections and to ease spasms and cramps. Place a few drops of its tincture in the ear to relieve earaches (when making the tincture, it's possible to use apple cider vinegar to extract its alkaloids). Because the lobeline contained within lobelia is similar to nicotine, lobelia is used in commercial smoking preparations to counteract the desire for tobacco (make yourself by including with other smoking herbs).

✿ LONGAN BERRIES

Euphoria longan; Sapindaceae   C
long yan rou

Part used: fruit

Energy, taste and Organs affected: warm; sweet; Heart, Spleen

Actions: tonify Blood

Biochemical constituents: adenine, choline, glucose, sucrose

Dose: 6-15 gms, decoction

Precautions: Dampness in Spleen or Stomach; Phlegm Fire

Other: Also known as *Arillus euphoriae longanae.*

Indications: *anemia, restlessness, anxiety, palpitations, insomnia, forgetfulness, dizziness*

Uses: These delicious berries quickly tonify Heart Blood (like no other herb I know), alleviating palpitations, anxiety, forgetfulness and insomnia, particularly due to overwork or from excessive thinking, studying, reading or talking (all of which use a lot of Heart Blood and blood sugar in the brain—these berries are high in glucose and sucrose, which quickly replenish blood sugar).

✿ LOQUAT

Eriobotrya japonica; Rosaceae   C
pi pa ye

Part used: leaf

Energy, taste and Organs affected: cool; bitter; Lungs, Stomach

Actions: relieve coughing and wheezing

Properties: antitussive, expectorant, anti-emetic

Biochemical constituents: neroldiol, farnesol, amygdalin

Dose: 4.5-12 gms dry, or 15-30 gms fresh, decoction; fry in honey to strengthen Lung-moistening properties, or in ginger juice to stop nausea and vomiting

Precautions: vomiting or cough due to Coldness

Indications: *cough with yellow phlegm, nausea, vomiting due to heat, hiccoughs, belching*

Uses: Loquat leaves are one of the best anti-cough remedies due to Heat. They redirect the Qi downwards, transforming phlegm and alleviating cough, nausea, vomiting, hiccoughing and belching. Loquat contains similar hydrocyanic glycosides found in apricot and peach seeds and wild cherry bark—all are used for coughs, but also as sources for the anticancer B17, or Laetrile. In fact, according to Michael Tierra loquat leaf tea (rub off hairs first as they're irritating to throat) is a folk medicine of Cyprus and Japan for the treatment of cancer.

✿ LYCII BERRIES

Lycium barbarum; L. chinensis; Solanaceae   C
gou qi zi

Part used: Chinese wolfberry fruit

Energy, taste and Organs affected: neutral; sweet; Liver, Lungs, Kidneys

Actions: tonify Blood

Properties: blood and nutritive tonic, hemostatic, antipyretic

Biochemical constituents: betaine, carotene, physalien, thiamine, riboflavin, vitamin C, linoleic acid

Dose: 6-18 gms, decoction

Precautions: Excess Heat, loose stools

Other: Grows in the Southwest as **wolfberry**; **lycii root**

bark (*di gu pi*) is used to cool the Blood, treating fever, cough, asthma, tuberculosis, nosebleed, childhood eczema and externally for genital itching. .

Indications: *anemia, dry eyes, dizziness, blurred vision, photosensitivity, night blindness, poor vision, impotence, nocturnal emission, pulmonary tuberculosis, sore back, knees and legs, low-grade abdominal pain, peri/menopausal complaintss*

Uses: This small red, sweet tasting berry tonifies Blood and Yin of the Liver and Kidneys, treating anemia, dizziness, poor eyesight, night blindness, blurred vision, sore back, knees and legs, impotence, seminal and nocturnal emission, tuberculosis and peri/menopausal complaints. Very high in beta-carotene, it promotes regeneration of liver cells, inhibits fat deposits in liver cells, lowers cholesterol, prevents artherosclerosis and enhances immunity. I always toss them in my hot cereals, soups or oatmeal cookies (instead of raisins), and frequently give them to patients as a snack. It is one of the best herbs to include in Kidney tonic formulas.

❧ MAGNOLIA

Magnolia officinalis (bark); M. liliflora (flower); Magnoliaceae   **C**
Bark: *hou po*; Flower: *xin yi hua*

Part used: bark, flower (bud)

Energy, taste and Organs affected: bark: warm; bitter, spicy; Large Intestine, Lungs, Spleen, Stomach; flower: warm; spicy; Lungs, Stomach

Actions: bark: aromatic stomachic; flower: warm and release Exterior

Properties: bark: stomachic, expectorant, carminative, antihypertensive, antibacterial antifungal; flower: diaphoretic, decongestant, expectorant, aromatic stimulant

Biochemical constituents: bark: magnolol, iso-magnolol, honokiol, machilol, eudesmol, magnocurarine; flower: cineol, methyl, citral, salicifoline, pinoresinol dimethyl ether, lirioresinol dimethyl ether, magnolin

Dose: 3-9 gms of bark or flower; decoct bark, infuse flower

Precautions: bark: pregnancy; don't use with **alisma**; flower: Deficient Yin with Heat; over-dosage can cause dizziness or redness of eyes

Indications: bark: *chronic digestive disturbances with gas, bloating, colic, chest and abdominal fullness, loss of appetite, vomiting, diarrhea, acid stomach, excess mucus, wheezing, cough, sensation of a lump in the throat;* flower: *nasal congestion, obstruction or discharge, loss of sense of smell, sinus problems due to Coldness*

❧ MARSHMALLOW

Althea officinalis; Malvaceae   **A, W**

Part used: root

Energy, taste and Organs affected: cool; sweet, mildly bitter; Small and Large Intestines, Lungs, Stomach, Kidneys, Bladder

Actions: tonify Yin

Properties: nutritive tonic, alterative, diuretic, demulcent, emollient, lithotriptic, antiinflammatory, vulnerary, laxative, expectorant, antispasmodic

Biochemical constituents: starch, mucilage, anthocyanidins, polysaccharides, pectin, bitter compound, saponins, sterols, asparagin, phenolic acids, flavonoids, saccharose, vitamin A

Dose: 6-15 gms; decoct 1 Tbsp./cup water; drink 3 cups a day; 30-60 drops tincture, 1-4 times/day

Precautions: diarrhea due to Cold Dampness,

Other: **Malvae** has very similar uses and may be substituted; the confectionery, marshmallows, were originally made from marshmallow root by the French.

Indications: *tuberculosis, cough, diabetes, dryness and inflammation of the lungs, kidney stones and inflammation, bladder infections, whooping cough, dry cough, colitis, internal bleeding, malnutrition, wounds, burns, skin eruptions, ulcers, gastritis*

Uses: Marshmallow is a wonderful antiinflammatory

herb, particularly for infections or inflammations of the mouth, throat, stomach, intestines, urinary bladder, kidneys or urethra. A wonderful demulcent that lubricates the body, protecting against irritation and dryness, it is a Yin tonic useful for wasting and thirsting diseases, such as tuberculosis and diabetes. It also settles acid indigestion, soothes dry cough, colitis and ulcers, lung inflammation, sore and irritated joints, gastritis, and the urinary system.

It is usually combined with other diuretic herbs to treat kidney and bladder inflammations, difficult or painful urination and kidney stones or gravel. Marshmallow stops bleeding in the urine, stool or nose, and vomiting or spitting of blood. It can be used with other laxative herbs for constipation due to Dryness or lack of roughage and heals irritations associated with diarrhea and dysentery. It also promotes lactation and treats inflammatory dry cough, colitis and ulcers

Externally, marshmallow is used as a poultice for inflammations and infections such as wounds, burns, boils, ulcers, abscesses, bruises, gangrene and blood poisoning. The tea can be gargled for sore or irritated throat. Ayurvedic medicine uses it as a rejuvenative tonic by decocting it in milk and adding a small amount of **ginger**. In this way it helps strengthen the body, thus prolonging a healthy life.

🌺 MILK THISTLE

Silybum marianum; Asteraceae   W

Part used: seeds

Energy, taste and Organs affected: cool; bitter, sweet; Liver, Spleen

Actions: clear Heat and toxins

Properties: hepatoprotective, hepatic tonic, bitter tonic, demulcent, galactogogue, demulcent, antioxidant, gastroprotectant

Biochemical constituents: flavolignans collectively known as silymarin

Dose: 20-60 drops tincture, 1-4 times/day; do not use

the seeds in tea form as they are not water-soluble—they may be eaten as desired, however

Precautions: none noted

Other: Also known as **St. Mary's thistle**.

Note: milk thistle doesn't extract in water (teas); it's best in whole, ground form

Indications: *liver congestion and disease, cirrhosis, jaundice, swelling and pain, toxicity; hepatitis*

Uses: Milk thistle seed extract inhibits the production of leukotrienes in the liver, one of the most damaging chemicals found in the body. As well it protects the liver against damage from other chemicals and toxins, including one of the strongest liver toxins known: the death cap mushroom (*Amanita phalloides*). But milk thistle not only protects the liver, it also helps regenerates it, making it extremely useful for treating an enormous variety of liver and gallbladder conditions, including chronic liver cirrhosis, necroses, jaundice, fatty liver, liver swelling and pain and hepatitis. It also lowers fat deposits in the liver. I have found it useful in alleviating chronic allergies due to Liver Heat and congestion, or stagnant Liver Qi.

🌺 MINT

Mentha haplocalyx, M. arvensis, M. piperita; Laminaceae
                                                      A, C, W

bo he (Mentha haplocalyx, M. arvensis); Sanskrit: *putani (M. piperita)*

Part used: leaves

Energy, taste and Organs affected: cool; spicy; Lungs, Liver

Actions: cools and releases the Exterior

Properties: diaphoretic, aromatic, carminative, calmative, mild alterative, antispasmodic

Biochemical constituents: volatile oils such as menthol and menthone, flavonoids, tannins, vitamin E

Dose: 2-6 gms; infuse 1 Tbsp./cup water, drink 3 cups a

day; 2 "00" capsules, 3 times/day; $^1/_2$-6 gms in formula; 10-30 drops tincture, 1-4 times/day

Precautions: severe chills, Exterior Deficiency, Deficient Yin with Heat signs; nursing mothers (can dry up milk); prolonged use by infants, in young children can cause a rash

Other: the Chinese use *Mentha haplocalyx* as *bo he; M. arvensis* is more common in India

Indications: *colds, flu, fever, headache, cough, sore throat, sinus congestion, earache, early stages of rashes and skin eruptions such as measles, red eyes and eye inflammations, indigestion, gas, colic, nausea, irritable bowel syndrome (IBS)*

Uses: One of the oldest medicinal herbs, mint is a cooling diaphoretic that opens the surface (pores) to release colds, flu, fevers and vent rashes, such as the initial stages of measles, all from Heat. It also eases indigestion, gas, colic and heartburn and counteracts nausea and vomiting. The Chinese use it to clear Heat from the head and eyes, treating sore throat and headache. As well, it regulates Liver Qi, treating tightness in the chest or flanks, emotional instability and gynecological problems. Mint oil can be applied externally to the forehead to relieve headache and ease insect bites, stings and itchy skin. A few drops may also be added to boiling water and inhaled for bronchitis, or general lung and nose congestion. Enteric-coated peppermint oil treats irritable bowel syndrome (IBS) since it bypasses the stomach to break down in the intestines, thereby having a direct effect on them.

✿ MOTHERWORT

Leonurus heterophyllus, L. cardiaca; Laminaceae   **C, W**
yi mu cao

Part used: above-ground parts

Energy, taste and Organs affected: slightly cold; spicy, bitter; Heart, Liver, Bladder

Actions: invigorates Blood

Properties: emmenagogue, cardiac tonic, diuretic, antispasmodic, antihypertensive

Biochemical constituents: leonurine, stachydrine, leonuridien, leonurinine, lauric acid, linolenic acid, oleic acid, oleanolic acid, sterol, vitamin A

Dose: 9-60 gms; infuse 1 Tbsp./cup water, drink 3 cups/day; 2 "00" capsules, 3 times/day; 20-40 drops tincture, 1-4 times/day

Precautions: do not use during pregnancy; Deficient Blood or Yin

Other: Literally translated, *yi mu cao* means "Good for Mother" attesting to its long respect in the treatment of women's ailments.

Indications: *menstrual disorders, amenorrhea, irregular menstruation, PMS abdominal pain, abdominal masses (fibroids, cysts, tumors), infertility from Deficient Blood, postpartum abdominal pain, edema, swellings, palpitations, angina pectoris, tachycardia and heart problems, PMS nerve tension, high blood pressure due to stress, herpes zoster or simplex nerve pain, nephritis, eczema, conjunctivitis*

Uses: An extremely useful and valuable herb, motherwort is a strong blood and uterine stimulant that also calms the nerves and protects the heart. Specifically, it treats menstrual disorders such as delayed, stopped or painful menses, amenorrhea and pain in the pelvic and lumbar region (a fomentation can be placed over the abdomen and the tea taken for these).

As an important cardiac tonic, motherwort is said to give courage and strengthen the heart. Indeed, it increases blood circulation in the coronary artery, decreases heart rate, improves microcirculation and prevents platelet agglutination. It should be taken regularly by those with angina pectoris, cardiac edema, palpitations and other heart conditions (it combines well with **hawthorn**). As well, it may be used to treat PMS nerve tension, high blood pressure due to stress, herpes zoster or simplex nerve pain, edema, nephritis, eczema and conjunctivitis.

The Chinese use motherwort (*L. heterophyllus*) for PMS abdominal pain, postpartum pain with clots, abdominal masses (hard and immobile fibroids, cysts and tumors), infertility due to Deficient Blood, irregular menses and to reduce swellings and promote urination, especially when there's blood in the urine. They often combine it with **dang gui** as a menstrual regulator. In ancient China the courtesans drank motherwort tea (called *I mu*) daily to prevent pregnancy.

✿ MUGWORT

Artemisia argyi, A. vulgaris; Asteraceae   **A, C, W**
ai ye; Sanskrit: *nagadamani (A. vulgaris)*

Part used: leaves

Energy, taste and Organs affected: charred is warm, raw is neutral; bitter, spicy; Spleen, Liver, Kidneys

Actions: stops bleeding

Properties: emmenagogue, vermifuge, cholagogue, hemostatic, antispasmodic, diaphoretic, mild narcotic, bitter tonic

Biochemical constituents: cineole, artemisia alcohol, camphor, borneol, linalool

Dose: 3-9 gms; char to enhance warming and stop bleeding properties; infuse 2-3 tsp./cup water, drink 1/2 cup, 2-3 times/day; 2 "00" capsules, 3 times/day; 10-30 drops tincture 3 times/day

Precautions: pregnancy; Deficient Blood or Yin; Heat in the Blood

Other: *Artemisia annuae* (**sweet annie**; *qing hao*), a related species, also stops bleeding and clears fevers, yet it specifically checks malarial disorders (and is used by the Red Cross around the world for this). In fact, it treats the Plasmodium falciparum parasite, the biggest mutated strain of malaria, by acting like a bomb when its two oxygen atoms break apart in the presence of iron, releasing lethal toxins that blow apart the parasite living in the blood. Take a dropperful of its tincture 1-2 times daily when traveling to prevent malaria. **Wormwood,** *A. absinthium* (yes, it's used to make absinthe, though this was outlawed in the States in the 1930s because it was considered to "drive you crazy" and "play with the mind"), is similar, though stronger in killing parasites (although not malaria).

Indications: *menstrual and abdominal pain, excessive menstrual bleeding, nosebleeds and spitting blood: all from coldness; habitual miscarriage, restless fetus, parasites and worms, colds, flu, cough, asthma, insomnia, nervousness, pain, non-healing sores*

Uses: While mugwort circulates Blood, especially through the lower abdomen and uterus, it also stops internal and external bleeding when charred (its ashes). It alleviates menstrual difficulties and cramps, leukorrhea, abdominal pains due to Coldness and calms a restless fetus, arresting threatened miscarriage (including any associated bleeding). When burnt it stops nosebleeds and excessive menstrual bleeding (put a teaspoon of ash in water and drink). As well, put the ashes on non-healing sores, even those related to diabetes. The Chinese also use it to treat infertility due to coldness in the womb and to relieve cough, asthma and resolve Phlegm.

As a bitter tonic, mugwort treats stomach disorders, improves digestion and cures and prevents parasites and worms (although wormwood, another *Artemesia* species member, is stronger for this). The Native Americans used it for colds, flu, bronchitis, fevers and sweating therapy. Mugwort is also a nervine and can be smoked, filling the lungs three to six times to ease nervousness and insomnia. Externally, apply as a liniment or wash to relieve itching, fungus and other skin infections, or as a douche for vaginal yeast infections.

Mugwort has several other interesting uses. The Native Americans called it "The Great Sage" and used it like incense in *smudging* rituals to purify the spiritual and physical environment (a process of burning sage with mugwort and using its smoke—see *Home Therapies*). It has also long been used in dream pillows by sewing its dried leaves into a pillow-sack and sleeping with it near the nose to intensify dreams and promote their recall (a caution in this: it can cause bad dreams in those who need detoxification!). Mugwort is also the prime ingredient in *moxibustion* (an extremely useful Chinese heat therapy—see *Home Therapies*), valued for its quick and high burning qualities and deeply penetrating heat. Burning moxibustion over a painful area increases blood circulation, relieves pain and quickly heals injuries and bruises. Make your own by rubbing aged, dried mugwort leaves, with stems removed, between your palms until a wooly consistency.

🦎 MULBERRY

Morus alba; Moraceae **C, W**

Fruit: *sang shen;* leaf: *sang ye;* twigs: *sang zhi;* root bark: *sang bai pi*

Parts used: fruit, leaf, twigs, root bark

Energy, taste and Organs affected:
Fruit: cold; sweet; Heart, Liver, Kidney
Leaf: cold; sweet, bitter; Liver, Lungs
Twigs: slightly cold; bitter, sweet; Liver
Root bark: cold; sweet; Lungs, Spleen

Actions:
Fruit: tonifies Blood
Leaf: cools and releases the Exterior
Twigs: dispels Wind and Dampness
Root bark: relieves coughing and wheezing

Properties:
Fruit: demulcent, nutritive
Leaf: diaphoretic
Twigs: antirheumatic, antispasmodic
Root bark: expectorant, antitussive

Biochemical constituents:
Fruit: carotene, thiamene, riboflavin, vitamin C, tannin, linoleic acid, stearic acid
Leaf: carotene, succine acid, adenine, choline, amylase
Twigs: mulberrin, mulberrochromene, cyclomulberrin, morin, cudranin, maclurin, cyclomulberrochromene, tetrahydroxystilbene, dihydromorin, dihydrokaempferol, fructose, glucose, arabinose, xylose, stachyose, sucrose
Root bark: morusin, mulberrin, mulberrochromene, cyclomulberrin, cyclomulberrochromene

Dose: infuse leaves, decoct the rest:
Fruit: 6-15 gms; often used in syrup form
Leaf: 4.5-15 gms; toast in honey for cough or Lung Dryness; external wash for eyes
Twigs: 10-30 gms; often the old stems are used
Root bark: 6-15 gms; honey-fry to stop coughing and wheezing

Precautions:
Fruit: diarrhea due to Spleen Deficiency
Leaf: none noted
Twigs: none noted
Root bark: excessive urination, cough due to Wind Cold

Other: Loranthus (*Loranthus parasiticus; sang ji sheng*), the mistletoe growing on the mulberry tree, is a Yin tonic used to treat low back and muscle pain, arthritis, rheumatism and hypertension.

Note: The mulberry tree is a pharmacopoeia in itself, and is amazing for how its many diverse parts are widely used for such different purposes (this may be due to the Chinese interest in the silk worm, which feeds on the tree, and since the Chinese are the major producers of silk in the world, they learned a great deal about the tree). The mulberry tree is an excellent study in how each part of a plant works uniquely, particularly when prepared in different ways. (It's also a lesson in Chinese: note how *sang* is the word for mulberry, while the words following it are names for each of the plant parts).

Indications:
Fruit: *dizziness, tinnitus, insomnia, premature graying hair, constipation due to Deficient Blood, wasting and thirsting disorder (diabetes, TB)*
Leaf: *fever, headache, sore throat, cough with thick, yellow phlegm, dry mouth, red, sore, dry or painful eyes, spots in front of eyes, vomiting of blood due to Heat in Blood*
Twigs: *edema, arthritis, rheumatism and painful joints, especially in the upper extremities*
Root bark: *coughing and wheezing due to Lung Heat (yellow mucus and inflammation), edema, facial edema, swelling of extremities, fever and thirst, difficulty in urination, hypertension*

🦎 MULLEIN

Verbascum thapsus; Scrophulariaceae **W**

Part used: leaves, flowers, root

Energy, taste and Organs affected: cool; bitter, astringent; Lungs, Stomach

Actions: cools and dissolves Phlegm and stops coughing

Properties: leaves: expectorant, astringent, diuretic, vulnerary, demulcent, emollient, antispasmodic; flowers: nervine, antispasmodic, sedative; root: astringent

Biochemical constituents: saponins, mucilage, two flavonoids (hesperidin and verbaside), rutin, aucubin, traces of essential oil

Dose: 3-9 gms; infuse 1 tsp. leaf/root, or 1Tbsp flowers/cup water; drink 1 cup every 2 hours until symptoms lessen; then drink 2 cups/day until problem heals; 10-40 drops tincture, 1-4 times/day; put 5-10 drops oil in ear every hour until earache is gone.

Precautions: do not use for clear to white phlegm, or Coldness

Other: It is said that figs wrapped in mullein leaves will not putrefy.

Indications: leaves: *coughs, whooping cough, asthma, pneumonia, colds, flu, bronchitis, mumps, earaches, stop smoking, lung or bowel bleeding, diarrhea, hemorrhoids, toothache, bruises;* flowers: *earaches, ear inflammation, eczema, bruises, hemorrhoids;* root: *sinus infections, lymphatic congestion, diarrhea*

Uses: An excellent lung herb, **mullein leaves and root** are useful for asthma, pneumonia, spasmodic coughs, colds, flu, bronchitis, hoarseness, and whooping cough. They expel yellow mucus, cleansing the bronchioles and lymphatic system and specifically alleviate mumps, earaches and glandular swellings. For all these conditions it can be taken as a tea, or the dried leaves can be smoked (which also soothes the throat and is a good tobacco substitute). As well, mullein stops bleeding from the lungs and intestines.

A poultice of mullein leaves can be locally applied to ease hemorrhoids, inflammations, wounds and toothache. One Native American teacher of mine uses the smoke from the burning root to successfully treat sinus infections. The root also clears lymphatic congestion and diarrhea. **Mullein flower oil**, strong in nervine, analgesic and antiinflammatory properties, is an important remedy for earaches, inner ear inflammation and discharge. As well, the oil treats frostbite, bruises, hem-

orrhoids, eczema of the external ear and canal, mucous membrane inflammations and hemorrhoids.

🎋 MYRRH

Commiphora myrrha, C. molmol; Burseraceae **A, C**
mo yao; Sanskrit: *Daindhava, Bola (Commiphora myrrh, C. molmol); guggulu (C. mukul)*

Part used: gum (resin)

Energy, taste and Organs affected: neutral; bitter; Heart, Liver, Spleen

Actions: invigorates the Blood

Properties: emmenagogue, expectorant, antispasmodic, disinfectant, stimulant, carminative, antifungal

Biochemical constituents: heerabomyrrholic acid, commiphoric acid, heerabomyrrhol, heeraboresence, commiferin, ergenol, cumin aldehyde, pinene, dipentene, limonene, cinnamic aldehyde, heerabolene

Dose: 3-12 gms, decoction; 10-40 drops tincture, 1-4 times/day; fry with vinegar to enhance its Blood-invigorating effects

Precautions: do not use during pregnancy or excessive uterine bleeding

Other: Another species of myrrh, *C. mukul,* called **guggulu,** or **guggul gum,** is a specific for lowering cholesterol and treating abnormal growths, tumors, cysts, arthritis, cancer, inflammation and glandular swellings.

Indications: *traumatic injuries, rheumatoid arthritis, painful and swollen joints, swellings, chest and abdominal pain, amenorrhea, abdominal cysts and fibroids, chronic nonhealing sores, carbuncles, inflamed sore gums, tonsillitis*

Uses: Like frankincense, myrrh wonderfully reduces pain due to stagnant Blood (fixed, boring and stabbing pain). It treats traumatic injuries, rheumatoid arthritis, painful and swollen joints and swellings, and works especially well when combined with **frankincense** and **corydalis** for these. I remember treating one elderly woman who had tremendous pain in her neck, down her entire back, into her hips and down one leg. While acupuncture helped tremendously, myrrh and frankincense finally alleviated the pain altogether.

Myrrh also promotes menstrual bleeding, treating amenorrhea and breaking up abdominal stagnant Blood masses, such as cysts and fibroids. Topically, it is used to promote wound healing, treat chronic nonhealing sores and carbuncles (use as a topical wash), and is one of the best topical remedies for inflamed sore gums and tonsillitis when its tincture is diluted in water, or as a mouthwash.

🦚 NEEM

Azadirachta indica; Meliaceae   **A**
Sanskrit: *nimba*

Part used: leaf, oil

Energy, taste and Organs affected: leaf: cold; bitter; Liver, Lungs, Large Intestine

Actions: clear Heat, clean toxins

Properties: antifungal, antibacterial, antiviral, parasiticide

Biochemical constituents: a bitter resin-margosin, volatile oil, gum

Dose: leaf: 1-2 gms, 2 times/day; 10-20 drops tincture, 2 times/day; oil: as needed

Precautions: do not use longer than 3 weeks as it excessively dampens digestion and cools Yang

Other: It is used in agriculture worldwide to repel insects on plants.

Indications: leaf: *skin conditions, dandruff, itching, vitiligo, parasites, scabies, lice, herpes, chicken pox, Candida, fever, sore throat, malaria, hepatitis A and B, mononucleosis, Epstein-Barr, fungal infections,* oil: *skin conditions, ulcers*

Uses: Neem is considered a "miracle cure-all" herb by many, not unlike garlic. And similar to garlic, it has a bad odor. However, its many uses make it well worth trying. A specific for all skin conditions, it treats dandruff, itching, skin diseases, vitiligo, parasites like scabies and lice, herpes and chickenpox (use in oil or liquid form). Internally, it also kills parasites and as an antifungal, is specific for Candida. As well, it is used for fever, sore throat, malaria, hepatitis A and B, mononucleosis and Epstein-Barr.

🦚 NETTLE

Urtica urens and spp.; Urticaceae   **W**

Part used: leaves, seeds, root

Energy, taste and Organs affected: cool; slightly bitter; Bladder, Kidneys, Lungs

Actions: drains Dampness

Properties: diuretic, astringent, hemostatic, galactogogue, expectorant, nutritive

Biochemical constituents: chlorophyll, indoles (histamine, serotonic), acetylcholine, silicic acid, vitamins C and A, silicon, calcium, magnesium, potassium, protein, fiber

Dose: 9-30 gms; infuse 1 Tbsp./cup water, drink 3 cups/day; 2 "00" capsules, 3 times/day; 10-60 drops tincture, 1-4 times/day

Precautions: use in smaller amounts during pregnancy

Other: Never harvest after flowers appear, or it may cause urinary tract infections; use nettle long term for best results.

Indications: leaves: *arthritis, rheumatism, asthma, eczema, skin eruptions, bleeding, low energy, stopped urine, gravel, kidney and bladder infections, edema, enlarged prostate, benign prostatic hyperplasia (BPH);* freeze-dried: *sinus infections;* seeds: *prostate and kidney disorders;* root: *prostate troubles*

Uses: Nettle certainly lives up to its common name, stinging nettle, for the tiny prickles on the underside of its leaves and stem sting intensely and seemingly indefinitely when touched (unless poulticed quickly with another green plant!). Yet, it is this same stinging quality that makes it an effective, though painful, remedy for arthritis where the person rolls (or brushes) the arthritic (or painful) area in a nettles patch, purposely causing the intense stinging. It has been said that this process can even cure arthritis, but use caution if you decide to try it as massive exposure to nettle plants causes severe shock symptoms in animals. If you don't need or desire arthritis therapy, be sure to wear gloves when picking the leaves! When made into a tea or cooked, the prickles 'wilt' and you may safely eat the leaves as a delicious and nutritious green, especially in spring (called a potherb).

Nettle treats lung mucus conditions, including asthma and excessive mucus discharge from the intestines, relieves skin complaints such as eczema and skin eruptions, and stops bleeding and hemorrhage. Its high iron content makes it useful for anemia (take with molasses for this). Cool nettle tea is a wonderful diuretic high in potassium, helping it effectively release excessive water and edema from the body without depleting potassium levels, as most diuretic medications do. This makes it useful for urinary problems such as stopped urine, gravel, bladder and kidney infections and enlarged prostate. As a daily tea (three times a day), nettle's high mineral content supports the energy and Kidneys. Nettle root is now being used to treat benign prostatic hyperplasia (BPH).

Freeze-dried nettle successfully treats sinus infections (it must be freeze dried as this process enhances nettle's formic acid content, the applicable ingredient here). Nettle seeds are used to treat prostate and kidney disorders.

🦎 OLIVE LEAF

Olea europea; Oleaceae   **W**

Part used: leaf (extract)

Energy, taste and Organs affected: cool; bitter; Large Intestine, Liver, Gallbladder

Actions: clears Heat and toxins

Properties: antiviral, antifungal, antibacterial, parasiticide, astringent, antiseptic, antihypertensive, antiinflammatory

Biochemical constituents: calcium elenolate, oleic, linoleic, palmitic and stearic acids

Dose: infuse 1 Tbsp./cup water, drink 2 cups/day; acute: 2-4 tablets, or 1 cup tea, every 3 hours

Precautions: none noted

Other: Widely used in cooking, olive oil is also wonderful for dry skin and dandruff.

Indications: *colds, flu, fever, mononucleosis, chronic fatigue, herpes, chickenpox, glandular fevers, shingles, Epstein-Barr, Candida, yeast and other fungal infections, high blood pressure, parasites*

Uses: I first learned about olive leaf extract several years ago after managing and teaching a week-long seminar when, in my usual fashion of overdoing it, I contracted a relentless lingering flu. So, dragging myself off to the local store to replenish the garlic and ginger I had just used up, I ran into a friend who manages the store's supplement department. He took pity on me and suggested I try olive leaf extract. I did, and the results were fabulous. Within the day I felt the flu lift and was over it completely in a few more days with no relapses. I learned about the wonderful antiviral property of this herb and realized it was just one more gift from the life-sustaining olive tree.

With more and more viruses appearing these days, I'm glad to know that there's a common and widely available herb ready to help. As a potent antiviral herb, olive leaf extract treats other viral conditions such as mononucleosis, chronic fatigue, herpes, chickenpox, glandular fevers, shingles and Epstein-Barr. As if this were not enough, it is also a valuable antifungal and antibacterial herb, treating Candida, yeast and other fungal infections. As well, it boosts immunity (and promotes energy as a result), lowers blood pressure, kills parasites and is a powerful antioxidant.

🦎 OPHIOPOGON

Ophiopogon japonicus; Liliaceae   **C**
mai men dong

Part used: tuber

Energy, taste and Organs affected: slightly cold; sweet, slightly bitter; Heart, Lungs, Stomach

Actions: tonify Yin

Properties: demulcent, expectorant

Biochemical constituents: ophiopogonin, ruscogenin, stigmasterol

Dose: 6-15 gms, decoction; fry in wine to reduce its cold properties

Precautions: diarrhea due to coldness or weakness, do not use with **coltsfoot** or **sophora**

Other: This ornamental grass is widely used in garden and tree borders, sometimes called **Japanese Turf Lily**, or **Mondo Grass**. Because its properties are similar to American ginseng and is a common, easily grown plant, it should be more widely used.

Indications: *dry cough, dry tongue and mouth, coughing up blood, irritability and feverishness worse at night, constipation from dryness, sore throat, mouth sores, diabetes*

Uses: Ophiopogon is a sweet and juicy root that wonderfully moistens the body's Yin. I'm always amazed at how effectively it alleviates dry, nonproductive coughs accompanied by weakness and tiredness. It also stops coughing of blood and treats dry tongue and mouth, irritability and fever (especially when worse at night) and constipation from Dryness. It is a specific for Deficient Yin signs arising after a fever (when Heat dries up the body Fluids). As well, it moistens the Stomach and treats diabetes.

❧ OREGON GRAPE ROOT

Mahonia spp.; Berberidaceae   **W**

Part used: rhizome and root

Energy, taste and Organs affected: cool; bitter; Liver, Gallbladder, Large Intestine

Actions: clears Heat, dries Dampness

Biochemical constituents: berberine alkaloid, palmatine, jatorrhizine, columbamine

Properties: cholagogue, alterative, hepatic, laxative, anti-inflammatory, bitter tonic, stomachic, antimicrobial, astringent

Dose: 3-9 gms, decoct 1 tsp./cup water, drink 2-3 cups a day; 10-60 drops tincture, 1-4 times/day; 2 "00" capsules, 3 times/day

Precautions: pregnancy since it stimulates the uterus

Other: This herb is at risk of becoming endangered, thus *only use the cultivated plant*, or better yet, choose **barberry** (*Berberis vulgaris*), the counterpart which grows in the Northeast.

Indications: *jaundice, hepatitis, enlargement of the liver and spleen, gallstones, acne, boils, psoriasis, dry eczema, skin diseases, conjunctivitis, fevers, cancer, tumors, constipation, arthritis, rheumatism, amoebic and bacillary chronic dysentery, diarrhea (yellow and foul-smelling), leukorrhea*

Uses: Oregon grape root is one of the mildest and best liver tonics known, more gentle in action than its other berberine-containing relatives such as **goldenseal**. It cleanses and regulates liver function and stimulates the flow of bile making it especially useful for jaundice, hepatitis, enlargement of the liver and spleen, gallstones and arthritis, especially when combined with **dandelion** and **fennel**. Its detoxifying action clears toxins and poisons, helping to heal acne, boils, psoriasis, dry eczema and other skin diseases, conjunctivitis, fevers, cancer and tumors. As a bitter tonic Oregon grape stimulates digestion, acts as a mild laxative, and clears the heat and toxins in arthritis and rheumatism. It is also useful for amoebic and bacillary chronic dysentery, diarrhea (yellow and foul-smelling) and leukorrhea.

❧ OYSTER SHELL

Ostrea gigas; Ostreidae   **C**
mu li

Part used: shell

Energy, taste and Organs affected: cool; salty, astringent; Liver, Kidneys

Actions: anchor, settle and calm the Spirit

Properties: sedative, demulcent, antacid, astringent

Biochemical constituents: calcium carbonate, calcium phosphate, magnesium, aluminum, potassium

Dose: 15-30 gms; decoct 1 hour; calcine to absorb acidity and prevent leakage of Fluids

Precautions: high fever with no sweating; do not use

with **fritillary**, **licorice**, **achyranthis**, **polygala**, **ephedra**, **asarum**; overdose may lead to indigestion or constipation

Indications: *palpitations with anxiety, restlessness, insomnia, irritability, dizziness, headache, ringing in ears, blurred vision, bad temper, heartburn, neck lumps (scrofula and goiter) spontaneous sweating, night sweats, nocturnal emissions, spermatorrhea, vaginal discharge, uterine bleeding due to weakness, peptic ulcers*

🐾 PARSLEY

Petroselinum spp.; Apiaceae   W

Part used: leaves, seeds, root

Energy, taste and Organs affected: leaves: warm; spicy; Kidneys; root: neutral; sweet; Kidneys

Actions: drain Dampness

Properties: diuretic, carminative, aperient, antispasmodic, antiseptic, expectorant, antirheumatic, sedative, emmenagogue (seeds)

Biochemical constituents: root: volatile oil, apiin, bergapten, isoimperatorin, mucilage, sugar; seeds: essential oil, apiole, myristicin, pinene, terpenes, flavone glycosides, furanocumarin, fatty oil, petroselinic acid; leaves: have similar but weaker constituents, vitamins A and C, calcium, iron

Dose: 3-9 gms; infuse 1 Tbsp. leaves or decoct 1 tsp. root or seeds/cup water, drink 3 cups/day; 10-30 drops tincture, 1-4 times/day

Precautions: pregnancy; parsley seeds in high dose can irritate the stomach, liver, heart and kidneys

Indications: *edema, frequent urination, bed-wetting, bladder and kidney infections, indigestion, gas, intestinal worms, stones, delayed menses, menstrual water retention and swollen breasts*

Uses: Best known as a culinary herb, parsley leaves and root are an effective diuretic useful for fluid retention, frequent urination, bed-wetting and bladder infections. A stronger diuretic, the seeds are particularly good for rheumatic complaints while the root specifically dissolves and eliminates stones and gravel (combine with

equal parts **gravel root** and a half part each **marshmallow** root and **ginger**). All three parts stimulate digestion and relieve bronchial and lung congestion. Parsley tea is an emmenagogue, promoting menses and dispelling premenstrual water retention from the abdomen, legs and breast. The leaf inserted into and retained in the vagina can bring on delayed menses. Because parsley is rich in vitamins, iron and minerals, be sure to eat your garnish! Drinking the fresh juice daily (2 tsp.) strengthens Kidneys and uterus.

🐾 PARTRIDGEBERRY

Mitchella repens; Rubiaceae   W

Part used: whole herb

Energy, taste and Organs affected: cool; bitter; Uterus, Liver

Actions: stabilize and bind

Properties: astringent, parturient, diuretic

Biochemical constituents: not known, probably some alkaloids, glycosides, tannins and mucilage

Dose: infuse 1 tsp./cup water, drink 3 cups/day; 10-40 drops tincture, 1-4 times/day; 2 "00" capsules, 3 times/day

Precautions: none noted

Other: Also known as **squawvine**, this herb is at risk of becoming endangered, thus *only use the cultivated plant.*

Indications: *excessive menstruation, delayed menses, scanty menses, amenorrhea, menstrual cramps, vaginal infections, leukorrhea, ovarian cysts*

Uses: Partridgeberry treats menstrual irregularities, particularly excessive menstruation (with bright red blood), delayed menses, scanty menses, amenorrhea and menstrual cramps. As well, it dries excessive vaginal secretions, treating vaginal infections and leukorrhea. I always include it in a bolus as well as give it with **raspberry** leaf for ovarian cysts (drink 3 cups tea/day for three months). As it tones the uterus and relieves uterine congestion, it is very effective for preparing the womb for, and easing, childbirth. Combine with two parts raspberry leaves and one part **black cohosh** root and take two weeks before delivery for best results. As well, partridgeberry treats postpartum hemorrhage (take with **shepherd's purse**). Include it in douches or boluses for vaginal infections.

❧ PASSIONFLOWER

Passiflora incarnata; Passifloraceae   **W**

Part used: leaves

Energy, taste and Organs affected: cool; bitter; Heart, Liver

Actions: calms the Spirit

Properties: mild sedative, hypnotic, antispasmodic, anodyne, hypotensive, nervine

Biochemical constituents: harmine alkaloids, the flavonoids apigenin and luteolin, sterols, gums, sugars

Dose: infuse 2 tsp./cup water; 10-40 drops tincture

Precautions: pregnancy, due to uterine stimulation

Indications: *insomnia, nervousness, Parkinson's, epilepsy, hysteria, neuralgia, shingles, anxiety, hypertension, restless agitation, exhaustion with muscular twitching or spasms, palpitations*

❧ PAU D'ARCO

Tabebuia heptaphylla, T. impetiginosa; Bignoniaceae   **W**

Part used: inner bark of tree

Energy, taste and Organs affected: cool; bitter; Liver, Lungs

Actions: clears Heat and toxins

Properties: alterative, antifungal, hypotensive, antidiabetic, bitter tonic, digestive, antibacterial, antitumor, lymphagogue, antiviral

Biochemical constituents: quinones, principally lapachol

Dose: decoct 1 Tbsp./cup water, drink 1 cup, 3-4 times daily in acute conditions, or 1 cup 3-4 times daily in chronic ones; 25-50 drops tincture, 1-4 times/day

Precautions: none noted

Other: The inner bark must be aged to maximize its effectiveness.

Indications: *cancer, tumors, leukemia, ulcers, ringworm, allergies, bronchitis, respiratory disorders, diabetes, lupus, polyps, prostatitis, leukorrhea, inflammations of the genito-urinary tract, arteriosclerosis, Hodgkin's disease, Parkinson's disease, colitis, cystitis, gastritis, gonorrhea, hemorrhage, lymphatic congestion, chronic fatigue, Candida, fungal and yeast problems*

Uses: Each part of the world has an herb that is treasured as a near "cure-all" because it treats an enormous variety of symptoms. Pau d'arco, or the Lapacho tree growing in Argentina, is this type of herb for the natives of South America. A specific herb for treating cancer, tumors and leukemia, it is also used for ulcers, ringworm, allergies, bronchitis and other respiratory disorders, diabetes, lupus, polyps, prostatitis, leukorrhea, inflammations of the genito-urinary tract, arteriosclerosis, Hodgkin's disease, Parkinson's disease, colitis, cystitis, gastritis, gonorrhea, hemorrhages, lymphatic congestion, chronic fatigue, Candida and other fungal and yeast problems (internally and externally).

❧ PEONY

Paeonia lactiflora; Ranunculaceae   **C, W**
bai shao

Part used: white peony root

Energy, taste and Organs affected: cool; bitter, sour; Liver, Spleen

Actions: tonify Blood

Properties: blood and nutritive tonic, emmenagogue, antispasmodic, astringent, antihypertensive, analgesic, sedative, anticonvulsive, diuretic, antibacterial

Biochemical constituents: paeoniflorin, paeonol, paeonin, albiflorin, triterpenoids, sistosterol

Dose: 6-15 gms; dry-fry to nourish the Blood

Precautions: diarrhea from Coldness and weakness; do not use with **dendrobium**, **mirabilitum** or **turtle shell**

Note: The "wild" **red peony** (*P. rubrae, P. veitchii; chi shao*) is used to invigorate Blood, break up Blood stagnation and clear Heat from the Liver, treating abdominal pain, abdominal masses, traumatic injury, dysmenorrhea and bleeding. Avoid if there is Deficient Blood (decoct 4.5-9 gm). The cortex of the **tree peony** root, or **Moutan** (*P. suffruticosa; mu dan pi*) is used to clear Heat and cool the Blood, treating high fevers, nosebleed, blood in sputum or vomit, profuse menstruation, amenorrhea, abdominal masses, headache, eye pain, flank pain, dysmenorrhea and topically for firm, non-draining sores (decoct 6-12 gms).

Indications: *menstrual irregularities, vaginal discharge, dysmenorrhea, uterine bleeding, anemia, pain in the chest, sides or abdomen, abdominal spasms, cramps or spasms in hands, calves or feet, headache, dizziness, spermatorrhea, spontaneous sweating, night sweats, ringing in the ears, diarrhea, dysentery, leukorrhea, nervous conditions, epilepsy*

Uses: White peony nourishes the Blood, preserves Yin and regulates menstruation, making it an important herb for anemia, menstrual irregularities, amenorrhea, cramps, dysmenorrhea, leukorrhea and uterine bleeding. As an antispasmodic it relaxes and calms emotional nervous conditions, muscle spasms, epilepsy, depression and PMS. It is a major herb added to formulas to relax muscles and tension, which enhances the effects of the other herbs and moves the deep blood circulation of the body.

Peony also eases stagnant Liver Qi and stops pain, treating flank, chest or abdominal pain and spasms in the hands, calves and feet. It relieves headaches (including hypertensive), dizziness, night sweats, ringing in the ears and spontaneous sweating due to Deficient Blood and Yin and rising Liver Yang. The Western eclectic herbalists used peony as an antispasmodic for epilepsy, spasms and various nervous complaints. I have successfully used it many times with Western **black cohosh** for epilepsy.

PLATYCODON

Platycodon grandiflorum; Campanulaceae　　　**C**
jie geng

Part used: root

Energy, taste and Organs affected: neutral; bitter, pungent; Lung

Actions: warm and dissolve Phlegm and stop cough

Properties: expectorant, demulcent, antiinflammatory

Biochemical constituents: polygalain acid, platycodigenin, glucosides, stigmasterol, betulin, platycodonin, platycogenic acid, glucose

Dose: 3-9 gms, decoction

Precautions: spitting up of blood; don't use with **gentian** (*long dan cao*) or **longan berries** (*Arillus euphoriae longanae)*

Other: Also known as the common garden ornamental **balloonflower**, this herb expels phlegm from the Lungs and upper body (joints and meridians, too) and is used for Wind Cold or Wind Heat, depending on the other herbs with which it's combined. As well, it acts as an envoy to direct other herbs to the upper part of the body. It is a common ornamental that is underutilized in the West.

Indications: *cough and phlegm in both hot and cold conditions, sore throat, loss of voice, lung or throat abscess, pus in the upper parts of body*

PLANTAIN

Plantago major; P. lanceolata (Western); *P. asiatica*　　**C, W**
(Chinese); *Plantaginaceae*
che qian cao (P. asiatica)

Part used: leaves, seeds

Energy, taste and Organs affected: cool; mildly bitter; Bladder, Small Intestine, Gallbladder

Actions: drains Dampness

Properties: diuretic, vulnerary, alterative, anti-inflammatory, antibacterial

Biochemical constituents: iridoids, aucubin, flavonoids, mucilage, tannins

Dose: 5-10 gms; infuse 1 Tbsp./cup water; drink 1-2 cups every 2 hours until symptoms subside, then 1 cup 2-3 times a day for about 3 days after all symptoms are gone; 15-40 drops tincture, 1-4 times/day

Precautions: none noted

Other: Also known as **ribwort**, there are two general species: narrow-leafed variety, or *P. lanceolata*, and a broad-leaved, preferred variety, *P. major.*

Indications: *urinary infections, insect bites and stings, wounds, burns, scrapes, hemorrhoids, infections and inflammations, ulcers, diarrhea, excessive menstrual discharge*

Uses: A "weed" growing on lawns and other "undesired" places, plantain has many medicinal uses, particularly for alleviating kidney and urinary bladder infections, water retention, hepatitis and bacillary dysentery. Its astringent property treats hemorrhoids, diarrhea, constipation and excessive menstrual discharge. Externally as a poultice, plantain is one of the very best remedies I've seen for poison oak.

As well, it is a seemingly miraculous poultice for stopping the pain of spider and snakebites, bee stings and other insect wounds and draws out their stingers and poisons. In fact, it can pull deeply imbedded splinters out if the poultice is left in place for a day or two (I know of someone who successfully used plantain poultices for 5 days to draw pieces of metal out of his hand). Plantain also heals wounds, burns, scrapes and cuts, its soothing effect is felt within minutes after applying to the skin.

The Chinese use *P. asiatica* as a diuretic and to treat furuncle, carbuncle, jaundice, gonorrhea, leukorrhea, acute dysentery and urinary infections. They also use the seeds (*che qian zi*) for edema, diarrhea, urinary infections, coughs with profuse phlegm, vertigo and red eyes and swelling.

🦎 PRICKLY ASH

Zanthoxylum americanum (Northern), *Z. clava-herculis* (Southern); **A, C, W**
Z. bungeanum (Chinese); *Rutaceae;*
chuan jiao (Z. bungeanum); Sanskrit: *Tumburu (Zanthoxylum spps.)*

Part used: bark

Energy, taste and Organs affected: warm; spicy; Spleen, Stomach, Kidneys

Actions: warms the Interior

Properties: stimulant, analgesic, alterative, anthelmintic, antirheumatic, astringent

Biochemical constituents: coumarins, alkaloids (including berberine), volatile oils, resin, tannin

Dose: 2-5 gms; infuse $1/2$ tsp./cup, drink in frequent small doses, totaling 2 cups/day; take 1 "00" capsules 3 times/day; 5-15 drops tincture, 1-3 times/day

Precautions: pregnancy; acute and heated conditions; if on blood-thinning medication

Other: Chinese prickly ash fruit (pepper), or *Z. bungeamum* (*chuan jiao*), is used similarly and to kill parasites, treat rumbling intestines (from Cold or parasites), diarrhea, vomiting, pain in the abdomen and Coldness. The peel (*hua jiao*) is used in the same way.

Indications: *cold hands and feet, joint pain, indigestion, diarrhea, rheumatism, arthritis, swellings, injuries, wounds, colic, cramps, toothaches, pyorrhea, receding gums, varicose veins, ulcer, chilblains, leg cramps, high blood pressure*

Uses: As a strong stimulant, prickly ash promotes peripheral blood and lymphatic circulation, restores vascular tone, promotes capillary circulation, warms the body, relieves cold extremities, joint pain and indigestion caused by coldness and stops diarrhea and vomiting. In addition, it treats rheumatism, arthritis, swelling, injuries and wounds that are slow to heal (take internally and rub on oil or liniment externally).

Prickly ash is very warming to the stomach, stimulating weak digestion and alleviating stomachaches, colic, gas, burping and cramps from Coldness. It also treats varicose veins, ulcers, chilblains (constriction of small arteries), leg cramps and lowers blood pressure, especially with a high systolic rate (the top number). Add to formulas as a stimulant for acute or chronic ailments. Externally, apply as a poultice to dry and heal wounds. Like **bayberry**, prickly ash powder can be used as a toothpowder for pyorrhea and receding gums (brush twice daily with it), or chew the bark for toothache relief. Ayurvedic medicine also uses it as a powerful detoxifier, particularly for the gastrointestinal tract and blood.

☙ PUERARIA

Pueraria lobata; Fabaceae   **A, C, W**
ge gen; Sanskrit: *bidari kand*

Part used: root, flowers

Energy, taste and Organs affected: cool; sweet, spicy; Spleen, Stomach

Actions: cools and releases the Exterior

Properties: antipyretic, diaphoretic, spasmolytic, demulcent, antihypertensive

Biochemical constituents: puerarin, puerarin-xyloside, daidzein, diacetyl puerarin, daidzin, beta-sitosterol, arachidonic acid

Dose: 6-12 gms, decoction; roast until yellow to treat diarrhea due to Deficient Spleen

Precautions: none noted

Other: Kuzu, or **kudzu**, is the starch of the root used as a thickener for sauces, particularly in macrobiotic and Japanese cooking (dissolve in cold water first before adding to prevent lumping). It was brought from the Philippines and planted to prevent soil erosion, but since growing wildly out of control, it is now the scourge of the South.

Indications: root: *colds, flu, fever, headache, dizziness, thirst, hypertension, ringing in the ears (tinnitus), diarrhea, measles and other skin eruptions, muscle aches and pains, tight neck and shoulders;* flower: *reduces alcohol cravings, relieves alcohol poisoning (nausea, vomiting, thirst and abdominal fullness)*

Uses: Pueraria has so many valuable uses that it forms the basis for dozens of formulas (especially for the Japanese, like **bupleurum** does for the Chinese). And similar to bupleurum, pueraria treats both the Exterior and Interior of the body, relaxing tight and sore muscles, particularly of the neck and shoulders (especially needed for those desperately trying to pull it out!), and releases the surface, treating fever, colds, flu (stomach and lung types), headache, thirst, sore throat and early stage of measles, all due to Heat. It also stops diarrhea due to Heat or Spleen deficiency, depending on its herbal combination.

I frequently use pueraria's muscle-relaxing properties coupled with its Exterior-releasing action to treat disorders lodged in the muscles, including stiff neck and shoulders, muscular tension, especially of the throat, neck and shoulder, and with other herbs to treat rheumatism. Because it neutralizes acidity, pueraria is useful for minor body aches and pains. Pueraria also treats hypertension with associated headache, dizziness and tinnitus, and alleviates thirst. **Pueraria flower** is extremely valuable for reducing alcohol cravings and relieving alcohol poisoning, treating nausea, vomiting, thirst and abdominal fullness. Ayurvedic medicine states it's a general tonic for health and long life.

☙ RASPBERRY

Rubus idaeus (Western); R. chingii (Chinese); Rosaceae
                                                    C, W
fu pen zi (R. chingii)

Part used: leaves, fruit

Energy, taste and Organs affected: leaves: cool; bitter; Spleen, Liver, Kidneys, reproductive organs; fruit: slightly warm; sweet, sour, astringent; Kidneys, Liver

Actions: stabilize and bind

Properties: leaves: hemostatic, astringent, mild alterative, uterine tonic in pregnancy, parturient; fruit: blood and nutritive tonic, refrigerant

Biochemical constituents: leaves: 1-2% organic acids of which 90% is citric acid, tannins, flavonoids, glycosides of kaempferol and quercitrin, pectins and sugar; fruit: citrus, malic, and salicylic acids; sugars, fragarin, vitamin C and niacin

Dose: leaves: 6-15 gms; infuse 1 Tbsp./cup water, drink 3 cups/day; take 2 "00" capsules 3 times/day; 10-60 drops tincture, 1-4 times/day; fruit: 9-15 gms, decoction

Precautions: fruit: Yin Deficiency with Heat signs; urinary difficulty

Other: The Chinese raspberry is yellowish green in color.

Indications: leaves: *childbirth, nausea, menstrual cramps, vaginal discharge;* fruit: *frequent urination, enuresis, spermatorrhea, premature ejaculation, wet dreams due to Deficient Kidney Yang, sore lower back, impotence and sterility due to Liver and Kidney Deficiency, premature graying of the hair, poor and blurry vision*

Uses: Raspberry leaves have long been used to strengthen and tonify uterine muscles for pregnancy and childbirth. Taken freely throughout the entire pregnancy (as tea or capsules), it definitely eases the process and pains of childbirth as well as relieves nausea and prevents hemorrhage, including postpartum. For the menstrual cycle, it eases cramps, and combined with other herbs such as **partridgeberry** and **uva ursi**, treats vaginal discharge and irregular and excessive menstruation. Like **blackberry** leaves, raspberry treats diarrhea and dysentery and is a general hemostatic for bleeding.

The Chinese use the yellowish-green **raspberry fruit** to astringe urine and semen, treating frequent urination, enuresis, spermatorrhea, premature ejaculation, wet dreams due to Deficient Kidney Yang, sore lower back, impotence and sterility due to Liver and Kidney Deficiency, premature graying of the hair and poor and blurry vision. Lab tests of the berries confirm estrogenic activity.

🦌 RED CLOVER

Trifolium pratense; Fabaceae   **A, W**
Sanskrit: *vana-methika*

Part used: flowers

Energy, taste and Organs affected: cool; sweet, salty; Liver, Heart, Lungs

Actions: clears Heat and toxins

Properties: alterative, antitumor

Biochemical constituents: coumarins, isoflavonoids (genistein, daidzein, biochanin, formononetin), flavonoids, resins, minerals, vitamins

Dose: 6-15 gms; infuse 1 Tbsp./cup water, drink 3 to 6 cups a day; 10-60 drops tincture, 3 times/day

Precautions: pregnancy; do not use if on blood thinner medication (and vice versa)

Indications: *non-healing sores, dry and scaly skin, eczema, psoriasis, fevers, arthritis, gout, cancer, tumors, hot flashes*

Uses: A good blood and lymphatic purifier and mild blood thinner, red clover's gentle action is beneficial for general and long-term consumption, including by children and the elderly. It clears skin conditions including non-healing sores, dry and scaly skin, eczema and psoriasis (use externally as fomentation, wash or poultice, and take internally). As well, it decongests the salivary glands and swollen, hard lymph nodes. Red clover also lowers fevers, heals inflammatory conditions such as arthritis and gout, and treats cancer and tumors (again, apply externally and take internally, frequently and in large amounts).

As a wonderful blood thinner (due to its coumarin content), it's too bad more people don't use this valuable herb rather than blood-thinning medications that cause side effects, such as tiredness. Further, it contains formononetin, a known phytoestrogen, and so has weak estrogenic activity that reduces hot flashes (in TCM this result is due to its Heat-clearing properties) and maintains bone health for many a grateful peri/menopausal woman.

🦌 REHMANNIA

Rehmannia glutinosa; Scrophulariaceae   **C**
shu di huang (prepared); sheng di huang (raw)

Part used: root of the Chinese foxglove

Energy, taste and Organs affected: prepared: slightly warm; sweet; Heart, Kidneys, Liver; raw: cold; sweet, bitter; Heart, Kidneys, Liver

Actions: prepared: tonify the Blood; raw: clears Heat and cools Blood

Properties: prepared: cardiotonic, diuretic, nutritive, demulcent; raw: antibacterial, antifungal, cardiotonic, diuretic

Biochemical constituents: prepared and raw: beta-sitosterol, mannitol, stigmansterol, campesterol, rehmannin, catalpol, arginine, glucose

Dose: prepared and raw: 9-30 gms, decoction; char to stop bleeding; give with **cardamom** or **citrus** to help counteract its heavy, cloying properties

Precautions: prepared and raw: caution in Deficient Spleen and/or Stomach, stagnant Qi, Phlegm; overuse can lead to abdominal distention and loose stools; raw: also do not use in pregnancy with anemia or Deficient Blood, or in those with Deficient Yang (coldness)

Other: It is prepared by stirring and steaming in red wine until both the inside and outside turn black and moist.

Indications: prepared: *pale face, palpitations, insomnia, irregular menstruation, infertility, uterine bleeding, postpartum bleeding, night sweats, nocturnal emissions, thirst, low back pain, ringing in the ears, dizziness, lightheadedness, diminished hearing, premature graying of hair;* raw: *high fever, thirst, hemorrhage, dry mouth, continuous low grade or afternoon fevers, constipation, throat pain, mouth and tongue sores, irritability, insomnia, malar flush*

Uses: Prepared rehmannia is one of the few herbs that tonifies Blood, Yin and Essence together. Its only drawback is a very dampening nature, causing difficult digestion with loose stools if taken to excess. Yet, rehmannia is extremely valuable in building Blood and alleviating symptoms of pale face, dizziness, palpitations and insomnia. As well, it treats gynecological problems such as irregular menstruation, infertility, uterine bleeding and postpartum bleeding and eases night sweats, nocturnal emissions and thirst.

Put in all Kidney-tonifying formulas, it strengthens bones and tendons, eases low back pain, ringing in the ears, dizziness, lightheadedness, diminished hearing and premature graying of hair, and is a tonic during pregnancy. **Raw rehmannia** clears Heat and cools the Blood, treating high fever, thirst, hemorrhage, dry mouth, continuous low grade or afternoon fevers, constipation, throat pain, mouth and tongue sores, irritability, insomnia and malar flush.

✤ REISHI

Ganoderma lucidum; Polyporaceae   C, W
ling zhi

Part used: whole mushroom

Energy, taste and Organs affected: slightly warm; sweet; Lungs, Heart, Spleen, Liver, Kidneys

Actions: tonify Qi

Properties: rejuvenative, antibacterial, antiviral, antitumor, immune tonic, antihypertensive, anticholesterol, antiinflammatory, antitussive, expectorant

Biochemical constituents: polysaccharides, triterpenes, sterols, adenosine, amino acids, albumin, protein (LZ-8), oleic acid, sulphur, essential oil, fat, saponin, ergosterol, enzymes, mannitol, vitamins

Dose: 3-15 gms; first break into small pieces (try using a hammer), then decoct 1 oz./quart water over low heat for 60 minutes, drink 1 cup 2-3 times/day; 40 drops tincture, 3 times/day

Precautions: Mold-sensitive individuals may have allergic reactions, yet I have usually seen reishi tonify their immune systems so they can handle it in lower doses and with meals.

Other: Its name means "Spirit Plant"; reishi is the Japanese name; it comes in many colors, but red is the most potent; several species grow in North America, such as *G. applanatum* and *G. oregonense*; many mushrooms are high in the polysaccharides that prevent and treat cancer, **shiitaki** among them, which is also a great herb for all liver diseases and is *antiviral, antitumor, anticancer, in-*

creases immunity, regulates blood pressure, reduces cholesterol, is high in B12, has all 8 essential amino acids and treats cancer, Candida, AIDS and frequent colds and flu.

Indications: *chronic fatigue, AIDS, cancer, tumors, heart disease, cholesterol, high blood pressure, allergies, bronchitis, asthma, dyspnea, pneumonia, rheumatism, insomnia, hepatitis, stress, liver diseases, weakness, dizziness*

Uses: Reishi mushroom, once a rare and secret plant revered by the ancient Taoists, was considered to be the elixir of life, even said to restore it, because of its amazing tonifying properties; no wonder it has been treasured more than gold! Entire books have been written about reishi alone (in fact, reishi is the first herb ever written about by the Chinese), and it's painted into numerous Chinese tapestries, paintings and the emperor's silk robes as a symbol of longevity. Indeed, reishi is the supreme immune tonic for such disorders as chronic fatigue (CFS), food sensitivities and AIDS, as it induces interferon production and raises the T cell levels (an index of AIDS and immune disorders). I have frequently treated people with extreme food sensitivities, some who could only eat eight foods, and they always improved with reishi and **astragalus**.

As well, reishi inhibits bacteria and viruses, treats and prevents cancer and tumors (officially listed as such by the Japanese government) and its adaptogenic quality protects the body against stress. It tonifies Blood along with Qi and is a bone marrow tonic. It also alleviates pain and relieves heart disease, reduces cholesterol and triglycerides, inhibits platelet aggregation, lowers high blood pressure and specifically nourishes the Spirit, treating anxiety, insomnia, nervousness arrhythmia and palpitations.

Calming and revitalizing at the same time, reishi increases inner stamina and strength. Strengthening to the Lungs, it relieves allergies (inhibits histamine release) and treats chronic bronchitis, asthma, dyspnea, chronic pneumonia and rheumatism. As well, reishi regenerates and protects the liver and decreases fatty accumulation there, treating hepatic necrosis, hepatitis and other liver diseases.

An anti-oxidant against free radicals, it protects against the effects of radiation and oxygenates the blood, helping against altitude sickness. Reishi is safe to take on a daily basis by most everyone and any time of year, and doing so is a great immune potentiator, preventing against colds and flu along with treating all the above conditions. An herb I give regularly, people often like the less bitter brown reishi rather than the stronger red variety.

🐾 RHUBARB

Rheum palmatum; Polygonaceae   **A, C**
da huang; Sanskrit: *amlavetasa*

Part used: root and rhizome

Energy, taste and Organs affected: cold; bitter; Heart, Large Intestine, Liver, Stomach

Actions: purgative

Properties: purgative, aperient, alterative, antibiotic, anthelmintic, vulnerary

Biochemical constituents: glycosides, tannic acids, gallic acid, catechin, tetrarin, glycogallin, cinnamic acid, rheosmin, fatty acids, calcium oxalate, glucose, fructose, sennoside A, B and C

Dose: 3-12 gms; decocting more than 10 minutes reduces its purgative effect; 20-60 drops tincture, 1-4 times/day; use raw as purgative, treat with wine or vinegar for blood invigoration; char to treat bleeding

Precautions: Deficient Qi or Blood, coldness, diarrhea, pregnancy, during menstruation, postpartum; contraindicated for nursing mothers; prolonged use weakens intestinal muscles, causing increased constipation and depletes potassium levels

Indications: *constipation, high fever, profuse sweating, abdominal distention and pain, delirium, jaundice, dysentery, painful urination, bleeding hemorrhoids, vomiting of blood, nosebleed with constipation, dysmenorrhea, amenorrhea, abdominal masses, swollen and painful eyes, hot skin lesions*

Uses: As this herb also invigorates stagnant Blood in the pelvic cavity, it is used for abdominal pain and masses, such as cysts and fibroids, dysmenorrhea and amenorrhea. Rhubarb is a great herb for constipation, but try simple remedies first, such as increasing dietary fiber and fluids while reducing meat and cheese.

❦ SAFFLOWER

Carthamus tinctorius; Asteraceae   **C, W**
hong hua

Part used: flower

Energy, taste and Organs affected: warm; acrid; Heart, Liver

Actions: invigorates Blood

Properties: circulatory stimulant, emmenagogue, lowers blood pressure, lowers cholesterol, analgesic, anodyne

Biochemical constituents: carthamin, carthamone, neocarthamin, palmitic acid, stearic acid, arachic acid, oleic acid, linoleic acid, linolenic acid

Dose: small dose: 0.9-1.5 gms; large dose: 3-9 gms; decoct for only 5 minutes in formulas, or steep 2 tsp./cup water; use raw to invigorate Blood; prepare with wine to break up Blood stagnation; with water to tonify Blood

Precautions: avoid during pregnancy; do not take during excessive menstrual bleeding; use with caution if taking anticoagulant medications

Other: In large doses this herb dispels stagnant Blood while in small doses it more gently moves the Blood.

Indications: *menstrual pain, delayed menses, blood clots, lower abdominal pains, amenorrhea, postpartum dizziness, abdominal masses (fibroids, cysts), nonsuppurative sores, carbuncles, the incomplete expression of rashes and measles, poor blood circulation, chest pain due to blood stagnation, traumatic injuries, enlarged liver and spleen, stops wound bleeding*

Uses: When Blood stagnates, it causes sharp, stabbing pains that can occur anywhere in the body. Safflower, similar to **calendula**, is a stronger blood-moving herb for breaking blood stagnation and alleviating this type of pain. It is particularly used for menstrual pain (dysmenorrhea), delayed menses, blood clots, lower abdominal pains, amenorrhea, postpartum dizziness and abdominal masses (fibroids, cysts). Further, it treats nonsuppurative sores, carbuncles and the incomplete expression of rashes and measles. It also improves poor blood circulation, alleviates chest pain due to stagnant Blood and treats traumatic injuries, stopping any pain, bleeding or swelling. As well, it treats an enlarged liver and spleen and may be used both internally and externally for this.

❦ SALVIA

Salvia miltiorrhiza; Laminaceae   **C**
dan shen

Part used: root

Energy, taste and Organs affected: slightly cold; bitter; Heart, Liver, Pericardium

Actions: invigorates Blood

Properties: vasodilator, anticoagulant, emmenagogue, sedative

Biochemical constituents: tanshinone I, IIA, IIB, cryptotanshinone, isotanshinone I, II, isocryptotanshinone, miltirone, tanshinol I, II, salviol, vitamin E

Dose: 6-15 gms; decoct 2 tsp./cup; fry in wine to enhance blood-moving properties; according to Bensky and Gamble in *Chinese Herbal Medicine Materia Medica*, do not use this herb long term in tincture form, as it can lead to pruritius, stomachache or reduced appetite

Precautions: pregnancy; when there is no blood stasis, patients who are taking anticoagulant medications, such as Warfarin, unless under direction of a qualified health-care practitioner

Other: *S. officinalis,* or **sage** leaf, is used to treat colds, flu, diarrhea, gum ulcers, sore throat, excessive perspiration and bacterial, strep and staph infections. Its smoke is used as *smudge* to purify by the Native Americans (another way of using its antibacterial properties).

Indications: *blood clots, angina pectoris, coronary heart*

disease, chest or epigastric pain, soreness in the ribs, palpitations, irritability, insomnia, painful menstruation, amenorrhea, endometriosis, abdominal masses, fibroids, cysts

Uses: Salvia, or red sage root, is one of the premier herbs for most all heart conditions, moving the blood, breaking up congestion and clots and regulating cholesterol and triglycerides. Because it is a cooling herb that moves Blood circulation (most are warming), it is extremely useful for a wide variety of blood stasis complaints in those with Excess Heat (such as inflammations) as well as those with Deficient Yin. It is especially applicable for angina pectoris, coronary heart disease, chest or epigastric pain (this is usually a sharp, stabbing type of pain), soreness in the ribs, palpitations, and menstrual pain.

In our Western culture where heart disease is a rampant killer, salvia is an important herb for preventing heart attacks and other heart ailments. I have seen it successfully relieve intense chest pains and prevent their return. Salvia's Heat-clearing ability also soothes irritability and treats insomnia. As well, it treats painful menstruation, amenorrhea, endometriosis and abdominal masses, such as fibroids and cysts. It is an important herb that is easily cultivated in certain areas of North America.

🦂 SARSAPARILLA

Smilax medica; S. officinalis, S. glabra and other spp.; Liliaceae
C, W

tu fu ling (S. glabra)

Part used: root

Energy, taste and Organs affected: cool; sweet, spicy; Liver, Stomach, Kidneys

Actions: clears Heat and toxins

Properties: alterative, antiinflammatory, antipruritic, diaphoretic

Biochemical constituents: saponins, parillin, sarsaponin, glycosides, sitosterol, stigmasterin, essential oil, resin, sugar, fat

Dose: 6-15 gms; decoct 1-2 tsp./cup water, drink 3

cups/day; 2-4 "00" capsules, 3 times/day; 10-40 drops tincture, 1-4 times/day

Precautions: pregnancy

Other: A traditional ingredient in root beers and soft drinks (smell it and you'll see why).

Indications: *skin diseases, herpes, psoriasis, arthritis, rheumatism, gout, venereal diseases, nervous disorders, epilepsy; S. glabra: joint pain, painful urination, jaundice, skin conditions*

Uses: Sarsaparilla is an excellent blood purifier, useful for skin disorders caused by blood impurities, acne, herpes, skin parasites, psoriasis, gout and rheumatism (use as tea or apply as wash or fomentation). Excellent for chronic liver disorders, it treats leukorrhea and venereal diseases such as gonorrhea and syphilis (for which it was introduced into Britain in the 17th century). It combines well with other alteratives, especially **yellow dock**, **sassafras**, **burdock** root and seed, **dandelion** and **red clover**. A hot decoction promotes profuse sweating, relieving colds, flu, fevers and mucus congestion, and powerfully expels gas from the stomach and intestines. The Chinese use *S. glabra* to treat joint pain, painful urination, jaundice due to Damp Heat and skin conditions from Damp Heat.

🦂 SASSAFRAS

Sassafras albidum, S. varifolium, S. officinale; Lauraceae **W**

Part used: root and root bark

Energy, taste and Organs affected: warm; spicy; Lungs, Kidneys

Actions: warms and releases the Exterior

Properties: alterative, diaphoretic, diuretic, carminative, antirheumatic

Biochemical constituents: essential oil, safrole, resin, tannin, alkaloids

Dose: 3-9 gms, decoct only 10 minutes; 10-30 drops tincture, 1-4 times/day

Precautions: while safrole itself may be toxic, when the whole herb is used it is quite safe

Indications: *acne, skin eruptions, eczema, psoriasis, poison oak, arthritis, rheumatism, colds, flu*

Uses: The original ingredient giving root beer its characteristic flavor, sassafras is a wonderful blood purifier natively used by rural folks in Southwest North America (Appalachia and the Ozarks). It clears most skin conditions, including acne, eczema, psoriasis and poison oak (internally and externally), and is normally combined with **sarsaparilla**, **dandelion**, **red clover**, **burdock** root and seed and **yellow dock** for these (many teens come to me for this formula with clear, smiling faces). It also effectively treats arthritic and rheumatic complaints, pains, ulcers, colds and flu.

🦎 SAW PALMETTO

Serenoa repens: Arecaceae　　　　　　　　　**W**

Part used: fruit

Energy, taste and Organs affected: warm; sweet, spicy; Kidneys, Spleen, Liver

Actions: tonify Yang (and Yin)

Properties: diuretic, expectorant, roborant, sedative, aphrodisiac, endocrine agent

Biochemical constituents: essential oil, fatty acids, carotene, polysaccharides, tannin, sitosterol, butyric acid, invert sugar, estrogenic substance

Dose: 3-12 gms; decoct 1-2 tsp./cup water; 2-4 capsules, 3 times/day; 10-60 drops tincture, 1-4 times/day

Precautions: pregnancy

Indications: *enlarged and debilitated prostate, low sex drive, impotence, frigidity, urinary tract infections, urethritis, interstitial cystitis, polycystic ovaries, helps weight gain, underdeveloped breasts, wasting of sexual organs, chronic cough*

Uses: Well known as a male reproductive tract tonic, saw palmetto is generally used to relieve prostate complaints, such as enlarged prostate, benign prostatic hyperplasia (BPH) and debilitated prostate (combine with **damiana** and **echinacea** for prostate complaints). Yet, it also tonifies Kidney Yang and to a lesser extent, Kidney Yin (the Kidneys rule the reproductive organs, thus the prostate connection). Saw palmetto also increases sex drive, alleviating impotence, frigidity and atony of the sexual organs, clears urinary tract infections and treats urethritis, interstitial cystitis, polycystic ovaries and chronic cough. As well, it normalizes weight and reputably enlarges breast size.

🦎 SCHISANDRA

Schisandra chinensis; Magnoliaceae　　　　　**C**
wu wei zi

Part used: seed

Energy, taste and Organs affected: warm; sour; Heart, Kidneys, Lungs

Actions: stabilize and bind

Properties: astringent, adaptogen, antitussive, expectorant, hepatoprotective, antioxidant

Biochemical constituents: sesquicarene, beta-bisabolene and chamigrene, alpha-ylangene, schizandrin, deoxyschizandrin, schizandrol, citral, stigmasterol, vitamins C and E

Dose: 1.5-9 gms; use 1.5-3 gms for chronic cough and 6-9 gms as a tonic; crush before using; decoct 1 tsp./cup water; 10-50 drops tincture, 1-4 times/day

Precautions: during colds, flu or fevers, Excess Heat; early stages of rash or coughs; may occasionally cause heartburn

Other: It contains all five tastes; this herb is sometimes spelled **schizandra**.

Indications: *chronic cough, wheezing, lung weakness, asthma, night sweats, excessive sweating, involuntary sweating, prolonged diarrhea, "daybreak" diarrhea, frequent urination, spermatorrhea, nocturnal emission, leukorrhea, nerve weakness, forgetfulness, insomnia, dream-disturbed sleep, elevated liver enzymes, hepatitis, stress*

Uses: Because this small, dark red berry has all five flavors (thus part of its Chinese name, *wu*, meaning five), it balances all bodily systems. As a tonic astringent, schisandra strengthens tissues, eliminates secretions and retains energy, Essence and leakages (good for all of you exhausted folks in physical and mental burnout). Thus, it treats chronic cough, wheezing, lung weakness, asthma, night sweats, excessive sweating (especially accompanied by thirst and a dry throat), involuntary sweating, prolonged diarrhea, "daybreak" diarrhea (early morning when the cock crows), frequent urination, spermatorrhea, nocturnal emission, leukorrhea and "nerve weakness" (neurasthenia—meaning weakness, fatigue and pallor).

As a calming herb, schisandra alleviates agitation, scatteredness, forgetfulness, insomnia and dream-disturbed sleep. It also protects and strengthens the liver and lowers elevated liver enzymes, useful in hepatitis and other liver ailments. Schisandra contains mild adaptogens that regulate various body functions, increase the ability to handle stress and relieve allergic skin disorders. It also regulates blood sugar, helps in the digestion of fats and treats acne and skin problems.

℞ SCUTE

Scutellaria baicalensis; Laminaceae   **C, W**
huang qin

Part used: root

Energy, taste and Organs affected: cold; bitter; Gallbladder, Large Intestine, Lungs, Stomach

Actions: clears Heat, dries Dampness

Properties: antiinflammatory, cholagogue, antihypertensive, expectorant, antipyretic, antibacterial, antispasmodic

Biochemical constituents: baicalein, baicalin, wogonin, wogonoside, neobaicalein, oroxylin aglueuronide, camphesterol, beta-sitosterol, benzoic acid

Dose: 6-15 gms, decoction; dry-fry to reduce cooling properties and to treat Heat in the lower abdomen and a restless fetus; wine-fry to treat the upper part of the body; char to enhance hemostatic properties

Precautions: Heat from Deficiency in the Lungs, Coldness; restless fetus due to Cold in the Blood; do not use with **moutan** or **veratri**

Other: Clears Heat, especially in the upper body; this is **Chinese skullcap**; for Western skullcap, see **Skullcap**.

Indications: *high fever, irritability, thirst, cough with thick, yellow mucus, hot sores and swellings, diarrhea, dysentery, bladder infections, jaundice, vomiting or coughing of blood, nosebleed, restless fetus, headache, red eyes, flushed face, hypertension*

Uses: A major herb in Chinese medicine, scute clears Heat, particularly in the upper body, treating high fever, irritability, thirst, cough with thick, yellow mucus, hot sores and swellings. Yet, it also clears Damp Heat from the Stomach and Intestine with diarrhea or dysentery with fever and a stifling sensation in the chest and thirst but inability to drink. As well, it treats bladder infections, jaundice, vomiting or coughing of blood, nosebleed, restless fetus, headache, red eyes, flushed face and a bitter taste in the mouth.

℞ SHEPHERD'S PURSE

Capsella bursa-pastoris; Brassicaceae   **C, W**
ji cai

Part used: above ground portions

Energy, taste and Organs affected: neutral; spicy, sweet; Liver, Stomach, Uterus

Actions: stops bleeding

Properties: hemostatic, antihemorrhagic, diuretic, urinary antiseptic, antipyretic, antihypertensive

Biochemical constituents: flavonoids, luteolin-7-rutinoside, quercitin-3-rutinoside, plant amino acids, choline, tyramine, diosmin, acetylcholine

Dose: 5-15 gms; infuse 1 Tblsp./cup water of fresh herb, drink 3 cups/day; 1 dropperful of tincture (only made from the fresh herb) every hour or two to stop bleeding; 20-60 drops, 1-4 times/day

Precautions: pregnancy

Other: This herb needs to be used fresh, or tinctured fresh.

Indications: *hemorrhaging, bladder infection, difficult urination, internal or external functional (rather than*

traumatic) bleeding, nosebleed, bleeding hemorrhoids, hypertension

Uses: Shepherd's purse is one of the most effective herbs to stop bleeding, including hemorrhaging of the stomach, intestines, lungs, uterus and other internal bleeding. It may also be used for excessive menstrual, postpartum and fibroid bleeding as it strengthens the uterus, thus helping it contract and stop bleeding. The tincture is a quick-acting and effective way to take the herb, although I think the charred herb would be more effective (charred herbs are more astringent and stop bleeding). Apply topically as a poultice to stop nosebleeds or bleeding hemorrhoids. A diuretic, too, it treats genito-urinary problems, bladder infection bleeding and difficult urination. The Chinese use this herb similarly, as well as for hypertension

❧ SIBERIAN GINSENG (ELEUTHRO)

Eleutherococcus senticosus; Araliaceae   **W**

Part used: root bark

Energy, taste and Organs affected: warm; sweet, acrid; Kidneys, Adrenals, Spleen

Actions: tonify Qi

Properties: adaptogenic energy tonic, antirheumatic, antispasmodic

Biochemical constituents: eleutherosides, polysaccarides, essential oil, resin, starch, vitamin A

Dose: 3-15 gms; for athletes to increase stamina, take 10-20 gms/day; decoct 1-2 tsp./cup water, drink 3 cups/day; 20-60 drops tincture, 1-4 times/day

Precautions: enhances action of antibiotics and effects of hexobarbital

Other: Commonly known as Siberian ginseng, this herb must now be legally called **eleuthro** (this name change was slipped through an agricultural bill in Wisconsin in late 2002) because eleuthro is not in the Panax ginseng family.

Indications: *low energy, vitality and endurance, chronic fatigue, exhaustion, weakness*

Uses: Eleuthro (Siberian ginseng) increases energy, vi-

tality, concentration and endurance and helps the body better withstand stress. In fact, tests on factory workers and athletes resulted in better workload capacities, faster running times and quicker recovery rates after exertion. Used year round, particularly to boost Kidney energy, it is an adrenal tonic that treats chronic fatigue, exhaustion and weakness, especially from over work or over exertion. Because it increases bone marrow activity (which then increases white blood cell production), it's useful during chemotherapy (take with **astragalus**).

❧ SKULLCAP

Scutellaria lateriflora; Laminaceae   **W**

Part used: above ground portion

Energy, taste and Organs affected: cool; bitter; Liver, Heart, Gallbladder, Large Intestine

Actions: calms the Spirit

Properties: nervine, antispasmodic, sedative, hypotensive

Biochemical constituents: volatile oil, scutellarin, bitter glycoside, tannin, fat, bitter principles, sugar

Dose: 3-9 gms; infuse 1 tsp-1 Tbsp./cup water, drink 3 cups a day; 2 "00" caps 3 times/day or 4 before bed; 20-40 drops tincture, 1-4 times/day

Precautions: much of what is sold as skullcap is actually **germander** (*Teucrium*); be sure to ask for the genuine herb

Other: Also spelled **scullcap**.

Indications: *restlessness, insomnia, anxiety, nervous conditions, debility and tension, excitability, hysteria, convulsions, epilepsy, nervous twitching and spasms, hypertension, nervous headache, PMS tension, neuralgia, addictions, drug and alcoholic withdrawal symptoms*

Uses: As a nervine high in calcium, potassium and magnesium, skullcap strengthens and quiets the entire nervous system, clearing restlessness, irritability of the nervous system and insomnia, especially restless sleep, in those with Excess or Deficient Heat. It also gives immediate relief in all chronic and acute nervous conditions and debility including nervous tension and anxiety with muscle spasms, twitching or tremors, worry, nervous fear, excitability, hysteria, convulsions, epilepsy, hypertension, nervous headache, PMS tension, neuralgia and nervous exhaustion and weakness (for those with nervous conditions from coldness, **valerian** is a better choice).

Skullcap is one of the best herbs to break addictions and ease drug and alcoholic withdrawal symptoms (take in half-cupful doses every hour or two, tapering off as symptoms subside). It can be combined with other nervines or antispasmodics, such as **passion-flower** or valerian, for a broader action. With **chamomile** it is a safe daily nervine.

Skullcap is a good brain tonic, calming the mind and aiding meditation (interestingly, its flower looks like a helmet that protects the skull). It also reduces hot emotions like anger, hatred, jealousy and irritability, as well as decreases excessive desires, promoting clarity, detachment and calm awareness. Chinese medicine uses *S. baicalensis* (**scutellaria**—see **Scute**) for headaches, irritability, red eyes, a bitter taste in the mouth, thirst and to calm a fetus restless from Heat.

☙ SLIPPERY ELM

Ulmus fulva; Ulmaceae • **W**

Part used: inner bark of tree

Energy, taste and Organs affected: neutral; sweet; Lungs, Stomach

Actions: tonify Yin

Properties: demulcent, nutritive tonic, expectorant, emollient, vulnerary

Biochemical constituents: proteins, mucins, amino acids, iodine, bromine, manganese salts

Dose: 9-30 gms of powder; decoct 1 tsp. cut root/cup water or 1 Tbsp. powder/cup cool water (then heat); 2 "00" capsules, 3 times/day

Precautions: pregnancy, Dampness

Other: As this tree is now endangered, *only use the cultivated herb*.

Indications: *indigestion, nausea, ulcers, colitis, sore throat, cough, bronchitis, lung bleeding, hyperacidity, sores, wounds, burns, tumors, boils, rash*

Uses: Slippery Elm is a highly nutritive and soothing food useful for digestive difficulties, stomach and intestinal ulcers, colitis, wasting diseases, sore and dry throats, coughs, bleeding from the lungs and bronchitis. It is also relieves inflammation of the respiratory and urinary tracts and of the mouth, throat, stomach, intestines and urethra. It is the same high content of mucilage that makes slippery elm soothing for skin disorders.

A paste (made by mixing the powder in cool water) may be applied to suppurating sores, bed sores, wounds, gangrene, burns, ulcers, tumors, boils, damaged tissues and inflamed and infected areas. Sprinkling the powder on my baby's diaper rash cured it and prevented further outbreaks. It also works well for skin disorders when combined with **echinacea**, **goldenseal**, **comfrey** and **marshmallow** root powders. Bandage in place and change dressing at least once daily.

Slippery elm may be taken in tea or capsule form, or made into gruel by slowly mixing cool water into powdered herb until a thick porridge consistency is achieved, then heating. Flavored with a little honey or a dash of **cinnamon** or **ginger**, this gruel is excellent to take for convalescence and when there is difficulty in keeping food down, even in infants. I have seen those who continuously throw up all food be able to eat and digest this gruel, which settles the stomach and gives much needed nutrition. It may also be decocted in milk as a nutritive tonic, for weight gain and to treat ulcers and hyperacidity. Supplement its tonic properties by preparing it with a tea of **ginseng** instead of water, a better choice for those with any Deficiencies.

☙ ST. JOHN'S WORT

Hypericum perforatum; Hypericaceae **W**

Part used: above ground portions; unopened flower bud is best

Energy, taste and Organs affected: cool; bitter, astringent; Liver

Actions: clear Heat, clean toxins

Properties: sedative, anti-inflammatory, astringent, antidepressant, antiviral

Active constituents: hypericin (which gives the tincture its beautiful red color), pseudohypericin, hyperforin, adhyperforin, essential oil, flavonoids such as quercitrin, amentoflavone, hyperin and xanthones

Dose: infuse 1-2 tsp./cup of water, drink 1-2 cups regularly morning and night; 2"00" capsules, 3 times/day; 1 tsp. oil, 2-3 times daily; 10-60 drops tincture, 1-4 times/day; homeopathic: 1-3 pellets, 3 times daily

Precautions: avoid in pregnancy, if using MAO-inhibitors, protease inhibitors (used for HIV and AIDS), or cyclosporine, theophylline, warfarin, digoxin, or if having anesthesia (must be off herb for five days before undergoing surgery)[5]; use cautiously in anxiety, or when taking pharmaceutical drugs (because it may lower their effects); it can create sun sensitivity and burning in fair-skinned people when taken internally for prolonged periods

Indications: *depression, nervous conditions, nervousness, nervous irritability, nervous tension, chronic tension headaches, menopausal tension, insomnia from restlessness, nerve pains, trigeminal neuralgia, sciatica, surgical trauma, rheumatism, wounds, burns, ulcers, skin irritations*

Uses: St. John's wort owes its name to the fact that it begins to flower around St. John's tide, the summer solstice. This pretty yellow flowering plant has several beneficial uses, the best known of which is the effective treatment of mild to moderate depression with few side effects (particularly when feeling isolated or disconnected), elevating the mood and increasing one's ability to cope. (It's extremely popular for this in Germany where physicians routinely prescribe herbal medicines.) This is because antidepressants are MAO-inhibitors and St. John's wort acts as one, blocking absorption of serotonin by post-synaptic receptors.

Interestingly, MAO-inhibitors prevent the liver from breaking down toxins, which means it then has a difficult time metabolizing cheese, nuts and alcohol. These very same foods (along with caffeine and fats) cause stagnant Liver Qi in TCM, which results in depression. I have found St. John's wort to work well for depression in those with Liver Heat, but not for depression caused by stagnant Liver Qi, and I've even seen it aggravate Candida symptoms in some.

Traditionally, St. John's wort is used to treat nervous conditions including nervousness, nervous irritability, nervous tension, chronic tension headaches, menopausal tension and insomnia from restlessness (it needs be taken several weeks to treat insomnia). It also effectively relieves any nerve pains such as neuralgia, trigeminal neuralgia, sciatica, surgical trauma, rheumatism, hemorrhoid pain and chronic pain with nervous exhaustion, and is a specific for treating diseases that directly affect the spine (homeopathic St. John's wort, called *Hypericum*, is specific for all types of nerve pain). St. John's wort is also one of the best wound-healing herbs. Take internally and/or apply externally for wounds, burns, ulcers, skin irritations and herpes sores (it is antiviral as well). As well, St. John's wort is a wonderful antiviral herb used for HIV and other viral conditions.

THYME

Thymus vulgaris; Laminaceae **W**

Part used: leaves and flowers

Energy, taste and Organs affected: warm; spicy; Lungs, Liver, Stomach

Actions: warms and clears Phlegm and stops coughing

Properties: expectorant, antitussive, carminative, antiseptic, spasmolytic, bronchodilator, antibacterial, antifungal, vermifuge

Biochemical constituents: essential oil with thymol, cavacrol, cymol, linalool, borneol, bitter principle, tannin, flavonoids, triterpenic acids

Dose: infuse 1 tsp./cup water; 10-30 drops tincture, 1-4 times/day

Precautions: none noted

Other: This is the garden, or common, thyme found in your kitchen.

[5] Tillotson, *The One Earth Herbal Sourcebook*, Kensington Publishing Group, 2001.

Indications: *acute and chronic respiratory problems, coughs, colds, gas, indigestion, diarrhea, whooping cough, bronchitis, spasmodic respiratory and urinary tract conditions, urinary tract infections*

🏵 TIENQI

Panax notoginseng, P. pseudoginseng; Araliaceae   C
san qi

Part used: root

Energy, taste and Organs affected: warm; sweet, slightly bitter; Liver, Stomach, Large Intestine

Actions: stops bleeding

Properties: hemostatic, cardiac tonic

Biochemical constituents: arasaponin A, arasaponin B, dencichine

Dose: 1-3 gms powder; 3-9 gms whole root, decoction; apply topically as needed

Precautions: pregnancy; Deficient Blood or Yin

Other: Also known as **pseudoginseng, notoginseng, tienchi, tien qi** and **tian qi**.

Indications: *internal and external bleeding, nosebleed, blood in urine, vomit, mucus or stool, traumatic injury due to falls, fractures, contusions and sprains, chest and abdominal pain, angina, coronary heart diseases, joint pain, hemorrhage, injuries, wounds, excessive menstruation, diabetic retinopathy*

Uses: Because of its ginseng-like energy, strengthening qualities, tienqi is called a "pseudo ginseng," yet this herb's special ability is to move stagnant Blood while stopping bleeding at the same time. It alleviates blood in vomit, urine or stool, nosebleeds, hemorrhaging, and internal and external bleeding with traumas, injuries, wounds and cuts (for this reason it is used extensively by martial artists). As well, it reduces swelling, alleviates pain and dissolves blood clots. I have seen it dissolve large blood clots and slow excessive menstrual bleeding and hemorrhage (high doses are needed for both).

In fact, tienqi should be used for any trauma from falls, fractures, contusions, or sprains since it quickly promotes blood circulation and stops bleeding. For these, it can be taken internally and externally placed on the wound in powder or liniment form. It is called *Yunan Bai Yao* (Formula #201) in its patent form, used to stop bleeding, including that from gunshot wounds. It may also be used for chest, abdominal and joint pain, excessive menstrual bleeding due to stagnant Blood and diabetic retinopathy. As well, it lowers blood pressure and increases coronary artery flow. Because of its tonic circulatory properties, it is one of the most popular of all herbs used by the Chinese.

🏵 TRIPHALA

Triphala is comprised of: A
Amla (Sanskrit)—*Emblica offincinalis;* **Indian Gooseberry** (Family: *Euphorbiacea*)
Haritaki (Sanskrit)—*Terminalia chebula;* Chinese: **he zi** (Family: *Combretaceae*)
Vibhitaki (**Bhibitaki**) (Sanskrit)—*Terminalia belerica* (Family: *Combretaceae*)

Part used: fruits

Energy, taste and Organs affected:
Amla: cool; sour, sweet, astringent; Heart, Lungs
Haritaki: hot (warm to Chinese); sweet, sour, astringent; bitter, spicy; Large Intestine, Heart, Liver, Kidneys
Vibhitaki: warm; sour, astringent; Lungs, Large Intestine

Actions: mild tonic laxative

Properties:
Amla: antioxidant, antitumor, anticholesterol
Haritaki: laxative, astringent, vermifuge, antimicrobial, antiviral, anticholesterol, antibacterial, adaptogenic
Vibhitaki: expectorant, antipyretic, anticholesterol, antifungal, antihistamine

Biochemical constituents:
Amla: vitamin C, bioflavonoids, tannin
Haritaki: anthraquinone glycoside, sennoside, tannins, ellagic and gallic acids, chebulinic acid, fixed oil, ethyl ester
Vibhitaki: tannins and other constituents

Dose: 2 gms powder, 2 times/day of each

Precautions: not for pregnancy

Other: Myrobalan refers to the use of these fruits in tanning; the Ayurvedic product, **gugglu**, is myrrh cooked in Triphala.

Indications for Triphala: *constipation, cough, asthma, bronchitis, intestinal problems, parasites, skin eruptions, ulcerous sores, herpes, wounds, inflamed eyes, blurry vision; promotes good health and longevity*

Uses: Amla, highly regarded as a heart tonic used for longevity, fever, cough, asthma, anemia, hemorrhage and alcoholism, it is not only a part of Triphala, but also forms about 80% of the Ayurvedic preparation, *Chyavanaprasha*, an ancient tonic "jam" that tonifies Qi and Blood. **Haritaki**, the strongest of the three fruits, promotes health and longevity and is a mild laxative that aids digestion and treats chronic diarrhea, dysentery and cough. It is regarded as the "king of medicines" in Tibet, while the Chinese use it similarly and for intestinal problems, worms, parasites, prolapsed rectum, gas, leukorrhea, seminal emission and excessive perspiration. **Vibhitaki** treats constipation, fevers, nausea from Dampness, cough, bronchitis, asthma, allergies and general inflammation. It also promotes hair growth and the fresh fruit pulp is applied to nontraumatic corneal ulcers.

In **Triphala**, these three fruits act together to balance *Vata* (Haritaki), *Pitta* (Amla) and *Kapha* (Vibhitaki). Triphala is so reliable and balanced that the common aphorism among Ayurvedic practitioners is, "when in doubt, use Triphala (Formula #97)." A mild, gentle and non-habit-forming laxative, Triphala is particularly beneficial for those with Deficiencies or for the elderly. It is taken as a weekly cleanser in India, usually at night, to purify the bowels, promote digestion, good health and longevity, protect the liver, and for its antioxidant, nutritive and antimicrobial properties. To increase its laxative action, combine with an equal part of **rhubarb**. As well, Triphala clears skin eruptions, ulcerous sores, herpes (as a wash) and may be applied topically to wounds. It is also used as eyewash for inflamed eyes and blurry vision.

🐉 TURMERIC

Curcuma longa; Zingiberaceae   **A, C, W**
Tuber: *yu jin*; Sanskrit: *haridra*; rhizome: *jiang huang*

Part used: tuber and rhizome

Energy, taste and Organs affected: tuber: cool; spicy, bitter; Heart, Lungs, Liver; rhizome: warm; spicy, bitter; Spleen, Stomach, Liver

Actions: invigorates Blood (and Qi)

Properties: emmenagogue, analgesic, cholagogue, antibacterial, antifungal, antiinflammatory

Biochemical constituents: tuber: camphor, curcumin, demethoxycurcumin, bisdemethoxycurcumin, turmerone, carvone; rhizome: turmerone, zingiberene, phellandrene, cineole, sabinene, borneol, curcumin, atiantane, glucose, fructose, arabinose

Dose: tuber: 4.5-9 gms; rhizome: 3-9 gms; decoct 1 Tblsp./cup water or use 3-9 gms, drink 3 cups a day; mix 1 tsp. per cup water, drink 2 cups a day; 10-40 drops, 1-4 times/day

Precautions: pregnancy, Deficient Blood or Yin, absence of stagnant Qi or Blood; tuber also: Deficient Yin from blood loss; do not use concentrated extract or oil in high doses, particularly if you have bile duct obstruction, gallstones, or stomach ulcers

Other: Often used as a dye, it gives the characteristic orange color to monks' robes.

Indications: tuber: *anxiety, agitation, seizures, mental derangement, hemorrhages, jaundice*, rhizome: *amenorrhea, dysmenorrhea, painful obstruction, shoulder pain, gastric or abdominal congestion and pain, gallstones, hepatitis wounds, bruises, traumas or injuries, toothache, hemorrhage, arthritis, cataracts, sports injuries*; both parts: *chest, abdominal, flank or menstrual pain and swelling from trauma*

Uses: Both the tuber and rhizome of turmeric stimulate blood circulation, yet because one is cool and the other warm, they have different uses. The **tuber** cools Blood, alleviating anxiety, agitation, seizures, mental derangement, hemorrhages and jaundice, and is applied topically to traumatic injuries and sores.

The **rhizome** (the spice used in Indian cooking) is antiinflammatory, antioxidant and purifies the blood and liver. It promotes menstruation, treating amenorrhea and dysmenorrhea due to Cold, and eases painful obstruction due to Wind and Dampness with stagnant Blood, particular for pain in the shoulders. Turmeric rhizome also strengthens digestion, improves intestinal flora, aids in digestion of protein, moves gastric or abdominal congestion and its related pain, and treats gas, colic and jaundice. It also detoxifies and decongests the Liver, dissolves gallstones, treats hepatitis and other liver issues, and may be combined with **barberry**, or **Oregon grape root** for releasing congestion in the Liver as effectively as Chinese **bupleurum**.

The blood-moving and antiinflammatory properties of turmeric make it useful for wounds, bruises and other traumas or injuries (including sports injuries), both externally and internally. As well, it is used for toothache, hemorrhage and arthritis, inhibits platelet aggregation and prevents cataracts. Both the **tuber and rhizome** move Qi along with Blood, treating chest, abdominal, flank or menstrual pain and swelling from trauma.

❀ USNEA

Usnea barbata; Usneaceae   **W**

Part used: whole plant (lichen growing on tree branches)

Energy, taste and Organs affected: cool; bitter; Lungs

Actions: clears Heat and toxins

Properties: antibiotic, antifungal, tuberculostatic, antibacterial, antispasmodic

Biochemical constituents: usnic acid, mucilage

Dose: 20-60 drops tincture, 1-4 times/day; externally as needed

Precautions: Coldness; Deficient Yang

Other: Also known as **beard lichen**.

Indications: *fungal, viral, respiratory, urinary and bacterial infections*

❀ UVA URSI

Arctostaphylos uva ursi; Ericaceae   **W**

Part used: leaves

Energy, taste and Organs affected: cool; bitter, astringent; Heart, Bladder, Small Intestine, Liver

Actions: drains Dampness

Properties: diuretic, urinary antiseptic, astringent

Biochemical constituents: arbutin, iridoids, flavonoids, oxytacin, tannins, volatile oil, ursolic, malic and gallic acids

Dose: 3-9 gms; infuse 1-2 tsp./cup water, drink cool, 3 cups a day; 10-60 drops tincture 1-4 times/day

Precautions: pregnancy; excessive use may cause nausea, vomiting, tinnitus and loss of consciousness

Other: Also known as **Bearberry**; Native Americans smoked it with tobacco and other herbs in the mixture called *Kinnikinnick.*

Indications: *bladder and kidney infections, stones, blood in the urine, postpartum hemorrhage and shrinking of uterus*

Uses: Uva ursi is a strong diuretic and urinary antiseptic useful for bladder and kidney infections, and when combined with **marshmallow** root, dissolves stones. It also strengthens and tones the urinary passages, clears blood in the urine, increases circulation in the kidneys and alkalinizes the pH of the urinary tract. Take cool to enhance its diuretic properties. The Native Americans used it after birthing to quickly shrink the uterus and to prevent infections. For this, both drink the tea and bathe in it. Alternatively, use the tincture to prevent postpartum hemorrhage and shrink the uterus as was done in many European hospitals.

❀ VALERIAN

Valeriana officinalis; Valerianaceae   **A, W**
Sanskrit: *tagara*

Part used: root

Energy, taste and Organs affected: warm; bitter, spicy; Liver, Heart

Actions: calms the Spirit

Properties: sedative, hypnotic, nervine, antispasmodic, carminative, stimulant, anodyne, hypotensive, anticonvulsant

Biochemical constituents: essential oil, valepotriates, alkaloids including actinidine and valerine, choline, flavonoids, sterols, tannins

Dose: 3-9 gms; infuse 1-2 tsp./cup water, drink 3 cups a day; 2 "00" caps, 3 times/day and 4 before bed; 1 tsp. tincture in 1/2 cup water taken as needed or 10-60 drops, 1-4 times/day

Precautions: it can cause insomnia in those with Heat conditions; potentiates action of barbituates

Other: It is best when used fresh, including tinctures from the fresh plant.

Indications: *pain, cramps, spasms, restlessness, anxiety, nervous disorders, nervous excitement, sleeplessness, palpitations, dizziness, menstrual cramps, neurasthenia, fainting, nervous headache, emotional disturbances, hysteria, hyperactivity, ADD, shingles*

Uses: Tranquilizing, calming and sedating, valerian is one of the best herbs for an individual with a Cold, nervous condition. It relieves pain, cramps, spasms and nervous disorders such as nervous excitement, restlessness, sleeplessness, anxiety, palpitations, dizziness, menstrual cramps, neurasthenia, fainting, nervous headache, emotional disturbances, hysteria, hyperactivity, ADD and shingles. Because it is heating, it can have an opposite effect on people with Heat conditions (this is a clear example of the need to choose herbs according to their energies rather than properties). For those with Heat conditions, **skullcap** is a better choice.

☙ VITEX

Vitex agnus-castus; *V. rotundifolia; V. trifolia; Verbenaceae man jing zi* **C, W**

Part used: berry

Energy, taste and Organs affected: cool; bitter, acrid; Liver, Spleen

Actions: regulates Qi (and Blood)

Properties: emmenagogue, vulnerary, galactogogue, amphoteric

Biochemical constituents: volatile oil, glycosides, castine (a bitter principle), flavonoids

Dose: 3-6 gms; infuse 1 tsp. crushed berry/cup water, drink 3 cups/day; 3-4 capsules or 20-75 drops to 1 tsp. tincture, 1-4 time/day, although taking it once/day in the morning on an empty stomach is usually sufficient; this herb should be taken long-term for optimum effects, 6 months or longer, although benefits may be felt after 10 days.

Precaution: pregnancy after the third month, as it could bring on the flow of milk too soon; it may counteract the effects of birth control pills and other hormone therapy

Other: Also known as **chaste tree berry**, the Chinese use *V. rotundifolia* or *V. trifolia* (*man jing zi*) for colds with migraines, cataracts, night blindness, arthritis and breast cancer.

Indications: *PMS, migraines, depression, cramps, edema in the legs, distended sensitive breasts, mood swings, endometriosis, herpes, infertility, dry vagina, hot flashes, dizziness, depression, amenorrhea, irregular menstruation, heavy bleeding, short menstrual cycle, withdrawal after the pill, fibroids, cysts, acne*

Uses: Vitex was frequently used as a symbol in Renaissance paintings to denote women's chastity, because at the time monks and nuns regularly took the chaste tree herb to curb sexual desires (one example of this is Titian's painting, "Venus of Urbino" in which the vitex, or chaste, tree stands outside the window). Before those times, it is said that ancient Greek and Roman priestesses also used it for the same thing. Now if you are a woman reading this, before you throw your vitex out the window or cross this plant off in your mind with a skull and crossbones, know that I have only met one woman who actually felt that vitex dampened her sex drive. In the meantime, all the many other women reported nothing but wonderful benefits from taking it.

In fact, vitex is a supreme female herb. It increases the lutenizing hormone that stimulates the release of progesterone, and inhibits FSH and prolactin[6] (prolactin inhibition is what lowers sex drive and, in men, also decreases sperm production). Thus, vitex regulates hormonal balance and the menstrual cycle, including normalizing estrogen along with progesterone. It treats PMS and its associated symptoms of migraines, depression, cramps, endometriosis, herpes, edema in the legs, distended sensitive breasts, acne and mood swings. I have seen it successfully clear severe PMS with intense food cravings and mood changes, but for this it must be used long-term, at least a year.

Vitex prepares the womb for implantation and when taken for many months, for infertility. It also alleviates problems associated with menopause such as dry vagina, hot flashes, dizziness and depression. As well, vitex treats amenorrhea, irregular menstruation, heavy bleeding or too short a menstrual cycle, fibroids, cysts and withdrawal after the pill (by regulating normal periods). It also treats acne in male and female teenagers. I have seen it work well for cysts and fibroids when taken in higher doses (1 tsp. tincture, 3 times/ day) along with **cotton root** and other Blood-moving herbs.

🦎 WALNUT
(Black Walnut; walnuts)

Juglans nigra, J. regia; Juglandaceae   **C, W**
hu tao ren (J. regia)

Part used: *J. nigra* (black walnut tree): fresh immature green hull, leaves, bark; *J. regia:* nuts

Energy, taste and Organs affected: leaves, bark and hull: cool; bitter; Large Intestine, skin; walnuts: warm; sweet; Kidneys, Large Intestine, Lungs

Actions: leaves, bark and hull: kills parasites; walnuts: Tonify Yang

Properties: leaves, bark and hull: antifungal, antiparasitic, antidysenteric; bark: mild laxative and alterative; walnuts: mild laxative, tonic

Biochemical constituents: juglandin, tannins; walnuts: fatty oil, linoleic acid, linolenic acid, oloeic acid, friglone, carotene, vitamin B2, protein

Dosage: leaves: infuse 2 tsp./cup water; bark and hull: decoct 1 tsp./cup water; hull: 1–10 drops tincture, 1–3 times daily; walnuts: 9–30 gms; peel skin off for constipation

Precautions: hull: local application in excess can cause irritation and blistering; internally, avoid in pregnancy or for extended periods of time; walnuts: yellow or red-tinged phlegm or cough due to Heat; Deficient Yin with Heat signs; watery stools; don't take with black tea

Other: Once considered a tree of life in France (like the olive tree in Italy), all parts of the tree were used. Today, NASA uses walnut shells to make thermal insulation for space craft and they're added to special sludges for leaks on oil rigs.

Indications: leaves, bark and hull: *athlete's foot, ring worm, fungal infections, Candida, pin or thread worms, tapeworm, Giardia, other parasites, skin diseases, eczema, herpes, psoriasis, hemorrhoids, constipation;* walnuts: *low back and knee pain, frequent urination, chronic cough, wheezing, constipation, increase body weight, urinary tract stones, dermatitis, eczema*

Uses: Black walnut **bark, leaves and hulls** are well known as antiparasitic, used to treat athlete's foot, ring worm, fungal infections such as Candida, pin or thread worms, tapeworm, Giardia and other parasites. For this to be successful, it is very important to take black walnut for ten days while eating a strict diet of brown rice and black, or Japanese adzuki, beans (raw garlic may be added). I have seen people take black walnut with dubious effects because they ignored the strict diet. Parasites can be difficult to get rid of naturally, yet it is possible and I have seen it work when black walnut is taken while fasting on brown rice for ten days. Black walnut also treats skin diseases such as eczema, herpes and psoriasis and for hemorrhoids and constipation. To treat Candida, eat a strict diet of animal protein, cooked vegetables and rice along with taking black walnut.

---

[6] Tilgnar, *Herbal Medicine from the Heart of the Earth*, Wise Acres Press, Inc. 1999.

The Chinese use **walnuts** to tonify Yang, strengthening the Kidneys and alleviating low back and knee pain and frequent urination. They also warm the Lungs and help the Kidneys to "pull down" Lung Qi, treating chronic cough or wheezing due to Deficient Lungs and Kidneys (this type of cough or wheezing is determined when it's harder to inhale than exhale, there's dribbling of urine upon sneezing, or there are accompanying symptoms of low back ache, frequent urination and/or nighttime urination).

Walnuts also act as a mild laxative, particularly in the elderly, anemic or those with Kidney Yang Deficiency. Constipation that doesn't respond to normal herbal laxatives in people who are tired, anemic, cold, have clear frequent urination, low back pain, low sex drive, lowered metabolism and/or edema of the legs usually responds to walnuts, since they lubricate the intestines and provide enough heat and energy to move the stools. Walnuts also increase body weight and dissolve stones in the urinary tract. In paste form and applied externally, they treat dermatitis and eczema.

❧ WILD CHERRY BARK

Prunus serotina; P. virginiana; Rosaceae   **A, W**
Sanskrit: *padmaka*

Part used: bark

Energy, taste and Organs affected: warm; spicy, astringent; Lungs, Spleen

Actions: stop coughing and wheezing

Properties: antitussive, expectorant, sedative, astringent, carminative

Biochemical constituents: hydrocyanic acid, isoamygdalin, amygdalin-like substance, gallic acid, prunasin, tannin

Dose: 3-9 gms; decoct in cool water as heat diminishes its cough-relieving properties; infuse 1 tsp./cup cool water, drink 3 cups a day; 2 "00" caps, 3 times/day; tincture, 10-15 drops, 1-4 times/day

Precautions: pregnancy; do not take in large doses or long term

Other: Also known as **chokecherry**.

Indications: *cough, asthma, nervous cough, whooping cough, chronic bronchitis, ulcers, gastritis, colitis, diarrhea, dysentery, irritated mucous membranes in respiratory, urinary and gastrointestinal tracts*

❧ WILD YAM

Dioscorea villosa (Western: American, Mexican);   **C, W**
D. opposita (Chinese); *Dioscoreace*
shan yao

Part used: root

Energy, taste and Organs affected: Western: warm; sweet, bitter; Liver, Gallbladder, Kidneys, Spleen; Chinese: neutral; sweet; Spleen, Lungs and Kidneys

Actions: Western: extinguish Internal Wind; Chinese: tonify Qi

Properties: Western: antispasmodic, antiinflammatory, cholagogue, diaphoretic, expectorant; Chinese: Qi tonic, nutritive, demulcent

Biochemical constituents: Western: steroidal saponins (mainly diosgenin); Chinese: starch, mannan allantoin, arginine, choline, diastases, saponin, mucilage, phytic acid, vitamin C

Dose: Western: 3–9 gms; decoct 1 tsp./cup water; 20–60 drops tincture, 1-4 times/day; Chinese: 9-30 gms, decoction; use raw to tonify the Yin; dry-fry to strengthen the Spleen

Precautions: Western: none noted; Chinese: Excess Heat, stagnation, Dampness

Other: Western: this herb forms the basis of the birth control pill and is now endangered in the wild, thus *only use cultivated western wild yam*; Chinese: Also called **mountain potato**, this delicious herb is eaten as a vegetable in both China and Japan. In those places menopausal symptoms are practically unknown along with fewer estrogen-sensitive tumors and cancers occurring.

Indications: Western: *PMS, mid-cycle spotting, painful menstrual cramps, morning sickness, endometriosis, spontaneous abortion, gall bladder pain and spasms, gallstones,* *arthritic and rheumatic pains, abdominal and intestinal cramps, gas, urinary pain;* Chinese: *diarrhea, fatigue, lack of strength, exhaustion, weakness, spontaneous sweating, lack of appetite, diarrhea, chronic dry cough or wheezing due to Lung weakness, spermatorrhea, nocturnal emission, leukorrhea, frequent urination, vaginal discharge, diabetes*

Uses: Western (American and Mexican): Wild yam is particularly noted these days for regulating female hormones (although it regulates low progesterone/high estrogen balance, recent research doesn't show that it binds to hormonal receptor sites)[7]. As such, it works fantastically well for a large array of hormonal issues: to lessen PMS symptoms, mid-cycle spotting, painful menstruation, morning sickness, breast and abdominal distension and pain, endometriosis and spontaneous abortion.

I remember one pregnant patient who tried everything to alleviate her morning sickness and nothing worked until she drank wild yam tea. The results were seemingly miraculous for her. Another patient I treated had a basketful of unrelated symptoms, even in TCM, and nothing helped her until she took wild yam. I know of a practitioner who gives it to most all her female patients and she says it has revolutionized her practice since it consistently helps them feel so much better. I also know some women who attempted a study using wild yam as a natural birth control herb. Yet, since it wasn't successful for all the women, don't try it yourself unless you're willing to get pregnant!

Traditionally, wild yam is used as a wonderful antispasmodic and cholagogue, treating spasms and pain of the gall bladder and gallstones, and other spasmodic or shooting, aching or shifting pains, including hip joint pain. For this, combine with **Oregon grape** or **barberry** root, **turmeric** root, **fringe tree** bark and **marshmallow** root. It also alleviates spasmodic, shooting and moving pains including menstrual cramps, arthritic and rheumatic pains, abdominal and intestinal cramps, gas and urinary pain.

Chinese: Usually called dioscorea by Chinese practitioners, this wild yam doesn't seem to have the phytoprogesterone activity of Western wild yam, although it hasn't really been tested for that use. Like other Spleen Qi tonics such as **ginseng, white atractylodes** and **astragalus**, dioscorea treats Spleen and Stomach Deficiency with symptoms of diarrhea, loose stools, fatigue, lack of strength, exhaustion, weakness, spontaneous sweating and lack of appetite.

Since Chinese wild yam is neutral in energy, it supports both the Yin and the Qi of the Lungs and Kidneys. Thus, it also treats chronic dry cough or wheezing and is most always included in Kidney tonic formulas to treat spermatorrhea, nocturnal emission, frequent urination, leukorrhea and vaginal discharge. It is also used for diabetes in daily doses of 250 mgs decocted as a tea. It is frequently combined with **astragalus**, **licorice**, **codonopsis**, **wild yam** and **ginseng** in tea or soup form and is quite bland to sweet-tasting when eaten. Whenever I make a Qi tonic formula or tonic herb soup, I always include this herb.

🎍 YARROW

Achillea millefolium; Asteraceae　　　　　　**A, W**
Sanskrit: *gandana*

Part used: above ground portions

Energy, taste and Organs affected: warm; bitter, spicy; Lungs, Liver

Actions: cools and releases the Exterior

Properties: diaphoretic, antiinflammatory, antipyretic, carminative, hemostatic, astringent, antispasmodic, stomachic, bitter tonic, antiseptic, antifungal, anodyne

Biochemical constituents: essential oil, cineol and pro-azulene, achilleine, achilletin, beta-iso-thujone, coumarins, chamazulene, apigenin, steroidal, beta- sitosterol

Dose: 3-9 gms; infuse 1 tsp./cup water, drink $1/2$ to 1 cup tea every hour or two until cold or fever breaks or bleeding stops; 10-30 drops tincture, 1-4 times/day

Precautions: pregnancy

Other: White or pink yarrow flowers are used medicinally while yellow is ornamental.

---

[7] Tilgnar, *Herbal Medicine from the Heart of the Earth*, Wise Acres Press, Inc. 1999.

Indications: *burns, cuts, bruises, hemorrhages, inflammations, wounds, hemorrhoids, leukorrhea, vaginal infections, bleeding piles, cramps, excess menstrual bleeding, internal hemorrhage, colds, flu, fevers, chicken pox, measles*

Uses: Yarrow has been used by many cultures and for thousands of years: the Chinese employed the stalks for divining the *I Ching*, an ancient Chinese book describing the laws of change and cycles; in Nordic countries yarrow substituted for hops in beer production; 16th century Germans used yarrow seeds as a preservative in wine barrels.

Its Latin name, *Achillea millefolium*, comes from the Greek hero, Achilles, who put yarrow directly on his soldier's wounds to stop them from bleeding. Achilles further recommended putting yarrow juice in the eye to take away redness. Europeans used it in dream pillows while reciting a poem to Venus, requesting a dream of one's future mate. The Native Americans used it for wounds too, and placed the rolled leaves in the nostrils to stop nosebleed. Interestingly, yarrow does contain a substance that hastens blood-clotting from injury, which explains its common name, *Nosebleed*.

Yarrow's astringent, antiseptic and hemostatic actions make it an invaluable remedy for healing burns, cuts, bruises, hemorrhages, excess menstrual bleeding, inflammations and other wounds, hemorrhoids and leukorrhea. It can be applied directly to wounds to stop bleeding and is used in a bolus or salve for vaginal infections and bleeding piles. Yarrow also causes sweating, relieving the first signs of colds, flu, fevers, chicken pox and measles (it helps eruptions come out faster). As well, it's a uterine astringent, protecting against uterine atony and treating cramps. One herbalist I know uses it for bleeding uterine fibroids in women 35 and over by having them sit in sitz baths of yarrow tea twice weekly, rubbing it on their abdomens and taking 2-3 dropperfuls tincture/day internally.

🦎 YELLOW DOCK

Rumex crispus; Polygonaceae   A, W
Sanskrit: *amla vetasa*

Part used: root

Energy, taste and Organs affected: cool; bitter, sweet; Liver, Large Intestine

Actions: clears Heat and toxins

Properties: cholagogue, alterative, mild laxative

Biochemical constituents: anthraquinone glycosides, rumicin, chrysarobin, tannins, oxalates

Dose: 3-9 gms; decoct 1 tsp./cup, drink $1/2$ cup, 2-3 times/day (its very bitter!); 1-2 "00" caps, 1-3 times/day; 10-40 drops tincture; 1 Tbsp. syrup, 2-3 times/day

Precautions: use cautiously if there's a history of oxalate kidney stones

Other: Also known as **broad leafed (or curly) dock**.

Indications: *skin diseases, eruptions, psoriasis, itching welts, eczema, anemia, jaundice, hepatitis, liver congestion, poor fat absorption, constipation. bleeding of wounds, hemorrhoids, swellings*

Uses: Yellow dock is an astringent blood purifier specific for acute and chronic skin diseases, including eruptions, psoriasis, itching welts and eczema. Because this herb helps the liver to use iron, it helps build Blood, but generally only when combined with a blood-nourishing agent, such as **lycii**, **longan** or **mulberries**, or blackstrap molasses (otherwise, its drying action depletes Blood). It may be used for anemia in this combination, even during pregnancy. Since yellow dock detoxifies the liver, it treats jaundice, hepatitis, liver congestion and poor fat absorption. As well, it stimulates bile secretion, causing a laxative action and relieving constipation without causing griping or pain. Externally, it is applied to stop bleeding of wounds, hemorrhoids and swellings.

PART II

Treating Illness

CHAPTER 5

Causes of Disease

F requently I am asked, "How did I get this problem?" or "I've always been well—why am I getting sick now?" These questions reflect the victim role we hold in the West: something happens to make us sick regardless of what we do. Rather, it is more useful to ask, "What factors in my life are causing illness? What am I doing to make myself sick?" as this more aptly addresses the real issue.

In TCM there are several categories encompassing the causes of disease: pathogenic factors (the Six Pernicious Influences of Wind, Cold, Heat, Damp, Dryness and Summer Heat), emotional issues (the Seven Emotions of Joy, Anger, Sadness, Grief, Pensiveness, Fear and Fright), lifestyle habits (diet, sexual activity, work and sleeping habits) and miscellaneous causes (inherited constitution, malnutrition, injuries, parasites and so on).

PERNICIOUS INFLUENCES

When wind, cold, heat, dampness or dryness penetrate the skin and enter your body, they cause illness. Called Pernicious Influences, there are six of these climactic factors: Wind, Cold, Heat, Damp, Dryness, and Summer Heat. Because we live and work in protected homes and artificial climates, we are less exposed to these influences today. When people lived nomadically, or in agri-

cultural tribes, they spent long hours, up to weeks and months at a time, exposed to the elements. Thus, invading External factors were a major cause of disease in the past while now, they usually invade after our bodies balances are upset from dietary indiscretions, overwork, insufficient rest, emotional extremes or inappropriate dress for weather changes.

The easiest way to understand Pernicious Influences is to think of their corresponding weather patterns. For instance, wind is fickle, moves things, changes direction and alternates intensity. Water is damp and heavy, sinks to low levels and creates sluggishness. Coldness contracts (like ice) and slows activity and movement. Heat circulates, activates and expands. Dryness evaporates moisture. Summer Heat scorches, rises and disperses. While this correlation between weather patterns and Pernicious Influences is metaphorical, it demonstrates how the microcosm in the body reflects the macrocosm in nature.

Illnesses from these External Pernicious Influences come on suddenly, acutely and are characterized by fever, chills, body aches, headaches, general tiredness and an aversion toward the particular Influence (such as fear of heat or cold, dislike of wind or dampness). While these Influences frequently attack through the back of the neck, they may also directly enter through the skin, mouth, nose, Organs, muscles or channels.

It is also possible for a Pernicious Influence to invade either singly or in combinations. Wind, Cold and Damp, or Wind, Heat and Damp frequently appear together. Likewise, Damp and Heat, or Heat and Dryness are typical mixtures. Further, it is possible for a Pernicious Influence to transform and change. For instance, pathogenic Cold can transform into Heat, Heat can change to Cold, and Summer Heat can consume Body Fluids (Yin), converting to Dryness.

When Pernicious Influences invade, they are called External Wind, External Heat and so on. Yet, these Influences may arise Internally, too, and when they do, they are termed Internal Wind (or just Wind), Internal Heat (or just Heat), and so on. (To better understand the following terms, see *The Energy of Illness*.)

Wind

Like wind in weather, pathogenic Wind creates movement, either Externally or Internally, and migrates through the body. It comes and goes, changes direction, location or intensity of symptoms, or periodically disappears altogether. Because Wind tends to rise, disperse and move upward and outward, it usually attacks the head, face, skin, muscles and Lungs, causing sudden onset of colds, chills, fever, stuffy nose, body aches and headache.

Of all Pathogenic Influences, Wind is the vehicle through which other climactic factors invade the body, readily creating combinations of Wind-Cold, Wind-Heat, Wind-Dryness and Wind-Damp. While generally associated with spring, External Wind invades any time there is overexposure to high winds, windy environments, or if dressed insufficiently for the weather. People often remember exposure to drafts before symptoms began.

Wind may also arise Internally, usually from Deficient Blood or Yin, Excess Liver Heat, or stagnant Qi, although Deficient Kidney Yin, a persistent high fever consuming Body Fluids, excessive eating of spicy, greasy, fatty and fried foods, excessive activity or stress, and insufficient rest may also cause Internal Wind. Wind especially injures Blood and Yin.

External Wind: Wind-Cold

sudden and rapid onset	slight fever
stronger chills	dull headache
aversion to wind and cold	body aches
stuffy nose	no sweating
itchy or slight sore throat	superficial cough
itchiness	

External Wind: Wind-Heat

sudden and rapid onset	high fever
slight chills	sweating
aversion to wind and heat	sharp headache
swollen, very sore throat	cough with yellow
red, itchy skin eruptions	sputum

Internal Wind

tremors	vertigo
dizziness	muscle spasms
paralysis	convulsions
numbness of limbs	tetany
convulsions	stiffness
itching	apoplexy
hemiplegia	twitching
upward turning of eyeballs	
rigidity and pain of neck and head	
deviation of mouth and eyes	
urticaria, itching skin eruptions that change locations	

Heat

Heat speeds metabolism, causing extreme activity in the body. It has a tendency to rise up and out, like heat from a fire, and when it does, it often moves other things with it, like Blood (high blood pressure, or blood in the mucus, stool and so forth), or the tongue (being loud and talkative). Excess Internal Heat is usually termed Fire.

External Heat

high fevers, mild chills	thirst
fear of heat	red skin eruptions
extreme sore, swollen throat	sweating
restlessness	yellow mucus
throbbing headaches	constipation

Internal Heat

constipation

aversion to heat

dark yellow or red urine

dark, scanty urination

irritability

sweats easily

yellow coated tongue

strong odors

strong appetite

infections, inflammations

dryness internally or externally

bloody nose, stools or urine

yellow mucus or urine

sticky, thick and hot-feeling excretions

swollen, red and painful eyes or gums

red face, eyes

thirst

craving for cold

hemorrhaging

fast pulse

burning digestion

high fever

red tongue body

preference for cold

burning sensations

restlessness

Extreme Heat

A more severe condition, it includes several of the Heat signs above plus:

delirium

shortness of breath

heat stroke

depletion of fluids

sudden high fever

coma

restlessness

disturbed mind

exhaustion

profuse sweating

Cold

Cold slows circulation and metabolism, creating contraction and constriction. Over time it can block the proper flow of Qi, Blood and Fluids in the body, causing dull, aching pains that are relieved by the application of heat.

External Cold

sudden onset of strong chills, mild fever

body aches

clear to white mucus

fear of cold

no sweating

mild sore throat

dull headache

no thirst

Internal Cold

clear to white copious bodily secretions

frequent and copious urination

loose stools or diarrhea

undigested food in stools

feelings of coldness

poor digestion

lack of appetite

hypoactive, depressed

dull, achy pains relieved by heat

wears lots of clothes

poor circulation

cold extremities

no thirst

no sweating

sleeps a lot

pale face, lips, nails

pale tongue body

sits hunched over

craving for heat

Dampness

Dampness is a condition of Excess Fluids in the body. Fluids include all fluidic substances in the body other than Blood: saliva, sweat, urine, tears, lymph, intracellular and cerebrol-spinal fluids, bodily secretions such as mucus, phlegm and so on. When Fluids collect and congeal, they form pathogenic Phlegm, a substance that is heavier than Dampness (but doesn't have its dirty, sticky or downward flowing characteristics), which collects in the joints, skin, channels, Lungs or Organs.

External Dampness

fevers not relieved by sweating

heavy vaginal discharge

oozing skin eruptions

fullness or constricted feeling in chest or abdomen

heavy diarrhea

no desire to drink

cloudy urine

Internal Dampness

a feeling of heaviness

abdominal distention

oozing skin eruptions

achy, sore, heavy or stiff joints

excessive leukorrhea

abdominal distention

edema

loose stools

chest fullness

nausea

sluggishness

lassitude

copious bodily excretions such as mucus or excessive vaginal discharge

secretions that are turbid, sluggish, sinking, viscous, copious, slimy, cloudy or sticky

Phlegm

thick, greasy secretions	cysts
soft lumps	nodules
numbness in limbs	tremors
coma	asthma
chaotic or erratic behavior	madness
muddled thought	tumors
cough with heavy expectoration of mucus	

Dryness

Dryness, characterized by dehydration, is a condition of Deficiency of Fluids. Generally invading during the heat of late summer or early autumn, it enters through the mouth and nose, impairing defensive Qi, the Lungs and Body Fluids. As well, it can arise internally due to Heat, or Deficient Blood or Yin.

External Dryness

fever, mild chills	headache
aversion to cold	dry skin
dry mouth, throat, nose	dry lips
extreme thirst	no sweating
cough with scanty or no sputum	
dry tongue with thin, white, dry coat	

Internal Dryness

dry, rough, chapped or cracked skin	dry stools
dry throat, nose, mouth or lips	unusual thirst
dry cough with little phlegm	dehydration

Summer Heat

Summer Heat only appears Externally and results from overexposure to extreme Heat, usually in summer or hot climates. In the West it is known as heat exhaustion. Summer Heat is an acute condition causing profuse perspiration, loss of Body Fluids and exhaustion.

Summer Heat

very high, sudden fever	dizziness
nausea	lassitude
extreme thirst	sudden fainting
heavy sweating	exhaustion
retention of fluids	delirium

loss of consciousness	coma
shortness of breath	flushed face

THE SEVEN EMOTIONS

There is a direct link between emotions and physical health. While appropriate emotional expression is healthy, if emotions are extreme, repressed or excessive, they cause disease. In TCM each Organ is associated with a particular emotion; that has a positive mental energy which can turn into a harmful emotion. Repeated or extreme expression of that emotion not only weakens its associated Organ, but an Organ imbalance causes its affiliated emotion to repeatedly arise. For instance, prolonged grief after a loved one leaves or dies causes susceptibility to pneumonia or asthma; while Deficient Lung Qi leads to feelings of grief and sadness with no apparent cause.

Thus, the Seven Emotions both cause as well as indicate an Organ imbalance, whereas the condition of your Internal Organs affects your emotional state. This is an important distinction, for recognizing the direct link of emotions to your body allows emotional imbalances, such as depression, to be treatable rather than only manageable with drug therapy.

There are seven main emotions: Joy, Anger, Sadness, Grief, Pensiveness (Worry), Fear and Fright (shock). As well, other emotions directly affect the body's health, such as love, anxiety, guilt, jealousy, hatred, desire and so on. Imbalanced emotions not only affect their associated Organs, but also injure the Heart, stagnate Qi and deplete Qi and Blood.

Joy

Normal joy is a beneficial state that settles the Mind, creating peace and relaxation. Injuring joy, characterized by over-excitability, excessive excitement, continuous mental stimulation and hard play (such as excessive intake of alcohol and drugs along with staying up too late), scatters and slows Qi. Injuring joy over-stimulates the Heart, making it larger and in time, leading to Heart-related problems such as palpitations, over-excitability, insomnia, anxiety, restlessness, muddled thinking, inappropriate crying, giddiness or laughter and, in extreme cases, hysteria and insanity. Sudden joy is akin to shock, causing Yang to float and blood vessels to dilate (this is why sudden migraines can occur after hearing good news, or sudden laughter can trigger heart attacks).

Transform injuring joy through compassion and taking care of yourself. Focus inwardly, spend time alone, relax, meditate, count your blessings, be thankful, take in Nature's beauty and practice Beingness.

Anger

Anger comes in many guises—resentment, frustration, irritability, rage, indignation, bitterness, animosity, pent-up grudges, feeling aggrieved. It often is a disguise for other emotions, such as guilt, fear, dislike of being controlled, weakness or an inferiority complex. Excess anger injures the Liver; likewise, a Liver imbalance can cause anger or a propensity to irrational outbursts, often without apparent cause or provocation. Because anger makes Qi rise, many of its symptoms manifest in the head and neck, such as headaches, tinnitus, dizziness, blurred vision, mental confusion, vomiting of blood and hypertension.

Anger also negatively affects digestion, causing nausea, vomiting, belching and burping or acid regurgitation. Anger 1-2 hours after a meal attacks the intestines, causing abdominal pain, distension or alternating constipation with diarrhea. Eventually, anger adversely affects the Heart (like all other emotions), causing Heart Fire (especially if you jog, hurry or exercise a lot) with symptoms of mouth and tongue ulcers, thirst, palpitations, mental restlessness, agitation, red or flushed face, bitter taste in the morning and hot, dark urine.

Long-standing stuffed anger causes depression, while long-term depression is frequently due to repressed anger or resentment (the person may look very pale, subdued, walk slowly and speak in a low voice). Resulting symptoms include pain in the ribs, a lump in the throat, PMS, swollen breasts before periods, irregular or painful periods and digestive upsets such as nau-

sea, poor appetite and pain in the stomach region. Ultimately, if anger isn't expressed, its Qi travels to the genitals through associated vessels and becomes expressed through sexuality and violence.

The Liver's positive mental power is dynamism, creativity and generosity. Thus, alleviate angry outbursts by focusing on life goals, performing acts of kindness, undertaking creative projects and acting decisively.

Sadness

Sadness, which includes regret, when the mind is constantly turned towards another time, crimps and agitates the Heart, which pushes towards the Lungs and stagnates Qi. Thus, sadness depletes Qi, leading to Deficient Lung or Heart Qi and in time, stagnant Qi. Symptoms include weak voice, tiredness, pale complexion, slight breathlessness, weeping, feeling of oppression in the chest, weakness and lowered resistance to colds and flu. In time, further symptoms can arise such as palpitations, dizziness, insomnia, anxiety and night sweats and in women, Deficient Blood and amenorrhea.

Dispel sadness by feeling joy and gratitude for what you have in life.

Grief

Grief, associated with the Lungs, depresses Lung Qi, damages the Heart and causes Phlegm accumulation. Grief stops the breath, causing shortness of breath, mucus, spontaneous sweating, tiredness, cough, susceptibility to colds, flu, allergies, asthma, pneumonia, bronchitis, emphysema and other lung complaints. Those with breathing difficulties often experience anxiety as well (Heart damage). It is not uncommon to develop bronchitis, asthma or pneumonia following the sudden loss of a loved one. Unexpressed grief adversely affects the Kidneys, causing poor Fluid metabolism.

The Lung's positive mental power is feeling confident and good about one's self. Further, time and space heal the Lungs (thus the adage, "All things heal in time."), especially if you healthily receive and let go in life.

Pensiveness

Pensiveness, expressed through worry, brooding and melancholy, is a constant dwelling on certain events or people; a nostalgic hankering after the past and intense thinking about life rather than living it. Ultimately, pensiveness leads to obsessive thoughts and behavior. As well, it includes excessive mental work or study, a type of obsession.

Pensiveness weakens the Spleen, causing Deficient or stagnant Qi and disrupts the Spleen's function of transforming and transporting food and Fluids. Results include tiredness, poor appetite, weak digestion, loose stools or diarrhea, abdominal pain or distention, fatigue, anemia, Dampness, an uncomfortable feeling in the chest, slight breathlessness, dry cough and pale complexion.

Eventually, the body weakens and immunity plummets, causing Deficient Qi and Blood. This is frequently seen in students and workaholics, especially if eating irregular meals on the run or while working or studying. Worry leads to constantly thinking or brooding about certain life events. It stagnates Qi, especially that of the Lungs and Heart, resulting in anxiety and breathlessness. On the other hand, those with a weak Spleen frequently worry or obsess.

The Spleen's positive mental power is the ability to think, concentrate and memorize. Release pensiveness and worry by nurturing or giving to others, feeling compassion, staying centered, counting your blessings and eating nourishing food.

Fear

Fear, insecurity and paranoia injures the Kidneys and adrenals, making their Qi descend (it is not uncommon to feel an uncontrollable urge to void the bladder when a fearful situation arises). Constantly living in a fearful situation eventually weakens the Kidneys, while individuals with weak Kidneys and adrenals tend to feel insecure, paranoid, easily frightened and generally more fearful (this is often seen in heavy marijuana users, since this plant weakens the Kidneys).

Resulting symptoms include bed-wetting in children, incontinence of urine or diarrhea in adults, frequent urination, chronic bladder infections, low back and knee pains, ear infections, premature aging signs and lowered immunity. Fear can also cause Deficient Kidney Yin with symptoms of night sweats, palpitations, a dry mouth and throat and malar flush. Chronic anxiety, a type of fear, similarly depletes and injures the Heart.

The positive mental counterpart of fear is flexibility, courage, wisdom and quiet endurance. As well, meditation, rest, sleep, drinking water and quiet time alone strengthen the Kidneys, dispelling fear.

Fright

Fright, different than fear, is sudden, alarming and unexpected, like shock. It scatters Qi, injuring the Heart and causing palpitations, breathlessness and insomnia, and damages the Kidneys, triggering urinary incontinence, night sweats, dizziness or tinnitus. Extreme shock "closes" the Heart, or makes it smaller (causing a bluish tinge on the forehead) and causes adrenal failure and chronic fatigue.

Disperse fright through compassion, taking care of yourself, meditating, resting and counting your blessings.

Other Emotions

While **love** is an emotion that opens and nourishes the Heart, if obsessive, such as jealously, or misdirected, such as loving someone who is physically or mentally abusive, then it injures the Heart and causes palpitations, red face, insomnia and mental restlessness. When cold and calculating malice is harbored for many years, **hatred** stagnates Liver and Heart Qi, resulting in chest and rib pains, insomnia, headaches, palpitation and body pain where the hatred is felt.

Craving (desiring) material objects or recognition and never being satisfied, depletes the Heart and scatters Qi, triggering palpitations, malar flush, dry throat, insomnia and mental restlessness. An extremely common emotion, **guilt** is self-blame for everything that goes wrong. This adversely affects the Heart and Kidneys and stagnates Qi in the chest, stomach region, or abdomen, causing symptoms of discomfort in those areas. **Jealousy** is similar to craving and can lead to anger, impairing the Heart and Liver. **Anxiety** injures the Heart, Kidneys and Spleen (likewise, an impairment of any of these Organs can lead to anxiety—this is true for all above emotions), producing palpitations, insomnia, urinary issues, low back pain or digestive problems.

LIFESTYLE HABITS

Lifestyle habits are considered neither External nor Internal causes of disease, yet they are major causative factors for illness. They consist of irregular diet, excessive sexual activity, overexertion (including over-working), inactivity and inadequate rest.

- Inadequate rest coupled with emotional stress and excessive sexual activity cause Deficient Kidney and Liver Yin, leading to Liver Yang rising and then Liver Wind. Ultimately, this leads to stroke, coma, mental cloudiness or paralysis.

- Irregular diet combined with physical overwork causes Deficient Spleen Qi, leading to Deficient Spleen and Kidney Yang and then to Heated Phlegm, eventually causing numb limbs, mental cloudiness and inability to speak.

- Excessive sexual activity coupled with inadequate rest causes Deficient Kidney Essence, leading to Deficient Blood and then stagnant Blood, creating arthritic and rheumatic aches and pains.

- Overexertion combined with inadequate rest weakens the channels and stirs up Internal Wind, leading to paralysis, Bell's palsy and wind-stroke.

Irregular Diet

Irregular diet, an increasingly significant causative factor for disease, includes both what and how we eat. Most foods eaten today were not available even a century ago. Since most food then was locally grown and only seasonally available, diet played a key role in helping to maintain homeostasis in one's geographic location, climate and lifestyle. Today, our diets are high in refined and processed foods, imported from all over the world and available any time of year. For example, cooling and moistening bananas are appropriate in hot climates, but since they are available year round everywhere, they cause Dampness in those living in damp, cold environments.

Furthermore, most foods are now adulterated with chemicals, such as preservatives, flavorings, colorings and emulsifiers. As well, air and water pollution cause residual chemicals in the food chain. Additionally, commercial meat contains hormones, and fish harvested from polluted coastal seas have dangerously high levels of heavy metals. As a result, many suffer from immune deficiency disorders, liver, colon and blood toxicity, chronic fatigue and degenerative diseases.

Irregular diet includes not only what we eat, but also how we eat. Here is a list of how our eating habits affect health.

Eating Habits:

- Overeating obstructs Stomach Qi and ultimately weakens Spleen Qi, leading to stagnant Qi and food causing acid regurgitation, stomach pain, belching, foul breath, poor digestion, weakness and tiredness.

- Under-eating, such as too strict a diet, malnourishment, fad dieting and so on, leads to Deficient Qi and Blood, causing dull stomach pain, tiredness and weak muscles.

- Eating too quickly, in a hurry, on the run, while watching TV (directs Stomach Qi to the eyes and can also cause forehead headaches), or while reading, studying, working or discussing business causes stagnant Stomach Qi and leads to acid regurgitation, stomach pain, belching and foul breath.

- Eating when distracted, going straight back to work after eating, or eating irregular amounts from day to day impairs digestion, eventually causing Deficient Spleen and Stomach Qi.

- Skipping breakfast causes Deficient Stomach Qi and, in time, Deficient Blood

- Eating when emotional causes stagnant Liver Qi.
- Eating irregularly (not at the same hours every day) or too late at night causes Deficient Stomach Yin.
- Slimming diets often lead to malnourishment, damaging Spleen Qi and causing poor digestion.

Food Choices:

- Excessive heating foods (curries, spices, pepper—white, black, red—red meat, alcohol, fried, fatty and greasy foods, caffeinated foods and drinks) cause Liver Fire and/or Stomach Heat, leading to Deficient Yin.
- Excessive cold and raw foods (juices, fruit, salads, bananas, cold or iced drinks, tofu, soy milk and frozen foods) create Cold and Dampness in the body, injuring Spleen Yang. In time this leads to stagnant Blood and Deficient Qi and Blood causing tiredness, poor digestion, anemia, weakness, dizziness, blurred vision, chronic fatigue, poor circulation and stabbing, fixed pains. While raw foods and juices are considered the epitome of healthy food by many, in excess they create a Cold, Damp Spleen, weakening digestion and causing poor appetite, mucus, loose stools, diarrhea, low energy, amenorrhea, runny nose and lowered immunity.
- Excessive dampening foods (greasy, fried or fatty foods, milk, cheese, butter, cream, ice cream, bananas, peanuts, sugar, flour products, avocados, nut butters) create Dampness, obstructing the Spleen and Lungs and causing sinusitis, nasal discharge, heavy and fuzzy head, dull headaches, mucus, cough, poor digestion and heaviness and cysts.
- Excessive salt (tinned or processed foods, salt, soy sauce, miso, bacon, sausage, cereals, smoked fish) depletes the Kidneys.
- Excessive sour foods (yogurt, grapefruit, green apples, pickles, vinegar, spinach, rhubarb, gooseberries, red currants) adversely affects the Liver, causing pain and contraction of tendons and pain.
- Excessive caffeinated foods and drinks (coffee, black tea, cocoa, colas, maté, chocolate) create Damp Heat in the Liver, Deficient Kidney Yang and Yin and acidity in the joints and muscles causing arthritis and rheumatism, resulting in headaches, migraines, low back pain, PMS, irritability, frustration, anger, irregular menstrual cycles, frequent urination, lowered libido, diabetes, impaired hearing and eyesight and poor memory.
- Excessive dairy causes Dampness, Phlegm (cough) and stagnant Qi, leading to lumps, cysts, fibroids, PMS, irregular menses, headaches, anger, irritability, nausea or dizziness.
- Excessive sweets and sugar cause overstimulation, Dampness and Heat in the Stomach with symptoms of poor focus, anxiety, blood sugar swings and diabetes.
- Excessive flour products (pasta, crackers, bagels, muffins, toast, breads, cookies, chips, pastries, pie crust, etc.) create Dampness and stagnate the Spleen function, injuring its ability to transform Fluids and resulting in mucus in the lungs or stools, vaginal discharge, loose stools or diarrhea and abdominal distention and fullness.
- Lack of fiber causes constipation and food stagnation.
- Smoking tobacco dries Lung Yin, causing initial symptoms of cough and wrinkles, and eventually, cancer.
- Excessive fried and greasy foods cause Dampness and Heat.
- Excessive supplements cause Dampness in the Spleen and obstruct the Spleen function.
- Excess bitter or downward-moving herbs (such as laxatives) injure Stomach Qi or Yin.
- Chemicals in food (MSG, additives, preservatives, food colorings, artificial flavorings and sweeteners) cause headaches and allergies.

Excessive Sexual Activity

Sexual activity causes a temporary loss of Kidney Essence. Usually restored quickly, if engaged in too frequently, or if you have a weak constitution, then Essence doesn't restore but causes Deficient Kidney Yang and Yin with possible uprising Liver Yang. Resulting symptoms include low back pain, knee weakness, dizziness, low energy, premature aging signs, teeth problems, tinnitus, loss of hearing and eyesight, dry throat, night sweats, malar flush, heat in the palms, soles and/or chest, coldness, frequent or nighttime urination and lowered libido.

Because excessive sexual activity specifically refers to ejaculation/orgasm, moderate sexual stimulation without ejaculation/orgasm actually promotes youthful vigor and, in some, smoothes stagnant Liver Qi. In fact, there are a number of ancient treatises promoting health and longevity through the practice of Taoist sexual yoga.

Excessive sexual activity is relative, depending on your constitution and inherited Essence. The stronger your constitution and health, the more sex you can enjoy without ill effects. However, if you have a weak constitution or poor health, curb sexual activity. How much sex is excessive? If you experience headaches, dizziness or insomnia following sex, that amount is definitely excessive. In general, men are more affected by excessive sexual activity than women because women absorb sperm (a nourishing fluid) through their vaginas.

Excessive sexual drive can indicate either Excess Yang or Deficient Kidney Yin. If Kidney Yin is severely Deficient, it's possible to have vivid sexual dreams with nocturnal emissions or orgasms. Heed the old Daoist saying: "Sleeping alone is better than taking 100 tonics!" On the other hand, lack of sexual desire with symptoms of impotence, premature ejaculation and frigidity, signifies Deficient Kidney Yang.

Inactivity

Before the advent of motor vehicles, day-to-day life encompassed a healthy amount of exercise to accomplish routine affairs and chores. Today's motorized conveniences and elaborate communication systems replace this need with widespread inactivity, resulting in stagnant Qi and Blood and leading to depletion of Yang with accumulation of Dampness. If you are inactive due to chronic tiredness or fatigue, this indicates Deficient Qi or Deficient Yang.

Various postures and movements benefit or injure each Organ. While sitting benefits the Spleen, if excessive, it impairs Spleen functions, leading to digestive problems. Excessive standing injures the Kidneys (one reason why we experience lower backache after prolonged standing). Moderate walking, especially outdoors, spreads Liver Qi smoothly and evenly, while excessive walking depletes Liver Qi, resulting in tiredness, irritability, frustration, headaches, tight neck and shoulders, mood swings, irregular or painful menses and dizziness. Reclining in moderation aids the Lungs, while if excessive, it injures them causing shortness of breath, cough and lung ailments.

Overexertion

Working long hours without adequate rest is the most common cause of Deficient Yin in the West. Over-activity has new meaning today in our fast-paced information-seeking global society. What took years previously we now accomplish in days, or even hours. While we experience many benefits, it also creates "burn-out," or Deficient Yin, like running a car without sufficient oil.

Stress from overexertion is recognized as a major cause of hypertension, heart disease and other debilitating ailments. Under normal circumstances, proper diet and rest easily replenish Qi used for daily activities. Even working hard for short periods, such as studying for exams or preparing for a special work presentation, can be restored within a few days.

However, if you work intensely for months, or even years, and without adequate rest or with excessive sexual activity, Qi is injured and forces the body to draw on its Essence reserves. Over time, this causes Deficient Kidney Yin, which eventually fails to nourish Heart

Yin, resulting in chest pain, palpitations, anxiety, insomnia and other Heart ailments. If you continuously push your limits of endurance, exhaustion that is hard to replenish results.

There are three types of over-exertion: mental, physical and overexercising. Mental over-work includes working long hours, often in confined spaces, with unreasonable deadlines, under stressful conditions and without sufficient rest or breaks. It also results in skipped, late or irregular meals, further contributing to Deficient Qi and Yin. Excessive computer work depletes Liver and Heart Blood and Kidney Qi, causing anxiety, palpitations, thinning hair, tiredness, headaches, insomnia, night sweats, five palm heat, malar flush and hot flashes.

Any type of physical overexertion without rest weakens muscles and the Spleen. Physical overexertion, such as excessive lifting, carrying or other physical activity without adequate rest, weakens Spleen and Lung Qi and Heart Blood, causing worry, anxiety, pensiveness, palpitations, anxiety, insomnia, tiredness, amenorrhea, anemia, and ultimately, Deficient Qi and Yin.

Overexercising depletes Qi, Blood, Yin and Essence. Excessive weight-lifting injures the Kidneys, while excessive jogging damages the tendons leading to Deficient Liver Blood or Yin and, in time, to Internal Liver Wind, causing rigidity, numbness and spasms of the legs. Among the most beneficial forms of exercise are Taoist Qi Gong, Tai Qi or Yoga, which combine slower meditative stretching movements with breathing. While aerobic exercise is beneficial in moderation, in excess it exhausts Yin.

Inadequate Rest

Staying up too late and getting insufficient sleep leads to chronic Deficient Qi and Yin, causing tiredness, weakness, lowered immunity, poor digestion, malar flush, night sweats, hot flashes, burning sensation in the palms, soles and chest, dry throat and eventually, adrenal exhaustion.

MISCELLANEOUS CAUSES

The miscellaneous causes of disease include weak constitution, malnutrition, childbirth, accidents, chronic illness, recreational drugs, old age, drugs, parasites and other conditions such as toxins, food poisoning, bites, stings and infected wounds.

Weak Constitution

Each of us is born with unique constitutional strengths, needs and deficiencies, determined by our parents' health at the time of birth. If parents' health is poor, or if our mother drinks alcohol, smokes, takes drugs during pregnancy or conceives when too old, we inherit weaker constitutions. Inherited constitutional strengths or weakness account for tolerance levels of dietary, emotional and lifestyle stresses.

Those with stronger constitutions can eat, drink and be merry their whole lives and suffer few consequences. Those with weaker constitutions experience greater sensitivity to dietary and lifestyle indiscretions. Genetic ancestry is also important, especially when considering diet. For instance, many Africans and Asians cannot digest dairy, while Scandinavians thrive on dairy. Similarly, certain dietary regimes, such as vegetarianism, are beneficial for some, while for others they are harmful. The following are signs of a weak inherited constitution affecting each Organ:

Spleen: physical weakness, tiredness, poor appetite, digestive problems, weak muscles, sallow complexion and in severe cases, childhood nutritional impairment

Lung: frequent colds and flu, respiratory infections, whooping cough, asthma, eczema, pale complexion, thin chest, weak voice

Heart: dream-disturbed sleep, nervousness, children under 3 waking up crying at night, newborns sleeping fitfully, crying during sleep, opening and closing eyes slightly during sleep, unexplained fevers, bluish tinge on child's forehead and chin (occurs from shock to pregnant mother)

Liver: myopia, headaches in childhood, greenish complexion, infertility or amenorrhea in women

Kidneys: nighttime urination, bed-wetting, fears in childhood, bluish color on the chin, poor bone or brain development, infertility, sterility, premature aging and graying of hair

Malnutrition

Malnutrition, an obvious cause of disease, exists not only in Third World countries, but also in slums, ghettoes and impoverished areas of wealthy countries. As well, those who eat diets full of empty calories, (sweets, sodas, chips, white flour products, canned, refined and processed foods), or who follow overly rigid diets (vegetarian, vegan, macrobiotic, high protein, high carbohydrate or diet fads), can also develop insidious nutritional deficiencies that damage metabolism. Following any extreme diet for a long time is detrimental for most people. Similarly, anorexic or bulimic people injure their Spleen Qi and immunity.

Childbirth

While childbirth is a normal life process, if too many children are birthed too close together (including miscarriages), then Deficient Blood and Qi arise along with Deficient Kidney Essence. Further, if the woman goes back to work too quickly after giving birth, it causes Deficient Liver Blood and chronic tiredness and depression. In general, childbirth weakens Kidney Qi, and women need to build Qi, Blood and the Kidneys by resting and eating well for at least a month or two after giving birth.

Accidents

Severe accidents and falls cause stagnant Blood, which may not show up for years. For instance, knee pain from a car accident or sports injury that is mistreated with repeated and prolonged application of ice[1] causes Cold and Damp obstruction to the deep underlying circulation. When the area is repeatedly exposed to Cold Damp climates, over time, this causes knee pain with limited movement and a predisposition to arthritic or rheumatic pains later in life. To prevent this, use moxibustion or other heat sources and/or liniments to promote circulation while healing the injury (see Moxibustion in *Home Therapies*).

Chronic illness

Protracted illness weakens Lung and Spleen Qi and results in other chronic issues such as tiredness, bronchitis, pneumonia, cough, poor appetite and weak muscles.

Recreational Drugs

Recreational drugs, such as cannabis, cocaine, heroine or LSD, weaken Kidney Qi, stagnate Liver Qi and cause Liver Heat. As well, they can lead to mental confusion, lack of memory and concentration, mental-emotional problems, tiredness, lethargy, sterility and infertility.

Old Age

As we age, Kidney Yang and Yin naturally decline and eventually fail to warm or nourish the Internal Organs. Thus, more problems arise at this time, such as feelings of coldness, poor circulation, failing senses, lowered energy and libido and so on. The more we take care of our bodies through proper nutrition, exercise and rest, the less we experience the effects of this decline.

Medications

Most all medications have known side effects that cause other conditions to arise. As one example, antibiotics actually lock residual pathogens (Wind, Cold, etc.) in the body, rather than releasing them, even though they destroy bacteria. Further, antibiotics kill beneficial bacteria as well, leaving the body weakened with propensities toward rheumatism, fibromyalgia and rheumatoid arthritis. While some individuals may need medications, many are able to reduce or eliminate them by using herbs, therapies, acupuncture (or other alternative healing methods) and diet.

---

[1] Ice is only beneficial for up to 15 minutes at a time. For best results, if ice is a must, alternate with heat applications and end with heat.

Parasites

Various parasites and intestinal worms, typically prevalent in tropical, humid climates, easily invade those who excessively consume greasy, sweet foods and flour products, since these cause Dampness, a parasite-friendly environment. Parasites can cause a plethora of problems (see Candida, in *Treatment of Specific Conditions* for symptoms and treatment).

Other Factors

Other factors causing disease include such issues as toxins (such as exposure to contaminated waste, heavy metal poisoning, herbicides and so forth), poisonous bites and stings, food poisoning and infected wounds. These lead to toxicity and stagnant Liver Qi or Liver Heat for starters, with many possible symptoms. While some of these are beyond our control, others we can manage or avoid by moving, being environmentally pro-active and/or immediately using herbs to detoxify the poisons after exposure.

CHAPTER 6
The Energy of Illness

✤

One of the marvels of life is that each and every one of us is created differently. While that may seem a ridiculously obvious statement, somehow it is forgotten when it comes to medicine and treating the human body. After all, most of us have a liver, heart, stomach, spleen and a pair of lungs and kidneys, not to mention cellularly each of us has the same microorganisms busily performing their multiple functions. From this perspective, it makes sense to diagnose every body as if it were the same.

Yet, if our bodies were this simply analyzed, then why can one person drink quantities of alcohol or coffee without ever seeming to get sick, while others get migraines, PMS or pain in the ribs as soon as they do so? Why can some people drink plenty of iced drinks and sit in air conditioning all day, while others get frequent colds, flu or bronchitis under the same conditions? And why can some people stay up until 3 AM, sleep five hours and then go all day while others soon get lowered immunity and fatigue when they do this?

Genetics play a role, yes, but it is more than this—constitutional energy, lifestyle factors, diet, emotions and spirit all combine to form your unique body's energies and determine your ability to stay strong, healthy and vibrant. Thus, when treating yourself or others, it is very important to remember that you are different than the next person and so need different treatment and herbs.

The coffee your mother drinks daily with apparent ease may be the very thing that causes your health problems when you drink it even one time a week. Burning the midnight oil might seemingly work for your husband, but may cause you serious maladies if you try to live the same way. Taking vitex helps your sister's PMS, but may not touch yours because you need something else to treat your unique body.

When I first studied Western herbs, I learned to apply them symptomatically. I used **echinacea** and **goldenseal** for colds, **valerian** for insomnia and **uva ursi** for bladder infections. Sometimes they worked, but not always. I was puzzled and couldn't understand why these herbs, which were supposed to be very effective, didn't always succeed for me. The clincher happened one spring when I came down with the Hong Kong flu. **Garlic** was the herb of choice, but no matter how much I took of it, I only got worse. Eventually I had to turn to Western drugs. They gave me nightmares, but I got over that awful flu.

For awhile I became discouraged with herbs. Then I learned how Traditional Chinese Medicine (TCM) matches the energy of herbs to that of the patient and the disease condition. Not only did this reveal a deeper understanding and more effective use of herbs, but it also explained why the herbs I used in the past didn't always work. Suddenly, the old adage, "it doesn't matter so much what disease a person has, as what person has the disease" made sense to me. I realized that I was using Western herbs similarly to the approach of Western medicine: I was treating illnesses and not the person who had the illness.

In *The Nature of Energetic Herbalism* we talked about the difference between using herbs symptomatically and energetically. When herbs are given symptomatically, the known use of an herb is matched with the symptoms of the illness, as I used **garlic** for my flu. When herbs are applied energetically, the individual characteristics of the herb are matched with the qualities causing the illness, and with the various traits of the person experiencing the illness. This energetic method is an approach of treating the person who has the disease rather than treating the disease itself.

When we experience illness, we are used to defining our condition in terms of its symptoms. For example, we define a cold as a stuffy nose, sneezing, possible cough, head congestion and low energy; a bladder infection as frequent and burning urination, possible blood in the urine and bloatedness; bronchitis as inflamed bronchioles in the lungs with mucus congestion and cough. Our treatment approach for these is to directly eliminate the symptoms with medications in order to "get rid of" the illness.

Both modern medicine and Western herbalism use this symptomatic treatment approach. It gives decongestants or expectorants for colds, antibiotics and diuretics for bladder infections and antibiotics or anti-inflammatories for bronchitis. In many cases this works, but in others it doesn't, making it a rather hit-or-miss approach. When it doesn't work, it can cause a prolonged healing process, a weakening of the body and/or a suppression of the true cause of the illness.

The reason the symptomatic treatment approach doesn't always work is because not every cold, bladder infection or bronchitis is the same. Further, not every body they manifest in is the same. A cold you have can be totally different from a friend's cold because both of you are different. Therefore, one overall treatment approach does not heal each type of cold, bladder infection or bronchial inflammation. Rather, each illness manifests with a different energy that varies according to the energy in each person's body.

ENERGETIC TREATMENT APPROACH

Just as herbs and foods have warm and cool energies, so do illnesses have various energies, such as warm or cool, excess or deficiency, damp or dry and so on. Which it is determines a different treatment approach. The energy of the illness varies for each person and it's analyzed according to various signs and symptoms. Once the energy of an illness is determined, we can choose the appropriate herbs and foods to heal it. If the energy of the illness is not determined before it is treated, then the problem can get worse, or reappear at a later date. In either case, the energetic cause of the illness still remains.

For example, one female patient, Kim, presented with recurring bladder infections. She first treated herself by drinking copious amounts of cranberry juice and taking **goldenseal** until the infection was gone. This worked, yet in another few weeks the infection returned. Repeating her treatment, the infection again cleared, yet re-manifested in another month. Kim then tried antibiotics, which didn't work either. She also felt continuously cold and ate lots of salads and fruit in her vegetarian diet.

Kim's bladder infection chronically recurred again and again because her overall condition was one of Coldness and her treatment approach was to give Cold cranberry juice (a Cold food), **goldenseal** (a Cold herb) and antibiotics (a Cold drug). Because an infection itself is Hot, the condition temporarily disappeared. Yet, this treatment only created more Coldness in her already cold body and metabolism. Thus, her body continued to manifest bladder infections.

My treatment began by giving Kim a warming diet. This was essential because the continued intake of cold food only negated the herbal treatment. Also, her body needed the warmth and strength of this type of food. I then gave her Warm herbs to build and heat her body along with more energetically balanced herbal antibiotics and anti-inflammatories. In time, not only did her bladder infection heal, but it has never returned. Not applying herbs energetically to an illness like this is often the reason that herbs seemingly "don't work." Rather, if herbs "don't work" it is usually due to their improper application or insufficient dosage.

FUNDAMENTAL PROPERTIES IN THE BODY

Before we learn how to treat illness, we must first examine the body's various energetic properties. These properties, such as Energy (Qi), Blood, Fluids, the Organs and so on, are seen so differently in Chinese medicine, that I will capitalize the Chinese terms to differentiate them from their Western meanings. Once we learn what these terms mean, then we can learn how disease arises in the body and what to do about it.

Because Chinese medicine originated around 5000 years ago when people lived in an agricultural society, its terms and theory reflect people's connection to and immersion in nature. All fundamental properties not only describe how things work in the body, but also how everything moves and functions throughout the very universe (the microcosm reflects the macrocosm and vice versa). If you keep this in mind while learning the Chinese system, it makes much more sense and is easier to grasp.

The theoretical foundation of Chinese medicine is based upon the concepts of Qi, Blood, Yin, Yang, Fluids, Essence, Shen, the Pernicious Influences and the Organs. Diagnosis and treatment is also founded on these ideas. Although strange at first to the western mind, repeated reading and application of the principles make them easier to grasp and in time, become a part of your world view and life habits.

QI

In its simplest form, Qi (pronounced chee) is energy, yet it is much more than that: Qi is the vital life force

that animates all sentient life.[1] It is formless, invisible and difficult to measure, although it can be palpably experienced and observed. Qi gives movement and heat to life. It is a precious commodity that is enhanced through breathing practices and proper nutrition. Qi has six major functions in the body.

Qi holds Blood in the vessels, adjusts the appropriate flow of sweat, urine and saliva and consolidates sperm.

Qi raises the Organs and keeps them in their proper places as well as lifts our spirits (keeping us positive, happy and even).

Qi protects us from the invasion of External Pathogenic Influences (such as Wind, Damp, etc.—see *The Causes of Disease*) so we don't get sick (Qi regulates the opening and closing of pores, for instance).

Qi transports Blood, Fluids and nutrients and provides the motive power behind metabolism.

Qi transforms what we eat and drink into usable Blood, energy and other substances such as feces, urine, tears and sweat.

Qi warms the body and provides metabolic digestive fires.

When imbalanced, Qi becomes either weak (Deficient) or congested (stagnated). Deficient Qi occurs when there isn't enough energy to perform the body's various functions. Symptoms include low vitality, lethargy, shortness of breath, slow metabolism, frequent colds and flu with slow recovery, low soft voice, spontaneous sweating, frequent urination, prolapsed organs, hemorrhoids and palpitations. Herbs that tonify Qi are used, such as **ginseng**, **codonopsis**, **astragalus**, **jujube dates** and **dioscorea**.

When Qi congests, flows improperly, or moves in the wrong direction (called *rebellious Qi*), it stagnates, just like cars piling up in a bad traffic jam. Symptoms of stagnant Qi include pains that come and go and change location and severity, distention in the ribs and ab-

---

[1] Because there is no exact English translation for the term Qi in all its meanings, it is more appropriate to simply use the word Qi, rather than energy.

domen, depression, moodiness, soft palpable lumps, frequent sighing, irregular menses, burping, belching, hiccuping, vomiting, nausea and shallow, non-productive cough. Herbs that move stagnant Qi are used, such as **cumin**, **cyperus**, **bupleurum** and **orange peel**.

BLOOD

Though similar to blood as we know it, Blood is a very dense and material form of Qi and, as such, is inseparable from it. Dense and fluidic in nature, Blood mainly functions to nourish, moisten and provide nutrients to the cells, Organs, brain, muscles, tendons, bones, skin, hair, eyes, sinews, tongue and so forth. It also warms the body. Blood is derived from both bone marrow and the food and fluids we ingest. This is why proper diet is so important in Chinese medicine.

There are three basic types of Blood imbalances: Deficient Blood, Heat in the Blood and stagnant Blood. **Deficient Blood** arises when there's isn't enough Blood in the body to perform its nourishing and moistening functions. Symptoms include dizziness, blurry vision, numbness, restlessness, anxiety, slight irritability, insomnia, scanty menses or amenorrhea, thinness or emaciation, dark spots in the visual field, dry skin, hair or eyes, lusterless, pale face and lips, tiredness, easily startled or overwhelmed and poor memory. Herbs that tonify Blood are used, such as **dang gui**, **lycii berries**, **cooked rehmannia**, **white peony** and **longan berries**.

Excess Heat in the body can cause **Heat in the Blood** that then pushes Blood out of the vessels, like erupting lava. The result is blood in the sputum, stools, urine or vomit, coughing up of blood, bloody nose, excessive menses, or red and hot skin eruptions.

Stagnant Blood occurs when circulation is slowed, or blocked, from too much Coldness, Heat, stagnant Qi or external injury. Symptoms include fixed, stabbing or boring pains, hard, immobile masses and lumps, hemorrhaging, clots, dark-colored menses, dark complexion, purple lips, nails, or tongue, tremors and swelling of the Organs. Herbs that move Blood are indicated, such as **angelica**, **safflower**, **myrrh** and **motherwort**.

FLUIDS

Fluids encompass all fluidic substances in the body other than Blood: saliva, sweat, urine, tears, lymph, intracellular and cerebrospinal fluids, bodily secretions such as mucus, phlegm and so on. Fluids moisten and nourish the skin and muscles, thin Blood and lubricate the joints, viscera, bowels, brain, marrow and spine. As such, they protect, such as the Lungs against harsh, drying air, the Stomach against burning hydrochloric acid, or the joints from abrading movement.

When Fluids collect and congeal, they form pathogenic **Phlegm**, a substance that is heavier than Dampness, but doesn't have its dirty, sticky or downward flowing characteristics. Phlegm can collect in the joints, skin, channels, Lungs or Organs.

Fluids can be Deficient or Excess. Deficient Fluids creates Dryness with symptoms of dry, rough, chapped or cracked skin, dry throat, nose, mouth or lips, dry cough with little phlegm, dry stools, dehydration and unusual thirst. Moistening herbs are used along with Yin tonics like **ophiopogon**, **Chinese asparagus root** and **lily bulb**.

Excess Fluids is the same as Dampness and is characterized by a feeling of heaviness, edema, loose stools, oozing skin eruptions, abdominal distention, chest fullness, nausea, sore, heavy or stiff joints and copious bodily excretions, such as mucus or excessive vaginal discharge. When Excess Fluids congeal and form Phlegm, tumors, cysts, soft lumps, nodules, cancer, numbness, tremors and paralysis result. Herbs that transform Dampness or resolve Phlegm are used, such as **fu ling**, **coix**, **fritillaria**, **platycodon**, **atractylodes** and **cardamom**.

ESSENCE

Essence, a highly refined fluid-like substance stored in the Kidneys, is the very foundation of life and the source of organic development. As such, it is considered a precious substance to be valued and guarded. Both nutritive and supportive, Essence is the basis of reproduction, development, growth, sexual power, conception, pregnancy and decay in the body. It forms our basic constitutional strength and vitality, including semen, reproductive capacity and hormonal secretions. Since Essence resides in the Kidneys, any imbalance of their functions may indicate an Essence dysfunction. Likewise, if the Kidneys become weakened or depleted from excessive working or sex, poor diet and/or lack of proper sleep, Essence also becomes depleted.

Essence is created from the innate energy we receive from our parents at birth. It can be likened to an inherited trust fund that determines our proper growth, development and maturation. This trust fund can never be added to, but is supplemented through food and drink we ingest and how we live. In other words, our inherited trust fund is the physical hand of cards we are dealt, while how we play the cards (how we eat and live) determines how slowly or quickly we age. Those of us with weaker Essence trust funds, or who spend their essence too quickly through fast living, insufficient rest or poor diet, experience illness earlier in life than those who inherit larger trust funds, or play their cards well.

We each are born with a fixed amount of Essence that naturally declines as we age, since its only pattern of disharmony is Deficient Essence. This normally occurs around age 49 in women (menopause) and age 64 in men (andropause), although it can transpire much earlier in life. Symptoms include premature aging, senility, bad or loose teeth, poor memory or concentration, brittle or softening of bones, weakness of knees and legs, thinning hair, premature graying of hair, low libido or impotence, habitual miscarriage or infertility and wasting of flesh.

In children, Deficient Essence results in late closure of the fontanel, improper or poor bone development, mental dullness or retardation, premature aging, or slowed physical growth. Herbs that nourish Essence are combined Yin, Yang, Blood and Qi tonics, such as **polygonati**, **he shou wu**, **cuscuta** and **epimedium**.

SHEN

Shen reflects the entire physical, emotional, mental and spiritual health of the body. It includes the capacity to think and act coherently and appropriately, the personality's magnetic force and the joy to live life. It is distinguished by the sparkle in the eyes, an overall vivaciousness and a will to live. Housed in the Heart, Shen is our enthusiasm, innate vitality and charisma. Spiritually, it is the dynamic faith, vitality and force of our personalities that are able to surmount obstacles and make things happen.

There are no disharmonies of Shen in and of itself, yet because it is connected with the Heart, Deficient Heart Qi or Blood can weaken Shen. This appears as a lack of joy or enthusiasm in life, dull eyes, dislike of talking, muddled thinking, forgetfulness, insomnia, lack of vitality, depression, unhappiness, confused speech, or excessive dreaming. In extreme, a Shen disharmony results in irrational behavior, incoherent speech, hysteria, delirium, unconsciousness, inappropriate responses to people or the environment, or violent madness.

Herbs that nourish the Heart also nourish Shen, such as **ziziphus seeds**, **biota seeds, polygala**, and **longan berries**. The true remedy for Shen problems, however, is addressing emotional and spiritual issues using counseling, prayer, affirmation, meditation, play, changing jobs, taking holidays and whatever else is needed to nourish the Spirit and Heart.

YIN AND YANG

Yin and Yang in the macrocosm represent the polarities of life: night and day, moon and sun, feminine and masculine, soft and hard and so on. Yin and Yang are so interrelated and interconnected that there is also some Yin in Yang and vice versa. As such, they are interdependent, so that one depends on the other to function properly. At their extremes, Yin can transform into Yang, and Yang into Yin, just as night turns to day and vice versa.

In the microcosm of the body, **Yin** is Blood and Moisture. Cooling, moistening and fluidic (like water) it embodies the ability to nurture, moisten and lubricate all aspects of the body. Physiologically, Yin represents the body's substance, such as muscles, flesh, organs, blood and fluids, while emotionally, it is the quiet, receptive, passive and inward expression of life.

In the body, **Yang** is energy and warmth. Warming, drying and stimulating (like fire), it signifies the capacity to circulate, transform and warm all aspects of the body. Physiologically Yang represents the body's organic functions and processes such as warmth, libido, appetite, digestion and assimilation, while emotionally, it is the active, stimulating and outward expression of life.

Yin and Yang are interconnected, as represented by the Yin-Yang symbol: there is always some Yin in Yang, and Yang in Yin. Physiologically, this translates as Yin (substance) being dependent on Yang (function) and vice versa. Yin moistens and anchors Yang, while Yang circulates and transforms Yin.

Excess Yin can be likened to too much Dampness in the body, with symptoms of heaviness, lethargy, edema, excessive secretions and excretions (such as copious mucus or vaginal discharge), flaccidity, copious urination, loose stools or diarrhea and no thirst. Herbs that drain or transform Dampness are used such as **fu ling**, **nettles**, **cardamom**, **elecampane** or **parsley**.

Deficient Yin is a lack of cooling, moistening Fluids with resulting depletion (fatigue, exhaustion, emaciation or thinness) along with specific types of Heat and Dryness signs: night sweats, malar flush (redness and burning heat along the cheeks and nose), five palm heat (burning sensation in the palms of the hands, soles of the feet and in the chest), afternoon fever or feelings of heat, restless sleep, dry throat or thirst at night, agitation, mental restlessness, dry cough, dry stools, and scanty dark urine. Herbs that tonify Yin are used, such as **ophiopogon**, **raw rehmannia**, or **Chinese asparagus root**.

Too much Yang, or **Excess Yang**, causes signs of high fever, thirst, red face, aversion to heat, restlessness, irritability, burning sensations, red eyes, scanty dark urine, yellow discharges and strong odors. Herbs that clear Heat are used, such as **dandelion**, **red clover**, **goldenseal** and **yellow dock**.

A lack of Yang, or **Deficient Yang**, arises when there isn't enough metabolic Heat, or fire, to warm the body, transform Fluids (Yin), or promote circulation. Symptoms include feelings of coldness, copious, clear urination, white, copious or runny discharges, pale, frigid appearance, cold limbs, lassitude, fatigue, edema, loose stools or diarrhea, nighttime urination, infertility, faint odors, impotence, frigidity and undigested food in the stools. Herbs that warm the Interior of the body and tonify Yang are used, such as **garlic**, **cinnamon bark**, **fenugreek**, **damiana**, **dipsacus** and **cuscuta**.

While **Excess Yang and Deficient Yin** are both associated with Heat signs, their symptoms arise from two entirely different causes and so their Heat is of very different types. Excess Yang is excessive Heat in the body, like how we feel under a blazing sun. Deficient Yin is a lack of cooling, moistening fluids causing apparent Heat and Dryness, such as a dry cough when there's insufficient fluids to moisten and protect the Lungs, or night sweats when Yin is depleted at the coolest time of "day". To treat Excess Yang, we use Heat-clearing herbs; to treat Deficient Yin, we use cooling Yin tonics.

Similarly, while **Deficient Yang and Excess Yin** are both associated with Dampness, their symptoms arise

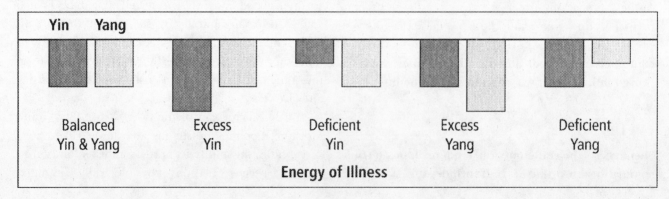

Yin Yang

Balanced Yin & Yang   Excess Yin   Deficient Yin   Excess Yang   Deficient Yang

Energy of Illness

from two entirely different causes. Deficient Yang occurs when there is insufficient Heat to metabolize, warm and transform Fluids. Coldness and tiredness result because the metabolic fires are too weak to perform their functions. Eventually Dampness arises from insufficient Yang fires to transform Fluids.

Excess Yin, on the other hand, causes stagnant Fluids and Excess Dampness. There aren't necessarily feelings of coldness or poor energy, but the overall body tends to look swollen and there's heaviness and copious discharges. To treat Deficient Yang, we give Yang tonics and herbs to warm the Interior of the body. To treat Excess Yin, we give herbs that drain or transform Dampness.

THE ORGANS

The Chinese view the Organs according to energetic rather than physical functions. They are seen as dynamic interrelated processes that occur throughout every level and cell of the body rather than as discrete, local organs with specialized functions. In fact, some of the Chinese Organs don't exist, or aren't considered "organs" at all, in Western medicine.

The Organs are divided into two types: the solid, or Yin, Organs that store and the hollow, or Yang, Organs that transport. The Yin Organs are vital while the Yang Organs are functional. Each Yin and Yang Organ is paired together in a system called "Husband-Wife" where each Organ interdependently performs its functions, yet mutually "communicates" and provides the other with energy. Because the Yin Organs are the vital ones, they are generally referred to rather than the Yang ones.

YIN ORGANS

HEART

The Heart is the supreme master of the Organs, as the emperor is of the people and like the emperor, the Heart links Heaven (the Spirit) and Earth (the body). It governs Blood and its vessels and smooth blood circulation throughout the body. It also houses Shen, or the Spirit—the power to exude joy, charisma, and enthusiasm—and the Mind—the capacity to clearly think, remember, comprehend and respond. Thus, thinking, long-term memory, sleeping and dreaming are all part of the Heart. The Heart produces sweat, appears as a bright sheen on the face, opens to the tongue and loathes Heat (since it's already a "warm" Organ from its Blood content).

When imbalanced, the Heart manifests symptoms of palpitations, chest pains, poor circulation, poor memory, insomnia, forgetfulness, poor long-term memory, dream-disturbed sleep or excessive dreaming, tongue sores and ulcers, excessive talking, inability to speak, incoherent speech, anxiety, mental restlessness, inappropriate behaviors; unclear thinking, unhappiness, lack of joy and mental disorders. Bitter herbs (that also help clear cholesterol from the veins and arteries) affect the Heart Organ. Other herbs, such as **zizyphus** and **biota**, calm the Spirit and nurture the Heart.

SPLEEN

The Spleen is responsible for transportation and transformation (assimilation) of nutrients throughout the body (metabolism). As this occurs on all levels, Spleen Qi not only controls food and fluid metabolism, but also cell respiration and other similar metabolic functions. The Spleen rules the muscles, flesh and limbs, keeps the Organs in place and the Blood in vessels, opens to the mouth and manifests in the lips. The Spleen hates to be Damp, as this interferes with its ability to transform and transport food and fluids.

A weak Spleen causes poor digestion, low appetite, gas, bloatedness, acid regurgitation, loose stools, undigested food in the stools, malnutrition, weakness in arms and legs, fatigue, poor muscle development, edema of abdomen, hips and thighs, blood spots under the skin, easy bruising, lack of sensation of taste, prolapsed organs, frequent bleeding, abdominal distension, obsession, worry, and anemia. Herbs that tonify Spleen Qi such as **ginseng** and **dioscorea (Chinese wild yam)**, warm or tonify Spleen Yang such as **psoralae** or **dried ginger**, or transform Spleen Dampness, such as **agastache** or **cardamom**, are used.

LUNGS

The Lungs govern respiration, receiving air and dispersing it throughout the body. They rule the skin and body hair, regulate the opening and closing of pores, control sweating, govern the voice and open to the nose. It is the only vital Organ with a direct link to the external environment and thus is quite sensitive and loathes Cold (air, temperatures).

Disorders of the Lungs cause symptoms of shortness of breath, cough, difficulty breathing, breathlessness, asthma, bronchitis, mucus, sore throat, colds, flu, lowered immunity, spontaneous sweating, allergies, rhinitis, soft, unclear or weak voice, grief, inability to give and/or receive, sadness and skin conditions. Warming or Cooling expectorants such as **mullein**, **coltsfoot** or **apricot seed**, Lung Qi tonics, such as **astragalus**, **ginseng** or **dioscorea**, or Lung Yin tonics such as **ophiopogon**, are used.

KIDNEYS

The root of Yin and Yang in the body, the Kidneys store Essence, regulate Fluid metabolism, dominate the hormonal (endocrine) system and open to the ears. As well, the Kidneys rule the bones (including teeth), produce bone marrow (thus, ruling the brain), manifest in the head hair and control the lower orifices (anus, vagina, urethra, sperm ducts). The Kidneys promote growth, development, reproduction and the deep underlying immune system. As well, they loathe dryness since they regulate Fluids. The Kidneys also rule the two "Extraordinary Organs", the uterus and brain.

Issues concerning fertility, sexuality, the urinary system, weakness, low back pain, nighttime urination, poor memory (especially short-term), weak knees, joint problems, swollen ankles, leg edema, early morning diarrhea, teeth problems, brittle bones, senility, fear, paranoia, hormonal issues, thinning hair or loss of head hair, lack of will power, ear and hearing problems and premature aging all signal Kidney imbalance. Salty and mineral-rich herbs (**nettles**) and diuretics (**uva ursi**, **parsley**), Kidney Yin tonics such as **Chinese asparagus root**, **marshmallow root**, **ligustrum (privet)** and **eclipta**,

and/or Kidney Yang tonics such as **fenugreek**, **damiana**, **ashwagandha** or **dipsacus**, are used depending on the condition.

LIVER

The Liver stores Blood and maintains the smooth flow of Qi in the body. It also opens to the eyes, controls the tendons and ligaments, manifests in the nails and harmonizes the emotions. The Liver directly links with the left side of the body, ribs, lower abdomen, external genitals and breasts. Pressure and emotional stress adversely affect the Liver, and it loathes wind since that disrupts its smooth flow of energy.

Liver imbalances include muscle spasms, cramps and tics, eye ailments, muscle tension, irregular menses and other menstrual problems, depression, mood swings, PMS, pain in the ribs, sighing, hiccups, feeling of a lump in the throat, lumps, cysts, fibroids, especially in breasts and abdomen, splitting headaches and migraines, difficulty falling asleep, tight neck and shoulders, nail issues, numb extremities, sluggish joint movements, difficulty in bending or stretching, alternating constipation and diarrhea, suppressed creative expression, lack of drive, anger, irritability, frustration and hypertension.

Sour herbs assist the Liver, while bitter ones stimulate the release of bile. Use herbs that regulate Liver Qi such as **bupleurum**, **cyperus** or **rose petals**, tonify Liver Blood such as **lycii berries**, **white peony** or blackstrap molasses, tonify Liver Yin such as **raw rehmannia**, **ligustrum** or **eclipta**, or clear Liver Heat such as **dandelion**, **yellow dock** or **burdock root**.

YANG ORGANS

SMALL INTESTINE

The Small Intestine partners with the Heart. It assists digestion by receiving food from the Stomach, separates the pure Fluids from the impure ones (the ability to discriminate), transports the pure fluids to various parts of the body and sends the impure ones to the Large Intestine. Disorders of the Small Intestine include constipation, diarrhea and some urinary disorders.

STOMACH

The counterpart of the Spleen, the Stomach receives food and drink and breaks them down, thus governing digestion. Imbalances result in lack of appetite, indigestion, vomiting, nausea, bleeding gums, bad breath, mouth sores and headaches across the forehead.

LARGE INTESTINE

The Large Intestine, pairing with the Lungs, is responsible for transporting waste products out of the body and governs the rectum. Constipation, dysentery, diarrhea and hemorrhoids are manifestations of Large Intestine disharmony.

URINARY BLADDER

The Urinary Bladder, the Kidney's partner, stores and excretes wastewater. Disharmonies of the Bladder result in edema and urinary disorders.

GALLBLADDER

The paired Organ to the Liver, the Gallbladder is in charge of storing and secreting bile. Because bile is the only pure substance in the body, it is considered responsible for a person's ability to make decisions. Imbalances manifest as digestive upset, timidity, indecisiveness, nausea and belching.

INTERRELATIONSHIP OF THE ORGANS

Rather than being discrete and independent, all the Organs interrelate, interact and inter-restrain; their functions directly influence, support and control each other. This is most easily seen in the system, **The Five Phases**, which outlines the specific ways in which the Organs relate. Sometimes called The Five Elements, the word

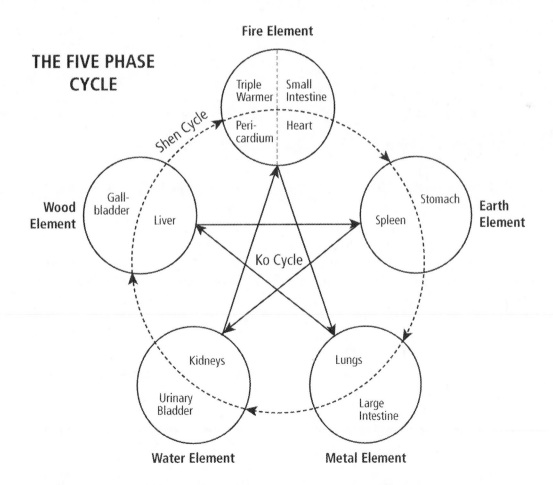

THE FIVE PHASE CYCLE

Fire Element

Shen Cycle

Triple Warmer | Small Intestine
Pericardium | Heart

Wood Element

Gallbladder | Liver

Earth Element

Stomach | Spleen

Ko Cycle

Kidneys

Urinary Bladder

Lungs

Large Intestine

Water Element

Metal Element

THE FIVE PHASES

Element	WOOD	FIRE	EARTH	METAL	WATER
Yin Organs	Liver	Heart	Spleen	Lung	Kidney
Yang Organs	Gallbladder	Small Intestine	Stomach	Large Intestine	Urinary Bladder
Opens To	Eyes	Tongue	Mouth	Nose	Ears
Sense	Sight	Speech	Taste	Smell	Hearing
Fluid	Tears/bile	Sweat/blood	Lymph/saliva	Mucus	Cerebrospinal fluid/sexual secretions
Rules	Tendons	Pulse	Muscles	Skin/ body hair	Bones/ head hair
Emotion	Anger	Over-excitement	Melancholy, worry	Grief	Fear
Sound	Shouting	Laughter	Song	Sobbing	Groaning
Color	Green	Red	Yellow	White	Black/dark blue
Taste	Sour	Bitter	Sweet	Pungent	Salty
Activity	Looking	Walking	Sitting	Reclining	Standing
Season	Spring	Summer	Indian summer	Autumn	Winter
Injurious Influence	Wind	Heat	Dampness	Dryness	Cold
External Manifestation	Nails	Complexion	Lips	Body hair	Head hair, anus

"phase" better describes the dynamic interchange of energies that occurs amongst the Organs.

Every Phase represents an elemental aspect of nature: Fire, Earth, Metal (air), Water and Wood (growth). Each Phase is comprised of two partner Organs, one more vital in function (the solid Yin—or *Zang*—Organs) and one more mechanical (the hollow Yang—or *Fu*—Organs). Each Organ Phase has specific traits and characteristics. The Five Phase system is important for diagnosis, as well as describes a healthy way of living life.

Looking at the Five Phases table, you can see the correspondences between the Organs and various influences that either positively or negatively affect them. For instance, in small amounts the sour taste tonifies the Liver, but in excess, it causes Heat in the Liver. Looking (using the eyes) is a Liver activity, but excessive looking (reading, watching TV, etc.), depletes Liver Blood or Yin. Overexposure to Wind aggravates the Liver, causing spasms or nervousness. Liver health can be viewed by examining the nails since they are its "secretion." Excess Liver disharmonies manifest in a shouting quality of voice. Anger aggravates the Liver while an imbalanced Liver makes us more easily irritated or angry.

Each Organ dynamically interconnects and influences every other Organ in one of two ways: nurturing or controlling (refer to the accompanying diagram, The Five Phase Cycle). In the Shen Cycle, every Organ nurtures the one following it (going in a clockwise direction), just as parents care for their children. The Heart nurtures the Spleen, the Spleen nurtures the Lungs, the Lungs nurture the Kidneys and so on. As well, each Organ controls every other Organ, called the Ko Cycle, like a grandparent watching the grandchildren while the parents are at work. Thus, the Lungs control the Liver, the Kidneys control the Heart, the Liver controls the Spleen and so forth.

The Organs' interactions are extremely useful in understanding the disease process and its causes. Because the Organs interrelate, an imbalance in one Organ usually causes an imbalance in another. For example, if there is a Kidney disharmony, it may adversely affect its child, the Liver, or its grandchild, the Heart. Thus, if the Kidneys are Deficient in Yin with symptoms of low back pain, tiredness, scanty, dark urination, night sweats and malar flush, Liver Yin eventually weakens because its "mother" (the Kidneys) can't nourish and support it. The result is migraines, insomnia (can't fall asleep or stay asleep), hot flashes, irregular menstruation and depression. However, Deficient Kidney Yin may cause Deficient Heart Yin instead, since depleted Kidneys may be unable to care for their grandchild. The consequence is palpitations, anxiety, mental restlessness, forgetfulness, especially long-term and insomnia (can't stay asleep).

These cycles can move the other way as well, so that an imbalance in a child Organ can drain its mother. Thus, weak Kidney's (child) can exhaust Lung Qi (its mother), causing breathlessness, shortness of breath, weak cough and frequent colds and flu. This occurs from different causes: either the child is too hyper (in an Excess state), or the mother is too depleted (in a Deficient state). Further, the grandchild Organ may be too unruly for its grandparent to control so that an unruly grandchild can overtake its grandparent, if it's too hyper or if the grandparent is too depleted. For instance, a "hyper" Heart (Excess Heart Heat) can overtake the Kidneys (its grandparent), causing low back pain, scanty, dark urination, exhaustion, dry mouth at night, mental restlessness, insomnia and dream-disturbed sleep.

How do you know which pattern is occurring? By reviewing the Organs' functions and symptoms of imbalance. Examine each Organ to identify which signs reflect your particular health imbalance symptoms. Then you'll know which Organs are involved in your particular illness. As well, there is an extremely useful system for identifying the energy of illness in our bodies, called The Eight Principles, as shortly follows.

INFLUENCES OF NATURE

In *The Causes of Disease*, we learn about the Pernicious Influences—Wind, Heat, Cold, Damp, Dryness and Summer Heat. When these Influences invade the body, they cause disease. However, when the fundamental properties or Organs of the body aren't functioning properly, these Influences may arise Internally as well. Thus, there is also Internal Wind, Internal Heat, Internal Dampness and so on. When these properties are referred to in their Internal aspect, they are just termed Wind, Heat, or Damp in relation to the Organs they influence, such as Liver Wind, Heart Heat (or Fire), or Spleen Damp. To review these Qualities, please refer to the section Pernicious Influences, in *The Causes of Disease*.

IDENTIFYING ILLNESS

In order to identify the energy of illness in the body, we need to look at how the Fundamental Properties (Qi, Blood, Fluids, Essence, Shen), Organs (Heart, Spleen, Lungs, Kidneys, Liver) and Influences (Wind, Heat, Cold, Damp, Dryness, Summer Heat) interact within the context of each person's energy and strength. A useful, easily understood system, called The Eight Principles, is a method of identifying the location, energy and severity of an illness in relation to the energy of the person experiencing it. When this system is applied, we understand what caused the disease and know the appropriate herbs to use for its treatment. The Eight

THE EIGHT PRINCIPLES

EXTERNAL	Surface of the body: colds, flu, fevers, skin eruptions, sore throats, headaches, injuries, acute arthritic conditions
INTERNAL	Interior of the body: conditions affecting the Qi, Blood, Fluids and Internal Organs; chronic digestive, eliminative, respiratory, urinary, reproductive and neurological diseases, such as constipation, gastritis, ulcers, urinary infections, low energy, weakness, diabetes, hypoglycemia, cancer, epilepsy, gynecological conditions, infertility, impotence
EXCESS	Stagnation of Qi, Blood, Fluids or too much Coldness or Heat in the body; obesity, constipation, hypertension, severe infections, sharp, stabbing pains
DEFICIENCY	A lack of Qi, Blood, Fluids, Yin or Yang in the body; thinness, fatigue, shortness of breath, cold intolerance, anorexia, dyspepsia, loose stools, frequent and clear urine, afternoon fevers, sensation of heat or burning of soles/and or palms, tiredness, weakness, weak digestion, low hydrochloric acid, hypothyroidism, hypoadrenalism, anemia, wasting diseases such as TB and AIDS
HOT	Overly active metabolism; high fevers, inflammation, infections, sensitivity to heat and hot weather, flushed complexion, yellow or blood-tinged discharges
COLD	Low metabolism; chills, lack of thirst, pale complexion, cold sensitivity, anemia, hypo-conditions, clear or whitish discharges
YANG	Body's capacity to generate and maintain warmth
YIN	Body's capacity to moisten and cool; the body's substance

Principles include the location of an illness (External or Internal), its energy (Hot or Cold), its severity in relation to the person's energy (Excess or Deficiency), and its overall state (Yang or Yin).

Location of Illness

External and Internal define the depth and location of an illness in the body. **External conditions** tend to be acute and are located on the surface of the body. They affect the nasal passages, mouth, throat, bronchioles and Lungs along with the skin and hair. These include colds, flu, fevers, skin eruptions, acute arthritic conditions and injuries. In general, inducing a sweat treats External diseases. Herbs with an outward and upward energy are used, such as diaphoretics, expectorants, and some stimulants and alteratives.

Internal syndromes describe conditions affecting the Qi, Blood, Fluids and Internal Organs. They can include such conditions as constipation, diarrhea, gastritis, ulcers, urinary infections, low energy, weakness, diabetes, hypoglycemia, cancer, epilepsy, gynecological

conditions, infertility, impotence and heart disease. Internal ailments are treated with herbs that have an inward, downward or tonic energy such as diuretics, laxatives, emmenagogues, tonics and some stimulants.

It is possible to have both an acute **External condition** and a **chronic Internal** one at the same time, such as a cold or flu, while dealing with poor digestion or menstrual irregularity. When this occurs, it is always necessary to treat the acute External condition first before attending to the Internal one.

Hot-Cold Energy of Illness

Hot and Cold refers to the body's innate metabolism. **Heat** causes extreme activity in the body with a tendency to rise up and out, like the heat from a fire. When it does this, it often moves other things with it, like Blood (high blood pressure, or blood in the mucus, stool and so forth) or the tongue (being loud and talkative). It is characterized by a fast metabolism, ruddy complexion, aggressive or overbearing manner, loud voice, thirst, constipation, dark yellow or red and scanty urine, craving

HEAT AND COLD SIGNS

HEAT SIGNS	COLD SIGNS
Thirst	No thirst
Dark yellow/red and scanty urination	Clear, copious and frequent urination
Craving for cold; dislike of heat	Craving for heat, dislike of cold
Yellow, sticky, thick and hot-feeling discharges, excretions and secretions	Clear, runny, copious discharges, excretions and secretions
Blood in any discharges	Poor circulation, cold extremities
Burning sensations	Dull, achy pains
Infections, inflammations	Low blood pressure
Dryness Internally or Externally	Dampness Internally or Externally
Red face, eyes	Pale face, lips, nails
Sweats easily	No sweating
Constipation	Diarrhea, loose stools
Irritability, hyperactive, aggressive	Depressed, hypoactive, quiet
Fever	Chills
Insomnia, restless, dream-filled sleep	Sleeps a lot
Strong appetite	Poor appetite
Red tongue body; yellow coated	Pale tongue body; moist or white coated
Fast pulse	Slow, deep pulse

for cold and aversion to heat, yellow mucus, stools, urine or vaginal secretions, blood in any discharges, burning digestion, infections, inflammations, dryness, red face or eyes, strong body odors, hemorrhaging, irritability, restlessness, sweating, strong appetite, high blood pressure, fever and all hyper-conditions such as hyperthyroidism or hyperadrenalism.

Coldness tends to congeal and contract, like ice. It causes a person to hunch over or curl up in order to minimize body surface and maintain inner warmth. With lack of Heat, activity in all forms slows. It is characterized by lowered metabolism, feelings of coldness, pale complexion, weakness, lethargy, poor digestion, lowered immunity, aversion to cold and craving for warmth, no thirst or sweating, slowness, diarrhea or loose stools, fluid retention, weak senses, timidity, being soft spoken, sleeping a lot, quietness, little body odors, poor circulation, low blood pressure, poor appetite, clear to white mucus, stools, urine or vaginal secretions, achy pain in the joints, frequent and copious clear urination, nighttime urination, frigidity, impotence, infertility, severe chills, lack of thirst, anemia and all hypo-conditions such as hypothyroidism, hypoadrenalism or hypoglycemia.

Look carefully at the chart, Heat and Cold Signs, for a clear delineation of each of these symptoms. Remember that this represents a continuum, so that a person may only have a few Cold signs and these may only occur occasionally or not be very pronounced. The same is true for someone with a few Heat signs.

Strength of Illness: Excess-Deficiency

Excess and Deficiency describe the strength of the disease in relation to the strength of the person. A person who is strong usually develops acute symptomatic reactions to stress, climate and foods, while a weakened person generally experiences chronic ailments. Excess or Deficiency is determined by looking at the root cause of an illness, not just its symptoms, and gauged according to the capacity of the individual to maintain a continued resistance to the onslaught of disease.

Excess represents too much, or a toxic congestion (stagnation) of Qi, Blood, Fluids, Coldness, Heat or food. Symptoms include obesity, constipation, hypertension, severe infections, purulent yellowish and smelly discharges and edema. Herbs used to treat Excess include those that dry Dampness, move congestion, detoxify and eliminate Heat and circulate Qi, Blood and Fluids. In general, Excess patterns are simpler to treat than Deficiency ones because it is easier and quicker to eliminate than to build.

Deficient states occur from a lack of Qi, Blood, Yin or Yang. An individual who is Deficient tends to have lowered immunity and hypersensitivity to stress, climate and foods. Conditions of Deficiency take a longer time to heal because the body needs to be strengthened. Example symptoms include tiredness, weakness, weak digestion, hypothyroidism, hypoadrenalism, anemia and wasting diseases such as TB and AIDS. Tonic herbs are used to strengthen the Qi, Blood, Yin or Yang of the body.

If we look at the body as a container that holds Qi, Blood and Fluids, we can view Excess and Deficiency in a different way. In an Excess condition the container is over-packed and bulging so that Qi, Blood or Fluid circulation slows and eventually stagnates. This overload increases until it needs release, like steam from a pressure cooker, eventually blowing holes in the container's sides. At that point, the vital eliminative systems malfunction. If it occurs long-term, the Organs overwork and become weak, or even fail in their functions. Thus, Excess needs to be eliminated to create a healthy container with easily and smoothly flowing contents. Many Western herbs tend to be eliminating in nature.

In a Deficient condition, the container is weakened and becomes porous, allowing the Qi, Blood, or Fluids to leak out, so less remains in the container. A person with a Deficient container tends to be weak, overly sensitive to stress, climate and foods and have a lowered immune system. Tonifying herbs and solid nourishment are needed to plug the holes and replenish the container's contents.

It is not unusual for Excess and Deficient conditions to coexist. In treating Excess conditions, especially acute ones, one should never tonify as this only feeds the disease rather than the body's normal energy. Elimination first needs to occur, even if there is weakness. After the first stages of elimination are complete, some tonifying therapy can be given concurrently, if appropriate. In treating Deficient conditions, it may be necessary to combine both tonifying and eliminative treatment in order to build the person's strength while clearing concurrent congestion. This may be done together in a single herbal formula.

Yang-Yin

Yang and Yin are a summation of the preceding aspects. Yang represents conditions that are External, Excess or Hot in nature. It is heating, circulating, activating and drying in energy. Yin encompasses conditions that are Internal, Deficient or Cold in nature. It is cooling, moistening and nurturing in energy.

Combinations of the Eight Principles

Disease is seen as a pattern formed from a combination of the Eight Principles. External and Internal conditions may coexist along with Hot and Cold, or Excess and Deficiency symptoms. Herbs are then given to treat the identified pattern. For example, a person may experience poor digestion with diarrhea, clear abundant urination and lowered immunity along with red skin eruptions at the same time. Treatment combines Internally tonifying and warming herbs that strengthen digestion, hold urination and tonify immunity with herbs that clear Heat from the External skin eruptions.

The following are symptoms of the various common combinations.

External-Excess-Heat: Skin eruptions, rashes, boils, eczema, strong body odor, possibly heavy, restless sleep, anxiety, yellowish mucus which may be red tinged with blood, loud and strong breathing, scanty, dark colored urination, high fever possible constipation or yellowish, foul-smelling diarrhea. Use cooling herbs that treat the Exterior and clear Heat, or cooling diuretics, antispasmodics, nervines, expectorants, purgatives or astringents.

External-Excess-Cold: Coldness, stiffness, lowered immunity, aversion to Cold, Wind and Damp, lack of sweating, lower fever with a tendency towards chills, pale, puffy and swollen complexion, drowsiness and sleepiness, clear or cloudy white mucus, strong and labored breathing, frequent urination that is clear to light-colored and normal to loose stool. Use warming herbs that treat the Exterior, such as warming diuretics, expectorants, aromatic stomachics and astringents.

External-Deficient-Heat: Frail, thin, restless, anxious, lowered immunity, aversion to Heat and Wind, thirst, spontaneous perspiration, night sweats, low grade fever, restless sleep, acute or chronic recurring sore throats, thin, yellowish urination with possible recurring bladder infections and watery, slightly yellowish stool or constipation. This is a Deficient Yin condition. Treat with Yin tonics and/or Externally cooling diaphoretics.

External-Deficient-Cold: Cold, frail, anemic, pale complexion, lowered immunity, clear or whitish mucus, no thirst, acute conditions that may arise quickly but with mild or subnormal fevers and chills, shallow breath, clear, copious urination, loose stools and tendency to sleep a lot. Use warming herbs that treat the Exterior, warm the body and circulate Qi, such as warming diaphoretics, astringents and Qi tonics.

Excess Yang (Internal-Excess-Heat): Strong odors, yellow discharges, rapid pulse, hypertension, high fever, red complexion, constipation, possible blood in the stool, urine, vomit or nose, strong body odors, aversion to Heat, irritable and aggressive temperament, active, energetic, restless with a tendency towards insomnia, loud, commanding voice, strong appetite, thirst, heavy coarse breathing, a tendency towards infections and inflammations, strong sexual drive, yellow or reddish colored eyes, dry and cracked lips, heavy menses which may be early and long-lasting, dark-colored urination, hard and solid stool, constipation, or hot, yellowish diarrhea. Use cooling herbs that clear Heat and Dampness and purgatives.

Excess Yin (Internal-Excess-Cold): Excessive fluid retention, plump or swollen appearance, coldness, pale complexion, flacidity, severe edema, slow moving but with adequate energy, aversion to Cold and Dampness, poor digestion, gas, bloating, clear or white mucus, allergies, cold extremities, short menstrual cycle, slow bleeding perhaps with dull pains, light-colored and copious urination with possible nighttime urination and loose stools. Treat with spicy, warming stimulants, aromatic stomachics, warming diuretics, and Yang and Qi tonics.

Deficient Yang (Internal-Deficiency-Cold): Lethargy, coldness, edema, poor digestion, lower back pain, the type of constipation caused by weak peristaltic motion, lack of libido, frail, cold, timid, low energy, hypothyroidism, hypoadrenalism, pale complexion, anemic, lack of thirst, recurring colds and flu, sleeps easily, thin, clear mucus discharges, pale and wet lips, shallow and weak breathing, aching lower back and joints, pale, light, late or irregular menstruation, frequent and copious urination with possible nighttime urination and loose stools. Here there is a lack of Heat and activity to perform adequate functions in the body. Use herbs that disperse Coldness, warm the Interior body and/or tonifies Yang.

Deficient Yin (Internal-Deficiency-Heat): Emaciation and weakness with Heat symptoms of night sweats, insomnia, a burning sensation in the palms, soles and chest (called "five palm heat"), malar flush, afternoon fever, thirst, restlessness, nervous exhaustion, dry throat, dry eyes, blurred vision, dizziness, nervous energy, talking fast but tiring quickly, little stamina, lowered immunity, thin constitution, low-grade infections and light and short menstruation but with some pain and irregularity. Treat with Yin tonics, astringents and cooling nervines, sedatives and calmatives. This type of Heat, sometimes termed "false heat", occurs because the cooling moistening Fluids (Yin) are lacking.

THE PATTERNS OF DISEASE

Now that we've learned the fundamental properties of the body and their functions, we can see how their imbalances cause disease. Through applying the Eight Principles to the fundamental properties of Qi, Blood, Fluids, Essence, Shen, Yin and Yang, with the Influences Wind, Heat, Cold, Damp, Dryness and Summer Heat, and the functions of the Organs, we can determine the patterns involved. It is the various combinations of these factors that create the Patterns of Disease (formally called differential diagnosis).

When determining which patterns of imbalance exist, be sure to examine *all* signs and symptoms occurring. Symptoms often have nothing to do with the disease label given by Western medicine, and it is not unusual for the symptoms to seem unrelated to the main complaint. Yet, to identify the correct pattern(s) of disharmony involved, it is necessary to consider all symptoms for accurate pattern identification.

For example, Neil thought nothing of his periodic burning stomach because of his severe, recurring headaches. Taking both symptoms into account, however, helps us better determine that his headaches arise from Stomach Heat rather than from Liver Heat or Deficient Blood, for instance. Then when we treat this pattern, both the headache and stomach upset disappear. Karen also complains of headaches, but she experiences periodic dizziness, frequent low back pain and night sweats. These additional symptoms identify a pattern of Deficient Kidney Yin, which requires a different treatment approach than that for Stomach Heat. When we tonify her Kidney Yin, not only is her headache cleared, but Karen's other symptoms wane as well.

At this point, things may seem so complicated that you may want to slam this book shut. To proceed, take a deep breath and remember that the patterns of disease are just combinations, or "conjugations," of the fundamental principles we discussed earlier. A simple review of these building-block elements will yield further understanding. Deficient Spleen Qi may sound exotic, but it simply means the energy (Qi) of the Spleen (Organ in charge of metabolism) is poorly functioning (Deficiency), thus causing signs of poor digestion, low appetite, gas, bloatedness and loose stools. Excess Stomach Heat may sound like a phrase turned sour, but it easily translates as too much Heat in the Stomach (the Organ responsible for digestion). Signs include hypermetabolism, inflammation, a desire for cold, a burning sensation in the Stomach below the ribs on the left side, extreme thirst, especially for cold drinks, constant and ravenous hunger, nausea, vomiting and sour regurgitation.

Let's look at it from another perspective. Weakness and tiredness indicate Deficient Qi, while frequent copious urination and low back pain indicate Kidney involvement. Put together, it forms the pattern, Deficient Kidney Qi. A sensation of heaviness, nausea and copious, cloudy discharges indicate the presence of Dampness. Frequently feeling cold, lack of thirst and loose stools signal Cold, or Deficient Yang. When these two combine with the further symptoms of lack of appetite, sweet taste in the mouth and stuffiness in the chest and epigastrium, all aspects signaling the involvement of the Spleen, we get the pattern, Deficient Spleen Yang.

When determining which pattern is involved, know that several symptoms appear in more than one category. Thus, there needs to be more than one symptom present in that same category to signal its involvement. For instance, a headache is a sign of *either* an External Pernicious Influence pattern *or* an Excess Liver Yang pattern (and several other possible patterns). If the headache is due to an External Pernicious Influence invading, there will also be chills and fever, sudden onset and body aches. If it is Excess Liver Yang, signs of dizziness, red face and eyes, thirst and dream-disturbed sleep can occur as well.

With this system we are not diagnosing and treating a specific disease as Western medicine does, such as diabetes or hepatitis. Rather, we are framing all the body's symptoms and signs within one or more co-existing and interrelating patterns of imbalance and treating that pattern.

For instance, rather than thinking of the disease, asthma, we identify several possible patterns causing the asthma, such as Wind Cold, Wind Heat, stagnant Liver Qi, or Deficient Liver and Lung Yin. Rather than seeing a person with hepatitis, we identify which pattern encompasses the symptoms of jaundice, fever, tiredness, weakness, nausea and pain under the right ribcage, such as Damp Heat in the Liver, stagnant Liver Qi, or Deficient Liver Yin.

In fact, any one of these patterns can manifest (cause) any number of different diseases. For instance, Damp Heat in the Liver can be involved in hepatitis, eczema, headaches, menstrual difficulties, insomnia, indigestion and constipation. Deficient Kidney Yin may underlie ringing in the ears, deafness, low back pain, tiredness, insomnia, headaches, constipation and menstrual difficulties. Thus, the disease does not matter, but the symptoms and what patterns they form do.

There are many advantages to this alternative diagnostic and treatment approach. "Untreatable" diseases now become treatable because we take them out of their discrete, labeled boxes and see further links within broader aspects of ourselves. We may now view ourselves as whole beings whose bodies, minds, emotions and spirits interconnect to bring us health or cause disease. We can also learn how to live healthily through diet, lifestyle habits, work influences, relationships and environmental choices to influence how we feel and heal. Further, we may remove ourselves from being machines in a body shop where our parts are examined, repaired or removed. Rather, we can see ourselves as the whole, interactive beings we are within the context of the entire universe.

In "real" life, few of us have symptoms that fit in just one of the patterns of disease. Rather, most of us experience mixed symptoms from a combination of these groups. There can be symptoms of half External–half Internal, part Excess–part Deficient and/or combined Cold–Hot. Simultaneous patterns of Deficient Kidney Yin with Excess Liver Heat and so on may also exist.

These types of conditions are not unusual and are treated by using integrated approaches. It is possible to treat the Exterior and Interior at the same time, or to simultaneously combine herbs that detoxify and tonify, or have cooling and warming natures. It is not only possible, but essential, to treat mixed patterns together, such as tonifying Kidney Yin at the same time as clearing Excess Liver Heat. In fact, the most powerful and effective formulas usually mix herbs of diverse energies and concurrently treat multiple patterns.

The major patterns of disease and their signs and symptoms are listed at the end of this chapter. Refer to those tables in determining which patterns are involved when investigating health issues.

ROOT AND BRANCH OF DISEASE

Each illness has two aspects: a root and a branch. The root is the underlying cause, while the branch is its symptoms. For example, a throat infection is the symptom, or branch, of a disease. Its underlying cause (such as Deficient Yin, Excess Heat, or Deficient Kidney Qi) is the root. A cough is the branch of a disease, while its underlying cause, or root, can be from Excess Lung Dampness, Deficient Lung Qi, Deficient Kidney Yang, or from an invading cold or flu. Because each cause is different, it requires a diverse approach.

If you only relieve the superficial branch when treating disease, such as the throat infection or cough, either the symptoms recur or other problems eventually develop because the root cause is still present. It is like weeding a garden: if only the leaves and stems are pulled, the weed grows back because the root remains. In order to eliminate the weed entirely, the entire root needs to be fully dug out.

Once you've identified which pattern(s) of disharmony are involved, you now know what herbs to use for treatment. For instance, if you want to treat Deficient Spleen Qi, then you use herbs that tonify Qi and whose energy goes to the Spleen. To quickly find these herbs, look at the beginning of the *Materia Medica*, and examine the herbal categories until you find Tonics, then look for Qi tonics. There you'll see a list of Chinese and Western herbs that tonify Qi. Reference each of these to see which go to the Spleen.

The protocol for treating illness then is to treat the root along with its branches. To do this, first look at the branch, or all the symptoms occurring, and determine which fundamental properties of the body are involved (refer to earlier sections in this chapter). Then determine which patterns these symptoms form. From the involved patterns, we can determine the root cause of the symptoms. This process is called determining the patterns of disease, or differential diagnosis.

As a note, when treating acute conditions it is important to treat the branch of a disease first. This is because acute conditions are critical and so need to heal quickly. Then the root, or original cause, of the condition can be treated. In chronic conditions, the branch and the root can be treated simultaneously.

DIAGNOSIS

Chinese diagnosis includes four methods of gathering information to determine the Patterns of Disease and, from there, the treatment principle and herbs used. These include looking, hearing (and smelling), asking and feeling. Asking questions is perhaps the most prevalent of the four, along with tongue and pulse diagnosis. At the beginning of *The Treatment of Specific Conditions*, a list of commonly considered areas to question is given in the chart Symptoms to Consider. Following is a brief description of tongue and pulse diagnosis.

Tongue Diagnosis

Tongue diagnosis is part of diagnosis by looking. It is considered a pillar of diagnosis because it provides clearly visible clues to a patient's pattern of disease. Since the tongue always reflects the basic, underlying pattern, it is extremely reliable, especially whenever there are conflicting manifestations. It also helps determine the predominant pattern when more than one is present.

Observation of the tongue is based on four areas: the tongue body color, the body shape, the coating and the moisture. Of these four, *the tongue body color is the most important* and its diagnostic indications help clarify the pattern of disease, especially when there are conflicting signs and symptoms. The body color indicates the condition of Blood, Qi and Yin Organs; body shape shows the state of Blood and Qi; tongue coating points to the condition of the Yang Organs; and moisture designates the state of Body Fluids. See the accompanying charts for each of their diagnostic indications.

Further, each area of the tongue reflects the state of specific Internal Organs (see diagram). Tongue color,

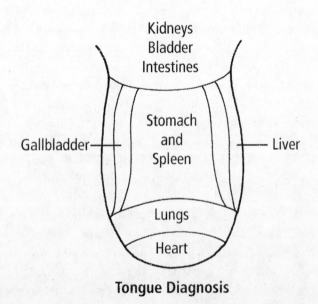

Tongue Diagnosis

TONGUE BODY COLOR

The tongue body color indicates the condition of Blood, Qi and Yin Organs

BODY COLOR	INDICATIONS
Pale	Deficient Blood, especially if also thin and/or slightly dry Deficient Yang, especially if also swollen and wet
Red	Heat; if with a full coat (especially yellow), this indicates Excess Heat; if with no coat (or a peeled coat), this indicates Deficient Yin
Deep Red	Same as red body color, only a more severe condition
Purple	Stagnant Blood; if reddish-purple, this indicates Heat and stagnant Blood; if bluish-purple, this is Cold and stagnant Blood
Blue	Cold causing stagnant Blood

TONGUE BODY SHAPE

The body shape indicates the state of Blood and Qi

BODY SHAPE	INDICATIONS
Thin	And pale indicates Deficient Blood And red with no coat or a peeled coat indicates Deficient Yin
Swollen	And pale indicates Dampness from Deficient Yang And red or normal-colored indicates Damp Heat Swollen edges or teeth marks indicates Deficient Spleen Qi
Stiff	Internal Wind And red indicates Heat injuring Body Fluids
Flaccid	And red indicates Deficient Body Fluids (Dryness, or Deficient Yin) And pale indicates Deficient Qi and Blood
Long	Heat, particularly Heart Heat
Short	And pale and wet indicates Internal Cold. And red with no coat or a peeled coat indicates extreme Deficient Yin, or Heat stirring Liver Wind
Cracked	Excess Heat or Deficient Yin Short horizontal cracks indicate Deficient Stomach Yin A deep and long midline crack reaching to the tip indicates a tendency toward Heart imbalances
Trembling	Deficient Spleen Qi
Crooked/Deviated	Internal Wind, generally Liver Wind, or External Wind invading
Curled up edges/sides	Stagnant Liver Qi
Strawberry/Red Spots	Heat toxins, stagnant Blood, or Heat in Blood
Swollen Sides	Liver Yang rising, or Liver Fire

TONGUE COATING

Tongue coating indicates the state of the Yang Organs

TONGUE COATING	INDICATIONS
Thick coat	Presence of an Internal or External pathogenic factor
No coat/peeled coat	Deficient Yin: on tip it's Deficient Heart Yin In front it's Deficient Lung Yin In center it's Deficient Stomach Yin In rear and if tongue is red all over it's Deficient Kidney Yin
White coat	Cold; if coat is thin and white, this is normal
Yellow	Excess Heat
Grey/Black	And wet indicates extreme Cold; and dry designates extreme Excess Heat.

TONGUE MOISTURE

This indicates the state of Body Fluids.

TONGUE MOISTURE	INDICATIONS
Wet	Dampness
Dry	And a coat indicates Excess Heat And no coat or a peeled coat indicates Deficient Yin
Creamy or Greasy	Retention of Dampness of Phlegm

shape, coating and moisture may vary in each of these areas and thus indicates the condition of imbalance or health in those corresponding Organs. For instance, if the tongue is pale on the sides, this indicates Deficient Liver Blood. If the tongue is purple in the center, this is stagnant Blood in the Stomach. If there's a thick yellow coat on the rear of the tongue, this indicates Damp Heat in the Intestines, Bladder or Uterus.

A normal healthy tongue is pale red in color, of medium thickness with a thin white coating and very slight moisture. It is best observed in outdoor light and no sooner than 1 hour after eating. If needed, use a flashlight to examine, taking into account any yellowish tinge cast by the light. Strange colors on the tongue usually reflect foods recently sucked or eaten.

Pulse Diagnosis

Pulse diagnosis is part of diagnosis by feeling (palpation). It gives detailed information on the state of Qi,

Blood, Yin, Yang, the Internal Organs and the person as a whole. Although the basic pulses can be learned fairly quickly and are quite useful diagnostically, pulse taking can also be quite complex.

Each position is usually felt at three levels: superficial (using very slight pressure), middle (using normal pressure) and deep (using strong pressure and pushing down to right above the bone). It is also felt in three locations—Front, Middle and Rear. Each pulse position reflects the state of Qi, Blood, Yin and Yang in each of the different Organs. Combined these indicate the status of all twelve Organs. Although there are different systems in taking pulses, what's offered here is one of the most commonly used today.

The pulse is taken on the radial artery right below the wrist. The person's arm should be horizontal and level with their heart (and no higher). To feel the pulse, place three fingers together at the base of the wrist. The forefinger is set closest to the wrist and is the Front Posi-

PULSE LEVELS AND THEIR INDICATIONS

LEVEL	ENERGY FELT	INDICATIONS	ORGANS
Superficial	Qi, Yang Organs	State of the Exterior	Heart and Lungs
Middle	Blood	Stomach and Spleen	Stomach and Spleen
Deep	Yin, Yin Organs	State of the Interior	Kidneys

PULSE POSITIONS AND THEIR INDICATIONS

POSITION	ENERGY	WARMER	LEFT SUPERFICIAL	LEFT DEEP	RIGHT SUPERFICIAL	RIGHT DEEP
Front	Qi	Upper	Small Intestine	Heart	Large Intestine	Lungs
Middle	Blood	Middle	Gallbladder	Liver	Stomach	Spleen
Rear	Yin	Lower	Bladder	Kidney Yin	Triple Warmer	Kidney Yang

tion; the ring finger is set furthest from the wrist and is the Rear Position; the middle finger is placed in between (on the small protruding bone there, called the styloid process) and is the Middle Position. Feel the pulse with all three fingers together to get a better idea of the general state of Qi and Blood.

Since the pulse is easily affected by such influences as climbing stairs, emotional upset or recent exercise, it can quickly change in the short-term. Thus, be sure to feel the pulse with the person at rest and ideally no sooner than one hour after eating or drinking. Further, the pulse changes according to the seasons, moving deeper in the winter and more superficial in the summer. As well, men's pulses are usually stronger on their left (the Yang side) while women's are stronger on their right (the Yin side).

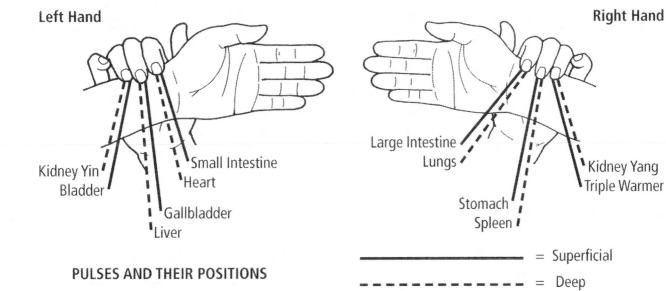

Left Hand

Kidney Yin
Bladder
Small Intestine
Heart
Gallbladder
Liver

PULSES AND THEIR POSITIONS

Right Hand

Large Intestine
Lungs
Kidney Yang
Triple Warmer
Stomach
Spleen

—————— = Superficial

- - - - - - = Deep

PULSE TYPES AND THEIR INDICATIONS

There are 28 pulses; the 12 primary pulses are given below.

PULSE TYPE	HOW PULSE FEELS	INDICATIONS
MODERATE (Normal)	Pulse has 4 beats (about 60 beats/minute) for each respiratory cycle and is relaxed, harmonious, forceful and almost slow.	Normal, healthy pulse
FLOATING (Superficial)	When pulse is felt with light finger pressure, it has a surplus; when pressing down, it is weaker; when pressure is released, it regains full strength.	Exterior Pattern: • Floating and tight indicates Wind Cold • Floating and fast designates Wind Heat. • Floating and Empty at Deep level indicates Deficient Yin
DEEP	Felt only at deepest level with heavy pressure, near the bone; cannot be detected with light or moderate pressure.	Interior conditions: • Deep and Weak indicates Deficient Qi and Yang • Deep and Full designates stagnant Qi or Blood, or Internal Heat • Deep and Slow indicates Internal Cold
FAST (Rapid)	Count the number of beats felt during one respiratory cycle of person, or count the number of beats for 15 seconds and multiply by four.	More than 5 beats (90 beats/minute) indicates Heat: • And Empty and Rapid designates Deficient Yin • And Full and Rapid indicates Excess Heat
SLOW	Count the number of beats felt during one respiratory cycle of person, or count the number of beats for 15 seconds and multiply by four.	Fewer than 4 beats (60 beats/minute) indicates Cold: • And Slow and Empty designates Deficient Yang • And Slow and Full indicates Excess Cold
FULL (Large-Excess)	Feels full, forceful, long, rather hard and has a surplus either Floating or Deep.	Excess pattern: • And Full and Fast indicates Excess Heat • And Full and Slow designates Excess Cold
EMPTY (Deficient)	Feels large but soft, slow, empty and forceless.	Deficient Qi
SLIPPERY	Feels smooth and rounded to touch; rolls or slides under the fingers, like pearls in a porcelain basin.	• Dampness, Phlegm • Stagnant food • Pregnancy or menstruation
CHOPPY	Feels rough with a jagged edge, like a caterpillar eating a mulberry leaf; pulse doesn't flow smoothly.	• Stagnant Blood • Deficient Blood • Exhaustion of Fluids
FINE/THIN (Thready)	Pulse is thinner and more narrow than normal, like a silken thread; weak and without strength.	• Deficient Blood • Internal Dampness with extreme Deficient Qi
WIRY (Bowstring)	Feels taut, tense and forceful, like pressing on a guitar or violin string.	• Liver disharmony • Pain • Phlegm
WEAK	Only felt at the deep level and is soft and fine.	Deficient Yang

The normal pulse should be relatively slow—4 beats per respiratory cycle (which is one inhalation and one exhalation), calm but with strength, neither too big or small, regular and felt clearly in the root positions. While there are 28 pulse qualities, the first six are the most important: *depth*—superficial or deep, *speed*—fast or slow, and *strength*—Full (Excess) or Empty (Deficiency). Get to know these six first before tackling any of the others. Next, learn Slippery (this is best learned by feeling the pulses of a pregnant or menstruating woman), Choppy, Fine/Thin, Wiry and Weak, as these are used in *The Treatment of Specific Conditions*.

After feeling the overall pulse with all three fingers to determine its depth, speed and strength, feel one position at a time with its individual finger to determine the relative energy of Qi and Blood in each of the twelve Organs. This is a further refinement of pulse taking that yields useful information in confirming the Patterns of Disease. Sometimes there are discrepancies in tongue and pulse diagnosis. If this happens, follow the tongue diagnosis first since it's extremely reliable and always reflects the basic, underlying pattern.

PATTERNS OF DISEASE CHARTS (Differential Diagnosis)

The **bold** symptoms are major indicators of that Organ imbalance. Only the most commonly seen Patterns of Disease are included here.

YIN ORGANS
HEART—EXCESS PATTERNS

STAGNANT HEART BLOOD	HEART FIRE (HEAT)	COLD DAMP OBSTRUCTING THE HEART	DAMP HEAT OBSTRUCTING THE HEART
Pain in heart region, which may radiate to inner aspect of left arm or shoulder	Mouth and tongue ulcers	Mental confusion	**Mental confusion, restlessness,** depression and dullness
Cyanosis of lips	Thirst	**Rattling sound in throat**	Incoherent speech
Palpitations	**Palpitations**	Lethargic stupor	Palpitations
Stuffiness; feeling of oppression or constriction of the chest	Mental restlessness; feeling agitated	Abnormal, inward, restrained and foolish behavior	Uncontrolled laughter or crying; shouting or muttering to oneself
Cyanosis of nails	Feelings of heat	Muttering to oneself	Rash behavior
Cold hands	Red or flushed face	Staring at walls	Agitation
	Hot, dark urine or blood in urine	Nausea	Tendency to hit or scold people
	Bitter taste in mouth in morning		Bitter taste in the mouth in the mornings
	Insomnia with feverish sensation; vivid dreams		Dream disturbed sleep; insomnia
Tongue: purple	**Tongue:** red, redder tip, yellow coat	**Tongue:** thick, sticky, slippery white coat	**Tongue:** red, yellow-sticky coat
Pulse: choppy	**Pulse:** fast and full	**Pulse:** slippery, possibly slow	**Pulse:** full, fast and slippery, or full, fast and wiry

HEART—DEFICIENCY PATTERNS

DEFICIENT HEART BLOOD	DEFICIENT HEART YIN	DEFICIENT HEART QI	DEFICIENT HEART YANG	COLLAPSE OF HEART YANG
Palpitations	**Palpitations**	**Palpitations**	**Palpitations**	Palpitations
Insomnia, with difficulty falling asleep, but then sleeps well	Insomnia with difficulty falling asleep and waking frequently	**Tiredness;** lethargy	Tiredness; lethargy	**Cyanosis of lips** (purple)
Excessive dreaming; dream-disturbed sleep	Dream-disturbed sleep		**Feeling of cold; cold limbs,** especially hands	**Cold limbs**
Forgetfulness and poor memory, especially long-term	Forgetfulness and poor memory, especially long-term; **mental restlessness**		Feeling of stuffiness or discomfort in heart region	Weak and shallow breathing
Dizziness	**Malar flush**	Shortness of breath on exertion	Shortness of breath on exertion	Shortness of breath
Anxiety	**Feelings of heat, especially in the evening**	Sweating	Sweating	Profuse sweating
Dull pale complexion	Easily startled	Pallor	Bright-pale face	Coma in severe cases
Easily startled	Anxiety, uneasiness, agitation			
Pale lips	Low-grade fever			
	Night sweating			
	Dry mouth and throat			
	Heat in the palms, soles and chest			
Tongue: pale, thin, slightly dry	**Tongue:** red with no coat; tip redder; deep midline crack reaching the tip	**Tongue:** pale or normal color	**Tongue:** pale, wet, swollen	**Tongue:** very pale or bluish-purple; short
Pulse: fine/thin or choppy	**Pulse:** floating, empty and fast, or thin/fine and fast	**Pulse: empty;** in severe cases superficially strong but empty underneath	**Pulse: deep** and weak, or choppy	**Pulse: Minute,** choppy, hidden

LUNGS—EXTERNAL PATTERNS

INVASION OF LUNGS BY WIND-COLD	INVASION OF LUNGS BY WIND-HEAT	COLD DAMPNESS OBSTRUCTING THE LUNGS	DAMP HEAT OBSTRUCTING THE LUNGS
Aversion to cold; Sneezing; Itchy throat	**Aversion to cold; Sore throat;** Swollen tonsils	**Chronic cough with profuse white sputum**	**Cough with profuse yellow or green sputum which is foul-smelling**
Slight fever; strong chills	**Fever;** slight chills	Wheezing or asthma with copious white sputum	Wheezing or asthma with copious yellow or green sputum
Stuffed or runny nose with clear-watery mucus	Stuffy or runny nose with yellow mucus	Chest and flank stuffiness, distension and soreness	Chest and flank stuffiness, distension and soreness
Body aches; aversion to cold	Body aches	Difficulty in breathing, especially when lying down	Difficulty in breathing, especially when lying down
Cough with thin, watery sputum	Cough with yellow mucus	Shortness of breath or breathlessness	Shortness of breath or breathlessness
Lack of sweating	Perspiration	White-pasty complexion	
Occipital headache (back of head)	Headache	Constipation	
No thirst	Thirst	Dark urine	
Tongue: thin white coat	**Tongue:** red on the sides or tip with a white or yellow coat	**Tongue:** thick, greasy white coat	**Tongue:** thick, greasy yellow coat
Pulse: floating	**Pulse:** floating and fast	**Pulse:** slippery, weak and floating or fine/thin	**Pulse:** slippery, fast or slippery, fast and floating

LUNGS—INTERNAL PATTERNS

DEFICIENT LUNG QI	DEFICIENT LUNG YIN
Shortness of breath	**Unproductive dry cough with little or no phlegm, or blood-tinged phlegm**
Weak voice	**Feeling of heat or low-grade fever in the afternoon or evening**
Bright-white complexion	Dry mouth and throat
Cough	Emaciated appearance
Watery sputum	Night sweats
Exhausted appearance and spirit	Malar flush
Low voice and lack of desire to talk	Low or hoarse voice
Weak respiration	Burning sensation in palms, soles and chest

(continued on next page)

LUNGS—INTERNAL PATTERNS *(continued)*

DEFICIENT LUNG QI	DEFICIENT LUNG YIN
Daytime sweats	Insomnia
Lowered resistance to colds and flu; aversion to cold	
Tiredness	
Tongue: pale or normal-colored	**Tongue: red, peeled,** dry; possible cracks in the Lung area
Pulse: empty and weak	**Pulse:** floating, empty and fast

SPLEEN—EXCESS PATTERNS

COLD DAMP INVADING THE SPLEEN	DAMP HEAT INVADING THE SPLEEN
Stuffiness of chest or epigastrium	**Loose stools with offensive odor**
Feeling of heaviness (in head, too)	**Low-grade fever constant throughout the day**
White vaginal discharge	Stuffiness of epigastrium and lower abdomen with some pain
Lack of appetite	No appetite
No thirst or desire to drink	Thirst without desire to drink, or desire to drink only in small sips
Lack of sensation of taste, or flat sweetish taste in mouth	Abdominal pain
Skin eruptions containing fluid	Feeling of heaviness
Watery or loose, thin stools	Scanty and dark-colored urine
Nausea	Nausea
Feeling cold in epigastrium, improved by application of warmth	Vomiting
Lethargy	Burning sensation of anus
	Headache
Tongue: thick, greasy, white coat	**Tongue: sticky, greasy, yellow coat**
Pulse: slippery and slow	**Pulse:** slippery and fast

SPLEEN—DEFICIENCY PATTERNS

DEFICIENT SPLEEN QI	DEFICIENT SPLEEN YANG	SINKING SPLEEN QI	SPLEEN UNABLE TO CONTROL BLOOD
	Chilliness; cold limbs	**Bearing down sensation in the abdomen**	**Bleeding**
No appetite	Lack of appetite	Prolapse of stomach, vagina, urinary bladder, uterus, anus	**Easily bruised**
Tiredness; fatigue and lethargy	**Tiredness**	Frequency and urgency of urination, or urinary incontinence	Subcutaneous hemorrhaging
Loose stools	**Loose stools**	Hemorrhoids	Blood spots under the skin
Poor digestion	Undigested food in the stools	Extreme chronic diarrhea	Blood in the urine or stools; bloody nose
Slight abdominal pain and distension relieved by pressure	Abdominal pain and distension relieved by pressure and warmth	Hemorrhage	Other signs of Deficient Spleen Qi
Gas and bloatedness	Gas and bloatedness	Other signs of Deficient Spleen Qi	Excessive menses
Sallow complexion	Sallow or bright-white complexion		Sallow complexion
Weakness of the limbs	Weakness of the four limbs		Uterine bleeding
	Edema		Shortness of breath
Tongue: pale or normal-colored with thin white moss; possible swollen sides	**Tongue:** pale, swollen, wet	**Tongue:** pale	**Tongue:** pale
Pulse: empty	**Pulse:** weak, slow and deep	**Pulse:** weak	**Pulse:** fine

LIVER—EXCESS PATTERNS

DAMP HEAT IN LIVER	STAGNANT COLD IN LIVER MERIDIAN	LIVER FIRE	INTERNAL LIVER WIND
Fever	**Hypogastric pain referring to scrotum** and testis, relieved by warmth	**Red face and eyes**	**High temperature**
Nausea	Straining of testis or contraction of scrotum	**Irritability**	**Convulsions**
Fullness and pain in chest and hypochondrium	In women there may be shrinking of the vagina	Propensity to outbursts of anger	Rigidity of the neck
Jaundice	Pain alleviated by warmth	Dizziness	Tremor of limbs

(continued on next page)

LIVER—EXCESS PATTERNS *(continued)*

DAMP HEAT IN LIVER	STAGNANT COLD IN LIVER MERIDIAN	LIVER FIRE	INTERNAL LIVER WIND
Vomiting		Dark, scanty urine	Tetany
Scanty, dark urine; possibly with burning upon urination		Tinnitus or sudden ringing; deafness	Coma in severe cases
Bitter taste in mouth		Dry mouth; thirst; bitter taste in mouth	Eyeballs rolling up
Abdominal distention		Tight neck and shoulders	
Loss of appetite		Temple headaches	
Pain, redness and swelling of the scrotum		Splitting headaches and migraines; dark scanty urine	
Vaginal discharge and itching		Insomnia; dream-disturbed sleep	
		Constipation with dry stools	
		Nosebleeds	
		Vomiting of blood	
		Coughing up of blood	
Tongue: red body with **sticky yellow coat**	**Tongue:** pale, wet, white coat	**Tongue: red body** with redder sides, dry, **yellow coat**	**Tongue: stiff,** deep red, thick yellow coat
Pulse: slippery, fast and wiry	**Pulse: deep, slow and wiry**	**Pulse:** full, wiry and fast	**Pulse:** full, fast and wiry

LIVER—EXCESS—STAGNATION PATTERNS

STAGNANT LIVER QI	STAGNANT LIVER BLOOD
Distension of hypochondrium and chest	**Dark and clotted menstrual blood**
Hypochondriac pain	Irregular menses
Depression, moodiness and mood swings	Painful menses
Sighing	Vomiting of blood
Hiccuping	Nosebleeds
Frustration; inappropriate anger	Abdominal pain
Feeling of a lump in the throat	Masses in abdomen, such as fibroids
Feeling of difficulty in swallowing	

(continued on next page)

LIVER—EXCESS—STAGNATION PATTERNS *(continued)*

STAGNANT LIVER QI	STAGNANT LIVER BLOOD
Unhappiness	
PMS tension and irritability; swollen breasts before periods; irregular periods; painful periods	
Nausea; vomiting; sour belching	
Abdominal pain	
Poor appetite	
Diarrhea or alternating diarrhea and constipation	
Churning feeling in the stomach	
Feeling of pulsation in epigastrium	
Abdominal distension	
Rumbling in intestines	
Lumps in the neck, breast, groin or flank	
Tongue: body color may be normal, or sides curled up	**Tongue: purple** with purplish spots, especially on sides
Pulse: wiry	**Pulse:** wiry

LIVER—EXCESS DEFICIENCY PATTERNS

DEFICIENT LIVER BLOOD	DEFICIENT LIVER YIN
Blurred vision	**Dry eyes**
Dull-pale complexion	**Dry throat**
Scanty periods, amenorrhea	**Night sweats**
Numbness of limbs	**Scanty menstruation;** amenorrhea
Pale lips	Muddled vision
Muscular weakness	Sallow complexion
Muscle spasms, cramps	Numbness
Withered and brittle nails	Dizziness
"Floaters" or black spots in the eyes	Blurred vision
Insomnia	Insomnia
Dizziness	Dream-disturbed sleep
	Malar flush

(continued on next page)

LIVER DEFICIENCY PATTERNS *(continued)*

DEFICIENT LIVER BLOOD	DEFICIENT LIVER YIN
	Afternoon fever
	Hot palms, soles and chest
	Nervousness
	Depression
	Nervous tension
Tongue: pale, especially on sides; dry	**Tongue: red, especially on sides; peeled**
Pulse: choppy or fine/thin	**Pulse:** wiry, fast and fine/thin, or floating and empty

LIVER—COMBINED EXCESS AND DEFICIENCY PATTERNS

DEFICIENT LIVER BLOOD GENERATING WIND	DEFICIENT LIVER YIN WITH LIVER YANG RISING AND GENERATING WIND	ARROGANT LIVER YANG
Shaking of head	**Sudden unconsciousness**	**Headache** in vertex, temples, eyes or lateral side of head
Tremors of limbs	**Convulsions**	**Irritability**
Tics	**Deviation of eye and mouth**	Dizziness
Numbness of limbs	Hemiplegia	Tinnitus
	Aphasia or difficult speech	Deafness
	Dizziness	Tight neck and shoulders
		Dry mouth and throat
		Irritability
		Insomnia
		Shouting in anger
Tongue: pale and deviated	**Tongue:** red and peeled, deviated	**Tongue:** red, especially on the sides
Pulse: choppy	**Pulse:** fast, floating and empty, or wiry and fine/thin	**Pulse:** wiry

KIDNEY DEFICIENCY PATTERNS

DEFICIENT KIDNEY YANG	DEFICIENT KIDNEY YIN	KIDNEY YIN, EMPTY FIRE BLAZING	DEFICIENT DEFICIENT KIDNEY ESSENCE	KIDNEYS FAILING TO RECEIVE QI
Cold and sore lower back	**Dry mouth at night**	**Malar flush**	**Weak knees** and legs	**Shortness of breath on exertion**
Copious, clear, pale urine	Dark, scanty urination	**Dry throat, especially at night**	**Weakness of sexual activity**	**Clear urination during asthma attack**
Cold limbs	**Night sweats**	Insomnia	**Falling hair**	**Sweating**
Fear of cold	Thin, shriveled	**Mental restlessness**	Premature aging or senility	Difficulty inhaling
Weak legs	Dry throat; thirst	**Feeling of heat in the afternoon**	**Poor bone development in children**	Rapid and weak breathing
Soreness and weakness of lower back	Dizziness; vertigo	Low-grade or afternoon fever	Softness or late closure of the fontanel	Mental listlessness
Cold and weak knees	Malar flush	Night sweats	Mental dullness or retardation in children	Cough; asthma
Bright, white or darkish face	Heat in palms, soles and chest	Scanty dark urine; blood in the urine	Bad or loose teeth	Cold limbs, especially after sweating
Lassitude, apathy	Ache in bones	Dry stools	Poor memory	Thin body
Edema of legs	Afternoon heat flushes	Soreness of the lower back	Brittle bones; softening of the bones	Soreness of the back
Poor appetite	Constipation	Excessive sexual desire	Premature graying of hair	Swelling of the face
Loose stools	Forgetfulness or poor memory	Nocturnal emissions with dreams	Soreness of the back	
Subdued, quiet manner	Tinnitus; poor hearing or deafness			
Sexual dysfunction	Weak and sore back			
Sterility or infertility	Premature ejaculation			
Premature ejaculation	Nocturnal emission			
Spermatorrhea	Little sperm			
Nocturnal emissions without dreams				
Chronic vaginal discharge or leukorrhea				
Loose teeth				

(continued on next page)

KIDNEY DEFICIENCY PATTERNS *(continued)*

DEFICIENT KIDNEY YANG	KIDNEYS FAILING TO RECEIVE QI	DEFICIENT KIDNEY YIN	DEFICIENT KIDNEY YIN, EMPTY FIRE BLAZING	DEFICIENT KIDNEY ESSENCE
Loss of hearing or deafness				
Nighttime urination				
Frequent and copious urination				
Clear urination				
Weak stream urination				
Dripping urine				
Urinary incontinence				
Tongue: pale	**Tongue:** pale	**Tongue: red, no coat,** cracks	**Tongue: red, peeled,** cracked, red tip	**Tongue:** red and peeled
Pulse: deep and slow	**Pulse:** weak, tight and deep	**Pulse:** floating, empty and fast	**Pulse:** floating, empty and fast	**Pulse:** floating and empty

YANG ORGANS
SMALL INTESTINE PATTERN

EXCESS PATTERN—HEAT IN THE SMALL INTESTINE
Abdominal pain
Tongue ulcers
Scanty, dark and painful urination; blood in urine
Mental restlessness
Pain in throat
Deafness
Heat sensation in the chest
Thirst
Tongue: red with redder swollen tip, yellow coat
Pulse: rapid and full

STOMACH PATTERNS

STOMACH EXCESS PATTERNS:				STOMACH DEFICIENCY PATTERN:
HEAT IN STOMACH	**COLD INVADING THE STOMACH**	**REBELLIOUS STOMACH QI**	**FOOD STAGNATION**	**DEFICIENT STOMACH YIN**
Burning sensation in the epigastrium	**Sudden pain in the epigastrium**	Nausea	Epigastric fullness	**Epigastric pain**
Thirst, especially for cold drinks	**Vomiting of clear fluid**	Vomiting	Sour regurgitation	**Dry mouth and throat**
Frontal headaches	Feeling cold	Hiccuping	No appetite	No appetite
Craving for cold drinks and foods	Desire for warmth, warm foods and liquids	Belching	Fullness and distension of the epigastrium which is relieved by vomiting	Fever or feeling of heat in the afternoon
Gum swelling, pain and bleeding; gum sores; mouth sores	Feeling worse after swallowing cold fluids, which are quickly vomited	Stomachache	Vomiting	Thirst but with no desire to drink or only small sips
Constant and ravenous hunger		Abdominal distension	Nausea	Feeling of fullness after eating
Constipation			Foul breath	Constipation with dry stools
Nausea; vomiting			Belching	
Sour regurgitation			Insomnia	
Feeling of dryness in mouth				
Dry lips				
Tongue: red with dry, thick, yellow coating	**Tongue:** thick, white coat	**Tongue:** no changes	**Tongue:** Thick coating, yellow or white	**Tongue: red and peeled in the center**
Pulse: full, slippery, and fast	**Pulse: deep, slow and tight**	**Pulse:** Tight in Stomach position	**Pulse:** full, slippery	**Pulse:** floating and empty in stomach position

LARGE INTESTINE—EXCESS PATTERN

DAMP HEAT IN THE LARGE INTESTINE	HEAT IN THE LARGE INTESTINE	COLD INVADING THE LARGE INTESTINE	LARGE INTESTINE COLD	COLLAPSE OF LARGE INTESTINE
Abdominal pain, worse with pressure or heat	**Dry stools**	**Sudden abdominal pain**	**Loose stools**	**Chronic diarrhea**
Diarrhea with mucus and blood in the stools	**Burning sensation in anus** and mouth	**Diarrhea with pain**	**Cold limbs**	**Prolapse of anus**
Foul odor of stools	Constipation	**Feeling of cold**	Rumbling intestines	Hemorrhoids
Burning of anus	Dry tongue	Cold sensation in abdomen	Dull abdominal pain	Tiredness after bowel movements
Scanty dark urine	Scanty dark urine		Pale urine	No appetite
Fever	Swelling of anus		Cold limbs	Mental exhaustion
Sweating which doesn't decrease with the fever				Desire to drink warm liquids and have the abdomen massaged
Thirst without desire to drink				Cold limbs
Feeling of heaviness of body and limbs				
Stuffiness of chest and epigastrium				
Tongue: red with greasy, yellow coat	**Tongue: thick yellow and dry coat**	**Tongue:** thick, white coat	**Tongue:** pale	**Tongue:** pale
Pulse: slippery and fast	**Pulse:** full and fast	**Pulse:** deep and wiry	**Pulse: fine** and deep	**Pulse:** deep ,fine and weak

GALLBLADDER PATTERNS

GALLBLADDER EXCESS PATTERN:	GALLBLADDER DEFICIENCY PATTERN:
DAMP HEAT IN THE GALLBLADDER	**DEFICIENCY OF GALLBLADDER**
Hypochondriac pain and distension	**Timidity**
Bitter taste	**Sighing**
Vomiting of bitter fluid	**Lack of courage** and initiative
Nausea	Nervousness
Jaundice or yellow complexion	Propensity to being easily startled
Poor digestion and absorption	Dizziness
Loss of appetite	Blurred vision
Nausea	
Belching	
Inability to digest fats	
Scanty and dark yellow urine	
Fever	
Thirst without desire to drink	
Tongue: thick, sticky yellow coat, either on both sides or **on the right side**	**Tongue:** pale or normal
Pulse: slippery and wiry	**Pulse:** weak

URINARY BLADDER—EXCESS PATTERNS

DAMP HEAT IN THE BLADDER	DAMP COLD IN THE BLADDER
Burning on urination	Pale and **turbid urine**
Dark yellow and/or turbid **urine**	**Feeling of heaviness in lower abdomen** and urethra
Difficult urination (stopping mid-stream)	**Difficult urination** (stopping mid-stream)
Frequent and urgent urination	Frequent and urgent urination
Blood in the urine	
Sand in the urine	
Fever	
Thirst	
Tongue: red; thick, sticky yellow coat on root with red spots	**Tongue:** white, sticky coating on root
Pulse: rapid and slippery	**Pulse:** slow and slippery

CHAPTER 7
The Process of Healing

❦

We all define health differently. Some feel a little stomach pain and think they're terribly ill. Others cheerfully live with diagnosed ulcers, as if nothing is wrong. Thus, it is difficult to define health. Traditional Chinese Medicine sees balance as the basis of health, and this is considered a dynamic process, not a static state.

Our bodies, minds and emotions constantly process our changing experiences. How well we handle these changes on all levels determines how healthy we really are. Some of these changes come externally in the form of climactic influences as our bodies adjust to climatic conditions, like sweltering heat or a blustery snowstorm. Others occur internally from harmful food and drinks, emotional issues, stress, or other miscellaneous factors that compromise the immune system. If our bodies can't cope with these conditions, illness develop (see *The Causes of Disease*).

When we maintain balance in all aspects of our lives, we keep ourselves well and prevent disease. The best way to achieve this is by eating the appropriate diet for your needs, living according to climactic influences, regulating lifestyle habits and moderating emotions. Living a balanced life does not need to be bland, boring and without risk. Rather, maintaining balance through simplicity in diet and lifestyle exercises our essential creativity as human beings.

In the West most of us grow up believing what we eat, drink, feel, express and do has little effect on our health, and then wonder why we "get" frequent colds or flu, chronic cough, low energy, high blood pressure, or recurring bladder infections. Instead, we undergo diagnostic tests, take the resulting prescribed medicines and hope for the best. This approach treats the body mechanistically, like a broken machine needing repair. As a dynamic, complex interrelated whole, the body is quite unlike a machine; treating it that way is like mistaking the carburetor for the car, or a single plant for the garden.

Thus, modern medicine is aimed at *curing*, not *healing*. When we take medications or herbs to eliminate our symptoms, we are looking for a cure, a quick fix. Healing is a deeper, more involved process that takes time, energy and effort (relative to a cure, at least). Healing treats not just the symptoms themselves, but also what created them in the first place: their root cause. Healing can delve to the core of your being and involve all aspects of yourself—mind, emotions and spirit as well as body.

INHERITED CONSTITUTION

Admittedly, making changes is more difficult for some of us than for others. On the other hand, many of us get sick more easily than do others, and so we are confronted repeatedly by our limitations. Frequently people

181

ask me: Why do I get sick after eating just a few cookies when my friend, or even Uncle George, can freely consume as much candy, sodas, alcohol or coffee as he wants? There are several answers to this complex question. First, are these people really well? Referring to our definition of health and wellness, do we agree that popping pills to feel well constitutes health? Do we consider those all-too-frequent outbursts of anger, depression or compulsive and addictive patterns of behavior to indicate wellness?

Perhaps we don't accept the way we physically or emotionally feel after eating a single fruit-juice sweetened cookie, while Uncle George doesn't recognize that eating two hamburgers, four beers, two cups of coffee and several pieces of cake causes his acid indigestion, recurring headaches, chronic tiredness or disturbing outbursts of anger. Nor does he consider these as signs of sickness!

The body is affected from this type of excessive behavior, however, and it ultimately does manifest illness. Seemingly "healthy" people who suddenly have cancer are examples. Because cancer and other degenerative diseases take years to develop, it's hard for us to connect disease with the poor habits or lifestyle factors that created it.

Another reason Uncle George can seemingly indulge without consequence may be due to his strong constitution. Each of us inherits a unique body that represents our potential for withstanding disease and sustaining life's stresses. Health and disease are part of the evolutionary process: balance is individual for all. We each inherit health imbalances and some of us help them progress. Eventually, each of us reaches a point where our bodies cannot sustain any more indulgences. Something must give. For some, this occurs later in life, for others, earlier.

While constitution affects health and longevity, it's not everything. Too often I have seen self-proclaimed and apparently healthy people suddenly die of a stroke or some terminal illness while seemingly weak and sensitive individuals who closely heed what they eat or do, live long, fruitful lives. In fact, it is more often the beef-eating, coffee-drinking, beer-swilling and sugar-addicted Uncle Georges who suddenly die of "unexpected" strokes, heart attacks or cancer.

It behooves those of us with strong constitutions to moderate our habits and those of us with weak ones to build ourselves so that we pass strength, rather than weakness, on to our children. When we don't, our children or grandchildren get sick earlier in life, or develop childhood diseases, such as immune weakness, asthma, or diabetes. If we understand this, perhaps we'll be motivated to make the needed changes to heal ourselves and strengthen our bodies.

Learn to recognize and honor any personal limits as extensions of your uniqueness. If tempted to explore and venture beyond your boundaries, recognize the early signs and take appropriate compensatory measures. For instance, if you stay up late at a party and enjoy food indiscretions, then the next several days may require more rest and a stricter diet than normal in counterbalance. Or if feeling on the verge of a cold, narrow your diet to only balancing foods for awhile, get more rest and curtail extra-curricular activities. When the cold or flu threat is gone, then broaden your dietary and lifestyle choices. In this way you can enjoy your desires and still maintain balance.

THE SEARCH FOR HEALTH

For those of us frequently falling ill, the search for balance needs a different approach than popping a pill and hoping the problem goes away. First, we need to recognize that something we are doing and/or ingesting is causing our illness and secondly, we must actively and personally undertake the appropriate measures for getting well.

This method goes beyond taking medications to patch symptoms, since drugs don't eliminate the original, or root, causes of illness but disturb the body's chemistry. For instance, antibiotics destroy important beneficial bacteria, leading to weak assimilation, elimination, immunity and consequently, a variety of illnesses ranging from chronic fatigue, allergies and

Factors That Weaken the Body and Predispose it to Illness

(How many of the following are factors in your life?)

- ↪ refined foods like white flour, white sugar, white rice, white pasta, refined salt
- ↪ chemicals and preservatives in food
- ↪ extensive use of canned foods
- ↪ frequent indulgence in "junk foods"
- ↪ polluted air and water
- ↪ proximity to major electrical wiring or power plants
- ↪ excessive noise
- ↪ stress-causing situations or conditions
- ↪ job stress or incompatibility
- ↪ relationship problems
- ↪ proximity to color TV and computer monitors
- ↪ extensive computer use without proper screening of the monitor
- ↪ living near toxic waste dumps
- ↪ frequent use of antibiotics
- ↪ synthetic fibers in clothing and home and office furnishings
- ↪ fast-paced life
- ↪ carcinogenic pollutants from materials built into the home or office
- ↪ side effects of drugs
- ↪ mercury amalgam fillings in teeth

How to Get Sick

There is so much focus on what one should do in order to stay well that I sometimes find switching the tables helps people gain a different perspective on how their habits invite sickness into their lives. Thus, I offer here the easiest ways to get sick. Have fun!

1. Eat all the ice cream, candy, pastries, desserts, caffeine and chocolate that you want, whenever you want.

2. Drink all the iced cold drinks that you desire.

3. Work all the time and definitely don't stop to rest or eat. Or if you must eat, be sure to do so while working, doing business, at your desk, standing up, or on the run.

4. Drink caffeine to wake up in the morning and to keep you going throughout the day.

5. Drink alcohol to relax every night.

6. Don't pay attention to your emotions, but assiduously ignore and stuff them.

7. Be sure not to laugh. Instead, feel resentful, bitter and critical. Definitely worry about everyone and everything.

8. Don't follow your heart's desires but follow your "shoulds." Avoid everything you really want to do and follow everyone else's opinions and advice.

9. Avoid making any changes that would bring you greater health, happiness and joy.

10. Sit all day and only travel in vehicles. Whatever you do, don't walk or exercise. Or if you must, exercise strenuously and to exhaustion.

11. Don't accept yourself, who you are, your unique body health needs or inner dreams.

12. Ignore any signs or symptoms indicating health imbalances. Wait until they are serious health issues before you seek help.

13. Work all the time and be productive. Don't stop to eat, rest, play, sleep or creatively express, or if you must, only do so quickly and then immediately return to work.

14. Don't follow your creative urges, but keep busy with work. There's always time for it another day (year…).

multiple food sensitivities, to premenstrual syndrome and Candida. Rather, identify what is causing your illness and correct those causative factors.

For true healing to occur, therefore, it is necessary to treat the root causes of illness and limit—or eliminate—the many ways we make ourselves sick. Diseases are simply the result of living out of harmony with our natural flow, such as inadequate sleep, poor dietary habits, overuse of harmful substances (sugar, alcohol, drugs and tobacco, for example), or unfulfilling jobs. It is easier to blame our discomforts and diseases on external causes rather than go to bed earlier, eat better meals, cut back on sugar, alcohol or tobacco, or alter careers. Yet, these are the very changes needed, and when done, many people "miraculously heal" their annoying conditions.

Often we ignore changing those things we know make us sick. For instance, despite having chronic fatigue or skin blemishes, we continue abusing sweets or eating chocolate. Even the threat of death is, in many cases, an insufficient motivator, such as continuing to smoke even though we know it causes lung cancer. Ultimately, we must choose between changing our habits or experiencing sickness. Illness-causing habits are not easy to change yet more serious conditions will occur if they aren't. What seems expedient to ignore in the present may cause more grief, pain and expense in the long run.

DESIRE TO BE HEALED

Many of us need to delve deeply into our whole beings to attain true healing. This means being honest with ourselves about our habits and underlying motives for getting sick. Paradoxically, many of us are not even sure that we want to feel better. Our illness may provide us with something that we can't have in any other way, such as attention, love, avoidance of situations, work, certain people, on doing things we don't want, indecision about something, or fear of confronting unresolved childhood issues.

We often use illness as an excuse to cover hidden motives. Despite our proclaimed intentions to heal, we may hide the true reasons for staying sick. For example, we may thrive on the sympathy we receive from others when we're ill. We may avoid going to hated work or school by being unwell. Thus, it's important to examine whether sickness is simply an excuse for attention, a poor substitute for love and affection, or satisfying some other need.

When we hide our reasons for staying ill, we often sabotage our efforts to get well. Rather than taking our herbs three times a day, we forget and take them sporadically. Instead of eliminating caffeine from our diets, we follow Uncle George who says that two cups of coffee every morning couldn't possibly cause any harm. Rather than going to bed by 11 PM, we continually stay up until 1 AM or later, saying that tomorrow night we'll definitely start going to bed earlier. All of these are tactics our hidden motives use to keep us sick.

For the healing process to occur then, we need to truly want to get well and willingly make the necessary changes. There are several questions we can ask ourselves which, when answered honestly, can reveal if we have hidden motives for staying ill (see the Self-Inquiry Questions and Emotions Checklist). Writing these questions and your answers in a journal may help reveal interesting understandings (refer to the section on Journal Writing in *Home Therapies*, for guidelines). As well, it may be beneficial to discuss these issues with a close and trusted friend, or speak them aloud into a tape recorder when alone.

While on one hand we frequently deny the true reasons we are sick, on the other we often claim our illnesses as a part of who we are, even putting them on the pedestal of our lives. It is important to not label ourselves or accept others' labels of us. Many people talk as if they proudly own their disease, saying things such as, "I'm asthmatic," or "No, I can't do that because of my chronic fatigue." This is a perfect way to continue your disease process and not heal. Because language is powerful, speak the truth you want to experience, especially in regards to your health.

Self-Inquiry Questions

Do I *truly* want to get better?

Am I ready to heal, to feel well and different than I am now?

And am I *willing* to do what is needed to make the necessary changes?

What would I do *without* this problem?

What would I *like* to do? Be? What are my *true* life dreams?

Do I try to sabotage my healing process? If so, why?

Why do I continue my harmful habits?

What do they give me that I don't get otherwise?

Do I have enough love in my life?

Do I get enough attention in my life?

Am I satisfied emotionally? Spiritually? Physically? Creatively? Mentally?

How important am I to me?

Do I feel good about myself? My life?

Do I allow the world to control and dominate me?

What unresolved issues from childhood or other times of life do I carry?

Do I like my work or my job?

Am I happy with my career?

Are my relationships satisfying?

What is my true heart's desire?

What is it I really want to do?

What do I need?

What changes can I make to follow my heart's desire?

What changes can I make to bring more satisfaction into my life?

What can I do to assure I follow the necessary changes for improving my health?

What specific help can I seek to make these changes?

Emotions Checklist

The following can be useful indicators for underlying emotional issues needing exploration in order to heal. As well, they can indicate imbalances in the body through their inner connections (refer to *The Causes of Disease*). Journal write on the following applicable questions. Do I:

- ↪ Have difficulty being present when another person is expressing his/her emotions?
- ↪ Have difficulty expressing my own emotions?
- ↪ Have difficulty expressing one particular emotion?
- ↪ Have a particular body part that becomes tense, tight or uncomfortable when a specific emotion or situation arises?
- ↪ Have a particular symptom arise when a specific emotion or situation occurs?
- ↪ Have a habit or behavior pattern regularly arise during emotional situations?
- ↪ Experience a flooding of thoughts, memories or fantasies during emotional situations, or when doing nothing? What are they?
- ↪ Experience 'no feelings' during emotional situations?
- ↪ Overreact to situations?
- ↪ Feel like a pressure cooker about to explode?
- ↪ Have difficulty laughing at myself?
- ↪ Feel trapped in an emotional situation?
- ↪ Have a body part that I'm out of touch with?
- ↪ Have a specific person, place or thing I can't stand seeing or being around?
- ↪ Spend most of my time in one particular emotion?

Healing with the Emotions

It is valuable to learn that our emotions, attitudes and self-perceptions are often physiologically rather than emotionally based. When Organs are imbalanced, their corresponding emotions either become exaggerated or repressed (refer to The Emotions in *The Causes of Disease*). Thus, when we heal the Organs, their corresponding emotion diminishes. These emotions may be used for healing in two ways: by cultivating virtues and by providing the Organs with their essential needs.

In ancient TCM times, physicians worked with patients to change their vices (adverse emotions) into virtues, called "culturing the virtue." You can do this as well by focusing on the corresponding virtues (beneficial emotions) to your excessively expressed or repressed emotions (the vices). Further, each Organ benefits from certain activities and qualities of being. (See the table, Healing with the Emotions).

METAPHORS FOR HEALING

Illness can be a useful metaphor for sleuthing what is actually going on deep inside of you. Both where it is located and the illness itself can give clues to underlying issues needing attention or correction. For example, poor digestion may actually be due to an inability to handle, or "digest", certain things in your life. When these "indigestible" issues or activities are identified and corrected, physical digestion usually improves. As another example, frequent bladder infections often signal the person is "pissed off" at certain people or situations. When these angry feelings are identified and released, the chronic bladder infections don't recur.

Louise Hay has done extensive work with metaphors and healing and written several books based on her experiences (refer to *Bibliography*). Below are a few to consider in your own healing process. These are not written in stone as the only possibilities; they are sug-

---

Metaphors for Healing

Body Parts:

Ears and eyes: that which we take in from the outside world and how we use it

Shoulders: taking on other's problems; not minding your own business; carrying too many responsibilities ("carrying the world on your shoulders")

Lungs: what we take in from the world, the ability to receive

Digestion: how we digest what we take in from the world

Thighs: childhood traumas

Knees: what stops you from moving or makes you bow or kneel to something?

Ankles and other joints: your ability to be flexible in life

Feet: energies being grounded

Skin: emotions erupting

Illnesses:

High blood pressure: succumbing to pressures

Diarrhea: difficulty collecting your energy

Bladder infections: "pissed off" about something or someone

Cough: rejecting something unwanted

Poor digestion: difficulty taking something in ("digesting" or assimilating something)

Asthma: congested life with difficulty in receiving and letting go; fear around loss

Frequent urination: wanting to empty out

Migraines: frustrated; plans not being made or followed

Fibroids: knotted emotions; what wants to be birthed?

Bulimia: what wants purging from your life (for example, a controlling, demanding person or situation)?

Stagnant Blood: unresolved issues

Dampness: unfinished lessons; issues you can't let go

HEALING WITH THE EMOTIONS

ORGAN	ESSENTIAL NEED	VICE/INJURING QUALITIES	VIRTUE/HEALING QUALITIES
HEART	Love, joy, beauty	Over-excitement, over-achieving, excess joy, fright (shock), sadness, unhappiness, excessive laughter, talking, partying and reading, excessive worrying/thinking, fear, anxiety, shock	Compassion, caring for yourself, following your heart's desires and spiritual path, love, working with your emotions, psychotherapy, joy, beauty, enthusiasm, joy of life, open-heartedness, laughter
LUNGS	Confidence, time and space	Exposure to cold, grief, sadness, criticism (from others or self), shallow breathing (you don't give yourself enough breath), unworthiness (don't feel worthy of living/breathing), reclining excessively, not living in the present but holding on to past sadness & hurts (pain in the present = hurt; pain in the past = anger; anger directed at self = guilt)—get the old hurt stuff out!	Protect yourself from cold (especially back of neck), conscientiousness, feeling good about one's self, creating room for yourself—enough time & space, confidence (its more important to act confident than to be confident), gratitude (it gets you breathing and allows things to come to you), being in the present
LIVER	Relaxation, peace, herbs	Anger, frustration, resentment, irritability, impatience, depression, annoyance, timidity, cowardice, excessive reading, repressing or stuffing your emotions, excessive and prolonged anger	Kindness, forgiveness, respect, esteem, service, benevolence, decisiveness, a healthy drive, creative expression, physical movement, appropriate emotional expression and release, naturally induced altered states, bravery, assertiveness, courageousness, herbs and medicines
SPLEEN	Nurturance, nutrition, giving to others	Obsession, worry, pensiveness, confusion, brooding, always caring for others without getting the care you need, dwelling on the past, eating on the run, while doing business or standing up, poor diet (especially excessive intake of cold and damp foods and drinks) and excessive sitting	Empathy, centeredness, right action, instinct, intuition, nurturance (being nurtured on all levels), good nutrition and giving yourself what you need (don't expect others to give it to you), quit giving it away (i.e., nurture yourself!)
KIDNEYS	Rest, quiet, sleep, meditation, drinking water	Fear, paranoia, worry, fright, apprehension, mistrustfulness, stubbornness, procrastination, excessive weight lifting, sitting on damp ground	Napping, meditation, resting, sleep, drinking water, cultivating wisdom (knowledge plus experience), and holding to a purpose in life—being resolute, determined, firm and enduring

gestions to trigger your own revelations. Make your personal connections and derive insights based on your unique body and individual needs.

DIALOGUE WITH YOUR ILLNESS

Sometimes it can be difficult to discover what underlying emotional issues or metaphors are connected with our illness. A useful technique I have found to work with such concerns is the *dialoguing process*. This is a simple method of "talking" with the diseased organ or condition in your body, either out loud to a tape recorder, or through journal writing (it must be one of these, for the process doesn't work if you just imagine it in your mind, internally).

By "talking" with the disease or illness, I mean asking it questions and then writing (or verbally saying) the responses. Possible questions to ask your ailment are: "Why are you here?" "What are you trying to tell (teach) me?" "What do you need in order to heal?" "What am I doing to cause you?" "What changes should I make to feel well again?"

Whatever questions you ask, sit silently a moment and listen. Then record the response you receive immediately. Don't try to make sense of it right then, or edit it with doubtful thoughts. Just let it flow as it comes. Then respond back to the answer with another question or comment. Listen and record the answering response again. Continue this process until it feels complete, which is usually obvious.

While the skeptic in each of us might balk at this strange idea, it is really a quite powerful and effective process (and is used in psychological therapies, such as psychosynthesis). Everyone I do this with receives some sort of response. Call it your own mind answering if you will, but the responses are generally quite wise and useful. You will be quite amazed at the experience. For journaling help, refer to Journal Writing in *Home Therapies*.

"GOING THROUGH IT"

Healing the root cause of an illness takes time and patience. Using alternative methods is usually slower than "magic bullet" cures. Yet, they provide a deeper healing approach with long-lasting change rather than a Band-Aid that masks. Because it is slow, we can lose confidence and trust in the process; we get impatient because we've been taught to expect fast results.

Therefore, it's necessary to remain confident and positive in the face of what may be minor "setbacks." Part of healing is elimination, and for most, this is a necessary step before the stage of rebuilding can occur. Just as it may be difficult to let go of old debilitating patterns, jobs or relationships, so it may be uncomfortable and inconvenient to alter patterns of sickness, old thoughts and emotions.

Certain types of elimination may occur during this healing process. Termed a "healing crisis," it manifests externally as an acute illness, such as a cold, fever, diarrhea, minor skin eruptions and other forms of elimination. It can also evoke emotional responses such as vulnerability, fear and anger. It usually comes quickly and lasts a short time. Afterwards, you feel better than you did before it began. A healing crisis is actually a very positive sign of improvement. When such symptoms arise they shouldn't be stopped, but dealt with as part of the entire healing process through using herbs and nutrition.

THE LAW OF CURE

Sometimes the healing crisis manifests as symptoms of an old illness. When this happens, it is called the Law of Cure. Samuel Hahnemann observed this law in the 1700s when founding his healing approach, homeopathy. The Law of Cure describes the healing progression: the body heals its most recent disease experienced first, then it works back through other diseases until the oldest one is healed. Also, symptoms first occur on the surface of the body and move from the top of the body down. Thus, the various symptoms that arise reflect the healing stage the body is experiencing.

For example, when naturally healing recurring bronchitis, you may experience a renewal of teenage chronic sore throat for a period of time. Then you might see your childhood eczema return. The eczema may start on the arms and then move down to the legs. If you persevere with natural remedies and appropriate diet, your body gathers enough strength and energy to throw it off entirely. These symptoms eventually disappear and a healing of your chronic bronchitis occurs. Through this process you heal the root cause of these conditions. However, if you return to your poor eating and living habits after healing, you will most likely get sick again. In order to distinguish a healing crisis from a genuine sickness, there are several guidelines. Refer to *Healing Crisis Characteristics* for these.

Other people experience what they think is a healing crisis when actually they take too many herbs or have minor allergic reactions to them. This is also important to differentiate from a true healing crisis. Overdosing with herbs or having allergic reactions usually appears soon after starting the herbs, and the symptoms don't let up after the "crisis" occurs. A healing crisis, on the other hand, takes longer to appear, the problem occurs for a short period amidst general improvement and the symptoms disappear after the healing is complete.

When going through the healing process it is most important to be gentle with yourself. Don't abandon play and humor. Remember how Norman Cousins literally laughed his cancer away by immersing himself in old comic movies. Note how Dr. Bernie Siegal helps many terminally ill people recover by learning to forgive themselves and renew their commitment to joy and love. Louise Hay helps AIDS patients live longer and have better lives, with some experiencing miraculous cures, by teaching them to develop positive self-images through the use of affirmations. These positive methods can definitely help make aches and pains easier to live with during recovery.

It's important to remember that natural healing takes time and effort; it is not a quick cure or fix, yet it yields longer lasting results as it aims at eliminating the cause of disease, rather than acting as a palliative to symptoms. Above all, don't berate yourself for being ill. Remember, life is a "terminal condition"; it is not a question of right and wrong, but of growing and learning.

Healing Crisis Characteristics

1. A healing crisis usually occurs in the midst of much greater improvement. Examine all symptoms experienced and look for genuine indications of health, such as increased energy and vitality. If these are also present, the disease symptom is part of the healing crisis.

2. A healing crisis is of relatively short duration and comes and leaves quickly.

3. The particular sickness or emotion expressed may occur for the last time. Old physical or emotional symptoms eliminated through healing crises usually don't return again.

4. Normally you'll feel better after a healing crisis than you did before it began.

5. Symptoms of old illnesses that you experienced during your teenage or childhood years may suddenly arise during a healing crisis.

6. Healing crisis symptoms usually move from the inside of the body outward, with surface ailments appearing first, such as skin eruptions, colds or flu. They also usually start from the top (head) and move downward to the lower body, so that a rash reappearing from childhood might first appear on the face, then move to the legs, disappearing as it goes.

HEALTH AND HEALING ROUTINES

Establishing a healing or health maintenance routine is incredibly supportive and beneficial to the healing process. It also serves as a preventative measure that over time, may become a way of life. Many cultures have specific living and eating routines or rituals for daily health. For example, the Chinese do Tai Chi in parks in the morning and the Indian yogis do Netibol before morning meditation (see *Home Therapies*). The ancient Egyptians, Greeks and Maltese built dream temples where the ill dreamed their cures, or became healed in their dreams. Many cultures pilgrimaged to sacred sites as a healing process.

Most of us have been cut off from such ancestral, ethnic and cultural roots. Reuniting with what is of value in our past heals tremendously. Rekindle a healthy lifestyle by creating your own daily routine based upon your personal needs. As a basic guideline, I suggest you include starting the day with a spiritual focus such as prayer or meditation, then do some form of exercise (such as aerobics, yoga, or Tai Chi), plan food for the day, and set out and/or prepare the day's herbs. Then, as the day progresses, these essential healing elements are not only handled, but also your food and herbs are easily incorporated into the rest of your busy day.

For instance, I find that if I plan and start my evening meal in the morning, then it takes little time or effort to complete when dinnertime arrives. If I don't do this, then in the late afternoon when I am often the busiest juggling home, business, children and answering the door and phone, I don't have time to make a good meal. I am also so hungry that I have little patience to prepare the food my family and I really need. Instead, I fix something quick. I find many patients learn these poor habits as well.

Over time these meals aren't nearly as satisfying or healing as those made with care, imagination and preparation. Cooking wholesome and nourishing food takes some time and effort. Popping a frozen dinner in the oven or microwave may be quick and easy, but it usually lacks the many essential and vital nutrients our bodies need. We eventually feel less energy, strength and ability to cope with life's demands. This is especially true if we've only had a quick cereal and sandwich previously in the day.

If you are single, or used to cooking for large families over the years, you may lack incentive to carefully cook meals for yourself. This situation can be improved if you take 1-2 hours two times a week to plan upcoming meals. During these times you can also cook a pot of rice (or other grain), a big pot of beans and a soup stock. These three items can be combined in many ways to prepare quick and delicious meals. You can easily add vegetables and more protein later.

Our mental state when we cook food is also important. In some way, we eat the thoughts and emotions of the cook. If angry or upset, the cook might hold the salt or spice shaker too long over the food, or if distracted, the food may get overcooked. If the cook is sad and lonely, then food may be made too sweet, in search for the needed emotional nourishment. Thus, how we feel when cooking food affects what we eat.

I have discovered that eating a full meal (like dinner) at lunchtime, or even breakfast, is tremendously health supportive for many people. Vegetables, grains, legumes and protein give us much more energy and strength to handle busy days than simple cereals, or toast, bagels, doughnuts or muffins. Each person's needs are different this way, yet, many find that switching to a more complete meal at breakfast and/or lunch makes all the difference in their energy and health.

Similarly, those who experience weak or poor digestion may need to carefully plan their meals throughout the day. Often symptoms of gas, bloating, abdominal distension, the need to sleep after meals, insomnia, or restless sleep occurs because we ate too late in the evening and went to bed on a full stomach. Over time, not only is sleep poor, but digestion becomes further impaired. For good digestion, assimilation and sleep, therefore, it is best to complete the evening meal at least three hours before going to sleep, usually by 7:00 PM. These benefits are further enhanced if this meal is light.

Since health and well-being are tremendously affected by the food we eat, it is quite useful to keep a **food diary** during the healing process. Many people find this an invaluable tool in discovering which foods cause their health problems and what ones are missing from the diet. It also teaches which meals work best for you and why and under what conditions you eat certain foods. Most importantly, it helps correlate foods eaten with your symptoms over time (we often don't feel the effects of many foods until 1-3 days later).

To keep a food diary, write down everything you eat on a daily basis. Include how much of each food you eat and when you eat it. Also note how you feel throughout the day, recording your symptoms when they occur. Review the diary after the first week, then alter your diet as you see necessary and keep the diary another week. If you follow your insights from doing this, eventually you will learn much about healing yourself with food.

How we eat is also important to health. Our digestion works best when we eat in a calm, slow manner. Eating standing up, in the car, or on the run creates bloating, nervousness, gas and, ultimately, poor digestion. Praying or meditating briefly before meals is calming to mind and body and slows us down. Rather than sleeping or working immediately after meals, it is more healthful to sit for 15 minutes and then take a relaxed walk.

Laughing and singing before and after meals enhance digestive fires and strengthen metabolism. Sitting with your legs folded under you (as the Japanese sit to eat) promotes digestion and alleviates gas and bloatedness. You can eat in this posture, or sit this way after the meal for 15-20 minutes.

It is also best to eat only when hungry. True hunger means the previous meal is digested. Likewise, avoiding between-meal snacks allows the digestive organs a rest. It also increases your appetite for healthy foods at mealtime. If you find snacks are frequently necessary, you are either not eating sufficient protein, or what you are eating is insubstantial for your needs. When the proper balance of protein, carbohydrates and fats is achieved, then snacks or another meal isn't needed for five or so hours afterwards (of course there are exceptions, such as strenuous exercising, poor metabolism, diabetes or emotional upset, which demand more nutrition).

It has been scientifically demonstrated that eating less is the best tonic for longevity. Overeating uses more energy to digest food than we ultimately receive (it also depletes and stagnates digestive energy). As we age we need less and less food. Yet, because we often eat for stimulation and sentimental reasons rather than for nutrition, we usually overindulge in food when under stress. It is important to determine the difference between a desire for food and a real physical need.

For good digestion, avoid extreme foods, such as those that are either too hot or too cold, or overly greasy or dry. Preferably, all food should be fresh rather than frozen or canned. Likewise, it is best to freshly prepare each meal before eating to receive the maximum amount of nutrients. Frequently eating reheated and canned foods causes symptoms such as gas, bloatedness and poor energy. Ideally, don't eat food that is more than two days old.

Overall, the most important thing to remember about food and eating is to be fully present with your food and give thanks for it. When you do this, you'll become more conscious of what you're eating and if it's proper for you. You'll also become aware of your eating habits and know what needs altering for good health.

Going to bed by 11 PM each evening is another important health habit to form. In Chinese medicine, the Wood element rules the body between 11 PM to 3 AM. This is the time the Liver is most active in its functions of storing and cleansing the Blood. If awake and active at this time, the Liver has less energy to perform these tasks. Many of us find we wake up refreshed and lively when we go to sleep by 11 PM, but don't feel as well if we go to bed later, even if we get the same amount of sleep. It is not always the length of sleeping time that matters, but the quality. This is affected by the time we go to bed.

Where we live and work also affects our health. Our local environment, climate, house and work place all influence how we feel. For example, those with Excess Dampness and symptoms of asthma, bronchitis, allergies, bloatedness, water retention and lack of taste should not live or work in damp locations, such as near the sea, rainy climates, or in concrete rooms or underground buildings, since all of these create more Dampness in the body. Instead, these individuals should live in dry, hot, sunny, even desert-type areas, houses above ground and upper stories of work buildings.

Likewise, those with too much Dryness and Heat dislike hot locations and feel better in wet, moist and cool areas, such as basements, the sea or places where it snows or rains frequently. As well, they should avoid extremely heated buildings, rooms at the top of buildings where the heat rises, the desert, sunbathing and other hot, dry activities or locations.

To live in environments which match your needs may mean moving or making a change in job locations. Even Western medicine often recommends those with severe allergies to live in desert areas. Usually we don't need to make such radical changes, but it's worth the effort if your environment negatively influences your health.

The seasons also affect how we feel. Living according to their various differences can tremendously influence health and illness. Each season requires different dressing, eating and lifestyle habits to stay in harmony and balance. Because this is so important, it is covered more extensively in *Living with the Seasons*.

The body undergoes biorhythm cycles during which certain activities are optimal for specific times each day. For example, defecation naturally occurs during Large Intestine time in the early morning hours between 5 AM and 7 AM. Eating a nutritious breakfast during Stomach-Spleen time between 7 AM and 11 AM in the morning when it digests most easily. Going to bed by 11 PM creates the most regenerative sleep since it is during Wood time, 11 to 3 AM, that the Liver cleans and replenishes the Blood.

Similarly, organic imbalances and weaknesses are likely to appear at certain times, making the body's biorhythms a useful diagnostic tool as well. For instance, it is common for people with Deficient Kidneys Qi to feel tired in the late afternoon, 3-7 PM, Urinary Bladder and

TCM BODY BIORHYTHMS

TIME	ORGANS	CORRESPONDING ACTIVITIES
3—5 AM	Lungs	Rise; perform breathing exercises and meditation/contemplation
5—7 AM	Large Intestine	Empty bowels; exercise
7—9 AM	Stomach	Eat a hearty breakfast, relax 15 minutes, walk 15 minutes after
9—11 AM	Spleen	Start work day
11 AM—1 PM	Heart	Eat lunch, relax 15 minutes, walk 15 minutes, rest 15—30 minutes
1—3 PM	Small Intestine	Return to work
3—5 PM	Urinary Bladder	Take a break, rest 15—30 minutes, light exercise, light snack
5—7 PM	Kidneys	Stop work
7—9 PM	Pericardium	Eat dinner, relax 15 minutes, walk 15 minutes, visit with people
9—11 PM	Triple Warmer	Visit with friends, wind down the evening, go to bed
11 PM—1 AM	Gallbladder	Be asleep no later than 11 PM
1—3 AM	Liver	Sleep

Kidney time. Further, people with Lung ailments or weakness often wake between 3-5 AM with breathing difficulties, or inability to go back to sleep. For more specifics, see the chart TCM Body Biorythms.

FEED THE COW SO THE SPIRIT CAN SOAR

An old Chinese adage states, "Feed the cow so the spirit can soar." While this may sound strange at first, it brings useful insight on further reflection. Cows need specific treatment in order to give the best milk possible. They must be milked at regular hours, put to pasture and brought in at certain times, given high quality feed and undergo frequent checkups. When this is followed, milk is rich and tasty; when disrupted, milk isn't as high quality. Likewise, each of us has specific needs that when supplied, the body and mind are happy and healthy, which allows our spirits to soar and accomplish their intended life goals.

What are *your* cow needs? What wants altering, regulating and/or healing in your life so *your* spirit can soar? Determining this demands reflection in all areas: eating, sleeping, supplementation, exercise, creative expression, emotional factors, relationships, career, spirituality and so on. For true healing to occur, all areas need tending and potential alteration. Create a healing plan based on these factors and stick to it. You'll be amazed at the outcome, not only in how you feel, but also with how freely your spirit flies as a result.

As well, it is extremely important to listen to your heart and follow your dreams. As Joseph Campbell so often said, "Follow your bliss." Doing so opens the heart, bringing important nourishment to the entire body. Dreams and passions are "cow" needs vital to a healthy existence, and not following them is the root cause of illness in many.

Too many of us work at jobs we hate, stay in unfulfilling or abusive relationships, loose contact with loved ones, or continuously postpone accomplishing desired creative projects or performing personal expressions. "I'll do that next week," or "Some day I'll get around to that," are typical words we tell ourselves. Delaying or ignoring our passions is a major reason so many suffer from heart disease, the number one killer in the West. Closing off our heart's dreams, desires and passions definitely leads to heart conditions. There is no better time than now to do what you love. As the ecstatic poet Rumi said: "There are a thousand ways to kiss the ground. Let the beauty you love, be what you do." I can't think of a better way to put it than that!

Most of us believe that we must be fully well and whole in order to follow our life's work and follow our dreams. Thus, we constantly strive to attain Perfect Health, and if we don't, we despair and fall back on old habits, thinking none of this "stuff" works for us anyway. However, there is really no such thing as Perfect Health; rather, when the body is *completely* in balance, all the elements comprising it separate and we die.

Thus, life is actually a continuing process of imbalance, or friction, change and adaptation. While we can't achieve Perfect Health, we can strive for our own personal highest possible state of health or balance. This means many of us may always live with diabetes, weak eyesight or infertility. Some conditions just cannot be healed (or eliminated) by physical means. However, it's still possible to lesson their impact on our daily lives and feel better in the process. It is the endeavor to feel the best we can with the bodies we have that constitutes true health.

CHAPTER 8
Treatment of Specific Conditions

We are a disease-based society in the West. We happily eat and do what we want, ignoring our bodies until something happens we can no longer ignore. Then we run to the doctor, expecting him/her to give a magic bullet and make us well. This is what most people ask of doctors: "Just make my problem go away so I can get on with my life." While drugs alleviate symptoms, they cause side effects, and the untreated root cause eventually appears as deeper, chronic issues. No wonder we eventually hear, "live with it, there's nothing more we can do, "or" you're crazy—go seek psychiatric help."

The reason this occurs is because Western medicine focuses on discrete, individual parts of a person and disease. This provides a useful, but limited perspective of the causes and treatment of illness. In contrast, TCM treats the whole person, seeing every aspect as interrelated and interdependent. Thus, diseases that are "incurable" in Western medicine become treatable in TCM because more possibilities are present, and these are also viewed from a broader perspective.

Of course, this holistic approach demands more of the patient—self-responsibility and awareness (this is also true of other wholistic healing systems, such as Ayurvedic, Tibetan and Unani Tib medicines, for instance). When taking responsibility for our bodies, we learn our individual health needs and disease prevention techniques. Ideally, this is what we should be ask-ing of our doctors—"Tell me what to do, how to live and what to eat so I can stay healthy."

In fact, the royal herbalist physicians in China were not paid if the emperor got sick. Rather, the healer was remunerated to keep the Emperor well. This shifts the focus of medicine to prevention rather than treatment of disease. There is a world of difference in this seemingly simple change.

This chapter is offered, therefore, to assist your personal search for health, both through identifying what is occurring in your body as well as what to do about it. Different than most herb books, here I'm going beyond what herbals usually offer and revealing advanced herbalist medicine practices. This is because most people have complicated conditions that need more than simple remedies. The roots of herbal medicine are old and deep, and it's just because herbs have been understood and used this way for so long that it is still so effective today.

HOW TO USE THIS CHAPTER

When determining your own health plan, begin your healing process with food changes, since an appropriate diet can clear up many, if not all, of your symptoms (refer to *The Energy of Food*, for specifics). Include herbs next, since as special foods they speed your healing course and correct the original underlying cause of the ailments. Then focus on lifestyle habits and emotional, mental and spiritual issues, because most chronic conditions that don't clear with diet or herbs are usually due to one of these, or to an inherited condition that cannot be completely healed with physical approaches.

In determining which herbs to use, start with the formulas or remedies given under the General Treatment section, particularly if dealing with a more simple case or issue. If you don't experience desired results and/or your condition is more complicated, then gather more diagnostic information by answering the questions in the sidebar, Symptoms to Consider. Next, look to one of the pattern tables included in most Sections (you may want to refer to TCM Fundamentals in *The Energy of Illness*, to brush up on terms such as Heat, Dampness, Liver, Blood and so forth).

Be sure to check all the patterns to find which best fit your symptoms. It may be helpful to first determine your condition according to the Eight Principles, as described in Identifying Illness, in *The Energy of Illness*, to see if it is External or Internal, Excess or Deficient and Hot or Cold in energy. Then read all the appropriate patterns and see which pattern(s) your symptoms are most like. You won't have all the symptoms given, and you may even have symptoms that are not listed. But usually you'll have two to three in one category that will identify its presence.

If there are multiple patterns involved in your condition, treat by combining formulas from all appropriate patterns. Some of the most powerful formulas mix heating and cooling, tonifying and stagnation-moving herbs together. If you experience more than one health issue at a time, look at the patterns underlying each ailment. Evaluate every one and its strength, then treat the most pressing problem first. If you have an acute condition, such as a cold, flu or bladder infection, treat it first; then treat any chronic conditions after.

Since TCM patterns have various symptoms, it is not unusual to find one pattern underlying most all your health issues, and when that pattern is treated, several different ailments also resolve. For example, if you have low energy, diarrhea and frequent colds and flu, you fit the patterns *Coldness*, in the Lungs, Spleen and Kidneys. The herbs to treat Coldness in each Organ are similar, and when used together, all three, and possibly even more, of your related symptoms will clear up. If not, you can better decide which herbal approach to follow from there.

If you're too confused to know where to begin your healing process, then heed what one of my Chinese teachers taught me: it's necessary to obtain restful sleep, strong digestion and regular elimination for complete healing to occur. Therefore, if you don't know where to start, correct these three first, then focus on other issues.

At the end of each pattern I have listed easily obtained formulas based on what Chinese herbalists typically use (and many of these formulas include Western herbs). Don't be intimidated by the formula numbers; they are easily referenced in the appendix *Formulas*, and may be purchased from sources located in *Resources*. Next a specific formula is listed that represents the herbs Western herbalists typically use (in some cases, Chinese herbs are included where there are no effective Western substitutes). If at all possible, seek out the prepared formulas and take with the suggested Western formula. While this represents 20 or more herbs, in difficult cases herbal treatment is most effective when many herbs are taken together over a longer period of time.

Although it's intended for you to use the formulas given, other formulas may of course be substituted. What's given here is intended for you to study and use as models to create your own formulas. I encourage you to personally tailor what's given by studying how the formulas are put together and each individual herb that comprises them. This is a great way to learn about herbs and healing.

When making the specific Western formula given under the Patterns, reference *Herbal Preparations*, for proper preparation. For instance, fresh **ginger** is added to many formulas as a carrier, so be sure to add 2-4 slices to the tea and simmer the last five minutes covered. Herbs too bitter to drink may be taken with the tea in tincture, tablet or capsule form. In fact, any formula given as a tea may have its bitter ingredients powdered and taken in capsule form along with a tea of the remaining herbs.

Formulas to tonify Blood or Yin may be mixed with blackstrap molasses and in fact, a delicious way to take these herbs is the following: make tea, strain and add 1 pint blackstrap molasses to resulting liquid (should be around 2 cups). Simmer together until 1 pint total remains (when water is evaporated). Bottle and refrigerate. Take 2 tablespoon, 2-3 times/day.

Once you've chosen an herbal treatment plan, take the herbs for three days. If after this time you experience a positive reaction, continue your plan until your symptoms are relieved. If you don't experience any changes, increase the dose and continue for another week, then re-evaluate your condition. Sometimes subtle changes occur slowly, which take time to feel. Other times you have the right herbs but need to take a higher dose for better results.

If you experience a mild negative reaction, cut down to a minimal dose (1 tablet or 10 drops tincture, 2 times/day) and continue for another three days. If the reaction continues, or if you experience a marked negative reaction, stop the herbs until the reactions disappear, then restart at a lower dose. If reactions recur again, you definitely know this is the wrong herbal approach and needs re-evaluation. Don't be discouraged if this occurs. Herbal medicine is a matter of strategy and herbalists often give a test formula or treatment to see if they have the right diagnosis. If an adverse reaction occurs, this may be used diagnostically to help reveal the correct treatment plan.

Treatment length varies according to the severity of the condition, how long it has been present, constitutional strength and how willing you are to make the needed changes. Most people experience some results immediately; others take longer. It may be necessary to follow your program for months, or even a year or so, to achieve full healing. As a rule of thumb, it takes one

---

Symptoms to Consider

- What is your major complaint? Other complaints?
- Chills and fever present?
- Is there sweating, or lack of sweating?
- Are there any headaches? (If so, where are they located and what is their quality?)
- Is there any pain? (Chest, abdominal, joint, low back, or other pain?)
- Is elimination regular? Quality of stools (hard or loose, for instance)? Frequency?
- How is urination? Frequency? Color? Amount? Nighttime?
- Is the appetite good or poor?
- How is digestion? Is there any gas? Bloatedness? Sleepiness after eating?
- Is there thirst, or lack of thirst?
- How is the mental condition (forgetfulness, poor memory)?
- How is the emotional state (depression, moodiness, a dominant emotion)?
- What are the sleeping habits? Is there insomnia (and if so, is it hard to fall asleep or stay asleep and what hours is person awake)? Or does person sleep excessively?
- Menstruation—amount and color of blood; regularity of cycle; PMS, pain, clots?
- Cough—dry or wet (if there's mucus, what is the color, amount, and thickness)?
- Are there other excretions or secretions present? Where, color and quantity?
- What is the quality of the skin—dry, puffy, or swollen?
- What is the quality of the voice—loud, shouting, soft?
- Is the person talkative, or doesn't like to talk?
- What is breathing like—loud, rapid, deep, or soft, shallow breath
- Is energy low, high or up and down?
- Are there any heart palpitations, or discomfort?
- Is there a preference for cold or warmth?

month to heal for each year you have experienced the condition. For example, a disease you have had for seven years could take seven months or more to heal.

The most "difficult" cases occur with people who don't want to do their part in the healing process (in other words, they don't want to change). These folks either don't believe what they eat, do, think or feel has any effect on their health issues, or they sabotage themselves ("oh, it won't hurt just this once"). Those who truly want to get well follow the guidelines and experience quicker and more sure results.

At the same time, be sure to follow the general dietary guidelines given in each section and in *The Energy of Food*. As well, once you determine which Pattern(s) you fit, look at Foods That Strengthen or Weaken Each Organ, in *The Energy of Food*, and incorporate those guidelines.

The conditions included here are the ones I frequently treat and are based on my clinical experience. The given remedies are the best I know at this time, although I'm always learning something new and additional products are being developed or discovered every day. And of course it must be said that if you have a serious health condition, it's necessary and important to consult a professional health practitioner. It can be hardest to see ourselves clearly, and consulting an herbalist can be extremely helpful as well as a valuable learning experience.

If you are currently on medication, review Herb/ Drug Interactions, in *Herbal Fundamentals*, before taking any of these herbs. In most cases, it is possible to take herbs while on medications, slowly reducing them as the herbs take effect. Of course, if your condition is complicated or serious, it's important to consult a professional health-care practitioner for guidance and monitoring.

❧ ARTHRITIS, RHEUMATISM, SCIATICA and JOINT PAINS

Arthritis encompasses joint inflammation while rheumatism includes inflammation, soreness and stiffness of the muscles and surrounding joints and structures.

Sciatica is sharp, shooting pain along the course of the sciatic nerve that starts in the hip or back of the thigh and runs down the back, inside or outside of the leg. While there are many types of arthritis and rheumatism, they, along with sciatica and joint pains, are all characterized by pain, swelling, possible redness and, in the case of arthritis, eventual deformity of the bone structure. In TCM, all these conditions come under the category Painful Obstruction, or *Bi*, Syndrome and are treated with the same approach.

General Treatment for Arthritis, Rheumatism, Sciatica and Joint Pains:

When Pathogenic Influences (Wind, Cold, Damp, and Heat) invade the body, they pass through the skin and penetrate the spaces between the skin and muscles, channels, sinews and/or bones. Lodging there, they stagnate and block the proper flow of Qi, Blood and Fluids, resulting in joint and muscle pain, swelling, ache, heaviness, heat and/or redness along with limitation of movement. Conditions such as tight or stiff neck and shoulders, frozen shoulder, carpal tunnel syndrome and sciatica may come under this category. Thus, Painful Obstruction Syndrome always involves Wind, Damp and Heat, or Wind, Damp and Cold, and may include stagnant Qi Blood or Fluids.

Treatment is quite effective for Painful Obstruction Syndrome and works quickly in acute conditions. Chronic conditions take extended treatment depending on how long it has been present. In either case, it's necessary to use topical remedies (moxibustion, cupping, liniments, oils, etc.) along with internal herbs.

The first thing to do for pain is apply moxibustion— it not only scatters Cold, but also dries Dampness and moves stagnant Blood. If you are using ice, stop (this is also true for *traumas*, *accidents* and *sports injuries*). Ice stagnates Blood, causing more Cold to enter the muscles and channels. Only if you have an acute trauma is ice helpful, and even then for no more than 15 minutes at a time (alternate cold and heat therapies ending with heat). While using ice alleviates pain, ultimately it causes

are extremely red and hot to the touch. Use moxa directly over the area of pain for 10-15 minutes, once or twice daily. The pain should improve fairly quickly. If it doesn't, or the area feels worse, then stop, as you now know there is Heat Painful Obstruction Syndrome.

Cupping relieves Damp, Cold, Heat, and stagnant Qi, Blood and Fluids specific types of Painful Obstruction while scraping alleviates all types, particularly Wind. Magnet therapy is also excellent for easing many types of pain. Treat Cold by placing the magnet's positive side against the skin. Treat all other types by placing it's negative side down. Leave continuously in place until pain is fully relieved. Periodically tap magnets for a minute to enhance their effects (for all therapies, see *Home Therapies*). Finally, castor oil packs are excellent for alleviating many types of pain (see *Herbal Preparations*), as are massage and the substance, DMSO (successfully used for pain in racing horses).

At the same time follow specific dietary guidelines. Avoid sour foods (yogurt, vinegar, oranges, grapefruit and pickles) as these over-stimulate the Liver, causing it to contract tendons and increase pain, and acidic foods (citrus, tomatoes, eggplant, peppers, potatoes, red meat, excess grains, alcohol, caffeine), which aggravate arthritis and acute pain. If experiencing acute pain, fast on simple soups, or in the case of Heat, red cherry juice.

If there is Wind, avoid prawns, shrimp, crab, lobster, spinach, rhubarb, mushrooms and caffeine. If Damp is present, avoid milk, cheese, butter, cream, ice cream, peanuts, bananas, flour products and greasy, fried and fatty foods. If there's Cold avoid raw foods, salads, fruit, juices, iced drinks/foods and melons. If Heat is present, avoid lamb, beef, game, spicy foods, alcohol and caffeine.

Several categories of herbs are effective for relieving Painful Obstruction Syndrome: surface-relieving herbs open the surface of the body to expel invading External Influences; herbs that relieve Wind-Cold-Damp and Wind-Cold-Heat Painful Obstruction Syndrome from the muscles, sinews, joints and bones (termed antirheumatics by Western herbalists); and Blood-moving herbs (disperse stagnant Blood).

stagnant Blood, setting up the perfect environment for future arthritic/rheumatic aches and pains.

Moxibustion isn't aggravating, even to most Heat conditions, although it may not be helpful for areas that

Differentiation of Arthritis, Rheumatism, Sciatica and Joint Pains:

Most cases of Painful Obstruction Syndrome have Wind, Damp and Cold factors involved, with one factor predominating over the others. In time, Heat Syndrome can arise, especially if there is underlying Deficient Yin. As well, the bones can be affected when Body Fluids turn to Phlegm, further obstructing joints and channels, leading to muscular atrophy and bone deformity.

The following list categorizes herbs according to their locations, and *the most specific ones are italicized*. Bear in mind that Wind accompanies all other factors for this condition, so herbs that expel Cold, Heat or Damp also usually expel Wind.

Rheumatic aches and pains—general: willow bark; Formulas #38, 59, 105

Neck and top of shoulder pain: *notopterygium, ligusticum gao ben, pueraria,* clematis, white peony, cyperus, dang gui, cooked rehmannia, cinnamon bark, salvia; Formulas #67, 98, and 155

Upper body pain: *notopterygium, angelica dahurica, turmeric rhizome, ligusticum, mulberry twig,* cinnamon branches, clematis; Formulas #38, 98

Shoulder joint pain: turmeric rhizome

Shoulder or elbow pain: *notopterygium, turmeric rhizome;* Formula #38

Upper limb pain: *cinnamon branches, notopterygium, turmeric rhizome,* clematis, Gentianna macrophylla, dang gui, white peony, cyperus

Lower body pain: *angelica (du huo), achyranthis,* clematis, eleuthro, Formulas #38, 59, and 187

Lower back pain: *polypody fern, eucommia, loranthus, epimedium* (Formula #51), *morinda, dipsacus, angelica du huo, chaenomelis;* Formulas #59, 187, and 264

Spine pain: *eucommia,* loranthus, dipsacus

Lower limb pain: *Gentianna macrophylla, achyranthis, chaeneomelis,* dang gui, salvia, notopterygium, white atractylodes, cyperus; Formula #59

Leg pain from Damp-Heat (hot, red, painful and swollen knee joint): black atractylodis, phellodendron; Formula #264

Knee pain: achyranthis, Formula #187

Joint swelling pain: *akebia, turmeric rhizome, mulberry twig*

Muscle pain: pueraria, cinnamon branches, white peony; Formula #155

Severe cramping pain: *chaenomalis*

General body aches and pains: *angelica du huo, ephedra* (also see Colds, Flu and Fevers); Formula #59

Degeneration of bones and surrounding tissues: *comfrey, dipsicus, bone marrow soup* (see Stocks under Recipes in *The Energy of Food*), mineral-rich herbs such as nettle, seaweeds, oatstraw and alfalfa, calcium

Nerve injury: *St. John's wort; California poppy*

Inflammation: echinacea, goldenseal, barberry

Rheumatoid arthritis: cuscuta; Formulas #155 with 261; 169

Traumas and Injuries: *Yunnan Paiyao* (capsules, powder or liquid), Formula #191

Stabbing, fixed pain: guggul, boswellia, corydalis

Further, certain herbs treat specific parts of the body, such as the neck, arms, legs and lower or upper back, and so should be chosen according to the locations of pain. For all types of Painful Obstruction Syndrome, except Heat, take herbs in tincture form, as alcohol specifically helps clear Wind, Damp and Cold and moves Blood. Further, liniments and plasters may be locally applied, such as wintergreen or pine oil, or Formula #38.

Guggul gum (a type of purified **myrrh**) and **boswellia** (purified **frankincense**) specifically relieve many

ARTHRITIS, RHEUMATISM, SCIATICA AND JOINT PAIN—ACUTE PATTERNS:

General formulas that may be used for any of the following conditions include Formulas #38, 59, 98 and 105.

WIND	DAMP	COLD	HEAT
Pain that moves from joint to joint	Fixed pain	Severe, fixed pain in one joint or muscle	Very severe pain
Soreness and pain of muscles and joints	Soreness, heaviness, swelling and numbness of joints and extremities	Possible feelings of coldness and preference for heat	Red, hot, swollen joints Joints hot to touch
Limitation of movement	Worse in damp weather	Limitation of movement	Limitation of movement
			Possible fever and sweating (usually due to Damp Heat)
Other possible symptoms:	***Other possible symptoms:***	***Other possible symptoms:***	***Other possible symptoms:***
Stiff neck and shoulders Muscle tics, spasms, cramps Itchiness Fear of wind Dizziness Stuffy nose	Turbid urine Loose stools; stools with mucus Sweetish taste in mouth Copious discharges that are cloudy, turbid or sticky No desire to drink, or only in small sips Feelings of heaviness Dizziness	No thirst No sweating Desire for warm drinks and food Desire to dress warmly Clear or white discharges and secretions Pale, frigid appearance Listlessness, slowness Little body odor Fear of cold	Sweating Dislike or fear of heat Desire for cold drinks and foods Desire for fewer clothes and covers Restlessness Irritability Ruddy, hot appearance Strong body odors
Tongue: trembles, or is deviated	***Tongue:*** possible coat on tongue	***Tongue:*** pale	***Tongue:*** red
Pulse: floating and slightly fast	***Pulse:*** slow and slightly slippery	***Pulse:*** tight	***Pulse:*** slippery and fast
Formulas: #67; tea of equal parts angelica, lovage, sarsaparilla and black cohosh with ½ part each fresh ginger and licorice	***Formulas:*** #164; tea of equal parts sassafras, sarsaparilla, black cohosh and kava kava with ½ part each fresh ginger and licorice	***Formulas:*** #187 or #200; tinctures or tablets of guggul and boswellia	***Formulas:*** #73, 264; tea of equal parts devils claw, meadowsweet, red clover, sassafras and black cohosh with ½ part licorice

types of Painful Obstruction Syndrome. Take them in tincture form along with trying this general formula: 1 part each **eleuthro**, **myrrh**, **yucca** root, **devil's claw**, **black cohosh**, **kava kava** and **prickly ash** and ½ part each **ginger** and **licorice**. For arthritis, also take a blood-purifying formula, such as equal parts **red clover**, **sassafras**, **sarsaparilla**, **burdock root**, **black cohosh** and **prickly ash**. Other formulas include Formula #38 for any type of Painful Obstruction Syndrome, Formula #98 for upper body pain and Formula #59 for lower body pain. Useful supplements include glucosamine sulfate and MSM sulfur (Formula #46).

Prevent arthritis, rheumatism, sciatica and joint pain by exercising regularly to circulate Qi and Blood,

ARTHRITIS, RHEUMATISM, SCIATICA AND JOINT PAIN—CHRONIC PATTERNS:

DEFICIENT QI, BLOOD, KIDNEYS OR LIVER	BLOOD STAGNATION	STAGNANT PHLEGM IN JOINTS
Chronic dull achy pain, especially of back and legs	Fixed, stabbing, boring pain	Painful joints with swelling and deformity of bones in joints
Dizziness	Purplish joint or skin area	Chronic condition
Blurry vision	Purple lips, nails	Limitation of movement
Tiredness		No thirst
Weakness		Contraction of tendons
Other possible symptoms: Insomnia, coldness, frequent urination, knee weakness and pain	**Other possible symptoms:** Dark menstrual blood; clots in menstrual blood; tremors	**Other possible Symptoms:** Heaviness of body; no sweating; cough with abundant-white sputum
Tongue: pale and thin	**Tongue:** purple	**Tongue:** thick, sticky white coat, possibly swollen
Pulse: pale and fine/thin	**Pulse:** choppy	**Pulse:** slippery
Formulas: #59 or 187; tincture or tablets of boswellia, ashwagandha and eleuthro	**Formulas:** #105 or 191; tinctures or tablets of guggul and boswellia, ginger and licorice	**Formulas:** #187; tinctures or tablets of guggul and boswellia with a tea of equal parts each kava kava, black cohosh and eleuthro and 1/2 part each fresh

keep the tendons and ligaments supple and prevent invasion of External Pathogenic Factors (especially stretching, such as yoga, which also "massages" Internal Organs). Avoid excessive weight lifting, jogging and aerobic exercises, as they put strain on the joints, easily leading to injuries.

Note that treating arthritis, rheumatism, sciatica and joint pain naturally requires patience and perseverance. These treatments are very effective and it is not unusual for rapid results to occur, but usually it takes time, even several months to a year depending on the severity of your condition and how long you've had it. If you are using the correct herbs and therapies, your symptoms should gradually improve.

☙ ATTENTION DEFICIT HYPER-ACTIVITY DISORDER (ADHD)

ADHD (also known as Attention Deficit Disorder, or **ADD**) is one of the fastest growing "diseases" today. A "new" ailment, mild forms of hyperactivity came to be seen as behavioral problems over the last thirty years of the 20th century, especially in the nineties, when up to 5% or more of all school-age children were diagnosed with ADHD (greater than 5 million children in 1995, over 25% higher than in 1985!). Since then, this number has continued to grow.

Tragically, many children are misdiagnosed, as their "misbehaviors" are usually due to concrete, changeable factors. However, Western medicine immediately puts children on Prozac or Ritalin anyway, regardless of negative effects on their bodies or psyches. This is very unfor-

Signs of ADHD:

These must be present for at least six months, in more than one setting (home, school, etc.), especially before the age of 7:

- Distractibility (inattention, inability to concentrate or focus)
- Impulsivity (poor self-control)
- Hyperactivity (excessive activity)

Causes of ADHD:

- Sugar, including juices and sugars that are hidden in most processed foods
- Caffenated substances (colas, chocolate, cocoa, black tea, coffee)
- Excessive intake of refined carbohydrate with inadequate protein
- Excessive intake of soy, especially in baby formulas (causes learning disabilities)
- Food allergies, such as wheat, dairy, peanuts, additives and preservatives (MSG, etc.)
- Inadequate sleep
- Insufficient physical exercise and activity
- Unexpressed and unresolved emotional issues from some type of stress or crisis (new baby, parent's divorce, death in the family, separation anxiety, traumas and more)
- Lead and heavy metal poisoning
- Head traumas
- Vaccinations
- Suppressed creativity
- Boredom at home or school
- Excessive TV, computer games
- Sleep deprivation (staying up too late coupled with getting up too early, insufficient rest time)
- Hormonal imbalances from diet (non-organic meats and dairy products)

tunate as many alternative treatments effectively correct "misbehaviors" without the need of any medications.

If we need to point a finger at causes for inattention, impulsivity and hyperactivity, it should be at our Western culture with its rampant sugar, excessive and violent TV and computer games, premature separation from working parents and poor diets, all of which cause over-stimulation, internally and externally. Unfortunately, children pay the high price of these cultural habits.

A high number of ADHD cases are actually due to a child's unresolved emotional issues around stress or crisis. Not able to express this, the child acts out instead. Problems paying attention or behaving properly are frequently due to an accumulation of emotional wounds, such as kids seeking attention to replace the void left by mothers and fathers prematurely separating from them.

This is especially true for boys (who comprise 90% of those diagnosed with ADHD) since they are taught the "boy code" early in life—"keep your chin up," "don't cry," or "hold it in" are common phrases used with boys when showing their emotions from infancy on. (Because it is expected for girls to be more emotional, their separation needs are treated differently.) As a result, boys frequently either withdraw (depression) or its opposite, act out (hyperactivity—although some forms of anger and aggression are really signs of depression, particularly in boys). (See the *Bibliography* for several excellent books on ADHD and emotional causes for this behavior.)

Of all the causes for ADHD, sugar alone is a major culprit. Sugar is hidden everywhere, even in the most unsuspecting places—baby formulas, cereals, juices, sodas, crackers, and most all canned, boxed and other processed foods used to make meals or snacks. Because sugar rapidly increases energy and blood sugar, it just as drastically drops within a short time, causing a roller-coaster ride of behavioral swings, alternating between bouncing off the walls with too much unfocused energy to deep depression. Soon the sugar cravings set in again, and another sweet snack is demanded and given, repeating the cycle continuously. It's no wonder children are unable to concentrate or sit still. I personally think this is one of the worst things we are doing to our children today: giving sugar (direct or hidden), then punishment or drugs.

While the sweet taste tonifies Spleen Qi in TCM, in excess it over-stimulates this Organ, weakening its Qi. Now look at the following connections—this is interesting: the Spleen is the Organ in charge of thinking and thought, providing the ability to concentrate, sit calmly, study, focus and memorize. When excessive sugar weakens the Spleen, concentrating, sitting still, focusing and learning are difficult or short-lived. Does that sound like ADD/ADHD to you? It does to me.

As if sugar weren't enough of a cause, there are many others. Combining caffeine with sugar, as in colas or chocolate, is a double stimulant guaranteed to feed children's "misbehaviors". Excessive use of computer games negatively affects the brain, reduces creativity and makes children erratic, just like the games themselves. Excessive TV watching leads to lack of exercise and restlessness, and stimulates children to act out the visual images of violence they "ingest" from the computer or TV shows.

It's also not unusual for children to be bored at school, especially if they have to continuously sit in a chair for hours at a time, or if the classwork is geared toward the slowest child in class. Boredom almost guarantees behavioral problems with most children. Furthermore, children often subconsciously act out what is going on in their environment—in fact, they are quite good barometers for stress levels at home, school and play areas. Thus, when children are hyperactive, they may actually be acting out the stresses that surround them rather than having a behavioral problem themselves.

Believe it or not, many teachers, and even parents, like to put their children on Ritalin or Prozac because it makes them easier to handle. It also allows teachers to obtain extended testing time on exams with children, since children sit longer when on these drugs. This is putting children into a "box" of expected behavior so they fit into the teacher's and parents' lives. After all, changing a child's diet or lifestyle habits means the parent and teacher must make similar changes, too. I find this very, very sad indeed. Now, this is not to say that some children's hyperactivity is caused by constitutional imbalances, or a hyperactive thyroid (it is worth getting this checked!). Yet, the vast majority labeled ADHD and put on drugs are actually victims of a poor diet and aggravating lifestyle habits.

General Treatment for ADHD:

The first approach for treating ADHD is talking with the child. Try to discover any underlying trapped feelings that may be causing him/her to withdraw or act out. Be patient and give the child extra attention until the feelings emerge. If they don't and you suspect trapped feelings are there, seek professional help. At the same time, turn to changing any dietary causes. Begin by eliminating all sugar from the diet. Use whole fruit for sweets and if you must give fruit juices, water them down substantially (remember, one small glass of apple juice is equivalent to about 6–8 apples, and without the fiber!). Alternatively, give vegetable juices. Be sure to remove other stimulants such as caffeine, found in colas, coffee, black tea, cocoa and chocolate.

Support concentration, focus and even energy by feeding a balanced diet of whole grains and legumes, animal protein as appropriate (protein increases calmness, alertness and prevents depression), lots of cooked and raw vegetables and baked fruit for desserts (cobblers, sauces, crisps or pies with cinnamon, walnuts and raisins satisfies most children's sweet desires). Particularly give a solid breakfast with protein, as this sustains level energy for many hours without the need (or desire) for sugary snacks. If necessary, include a vitamin and mineral supplement and essential fatty acids (**flaxseed**, **borage**, **evening primrose** or fish oils).

Just to make this point clear, the following are poor breakfasts guaranteed to create a hyperactive child: pancakes or waffles with syrup; sugary cereal with cold milk and orange juice; muffins/bagel/toast with jam; toast and orange juice. Here are some balanced breakfasts to try instead: pancakes or waffles with yogurt and fruit; scrambled eggs with toast; bean and cheese burritos; oatmeal or other whole grain cooked cereal with milk or yogurt (add in raisins, apples or other fruit if desired); soups; left-over dinner; rice and eggs scrambled with vegetables.

Next, limit TV/computer game time and make sure your child is getting enough physical activity and exercise. Nourish the child's interests and channel excess "energy" into something beneficial, such as a sport, martial art or other physical release. If there are stressful issues at home or school, help your child deal with them. (Look at yourself and see how you may be directly contributing to your child's behavior as well. Journal writing can be useful here.) Consider alternative schooling options if your child is bored or not getting sufficient attention.

In the meantime, there are many useful herbs that specifically help children relax, focus, handle stress and sleep better. One of the best is **chamomile**, which treats tension, restlessness, crying, nervousness, irritability and a bad temper. **Lemon balm** is also useful as it nourishes the nervous system and treats restlessness, crying, whining, sadness and depression. Both herbs help improve sleep.

A wonderful ADHD/ADD formula is equal parts **chamomile, lemon balm, gotu kola, zizyphus** and **hawthorn**. Powder herbs and mix with enough honey to form a paste. Give $1/2$-1 teaspoon, 2-3 times/day in this case honey is used medicinally and the herbs counteract any negative effects of the sugar.) A calcium/magnesium supplement may be added for further calming and relaxing actions. Alternatively, give Formulas #15 and 16 in tablet or syrup form. If there is difficulty sleeping, try a tea of equal parts **chamomile, lemon balm, hops** and **passionflower**.

If a child acts angry, irritable, easily frustrated or aggressive, there is also Heat and/or congestion in the Liver. Reduce or eliminate cheese, pizza, red meat, nuts and nut butters, turkey, fried and fatty foods (french fries, etc.), caffeine (coffee, black tea, colas, cocoa), chocolate and vinegar (use lemons), as these create Excess Heat and stagnation in the Liver. If you think this is

too difficult or impossible, then obviously the child is already getting too much of these foods!

Instead, emphasize vegetables, vegetable juices and greens along with white meats for animal protein, whole grains, legumes and some fruit. Make a "coffee" out of 1 part **dandelion** and $1/2$ part **chicory** (this clears Heat and congestion from the Liver), or "soft drinks" out of **sarsaparilla, fennel, licorice** and **ginger** (make herb tea, add an equal amount of carbonated water, if needed, and sweeten with a little raw, unrefined sugar).

Be careful of excessive carbohydrates in the form of processed foods and flour products, such as breads, toast, muffins, crackers, pasta and chips. These quickly metabolize into sugar, setting up blood sugar swings and subsequent cravings. Instead, give snacks balanced in protein, carbohydrates and fats. Protein without sugar improves concentration.

If there is a lot of stress in the environment, give **eleuthro** ($1/4 - 1/2$ tsp. tinctures, 2-3 times daily) as this will help your child handle stress (and take some yourself!). **Ginkgo** and **gotu kola** improve memory and mental clarity while **oatstraw, skullcap, lemon balm** and **oatmeal** soothe nerves. Try **St. John's wort** or **albizzia** if there is any depression and **gotu kola** for more focus. Also try Formulas #88, 90 and/or 92 for calming hyperactivity and treating depression.

Bladder Infections: see Urinary Bladder Infections

❦ COLDS, FLU and FEVERS

In the West when someone "catches" a cold or flu, we mean that "germs" or viruses have passed from one person to another. This is seen differently in Chinese Medicine. People don't succumb to colds or flu if their immunities are strong, even if it is a "catchable" virus, but if immunity is weakened for whatever reason, or the virus is particularly strong, an Exterior "evil", or pathogen, can invade the body, causing a cold, flu or fever. Typically these pathogens are carried by Wind (like wind as we know it) and invade the body at the back of the neck. That is one reason why Asian people cover their necks with high collars (scarves work well, too).

Causes for Colds, Flu and Fevers:

The following weaken immunity, bringing on colds, flu and fevers:

- ✤ Overworking for long hours under stressful conditions without getting sufficient rest or nourishing food (weakens Kidneys and immunity)
- ✤ Emotional stress of any sort, especially grief or sadness (weakens Lungs)

- ✤ Excessive sexual activity, caffeine, sugar and alcohol (weaken Kidneys and immunity)
- ✤ Sugar (weakens immunity as much as 50%—normally the body can tolerate this unless weakened by other factors or eaten to excess; also weakens Kidneys and Spleen)
- ✤ Exposure to cold, windy days when improperly dressed (allows for invasion of External Influences)

External pathogens causing colds, flu and fevers quickly develop and move to the Interior of the body, or get stuck between the Exterior and Interior layers, lingering for weeks or months. When either of these occur, you'll no longer have obvious symptoms of a cold, flu or fever, but still experience low energy and possible cough, and not feel well or normal. If a cold, flu or fever is improperly treated, such as with antibiotics, the pathogens are suppressed and pushed deeper into the body (repeated doses of antibiotics also weaken the body until it is no longer responsive to them). Eventually it may manifest as a serious issue, such as chronic fatigue, Epstein-Barr or rheumatoid arthritis, for example. To clear the trapped pathogen then, it becomes necessary to push it out to the body's surface where it can be released. In the meantime, the weakened body becomes susceptible to other seemingly unrelated illnesses. Thus, it is very important to properly treat colds, flu and fevers to prevent more complications.

General Treatment for Colds, Flu and Fevers:

Colds, flu and fevers can change very quickly, even within hours. Try to catch one at its *very beginning stage* by taking the extremely effective homeopathic remedy, *Oscillococcinum* (found at health food stores—put 3-5 pellets directly in your mouth three times daily, let dissolve and do not eat or drink anything within 15 minutes before or after taking the remedy). **Echinacea** has recently been used to treat beginning stages of colds, flu and fevers from Heat (see Patterns for Heat symptoms).

Take a dropperful of echinacea tincture (Formula #28). or 2-4 tablets, every two hours (Formula #29). As soon as you take echinacea, exercise for a half-hour, especially anaerobic exercise, as this seems to potentiate its effects. (However, echinacea's effectiveness seems to diminish within ten days.) Alternatively, drink 1-2 cups of strong **sweet basil** tea, or try Formula #109.

Ginger and **garlic** work well at fending off beginning stages of colds, flu and fevers from Coldness (see Patterns for Symptoms of Coldness). Drink several cups of fresh ginger tea and eat 3-6 raw cloves garlic daily. Take a hot bath for 20 minutes in which you've added 2 tsp. **cayenne** pepper and 2 tablespoons **turmeric** powder. Then immediately dress in warm clothes and get in bed under several layers of blankets and sweat. Take one of the herbs above, or drink 1/2-1 tsp. **cayenne** mixed in 1 cup hot water. After a half-hour, quickly sponge off with cool water, dress in dry clothes, eat some light soup and go back to bed.

To open nasal and sinus passages, do a facial steam with **eucalyptus**, **mint** or **thyme**, do a nasal wash, and/or tape a magnet on either side of the nose with the negative pole pointing down. Leave in place until the cold or flu is gone (see *Home Therapies*, for nasal wash and magnets).

Because colds and flu (and many resulting fevers) are due to a virus, it is extremely helpful to dose yourself with antiviral herbs now (as well as during any stage of a cold or flu). Luckily, there are many great antiviral herbs, such as **olive leaf**, **isatis**, **andrographis**, **lemon balm** and **elder**, all of which are commonly available on the market (Formula #34 includes most of these; also good are Formulas #32, 36, 142 and 103—children love this latter one!).

Once a cold, flu or fever has entered, you can quickly get rid of it if you *immediately* treat it. A tea made of equal parts **yarrow**, **elder**, **angelica** and **lemon balm** with ¹/2 part fresh **ginger** treats colds, flu and fevers due to Heat or Cold (Chinese patents work well now, too—see Patterns for specifics). Drink several cups throughout the day while resting, drinking water and eating light soups or cooked cereals. Alternatively, try Formulas #109 or 110 (or see Patterns). Be sure to take herbs every 2 to 3 hours for acute conditions.

Sweating therapy is appropriate for those who have colds, flu or fevers from Heat, and Formula #172 is appropriate. While those who are Deficient should avoid this therapy, if sweating occurs after taking herbs, such as Formula #160, eat a bowl of rice to replenish energy. In general, use this time to detoxify the body and rest. For headaches, see the section Headaches.

Prolonged colds and flu need a different approach. Once the acute stage passes, the pathogen penetrates deeper into the body. At this point, acute symptoms are gone (fever and headache), but there is still mucus, low energy and/or no appetite. In fact, it may be possible for you to go back to work, though you still feel lousy. Now antiviral herbs are definitely needed (if they haven't been taken yet—see these listed above). Further, since the condition is partly External and partly Internal, herbs are used to release the Exterior and clear the Interior manifestations, generally a **bupleurum**-based formula, such as Formula #241, or 173 if there's also constipation (see Half External-Half Internal Pattern).

Recurring colds, flu, sore throats and sinus infections are generally due to pathogenic bacteria lodging internally between the upper bridge of the nose and the throat. The best way to naturally destroy bacteria there is through nasal wash, by pouring saltwater up the nose and draining it down and out into the mouth, two times daily. At the same time, be sure you are taking antiviral herbs, listed above. Also regularly take Formulas

#4 & 31. For **cough** with colds and flu, see the section Coughs.

Those who experience *frequent colds/ flu and fever* have Deficient Lung Qi. **Astragalus** is the best herb for building defensive Qi and should be taken preventatively as a daily tea, or cooked in soups, grains or hot cereals (Formula #4 may be used). Other useful herbs include **codonopsis**, **schisandra**, **reishi**, **American ginseng** and **eleuthro**. A **ginger** fomentation over the Kidneys boosts immunity as well. At the same time, it's important to eat a balanced diet, eliminating excessive meat, sugar, dairy, salads, juices, raw foods, alcohol and caffeine. Get plenty of rest, cut back on your work and social schedule, and exercise. Journal write about what is being suppressed in your life or any inner "crying" over something you feel you can't do anything about. Keep this routine well in place until you no longer experience recurring colds/flu or fevers.

Summer colds, flu and fevers take a different approach. If the usual herbs don't work, it's necessary to warm the Interior of the body in order to reduce the fever, because in hot weather Internal Heat is pushed to the Exterior, leaving Coldness in the Interior. There may also be accompanying symptoms of diarrhea, loss of appetite, stomachache, nausea and vomiting. Formula #236 works very well for summer colds and flu.

Treat *fevers* the same way as colds and flu, since diaphoretic herbs treat fevers, too. **Boneset**, one of the best antipyretic herbs, is quite nasty tasting, but breaks fevers quickly and resolves colds and flu symptoms. Other good herbs include **yarrow**, **elder**, **mint** and **ginger**. Acute high fevers without cold or flu symptoms are due to Internal Heat in the Lungs, Stomach and/or Intestines (see Patterns for appropriate herbs). As these fevers can be serious, be sure to monitor temperatures— if it goes above 105 degrees F (less for elderly patients or those with heart conditions), take steps to directly control the fever. Sweating therapy works well to break fevers in the safe range, as does a cold sponge bath or cold sheet treatment (see *Home Therapies*). There are two unique fever situations—Deficient Qi and Deficient Yin. See Patterns for symptoms and treatment.

Children frequently get fevers without cold or flu symptoms. This is the body's natural immune response to fighting pathogens. It is best to let the child's body go through the fever, if at all possible, as this builds a strong immune system (of course this is only appropriate if the temperature doesn't linger at 104-5 degrees F). At the same time, be sure to keep the head, along with male genitals, cool and feed only simple foods, such as soup.

When children (or adults) take aspirin or antibiotics to relieve colds and flu, it only masks the symptoms and pushes them deeper. Eventually such problems as asthma or wheezing can arise. Results from repeated antibiotics aren't usually seen for ten to twenty years or more, but symptoms do occur along with a weakened immune system. Instead, give **willow bark** tea and/or bath, the herbs listed in this section or from one of the Patterns, cold sponge baths, lots of water (avoid sugary drinks as sugar feeds infections) and light soups. Normally such fevers break on their own within three days, **but if the fever gets too high (104-105 degrees F), then seek medical attention.**

Sore throats frequently accompany beginning stages of colds, flu and fevers and may be quite severe in Heat conditions. Suck on zinc or **slippery elm** lozenges, or a small piece of **licorice** root; drink hot water with honey, lemon and a pinch of **cayenne** pepper (this is a good *formula for singers*); gargle with saltwater, or squirt **echinacea** tincture on the throat every hour. Sore throats from Heat respond well to **echinacea, honeysuckle, raw rehmannia, burdock seed, scrophularia** or **slippery elm.** Also, repeatedly pinch throat skin until red to move out toxins and flush new blood through the area.

Severe sore throats, including *strep throat*, need strong Heat-clearing herbs, such as **goldenseal, honeysuckle, gardenia, echinacea, scutellaria, coptis** or **baptisia.** *Tonsillitis* responds to the same herbs and Formula #196.

Sore throats from Coldness resolve with **ginger, cayenne, bayberry, garlic, licorice** or **cinnamon,** a **ginger** fomentation over the throat and moxibustion over the lower back, level with the waist, covering a line that includes the area between three inches on either side of the spine (Chinese Kidney area).

Chronic, recurring sore throats with no other acute symptoms are usually due to Deficient Kidney Qi. This is a signal that you are overworking, resting insufficiently and not eating right. To heal this type of sore throat, slow down, rest and eat properly (there is no substitute for these). Frequently, emotional issues block the throat, such as problems with self-expression, creativity, words not being said, or not speaking one's truth. Explore these through journal writing and release as appropriate.

Earaches (including swimmer's ear) respond extremely well to **mullein, St. John's wort** and **garlic** (also rue) oil used as eardrops (see *Home Remedies*), especially when used immediately. For *swimmer's ear* also try $1/2$ part white vinegar mixed with $1/2$ part rubbing alcohol, putting 1-2 drops in ears immediately after leaving water. Frequent, recurring earaches, especially those in children, almost always signal lowered immunity and Deficient Kidney Qi from too much sugar in the diet (sweets, chocolate, soft drinks, juices), not enough rest, excessive caffeine and/or insufficient dietary nourishment. Instead, use eardrops, change the diet, get plenty of rest and take herbs to tonify the immune system, like **eleuthro** or **astragalus.**

Chronic earaches, particularly in adults, may signal hypothyroidism (see the section Tiredness, for information on this). Using antibiotics to treat earaches only masks these true causes, weakens immunity and destroys important favorable bacteria, making it easier for ear infections to recur again and again. (However, if an ear infection isn't treated immediately, or doesn't respond to herbs, do seek medical attention.)

Sinus infections can be brought on with, or from similar causes to, colds, flu and fevers. One of the best remedies I've found for sinus infections with Heat (yellow mucus, throbbing headaches, thirst) is a nasal spray of grapefruit seed extract. If the sinus infection is from Coldness (feelings of being cold, dull headache, no thirst, white to clear mucus), mix equal parts of **black pepper, ginger** and **anise** powders (**bayberry,** too) with enough

RELATED AILMENTS:

Be sure to look up the energy of each herb to choose the right ones for you.

SWOLLEN GLANDS	MUMPS	TONSILLITIS	HOARSE VOICE	LARYNGITIS
Red clover, yarrow, mullein, echinacea, garlic oil	Echinacea, isatis, coptis, mullein	Echinacea, burdock seed, comfrey, gotu kola, baptisia, coptis, isatis, scutellaria, gardenia, honeysuckle	Coltsfoot, mullein, marshmallow, licorice, cardamom	Goldenseal, chamomile, cayenne, coltsfoot, licorice, isatis, slippery elm, echinacea, honeysuckle, gardenia
Formula: #73	**Formula:** #73	**Formulas:** #73 and 109	**Formulas:** #73 and 109	**Formulas:** #73 and 109

COLDS/FLU/FEVERS PATTERNS:

As these conditions change rapidly, regularly monitor symptoms and alter herbs accordingly. When properly treated, acute conditions respond quickly, even within the day. If there is no response within 24 hours, change your herbal approach.

ACUTE COLDS/FLU/FEVER—EXTERNAL PATTERNS:

This is your typical cold/flu condition with fever, chills, body aches, runny nose and cough.

EXTERNAL WIND HEAT	EXTERNAL WIND COLD
Stronger fever than chills	No or low fever, strong chills and shivering
Aversion to heat	Fear of cold
Thirst	No thirst
Sweating	No sweating
Body aches	Body aches
Strong sore throat, swollen tonsils	Stiff neck; possible mild sore throat
Headache	Headache at the back of the head (occiput)
Runny nose with yellow discharge	Runny nose with white discharge, sneezing
Possible cough with yellow mucus	Possible cough with white mucus
Slightly dark urine	Pale urine
Tongue: no change initially	**Tongue:** slightly red on sides and/or front
Pulse: floating and tight (like a rope)	**Pulse:** floating and fast
Formulas: #110; tincture, tablets or capsules of boneset with a tea or equal parts yarrow, mint or lemon balm, elder and ¼ part fresh ginger.	**Formulas:** #41, 160 or 234; fresh garlic or garlic juice along with a tea of 1 part hyssop and ½ part each bayberry and fresh ginger.

FEVER DUE TO DEFICIENT QI

Fever due to Deficient Qi is different in that there is concurrent weakness. This is the only case in which some tonics, such as ginseng, may be taken during an acute condition.

Fever that can be high; aversion to cold; no sweating; headache; neck pain
Muscle aches; cough with mucus; sensation of fullness in chest and stomach region
Shortness of breath; fatigue; poor appetite; loose stools; stuffy nose
Tongue: Pale   **Pulse:** Empty
Formulas: tea of equal parts eleuthro, lemon balm, elder and fresh ginger

ACUTE COLDS/FLU/FEVER—INTERNAL PATTERNS:

These colds/flu typically have acute high fevers as their major symptom.

LUNG HEAT	STOMACH HEAT	STOMACH AND INTESTINES HEAT
High fever	High fever	High fever, worse in afternoon
Feeling of heat	Feeling of heat	Faint feeling
Cough with yellow mucus	Possible dry cough	Constipation
Thirst	Intense thirst	Thirst
Restlessness	Restlessness	Restlessness
Sweating	Profuse sweating	Possibly no sweating
Possible breathlessness	Coarse breathing	Burning sensation in the anus
Extreme sore, or strep, throat	Extreme sore, or strep, throat	Delirium
Swollen glands		Abdominal pain and fullness that is worse with pressure
Tongue: red with yellow coat	**Tongue:** red with dry, yellow coat	**Tongue:** red with dry, thick yellow, brown or black coat
Pulse: overflowing and fast	**Pulse:** overflowing or big	**Pulse:** deep, full and fast
Formulas: #142; tea of equal parts sweet basil, mullein, red clover with ½ part licorice and ¼ part lobelia.	**Formulas:** #197; 2 capsules each of boneset and goldenseal with tea of equal parts marshmallow, red clover, dandelion and ½ part licorice.	**Formulas:** #173; 2 capsules of goldenseal and rhubarb with tea of equal parts dandelion, chamomile, sweet basil and ½ part licorice.

honey to form a paste, taking ½ teaspoon several times daily (alternatively, take Formula #84 or 94).

For chronic sinus infections it is necessary to also detoxify the Liver. Take **milk thistle** (Formula #83), or take Formula #12. As well, nasal wash and facial steams with **eucalyptus**, **mint** or **thyme** (see *Home Therapies*) are beneficial. An effective Chinese patent for sinus infections include Formula #135, and specific sinus herbs include **eyebright**, **nettles** (only freeze-dried works here), **echinacea**, **goldenseal**, **horseradish**, **pueraria**,

ACUTE OR CHRONIC COLDS/FLU/FEVER—HALF EXTERNAL/HALF INTERNAL:

These occur after acute stage of colds or flu, lingering for weeks to months at a time.
You may lead a normal life, but feel tired and not fully well with any of the following symptoms:

Alternating between feeling hot and cold and fever and chills; bitter taste in mouth
Irritability; tiredness; nausea or vomiting; dry throat
Pain, oppression and distension in rib area; possible lingering cough with yellow or white mucus

Tongue: white coat	**Pulse:** wiry and fine

Formulas: #241, or #173 if there's constipation; tea of equal parts Chinese black cohosh, sassafras, elder, mint or lemon balm and ½ part each licorice and fresh ginger

FEVER DUE TO DEFICIENT YIN

Low-grade fevers are generally due to Deficient Yin and are treated differently. These may occur with acute conditions, but may also be chronic. After the fever is gone, take the herb American ginseng to restore Yin (traditionally the Chinese use e jiao, or gelatin derived from donkey skin).

Low-grade or tidal fever (rises late afternoon or evening and drops at other times); thirst; scanty, dark urine; dry cough; hot flashes; night sweats; insomnia; restless sleep
Burning in the palms, soles and/or chest; burning sensation over the kidneys
Dizziness; tinnitus; aching lower back and knees

Tongue: deep red without coat; dry	**Pulse:** fine/thin and fast

Formulas: #130; tea of equal parts American ginseng and ophiopogon with ½ part licorice

ephedra, **magnolia flower**, **angelica dahurica**, **cinnamon twig**, **white peony**, **asarum** and **ligusticum**. A useful combination is equal parts **eyebright**, **yarrow**, **burdock** and **dandelion**. For a simple *blocked nose* try a facial steam with **eucalyptus** or **mint**, and take **horseradish** and **eyebright** internally.

Allergies and *hay fever* are due to similar causes and patterns as colds, flu and fevers, although they have more Wind involved. Treat with herbs such as **nettle**, **milk thistle**, **schizonepeta**, **siler**, **chrysanthemum**, **magnolia buds**, **ephedra**, **apricot seed**, **wild cherry**, **turmeric**, **xanthium** and **pueraria**. A useful Chinese patent is Formula #135. As well, cleanse the liver and use nasal wash (see *Home Therapies*) and facial steams. Many have also found tremendous benefit from using 200-500 mg of the sup-

plement quercetin 2 times/day (if possible, start taking it one month before allergy season), taking 5 drops daily of **castor** oil, or sucking on a pinch of Celtic sea salt (no other kind of salt seems to work).

☙ COUGH

There is a wide range and variety of coughs: inflammatory with yellow blobs of phlegm; productive with watery to white phlegm; dry and non-productive; and spasmodic, such as whooping cough, wheezing and asthma. Some coughs accompanying colds or flu have mucus dripping into the bronchioles and lungs. Others can be chronic, like bronchitis.

In TCM, the natural flow of Lung Qi is to descend and disperse throughout the body. When the descending function is impaired, it ascends instead, causing a cough. At the same time, Kidney Qi rises to grasp Lung Qi, helping it descend. If Kidney Qi is weak, it cannot grasp Lung Qi and cough results. To tell the difference: if it is more difficult to inhale, Kidney Qi is Deficient; if it is harder to exhale, Lung Qi is Deficient; if neither, there is Lung Qi Deficiency or another cause, such as Dampness.

General Treatment for Cough:

To treat a cough, first eliminate phlegm-producing foods: dairy, flour products (breads, pasta, chips, cookies, crackers, pastries, etc.), iced drinks and foods, raw foods, juices, wheat, oats, potatoes, soy milk, tofu and excessive intake of fruit. These dampening foods congest digestion, resulting in poor absorption and assimilation along with congestion, causing Lung and Spleen Dampness. For this reason, it is a good idea to cook food with spices that promote digestion, such as peppers, **coriander**, **cumin**, **fenugreek**, **mustard seeds**, **asafoetida**, **thyme**, **basil**, **garlic**, **cinnamon**, **cardamom** and **oregano**.

Useful therapies for coughs include cupping over the back and chest (this can be done daily, see *Home Therapies*), facial steams of **eucalyptus**, **wintergreen** or **pine**, smoking herbs, such as **coltsfoot**, **mullein** and **licorice**, a mustard plaster or onion poultice over the chest and deep breathing exercises. Journal writing is useful for chronic Lung (and skin) issues, particularly when focusing on any loss, the inability to receive or give, or any limitations being felt (the Lungs need time and space).

The next approach is to take appropriate herbs for the type of cough you have (see Patterns—if there is an accompanying cold or flu, also see the section Colds, Flu and Fevers). One of the best all-round herbs for most coughs with mucus, especially those with white to clear phlegm, is fresh **garlic**. It may be eaten straight, or minced and chopped in olive oil and spread on bread. The best form is garlic juice (which may often be purchased in the spice section of grocery stores), taking a

> ### *Causes for Cough:*
>
> - Coughs that are acute and come with a cold or flu are considered Exterior coughs due to Wind-Cold, Wind-Heat, or Wind-Dryness invading the Lungs
> - Emotional stress, especially sadness or grief injure the Lungs (I have known several people who came down with bronchitis, pneumonia, or coughs after losing a loved one)
> - Prolonged anger, frustration or resentment (stagnate Liver Qi which then attacks the Lungs)
> - Excessive consumption of sweets, dairy, greasy foods, flour products, iced drinks and foods, juices and raw foods (cause Damp and Phlegm to settle in Lungs—these usually cause profuse expectoration with cough that's worse after eating)
> - Excessive intake of alcohol, spicy or greasy foods (lead to Phlegm and Heat settling in Lungs, producing cough with yellow Phlegm)
> - Chronic illness (weakens Lung Qi and Yin, causing chronic coughs)

teaspoonful every 2-3 hours. Do not choose garlic in capsules or tablets in which volatile oils have been removed, as this active ingredient is needed here. Another beneficial cough herb is **thyme** in syrup or tea form.

A great formula that treats most coughs, including *bronchitis*, is equal parts **mullein**, **coltsfoot**, **wild cherry bark**, **thyme** and **elecampane** and $1/2$ part **licorice**. Drinking 3 cups tea daily is best, although it may be taken in powder form, mixed with honey and eaten in teaspoon doses, 3 times daily. There are several great general formulas for coughs: Formula #21 is specific when it's harder to inhale; Formula #64 is best if harder to exhale. The more chronic the condition, the longer the formula needs be taken. If there is accompanying fever, see the section Colds Flu and Fevers. Cough syrups are useful here as well, such as Formulas #68, #36 for coughs from viral conditions or colds, #171 for coughs with thick yellow phlegm, or a simple syrup of fresh **garlic** and fresh grated **ginger** in honey, using 1 tablespoon of any syrup every 1-2 hours or as needed.

Pneumonia can be a serious condition that may be acute, or "chronic", as in walking pneumonia. If there is a fever present, this condition requires similar treatment as Colds, Flu and Fevers (see that section). Take great care and monitor the condition, and **if you don't see improvement within 2-3 days, then definitely seek medical help.** However, many people have found **scute** and **usnea** to be useful if there is yellow phlegm, or **ginger, cayenne, licorice** and **cinnamon** if there is white phlegm. Either type benefits from an onion poultice over the chest, an herbal steam of **eucalyptus** or **mint**, a tea of 1 part each **pleurisy root, yerba santa, scute** and **eucalyptus** and ¼ part each **licorice** and **ginger** and frequently taking **garlic** raw or in juice or syrup form. If there is Deficient Kidney Yang present (it is harder to inhale), also use **cordyceps** in your formula (Formula #21).

Asthma and *wheezing* are treated differently in TCM. Asthma is caused by a type of trapped Wind that is neither External nor Internal, but a kind of chronic External Wind locked in the bronchi. When triggered, the Wind causes bronchospasm. (The TCM idea of Wind in this case may be compared to the Western concept of allergens.) This is why x-rays have no diagnostic value in asthma—because Wind is non-substantial. It also points to why acupuncture is remarkably effective in stopping acute asthma attacks. Phlegm may arise from asthma, especially over the long term, however it does not cause it. On the other hand, wheezing is caused by hidden phlegm stored in the lungs that blocks the airways. This is a constant condition until the phlegm is eliminated. Diet is very important in treating both and dampening foods must be reduced or eliminated in order for the herbs to be effective.

For either asthma or wheezing, take a dropperful of **lobelia** for acute attacks. When treating acute asthma, it's also important to calm the Mind and treat possible invasion of External Wind (there may be aversion to cold, shivering and possible fever). For chronic asthma, differentiate and treat the underlying Deficiencies (Lung, Spleen and/or Kidneys—see Patterns). The best herbs for asthma are **ephedra, coltsfoot, apricot seed** and **siler**. A general asthma formula includes 2 parts ephedra, 1 part each **thyme, coltsfoot** and **apricot seed** and ½ part **licorice**. Other beneficial herbs include **nettles, mullein** and **plantain** for yellow phlegm, or **ginger, cardamom, garlic, elecampane, schisandra, thyme, horseradish** or wild cherry bark for white phlegm. Also try Formulas #64 or 171. *For asthma due to allergens*, try formula #199. The best herbs for wheezing are **lobelia, mullein, coltsfoot, platycodon, wild cherry bark, garlic, elecampane** and **apricot seed**.

The Liver is frequently involved in asthma, particularly adult onset, or in early onset if there is emotional stress. This may occur when stagnant Liver Qi or Liver Fire rebels upwards and obstructs descending of Lung Qi, or when Deficient Liver Yin fails to nourish the Kidneys, leading to Dryness in the Lungs and/or Kidneys not grasping Lung Qi. In this case, herbs that regulate Liver Qi (**cyperus**), clear Liver Heat (**goldenseal**) or tonify Liver Yin (**raw rehmannia**) should be added to the asthma formula.

Differentiation of Coughs:

- A weak-sounding cough indicates Deficiency.
- A loud-sounding cough indicates Excess.
- A barking cough indicates Heat.
- A loose, rattling cough indicates Phlegm.
- Coughs worse in the morning are usually due to Phlegm.
- Coughs in the late afternoon or evening indicate Deficient Yin.
- Coughs without sputum indicate Deficiency or Heat.
- Coughs with abundant sputum are due to Phlegm.
- Yellow sputum indicates Heat.
- Dilute white sputum indicates Coldness.
- Sticky white sputum indicates Dampness and Phlegm.
- Blood-tinged sputum indicates Excess or Deficient Heat.
- Green sputum indicates Heat.

Coughs with Yellow Phlegm: These coughs are due to Damp Heat in the Lungs with possible symptoms of dry mouth and throat, sore throat, fever, sweating, thirst, blood-tinged sputum, acute tonsillitis or another infection such as pneumonia. The best herbs to use are **horehound, lungwort, mullein, mulberry leaf, pleurisy root, nettles, fritillary** and **bamboo**. Also try Formulas #68, 141 or 171. If there is an accompanying infection, take **echinacea** tincture hourly and/or 2 capsules of **goldenseal** powder every 2-3 hours.

Coughs with White or Clear Phlegm: Due to Cold Damp in the Lungs, these coughs may have symptoms of cold-ness, chills, no sweating or thirst, low fever, poor appetite and white, copious, runny Phlegm. Beneficial herbs cough include **coltsfoot, elecampane, garlic** (raw, syrup or juice), **wild cherry bark, hyssop, thyme, black pepper, pinellia, platycodon** and **ephedra**. Honey is a good carrier for these herbs as it's warming energy clears Cold mucus. Also try Formula #64.

Dry Coughs: Since dry coughs are generally due to Deficient Yin, it's necessary to moisten the Lungs in order to produce and expectorate the Phlegm. A delicious remedy is baked pear with rock sugar and/or honey. Herbally, take **ophiopogon, slippery elm, marshmal-**

ACUTE COUGH—EXTERIOR PATTERNS:

INVASION OF WIND-COLD	INVASION OF WIND-HEAT	INVASION OF WIND-DRYNESS
Cough	Dry cough with tickling sensation in the throat	Dry and ticklish cough
Aversion to cold	Aversion to heat	Aversion to wind and slight aversion to cold
Slight breathlessness	Sore throat	Dry, itchy sore throat
Sneezing	Sneezing	
Runny nose with white discharge	Runny nose with yellow discharge	Stuffy nose
Headache	Headache	Headache
No or low fever, stronger chills	Fever, slight chills	Slight shivers
No sweating	Slight sweating	Dry lips
Body aches	Body aches	Dry mouth
No thirst	Thirst	Sore sensation in upper chest
Stiff neck	Possible stiff neck	
Pale urine	Slightly dark urine	
Tongue: possibly no change	**Tongue:** slightly red sides and/or front	**Tongue:** slightly red sides and/or front
Pulse: floating and tight	**Pulse:** floating and fast	**Pulse:** floating
Formulas: #64, 68; 10 drops lobelia tincture with fresh garlic or garlic juice and a tea of thyme, wild cherry bark, elecampane, yerba santa and citrus peel (orange, tangerine or grapefruit) with ½ part fresh ginger and ¼ part licorice	**Formulas:** #64, 68; 10 drops lobelia tincture with tea of equal parts mullein, eyebright, coltsfoot, elder and wild cherry bark. Suck on horehound cough drops, or include tincture in tea	**Formulas:** #68; tea of equal parts wild cherry bark and ophiopogon

low, **Iceland moss** and **Irish moss**, or Formula #168.

Spasmodic Coughs: Use antitussive herbs that relieve difficult breathing and lessen coughs, such as **coltsfoot** and **thyme** (both of which are also specific for *whooping cough*), **apricot seed**, **yerba santa**, **lobelia** (10 drops when needed), **wild cherry bark**, **loquat leaf**, **grindellia** and **mullein**.

Dry Throat from Coughs: Suck on a **licorice** stick or **slippery elm** lozenges, or their powders mixed in honey.

Whooping Cough: These herbs work very well: **coltsfoot**, **thyme**, **lobelia**, **wild cherry bark**, **mullein**, **grindelia** and **yerba santa**.

Emphysema: **wild cherry bark**, **lobelia**, **thyme**, **mullein**

ACUTE COUGH—INTERIOR PATTERNS:

LUNG HEAT	LUNG PHLEGM-HEAT
Barking cough with small amounts of yellow sputum	Barking cough with profuse expectoration of sticky-yellow sputum
Chest pain, breathlessness	Feeling of heat and oppression in the chest
Fever	Fever
Thirst	Thirst
Sweating	Sweating
Restlessness	Restlessness
Aversion to heat	
Tongue: red with yellow coat	**Tongue:** red with stick, yellow coat
Pulse: fast and overflowing	**Pulse:** fast and slippery
Formulas: #64, 134; 10 drops lobelia tincture with tea of equal parts sweet basil, mullein, coltsfoot, red clover, platycodon and ½ part licorice.	**Formulas:** #68, 141; 10 drops lobelia tincture wth tea of equal parts mullein, coltsfoot, platycodon and ½ part licorice.

CHRONIC COUGH—EXCESS PATTERNS:

DAMPNESS IN THE LUNGS	PHLEGM-HEAT IN THE LUNGS	LIVER FIRE INSULTING THE LUNGS
Frequent coughing attacks	Frequent coughing attacks	Sudden bouts of cough with a red face; comes on by emotional stress
Profuse expectoration of white, sticky phlegm	Profuse expectoration of yellow or blood-tinged sputum	Expectoration of scanty phlegm
Worse in the mornings and after eating	Red face	Pain on coughing
Breathlessness	Breathlessness	Dry throat
Sensation of oppression in the chest	Sensation of oppression in the chest	Pain an distension under the ribs
Feeling of fullness in the stomach region and diaphragm	Dry mouth	Dry mouth
Nausea	Thirst	Bitter taste in the mouth

(continued on next page)

CHRONIC COUGH—EXCESS PATTERNS: *(continued)*

DAMPNESS IN THE LUNGS	PHELGM-HEAT IN THE LUNGS	LIVER FIRE INSULTING THE LUNGS
Poor appetite	Poor appetite	Dark urine
Tiredness	Tiredness	Irritability
Feeling of heaviness	Feeling of heat	Feeling of phlegm in the throat
Loose stools	Rattling sound in the throat	Dry stools
Tongue: pale or normal with sticky thick, white coat	**Tongue:** red with sticky, yellow coat	**Tongue:** red with redder sides, dry, yellow coat
Pulse: slippery	**Pulse:** slippery and fast, or weak, floating, slightly slippery and fast	**Pulse:** wiry and fast
Formulas: #64, 68; Trikatu: (equal parts powdered black pepper, ginger and anise mixed with enough honey to form a paste)—take 1 tsp. every 3-4 hours.	**Formulas:** #68 & 64 or #141; 10 drops lobelia tincture with tea of equal parts mullein, coltsfoot and platycodon with ½ part licorice.	**Formulas:** #64 or 141; 10 drops lobelia tincture with 2 capsules goldenseal and tea of equal parts mullein, coltsfoot and loquat with ½ part licorice.

CHRONIC COUGH—DEFICIENCY PATTERNS:

DEFICIENT LUNG QI	DEFICIENT LUNG YIN
Slight cough with low sound	Dry cough in short bursts with a low sound
No phlegm	No phlegm or scanty phlegm
Spontaneous sweating	Blood-streaked sputum
Easily catches colds and flu	Dry throat
Weak voice	Feeling of heat in the evening
Tiredness	Burning sensation in the palms, soles and/or chest
Pale face	Night sweats
	Thin body
Tongue: pale	**Tongue:** red without coat, dry, cracks in Lung area
Pulse: empty	**Pulse:** floating and empty
Formulas: #77, 176; tea of equal parts American ginseng, schisandra, astragalus, elecampane and ½ part each licorice and fenugreek.	**Formulas:** #168; tea of equal parts Iceland moss, Irish moss, ophiopogon, slippery elm, marshmallow and American ginseng and ½ part each licorice and fenugreek.

❦ DEPRESSION

Depression is a state of mind ranging from mild, temporary sadness, to intense states of despair, possibly even suicide. Manic depression is a condition of alternating moods between extreme depression and elation. While short-term depression from disappointment or loss is normal, repeated occurrence for no apparent reason, or lasting longer than reasonable, means an imbalance needs correcting.

These symptoms may be expressed in any number of ways, such as increased irritability and dissatisfaction, withdrawal from others, crying spells, moodiness, nervousness, anxiety, unwillingness to get out of bed in the morning, tiredness, insomnia, headaches, muscle aches and pains and/or palpitations. Depression may also be expressed through "sudden" anger and aggressive behavior, especially in boys and men (because of the Western "boy code"—keep your chin up, don't be a crybaby—males are more often taught to hide their emotions).

Depression has become so widespread, particularly in the U.S., that Europeans call this country the "Prozac Nation". Indeed, it is very common for these people to use antidepressants, and it is becoming more and more common in children (see section Attention Deficit Hyperactivity Disorder) and teenagers as well (take any comments about "ending it all" seriously). Further, it is not unusual for women to experience mild depression before or during menses, after childbirth or through peri/menopausal years. Severe depression and depression due to inherited causes or childhood factors usually need professional guidance and counseling. However, such treatment may be coupled with herbs and diet for more efficient results.

In TCM, there are actual physiological causes for depression that can be treated and improved. This is a tremendous boon since using drugs only applies a Band-Aid to mask underlying symptoms.[1] Thus, it is important to determine and correct the root cause of depression. While there are many patterns and causes for depression in TCM, the most common is stagnant Liver Qi.

Just as a tree spreads out freely in all directions, so does the Liver promote unrestrained and regular

---

[1] This is not to say that antidepressants aren't applicable in certain circumstances, or can't help someone get over an extremely difficult time in life. Yet, the underlying causes and imbalances need correcting, and when they are, drugs are usually not needed.

Symptoms of Depression:

The following is a list of symptoms that define depression according to the American Psychiatric Association:

- Loss of interest or pleasure in usual activities and pastimes
- Increased or decreased appetite with noticeable weight change
- Excessive sleepiness or sleeplessness (insomnia)
- Hyperactivity or slowed activity
- No interest or pleasure in normal activities, with possible inability to get out of bed in the morning
- Reduced sex drive
- Fatigue or lack of energy
- Feelings of guilt, self-reproach, or lack of personal worth
- Impaired mental abilities
- Preoccupation with thoughts of death or suicide; attempted suicide

movement of Qi and Blood throughout the body. In its ideal state, Qi flows smoothly and disperses and circulates freely. When imbalanced, its flow is irregular and Qi doesn't flow smoothly, evenly, or in the right directions. This can occur in most anyone—male, female, young, or old—but because the Liver is so intimately involved with women's monthly cycles, menstruating women tend to experience it more often (this is probably why more women feel depressed). When Liver Qi stagnates, it has far-reaching effects, many of which co-exist with depression: pain and distension in the ribs, breasts and lower abdomen; movable or fixed cysts, fibroids and other lumps in the abdomen and breasts with little to extreme stabbing pain; irregular menstruation, dysmenorrhea or amenorrhea; belching, sour regurgitation, nausea, vomiting, chronic diarrhea, abdominal distension, loss of appetite, or jaundice.

Smooth Liver Qi harmonizes emotions with the Mind by keeping a happy state, sensitivity, ability to

Causes for Depression:

While some of the following are commonly acknowledged Western causes for depression, others are those according to TCM. Most depression results from a combination of the following:

- Hypothyroidism (see section Tiredness, for more details)
- Suppressed, unexpressed and unreleased emotions, particularly anger, frustration and resentment, though it can be any long-term repressed emotion (stagnates Liver Qi)
- Sudden emotional extremes, such as those from shock or crisis (depletes Kidneys and Heart)
- Genetic predisposition or inherited weak nervous system (weakened Kidneys and/or Liver)
- Difficult childhood, such as abuse, deprivation or neglect (stagnates Liver Qi)
- Extreme stress, especially if feeling an inability to cope, such as the death of a loved one, divorce, loss of job, abuse, neglect, financial collapse, mid-life crisis (weakens Kidneys, stagnates Liver)
- Excessive use of alcohol, caffeine (coffee, black tea, colas, maté, cocoa and chocolate) or drugs (recreational or medical)—(stagnates Liver Qi, weakens Kidneys)
- Excessive intake of dairy, nuts and nut butters, turkey, avocados, fried and fatty foods, chips and oily, greasy foods (stagnates Liver Qi)
- Long-term chemical exposure, such as herbicide sprays or metalworking (stagnates Liver Qi)
- Suppressed creativity (stagnates Liver Qi)
- Suppressed desires and dreams for one's life (stagnates Liver Qi, depletes Heart)
- Overworking combined with irregular diet and excessive activity or sex (weakens Kidneys)
- Lack of exercise (stagnates Liver Qi)
- Not liking one's work or job (stagnates Liver Qi, weakens Heart)
- Long-term chronic disease (weakens Kidneys and Spleen)
- Birthing too many children too close together (weakens Kidneys)
- Low or imbalanced blood sugar levels (weakens Spleen)
- Low energy, tiredness (weakens Spleen and Kidneys, stagnates Liver Qi)
- Unresolved stress (stagnates Liver Qi)
- Continuously not feeling well (weakens Kidneys and Spleen)
- Unhappy or unfulfilling relationships (stagnates Liver Qi, weakens Heart)

reason, an even disposition and a sense of ease. Thus, obstructed Liver Qi adversely affects emotions, causing emotional swings, irritability, frustration, and depression. It also triggers breast distension, a sensation of oppression or pain in chest or under ribs, sighing, a feeling of a "lump" in the throat and PMS symptoms.

As well, the Liver is associated with the Ethereal Soul (Hun) in TCM, the part of us that dreams, plans, envisions, creates and imagines. It is the vehicle through which images, ideas and dreams emerge into our conscious mind from our subconscious (and from the collective unconscious, to use Jung's terminology). If the Ethereal Soul is unsettled, Mind (Shen) is cut off from the Universal Mind, resulting in a lack of direction in life, feelings of aimlessness, and unrealized dreams and plans. Such "isolation" leads to moodiness, sudden outbursts of anger or aggression and depression.

General Treatment for Depression:

At first signs of depression, physically move your body. While this may be the last thing you feel like doing, it is the easiest and most efficient way to move stagnant Qi and change emotions. Do whatever is easiest and most satisfying—walk, run, dance, pound pillows, garden, or do yoga, Qi Gong or something similar—just so you move your body. After five or ten minutes, you'll feel better. Now move some more. A half-hour is ideal, but if five minutes is all you can do, even that makes a difference. Moving in nature is even better, as nature is powerfully healing.

In general, daily exercise is beneficial for preventing and treating depression, as it keeps Liver Qi healthy and stimulates production of endorphins, natural mood-elevating chemicals. Having little need for natural exercise in our modern lives, we substitute with gyms, exercise equipment and videotapes, yet this does not compare to the amount of walking, lifting and carrying that was a normal part of life before motor vehicles and appliances. In fact, one of the best expressions of frustration, anger and resentment is constructive movement. Anger is energy, so clean up the kitchen, unload old drawers/closets, or run around the block—all help to express and release this energy in healthy ways.

Since stagnant Qi results from any long-term suppressed or repressed emotions, it is now important to discover their underlying causes and outlets. Above all, do not repress or stuff emotions, as this creates more depression. Rather, long-term suppressed emotions may be moved through many ways. Appropriately express and release emotions (do not hesitate to get help from a friend or professional if needed). Journal write, as this unloads repressed feelings, moving energy and inviting insights, solutions and ideas that may help sort through painful emotions and clarify decisions. Go on a retreat or vision quest.

Take time off and explore what is not working in your life so you can come up with a plan for change. Identify stressful factors in your home and work environment and modify them. Put energy into creative outlets since creativity opens doors to your subconscious mind, allowing energy to flow again. It doesn't have to be a big or "important" project—simple activities such as rearranging furniture, decorating, building a carpentry project, planning a new garden area, playing a musical instrument, or singing are all beneficial. In fact, any form of appropriate self-expression moves stagnant Qi.

To relieve depression, it is extremely important to refine your diet by eliminating depression-causing foods and including stagnation-moving ones. Foods that congest Qi are, unfortunately, very prevalent in the Western diet. On the other hand, it explains why depression occurs, and their removal quickly aids in the body regaining balance. In severe depression, it is essential to completely eliminate the following foods to get best results: fried, greasy and fatty foods, nuts and nut butters, avocados, cheese and dairy, chips of all kinds, turkey and red meats, alcohol, caffeinated foods and drinks (coffee, black tea, maté, cocoa, colas and chocolate) and recreational drugs. Beneficial decongesting and Liver-aiding foods include vegetables, lemons, dark leafy greens such as kale, collards, **dandelion**, mustard, beet and other bitter foods.

Lastly, reflect on your lifestyle habits and balance them as appropriate. Excessive activity, sex, or exercise deplete Qi, as do keeping late bedtimes (after 11 PM), working at jobs one doesn't like, overworking physically and mentally, and insufficient physical activity. Ultimately, such depletion leads to depression. To rebalance the Liver, go to bed before 11 PM at the latest, get plenty of physical exercise, find enjoyable and fulfilling work and jobs and alternate work with rest and play. Regularity of habits regulates Liver Qi.

When Qi is stagnant, do not give tonifying herbs, unless you also take Qi-moving herbs, as they only create more stagnation, like adding cars to a bad traffic jam. In fact, Chinese herbal masters often first gave Qi moving herbs, or Qi-regulating Herbs, before following any other herbal therapy. In Western herbalism, these herbs are fairly equivalent to carminative herbs. Examples of herbs that regulate Liver Qi, moving stagnation and easing depression include **vitex**, **citrus** (tangerine peel, both the ripe and unripe and the unripe fruit of the bitter orange), **cyperus (sedge root)**, **sandalwood**, **Chinese chive**, **rose petals**, **mint**, **lemon balm** and **cumin**, as well as the Chinese herbs **bupleurum** and **saussurea**.

St. John's wort has become very well-known for treating mild to moderate depression, particularly in Europe where it's effectively used in clinics for mild to moderate depression with few side effects (Formulas #89, 90). In some cases it works well, but in those with stagnant Liver Qi, I have not seen it be effective. It seems to work best for those with Liver Heat. For depression related to the hormonal cycle, try **wild yam** and **vitex** (Formulas #102, 104). Also refer to PMS under the section Menstrual Issues. Some Chinese herbalists consider **albizzia** (mimosa tree) bark (or flower) an herbal Prozac, particularly for emotional trauma or sudden loss, or with accompanying anger and anxiety.

The best herbal formula I have found to relieve most depression cases is Formula #12 (or 153). Normal dosage is 8 pills (or 2 tabs), 3 times/daily, but in extreme cases take 16-24 pills (or 4 tabs), 4-6 times/daily, until symptoms subside; then taper down dosage. This formula is fabulous for moving stagnant Liver Qi and harmonizing the Liver and Spleen, successfully alleviating mood swings, PMS and depression. If there is also anger, irritability, frustration, a throbbing headache, red eyes, thirst or other Heat signs accompanying depression, take Formula #154, using the same dosage. Also consider taking Formula #92 to increase stress-handling ability, thus alleviating depression.

Lastly, it is not uncommon for depression to be caused by hypothyroidism. If you suspect this is the case, or if what is offered here doesn't work, check the section Tiredness, for symptoms and details on determining and treating hypothyroidism. For anxiety, see the section Insomnia.

DEPRESSION PATTERNS:

Refer to PMS under Menstrual Issues, for other possible patterns (even if you are male). For related symptoms, such as insomnia (including palpitations), poor memory or tiredness, refer to those sections.

DEPRESSION—EXCESS PATTERNS:

STAGNANT QI	LIVER FIRE	STAGNANT HEART BLOOD	STAGNANT LIVER BLOOD	HEAT AND PHLEGM BLOCKING THE MIND
Depression	Depression	Depression	Extreme depression	Depression alternating with confusion and elation
Moodiness	Similar signs to Qi stagnation but with more Heat signs	Palpitations	Severe mood swings	Manic depressive; lack of mental clarity
Mental confusion	Speaks in a low voice	Insomnia	Intense irritability	Anxious
PMS	Subdued behavior	Nightmares	Propensity to be violent	Agitated; weeping
Irritability, frustration, annoyance, impatience	Irritability, frustration, anger, hatred churning within	Suffocating sensation in chest	Obsessive jealousy	Tendency toward suicide
Sighing		Irritability	Outbursts of anger	Dizziness
Belching		Mood swings	Manic-depressive	Dull headache
Tiredness		Excitable		Nausea
Pain in the ribs or side		Psychosis in extreme cases		Desire to lie down

(continued on next page)

DEPRESSION—EXCESS PATTERNS: *(continued)*

STAGNANT QI	LIVER FIRE	STAGNANT HEART BLOOD	STAGNANT LIVER BLOOD	HEAT AND PHLEGM BLOCKING THE MIND
Feeling of tightness in the chest				Feeling of oppression in chest
Irregular periods				Poor appetite
Clumsiness				Tiredness
Breast distension				Poor concentration
Tongue: possibly no change	**Tongue:** red with redder sides	**Tongue:** purple	**Tongue:** purple on sides	**Tongue:** swollen with sticky coat
Pulse: wiry	**Pulse:** wiry and fast	**Pulse:** wiry or choppy	**Pulse:** wiry or choppy	**Pulse:** slippery and wiry
Formulas: #12 or 153; 4 capsules of equal parts powdered vitex, lemon balm, white peony, dang gui, cyperus, lycii and bupleurum with 1/2 part green citrus. Eat rose petal paste as well.	**Formulas:** #12 with 13, or #154; 4 capsules of equal parts powdered bupleurum, white peony, lycii, gardenia, zizyphus, St. John's wort, scutellaria and 1/2 part green citrus peel. Take with lemon balm tea.	**Formulas:** #113 or 182; tablets of boswellia and guggul with tea of equal parts mother-wort, salvia, dang gui, zizyphus and albizzia.	**Formulas:** #113 or 182; tea or 4 capsules powder of equal parts ligusticum, gardenia, turmeric, dang gui, white peony, zizyphus, he shou wu vine and cyperus.	**Formulas:** #13 with 64; tea of equal parts fu ling, citrus peel, polygala, bamboo leaves and 1/2 part licorice and coptis.

DEPRESSION—DEFICIENT QI, BLOOD AND YANG PATTERNS:

DEFICIENT QI	DEFICIENT BLOOD	DEFICIENT YANG
Depression	Vaguely depressed	Depression
Extreme tiredness	Tiredness	Mentally/physically exhausted
No desire to speak/talk	Anxious	Lack of will power
Lack of motivation	Easily startled	Lost of interest in life
No appetite	Palpitations	Loss of initiative
Restless sleep, unpleasant dreams	Pale, dull complexion	Everything takes too much effort
Loose stools	Dull eyes	Hopelessness
Slight breathlessness	Dizziness	Low back ache
Weak voice	Blurred vision	Weak knees
Pale, shiny face	Numbness in limbs	Poor memory
Obsessive thinking	Hard to fall asleep	Cold legs and back
Poor concentration	Poor memory	Frequent and pale urination

(continued on next page)

DEPRESSION—DEFICIENT QI, BLOOD AND YANG PATTERNS: *(continued)*

DEFICIENT QI	DEFICIENT BLOOD	DEFICIENT YANG
	Timid	Nighttime urination
Tongue: pale	**Tongue:** pale and thin	**Tongue:** pale and swollen
Pulse: empty or weak	**Pulse:** choppy	**Pulse:** deep and slow
Formulas: 4-6 tablets #77 with 138; tea of equal parts astragalus, reishi, codonopsis, albizzia, longan and jujube dates.	**Formulas:** #106 or 159; tea of equal parts cooked rehmannia, white peony, dang gui, longan, jujube dates, albizzia, reishi and schisandra.	**Formulas:** #75 or 180; 1 tablet deer antler (#1), or 1 capsule dried ginger and cinnamon bark, with tea of equal parts cooked rehmannia, Chinese wild yam, polygala, lycii and ashwagandha.

DEPRESSION—DEFICIENT YIN PATTERNS:

DEFICIENT HEART YIN	DEFICIENT LIVER YIN	DEFICIENT KIDNEY YIN
Depression	Depressed	Depression
Very anxious	Lacks sense of direction in life	Very anxious
Restlessness	Mentally restless	Mentally restless
Palpitations	Wakes up frequently during night	Low back pain
Dispirited	Restless dreams	Fitful sleep
Dry eyes	Tiredness	Lack of willpower
Tongue: red without coat with redder tip	**Tongue:** red without coat, especially sides	**Tongue:** red without coat with redder root
Pulse: floating and empty	**Pulse:** floating and empty	**Pulse:** floating and empty
Formulas: #136; tea of equal parts he shou wu vine, albizzia, zizyphus, lycii, ophiopogon, American ginseng and schisandra.	**Formulas:** #74, 169 or 190; tea of equal parts he shou wu vine, lycii, ophiopogon, raw rehmannia, zizyphus, white peony and albizzia.	**Formulas:** #74 or 230; tea of equal parts he shou wu vine, lycii, ophiopogon, raw and cooked rehmannia, American ginseng, ashwagandha, schisandra and albizzia.

❦ DIGESTIVE DISORDERS

There are many possible digestive orders. Here I cover Candida, constipation, diarrhea, gluten intolerance (celiac disease) and gastroesophageal reflux disease (GERD).

CANDIDA

Candida albicans is a condition of yeast overgrowth in the intestines that may also manifest as fungus in the vagina, external genitalia, nails, under the breasts, folds of the groin, armpits and fingers, or in the mouth and throat (called thrush). In rare conditions, it can spread systemically throughout the body (I say rare because many signs of Candida are actually indicative of a toxic colon, leaky gut syndrome, gluten intolerance, celiac disease, or hyperacidity of the body). While yeast is a natural and necessary part of the intestines that aids digestion, when it grows out of control many uncomfort-

Candida Signs:

Chronic fatigue, weakness, tiredness, light to profuse vaginal discharge (that is itchy and has a white to cream-colored thin or clumpy consistency), anal itching, thrush, food allergies, moodiness, gas, bloatedness, depression, extreme PMS, dizziness, headaches, fuzzy thinking ("fog brain"), poor memory and concentration, cold sweats, night sweats, muscle and joint pains, chronic sore throat, low-grade fever, constipation or diarrhea, yeast rashes, fungal infections, itchy red skin spots, loss of sex drive, sugar and carbohydrate cravings.

Causes of Candida:

These factors either lower immunity and/or create a Candida-friendly environment:

- Excessive use of antibiotics and NSAIDs (aspirin, ibuprofen, etc.)
- Birth control pill, multiple pregnancies and progesterone in HRT
- Stress (weakens immunity and stagnates Qi)
- Immunosuppressive agents, such as cytotoxic drugs and corticosteroids (weaken immunity, allowing yeast to grow unchecked)
- Low thyroid function (causes a yeast-friendly Damp environment—see the section Tiredness, if you suspect hypothyroidism)
- Excessive eating of Dampening foods such as raw foods, most fruit, fruit juices, iced drinks and foods, dairy, soy milk, tofu, flour products, refined and processed foods and sugar
- Transfats, saturated fats and excessive sugar intake (especially refined sugars)
- Exposure to toxic substances and environmental toxins
- Common food allergens such as dairy, eggs, gluten grains (wheat, oats, rye), corn, beans, soy products and nuts (lower immunity and create stagnation, congesting digestive functions—interestingly, those with dairy and wheat allergies tend to do fine with cultured dairy and non-hybridized wheat, such as kamut or spelt)
- Leaky gut syndrome
- Stress, emotional strain, long-term suppressed emotions (cause stagnant Liver Qi), or lack of self-esteem and confidence (depletes Spleen Qi, causing poor transformation of fluids, resulting in Dampness)
- Excessive physical work, including sports (weakens Spleen Qi, causing poor transformation of fluids, resulting in Dampness)
- Overwork, especially without adequate rest or diet (depletes Liver and Kidney Yin)
- Poor digestion and incomplete assimilation
- Parasites

able symptoms result. It's not uncommon for people to have yeast overgrowth and not even know it.

Typical testing for Candida is done through stool samples, but even then it may not show up for various reasons. The most dependable test is an anal swab test. Others find live blood cell analysis useful. Most tests indicate the level of abnormal yeast present and substances most effective for its elimination. This can be helpful because not everyone is responsive to the same substances.

The list of effective substances for eliminating yeast overgrowth range from garlic to berberine-containing herbs (**Oregon grape**, **goldenseal**, **scutellaria**, **gentian**, **grapefruit seed extract**), caprylic acid, undecylenic acid and medications such as Diflucan and Nystatin, to name a few. Many people are able to control their yeast overgrowth with any one or a combination of these substances. However, they are only doing that, controlling it, and not healing the body so the Candida doesn't return. Rather, it is common for yeast overgrowth symptoms to recur again and again, even if it is years before their return.

While the medications given to treat Candida can be very effective for some people, in others they can cause side effects, such as liver toxicity. Further, it is still possible (even probable) to experience a recurrence of yeast overgrowth symptoms as frequently as do those who use herbs. The reason these symptoms rear their ugly heads over and over again is because most approaches only cure the symptoms rather than treat the original root cause of the yeast overgrowth. So what is the root cause? Simply put, it is poor digestion.

Poor digestion results from either lack of Qi, insufficient metabolic Heat and /or congestion blocking efficient digestive function. Many commonly eaten foods actually squelch digestive fires, which is like turning the burner down on your stove. This occurs through excessive intake of foods that are Cooling (soy milk, tofu, iced drinks and foods, raw foods, salads, juices), Dampening (same as Cold foods with flour products, processed foods, dairy and fatty, sugary and greasy foods as well), and/or from poor digestion. The result is sluggish digestion with poor assimilation, causing stagnation in the intestines and a swamp-like environment that slows or blocks movement. Then just like a swamp, harmful bacteria and yeast breed to eventually outweigh important beneficial bacteria.

At this point, the murky swamp festers and Heat signs arise, such as red itchy skin spots or burning and itchy vaginal discharge. Ultimately, it's possible for someone with Candida to experience symptoms of both Heat and Coldness. Unchecked harmful bacteria eventually create inflammation and eat away intestinal walls, creating permeability through which undigested food particles leak into the bloodstream and circulate throughout the body. Termed leaky gut syndrome, this is a common occurrence in those with chronic or systemic Candida (and in those without Candida who have a toxic or congested colon and liver) causing a vast array of symptoms. Taking herbs and drugs to treat Candida only clears excessive yeast. If intestinal permeability isn't healed, sooner or later the problem reappears.

General Treatment for Candida:

Some people who think they have Candida actually have poor digestion (meaning there is Deficient Spleen Qi and Dampness), since signs of both are similar. If so, results come quickly by following the table Foods to Avoid and Eat for Candida and taking Spleen Qi tonics such as **ginseng**, **astragalus**, **baked licorice**, **white atractylodes** (or Formula #43) along with Dampness clearing herbs, such as **asafoetida**, **cumin**, and **ginger** (or Formula #17), and blood cleansers, such as **red clover**, **pau d'arco**, **red clover**, **dandelion root** and **burdock root** (or Formula #70).

True Candida overgrowth can be very difficult to eliminate for good, taking time and effort along with adherence to a strict protocol, for it is necessary to both heal the intestinal holes as well as strengthen the digestion. This is true for leaky gut syndrome as well. Feeding beneficial flora to the intestines is useful to heal wall membranes by boosting the level of favorable bacteria to eat up the harmful ones. Products containing multiple strains of acidophilus and bifidus are readily available and should be a daily part of the diet in any who have Candida.

Acidophilus generally benefits the large intestines and bifidus the small intestines (an excess of acidophilus can cause loose stools while an excess of bifidus can result in constipation). Normal dosage for this condition is anywhere between 1 tsp. to 1 Tbsp., 3 times/day with meals. When first starting acidophilus and bifidus, you may experience gas, bloatedness, diarrhea or constipation, a result of the intestinal congestion and die-off of unfavorable bacteria. Back down on your dose and perhaps take every other day until the symptoms stop. Then gradually increase again.

By itself, acidophilus wonderfully boosts the immune system as it enhances colon immunity, the second line of defense in the body (in fact, if you feel the onset of a cold, you can often fight it off by taking large quantities of acidophilus throughout one day—up to 2-4 oz). Another immune-boosting product I have found very useful for Candida is colostrum. Naturally found in mother's milk, this powerful immune system stimulant works particularly well for those with Candida or leaky gut syndrome (take 4 capsules, twice a day with meals). Further, L-glutamine is used to heal leaky gut syndrome in the stomach while N-A-glucosamine heals leaky gut in the intestines.

Acidophilus and bifidus may or may not heal the intestinal holes, depending on your ability to follow a strict diet and improve your digestion. Most people aren't patient or strong-willed enough to do what this takes. After all, it's not much "fun" and having fun with foods like sugar, alcohol and flour products is what helped create the problem in the first place. Thus, something stronger is needed, and the best I've found is soil-based organisms (for products with these organisms, refer to *Resources*). These beneficial bacteria found growing in the soil actively attach to intestinal walls and quickly proliferate down the intestinal tract.[2] There they feast on the harmful bacteria and close leaky gut holes, healing the intestines and resulting in overall increased health and immunity. This process takes from two to six months, depending on the severity of the condition, and the diet needs to be particularly strict during this time

Next, strengthen your digestion by changing your food choices and taking herbs. While many books proclaim varying diets beneficial for healing Candida, TCM holds a unique perspective. In TCM, the Stomach is in charge of physically breaking down and mixing food, while the Spleen is responsible for transforming and transporting this mash into Blood and Qi. Thus, foods impairing Spleen and Stomach function must be eliminated, while foods and herbs that strengthen these Organs need be taken (see the table, Foods to Eat and Avoid for Candida).

Interestingly, I find most people who develop Candida have O-Blood types and northern climate ancestries, which create a higher physical demand for protein than any other type. Yet, they frequently become vegetarian, macrobiotic or vegan. Over time, lack of dietary protein accompanied by excessive grains, flour products, sugar, raw foods, fruit juices and soy weaken digestive fires and create food stagnation, the perfect intestinal swamp in which Candida best thrives.

While fermented products supply favorable bacteria, they frequently exacerbate Candida symptoms because of increasing pathogenic Heat. Thus, eliminate these foods until the intestinal walls are healed and yeast overgrowth is cleared. While mushrooms normally worsen Candida, I've found medicinal mushrooms are fine, such as **fu ling, shitake** and **reishi**, because they strengthen immunity, giving the energy boost needed to effectively clear yeast overgrowth symptoms.

A good general program is as follows: take an herbal formula, such as 3 parts each **coix** and **agastache**, 2 parts each **hawthorn berries**, **oregano**, **spilanthes**, **asafoetida**, **eleuthro**, **astragalus** and **dioscorea**, 1 part each **citrus** and **fu ling**, and ¹/₂ part **goldenseal** (alternatively, use 4-6 tablets, 3 times daily of Formula #17). Include immune-tonifying herbs, such as **astragalus**, **reishi** and **ginseng** (Formula #77), **grapefruit seed extract**, colostrum, soil-based organisms and one or more of the suggested supplements. Follow the Candida diet, including raw **garlic** daily (Formula #39). Stick to this program for three to six months. Of course, it is also important to eliminate antibiotics, birth control pills, progesterone and other yeast-proliferating factors from your routine.

Your symptoms may worsen as the Candida dies off during this process. This is actually a good sign that Candida is being eliminated. Since the die-off of harmful bacteria creates acids in the body, eat more alkalinizing foods, take 1 teaspoon of baking soda in a glass of water daily along with the supplements N-A-G and L-glutamine, and include a few immune tonics to ease die-off symptoms.

As well, use this time to rest, reflect on your life and make any changes needed for your healing. If your symptoms are too overwhelming, then back down doses of herbs and soil-based organisms and proceed at

---

[2] Interestingly, in our "cleanliness is next to godliness" culture, we have managed to wipe out favorable bacteria normally found growing on our fruits and vegetables. We used to obtain an abundance of these favorable organisms this way and now don't get enough. In fact, I remember reading a fascinating article published in a national natural health magazine in the 1980s which discussed the abundance of B vitamins found in Indonesian made tempeh versus the notable lack of B vitamins found in tempeh manufactured in sterile (but clean!) Western kitchens!

FOODS TO AVOID AND EAT FOR CANDIDA:

CANDIDA-CAUSING FOODS TO AVOID: It is usually an excessive intake of the following combinations of foods that creates poor digestion and food stagnation:	CANDIDA-HEALING DIET TO FOLLOW: These foods create a balanced diet and aid digestion:
Sugar in all forms, including dried fruit and alcohol	Sufficient protein for your body's needs
Possible food allergens such as dairy, eggs, gluten grains (wheat, oats, rye), corn, beans (especially soy), sugar and nuts	Lots of mostly cooked vegetables (except carrots, peas and potatoes) with a large variety and of all colors.
Flour products (bagels, muffins, bread, toast, pasta, chips, crackers, cookies, pastries, pies, cakes, etc.)	A moderate amount of whole grains and legumes, soaked 12–24 hours and well cooked, as appropriate for your body type
Cooling foods (bananas, melons, shellfish, raw foods, iced drinks, ice cream, fruit juices, melons, bananas, soy milk and tofu)	Periodic small amounts of cooked seasonal fruit with spices added to aid in digestion (ginger, cardamom, cinnamon)
Chlorinated water	Water, herb teas, green tea and lemon water are the best drinks
Fruit and/or fruit juices, iced drinks, ice cream, dairy	Dark leafy greens, such as collards, kale, mustard, bok choy
Raw foods, including salads	Eat all cooked foods and cook with spices such as garlic, ginger, cumin, basil, turmeric, coriander, asafoetida, dill, etc.
Acidic foods: flour products, excess of red meats and grains, citrus—except lemons and limes—tomatoes, green bell peppers, caffeine, chocolate, nuts and seeds, heated oils and fats, dairy, gluten	Alkaline foods such as lemons, limes, millet, amaranth, quinoa, umeboshi paste and vegetables (except tomatoes, green bell peppers, potatoes, and eggplant) alkalinize the body; also take red marine algae or 1 tsp. baking soda in 1 glass of water every day for a week to alkalinize
Insufficient or excessive protein for your body's needs	Seaweeds for minerals
Dairy	Cultured dairy in small amounts as needed (yogurt, cottage cheese, etc.)
Ice cream, popsicles, frozen yogurt, etc.	Mostly cooked and warm foods and drinks
Vinegar-containing foods (salad dressings, sauerkraut, green olives, pickled vegetables, relishes)	
Fermented foods, including soy sauce	Cultured foods and salt-pickled foods
Mushrooms (except medicinal)	Shiitake and reishi mushrooms
Other mold-aggravating foods such as raw and roasted nuts and seeds, barbecued foods, commercial soups, yeast and yeast-containing products, pork products, soft drinks, dried and smoked meats	

a slower pace. As you re-stabilize, slowly increase them again. After this process is complete, the body won't develop Candida again as long as good digestion and a healthy diet are maintained. Preventatively, include acidophilus and bifidus regularly in the diet and take soil-based organisms for one month every year while eating an especially healthy diet.

As a further note, many people who have Candida also have hypothyroidism. In fact, low thyroid is often what allowed yeast to overgrow in the first place. See the

CREATE AN INDIVIDUAL HERBAL FORMULA TO TREAT CANDIDA:

There are many beneficial herbs to improve digestion and clear Candida. Create an individual formula for your particular needs by choosing herbs from the following categories, emphasizing those most particular to your condition:

Strengthen Digestion	Eliminate Dampness	Clear Food Stagnation	Regulate Qi	Clear Damp Heat	Tonify Immunity	Antifungal Herbs	Supplements
Signs: gas, bloatedness, sleepiness after meals, poor appetite, loose stools, fatigue, weak limbs, low energy	**Signs:** Feelings of heaviness, lack of appetite, no thirst or desire to sip only small amounts, edema watery stools, nausea, stuffiness of chest or stomach region	**Signs:** foul gas, bloatedness, fullness and stuffiness around diaphragm region, nausea, foul breath, sour regurgitation, belching, vomiting	**Signs:** pain in ribs, depression, irritability, moodiness, frequent sighing, feeling of distension under ribs, hiccuping, PMS, alternating constipation and diarrhea	**Signs:** bitter taste, yellow vaginal discharge and itching pain, diarrhea with mucus in stools, burning of anus, genital itching	**Signs:** lowered resistance, tiredness, Candida signs, frequent colds and flu	**Signs:** Candida signs	Take as desired and needed
Herbs: ginseng, astragalus, dioscorea, jujube date, licorice, codonopsis, white atractylodes, psoralea	**Herbs:** coix, fu ling, cardamom, agastache, black atractylodes, asafoetida, caraway, dill, magnolia bark	**Herbs:** hawthorn berries, radish seeds, sprouted rice and barley, asafoetida, cyperus, green citrus	**Herbs:** citrus peel, fennel, saussurea, aquilaria, chive bulb, cyperus, star anise, anise, cumin	**Herbs:** coptis, scutellaria, phellodendron, goldenseal, Oregon grape, gentian, barberry	**Herbs:** astragalus, schisandra, eleuthro, reishi, codonopsis	**Herbs:** garlic, oregano, pau d'arco, grapefruit seed extract, spilanthes, usnea, tea tree oil, olive leaf extract, black walnut hulls, calendula, neem	Caprylic Acid, Undecyl-Enic Acid, L-glutamine, N-A-glucosamine

ailment Tiredness, for more on this. For those who have vaginal discharge and itch, see the ailment, Vaginal Infections and Discharge, under the section Menstrual Issues.

Leaky gut syndrome occurs when the small intestine becomes inflamed and irritated, increasing the permeability of the intestinal lining to metabolic and microbial waste ("toxins"). Some of this waste is comprised of undigested nutrients, and when they filter into the bloodstream the body's immune system responds by tagging certain ones as foreign irritants. This causes an allergic response to those particular foods so that every time they touch the intestinal lining, they cause further damage and inflammation, resulting in symptoms of food allergies, asthma, chronic sinusitis, eczema, migraines, irritable bowel, Epstein-Barr, chronic fatigue syndrome, fungal disorders (Candida, etc.), pollen or food allergies, lowered immunity, lupus, diabetes, Crohn's disease, weakness, fatigue, fibromyalgia and inflammatory joint disorders, including rheumatoid arthritis. Common food allergens include dairy, eggs, gluten grains (wheat, oats, rye), corn, beans (especially soy), sugar and nuts.

These leaked "toxins" stress the immune system in three ways: at the site of the intestinal lining, the liver and lymphatic system, and the kidneys and adrenals.

CANDIDA

EXCESS PATTERN:	DEFICIENCY PATTERNS:	
DAMP HEAT IN LIVER CHANNEL	**DEFICIENT SPLEEN QI AND DAMPNESS**	**DEFICIENT LIVER AND KIDNEY YIN**
Intense vulvae/vaginal itching	Vulvae/vaginal itching	Slight itching of vulva/vagina with slight burning sensation
Yellow vaginal discharge	Slight white vaginal discharge	Dryness of vagina
Pain on intercourse	Tiredness, lethargy	Heat in palms and/or soles of feet and chest
Mental restlessness	Loose stools	Dizziness
Irritability	Bloatedness, gas	Tinnitus
Insomnia (hard to fall asleep)	Weakness of arms and legs	Feeling of heat in afternoon
Dark urine	Cloudy urine	Dark, scanty urine
Tongue: red with redder sides and sticky, yellow coat with red spots on root	**Tongue:** pale with sticky, white coat	**Tongue:** red without coat
Pulse: slippery or wiry	**Pulse:** weak and slightly slippery	**Pulse:** floating and empty
Formulas: #13 or 170; 4 capsules, 3 times/day of equal parts powdered goldenseal, gentian, phellodendron, barberry, fu ling and wild yam with ½ part each fennel and fresh ginger.	**Formulas:** #17 with 43, or #185; 1 capsule or tablet of dried ginger (#40) with tea of equal parts codonopsis or ginseng, cardamom, astragalus, fenugreek, asafoetida or agastache and ½ part citrus peel and licorice.	**Formulas:** #74 or 169; tea of equal parts American ginseng, astragalus, raw rehmannia, lycii, ophiopogon and schisandra with ½ part white atractylodes and cuscuta.

Further, as immune response diminishes, more microbes multiply (such as viruses, bacteria and fungi), causing a chronic state of infection. To treat, it is necessary to heal the intestinal lining, cleanse and decongest the lymphatic system and liver, boost immunity, strengthen the Spleen and Kidneys, and, of course, remove irritating foods. Following the same protocol (diet, herbs, and supplements) as that for Candida usually effectively treats leaky gut syndrome.

For those who experience *anal itch* include the herbs **gentian**, **barberry**, **dandelion** root, **gardenia** and/or **Oregon grape**. Some respond to a wash of apple cider vinegar (this type is usually not due to yeast). *Nail fungus* responds extremely well to **tea tree** or **neem oils**; apply liberally throughout the day and/or at night, wrapping the area in a plastic bag to keep the area saturated all night. *Athlete's foot* may be treated with tea tree oil, **calendula** oil, **neem** oil, **black walnut** hull tincture and/or **garlic juice** (treat like nail fungus). To prevent its return, keep the area dry and wear shoes that breathe.

Others may experience co-existing *parasites*. Acute symptoms include abdominal distress, diarrhea that can be urgent and with burning sensations and extreme fluid loss. Chronic symptoms add in bloating, gas, cramps, maldigestion and malabsorption, alternating periods of constipation and diarrhea, abdominal distension, bloating, intestinal cramping followed by burning sensations, abrupt urge to eliminate, sudden food cravings, extreme emaciation or overweight, blood sugar fluctuations, fatigue, allergies, nausea, memory loss, brain fog, irritability, poor coordination, skin disorders, pain and muscle problems. Less frequent symptoms include intestinal bleeding, irritable bowel syndrome, ulcerative colitis, leaky gut, excess intestinal mucus secretion, fever, headache, immune deficiency, insomnia, weight changes, respiratory and hepatic symptoms and peritonitis.

As is obvious, parasites can cause a plethora of symptoms. Usually, stool tests can verify the presence of parasites, although because of their cyclical nature, it may be necessary to test repeatedly to be sure. If you suspect parasites, it's important to get a stool test to confirm, as taking some of these herbs (like black walnut) when not needed can imbalance your body.

On the other hand, having these symptoms is not necessarily an indication of parasite infestation. Many of these problems indicate Organ imbalances, such as Deficient Spleen Qi and stagnant Liver Qi, or other health imbalances, such as Candida. In fact, there is literature available that offers the extreme view that all health problems are caused by parasites. Thus, if you are unsure, get several stool tests, including anal swab tests, to verify or eliminate this possibility.

There are many types of parasites and they can be quite stubborn to eliminate. Yet many herbs effectively treat them, such as **black walnut** hulls, **clove**, **garlic**, **mugwort**, **wormwood** and **asafoetida**. The quickest and most successful treatment for parasites I've seen is a ten-day fast, eating only 1-2 tablespoons of raw brown rice in the morning (powder first) and kicharee the rest of the day. At the same time, take the listed antiparasitical herbs. Some people need to take the herbs for three months to completely eliminate all parasite infestation.

CONSTIPATION

Whether people admit it or not, constipation is one of the most common ailments in the West. In fact, the best-selling formula of one major herbal company I know is their laxative product. Interestingly, people's conception of constipation varies tremendously. One

---

Causes for Constipation:

- ⇝ Excessive consumption of heating foods, such as red meat and spicy, fried, fatty or greasy foods (dries up intestinal fluids)
- ⇝ Excessive intake of cooling foods such as melons, raw foods, juices, soy milk, refrigerated foods and drinks, iced drinks and foods, bananas, crabmeat and shellfish, especially without sufficient protein (these cause Coldness and contraction of intestines)
- ⇝ Excessive intake of refined and processed foods, including wheat, dairy, flour products and sugar (cause Damp stagnation)
- ⇝ Lack of fiber in the diet
- ⇝ Insufficient bile secretion (affects proper intestinal peristalsis)
- ⇝ Drinking insufficient amounts of water
- ⇝ Habitual use of laxatives
- ⇝ Lack of intestinal nerve force
- ⇝ Overweight condition
- ⇝ Stress
- ⇝ Prolonged anger, frustration and/or resentment (stagnate Qi)
- ⇝ Excessive mental work, thinking, worrying and brooding (slow food transportation and elimination)
- ⇝ Insufficient exercise
- ⇝ Physical overwork, especially without sufficient rest (weakens Spleen Qi, injuring the muscles and Kidney Yin, causing dry, difficult stools)

---

client thought she was constipated if she didn't have a bowel movement at least three to four times daily. Another patient felt elimination once a week was normal, and he wasn't happy when his bowel movements became daily!

Chinese medicine defines normal bowel movements as once to twice daily (Stools more frequent than that may actually be diarrhea—see that section.). Stools should be well-formed, light brown in color, cylindrical in shape and many inches long. Stools that don't occur daily, are abnormally shaped, small, dry, or difficult to expel, constitute constipation.

There are many causes for constipation, the most common being excessive consumption of red meat, alcohol, sugar, flour products and other congesting foods that cause Excess Heat. Yet, it's also possible for vegetarians to be constipated from Deficient Qi or Yang (insufficient energy or heat, causing a lack of nerve force to move the bowels). Further, it's possible to have a blockage of some sort (stagnant Qi or Blood), not enough moisture to smooth the elimination process (Deficient Blood or Yin), or Coldness contracting the intestines, making bowel movements difficult.

General Treatment for Constipation:

The best treatment for chronic constipation is to change your diet and regulate your lifestyle. If a meat-eater, reduce intake of red meat (eat fish and chicken instead), processed foods, sugar and refined flour products. Increase fiber intake from sources such as vegetables, fruits, whole grains and bran. Drink 6-8 glasses of water daily. If a vegetarian, reduce salads, raw foods and juices, include some fish (and chicken, if possible) and eat only cooked foods. Include fermented foods and 1 tsp.-1 Tbsp. acidophilus, 2-3 times/day with meals.

Natural elimination promoting foods for either type include prunes, figs, tomatoes, rhubarb, buttermilk, **flaxseed**, hemp seed, olive oil, bee pollen, honey, wheat and oat brans, apples, whey powder, sunflower and pumpkin seeds, yogurt, apricots and lemons (the European "constitutional" used to be hot lemon water first thing every morning). Consume 6-8 gms of fiber daily (but add in gradually to avoid intestinal gas and bloating).

Be sure to get plenty of exercise as this helps bowel peristalsis and regularity (walking is excellent). When you feel nature calling, go; don't wait until you've read the next paragraph, finished a phone call or completed computer work. While this may seem obvious, it's not uncommon for people to hold back bowel movements until ready to give it due attention, but by then the urge may have passed. Over time, this habit breeds constipa-

tion. Thus, establish regularity in relaxed bathroom visits, sleeping, eating and exercise. Perform breathing exercises (see *Home Therapies*), as in strengthening the Lungs, they assist their partner, the Large Intestine. Only use enemas and laxatives to unblock bowels, as long-term laxative use leads to habituation and addiction so the body can't eliminate on its own.

Simple non-addictive constipation remedies that also nourish include **psyllium seeds**, **fennel**, **fenugreek**, **olive oil** and **cannabis seeds**. Psyllium seeds may be soaked overnight in water, then eaten in the morning. Fennel and fenugreek make wonderful teas, or cooked with food, and are especially beneficial for constipation due to Coldness. For constipation due to Dryness, use olive oil or cannabis seeds. For constipation due to Heat, use **turmeric**, **gentian**, **yellow dock**, **dandelion** or **Oregon grape**. In fact, a simple formula like yellow dock, dandelion and Oregon grape works well for constipation because although these aren't laxatives "technically", they are cholagogues, which clear Heat from the Liver and release bile from the gallbladder, thus stimulating proper peristalsis in the bowels and movement of stools.

A great formula for chronic constipation of all types is the Ayurvedic product **Triphala**, because it works on the entire digestive tract. A combination of three myrobalans (fruits), this promotes bowel regularity, gently eliminates excess and doesn't create dependency (try Formulas #95, 97). It can be varied to one's needs by altering the proportion of each fruit. If constipation is severe or habitual, it may be necessary *for a very short time* to use a laxative such as **rhubarb**. Since there are many root causes for constipation, a wide variety of laxatives exist to choose from (see Patterns).

Hemorrhoids frequently appear with constipation. To treat, apply witch hazel or horse chestnut cream (Formula #52) externally and take internally (Formula #53). Alternatively, if hemorrhoids are due to Heat (burning sensation in anal area, scanty urination and other Heat signs with or without bleeding, use Formula #188). If due to Deficient Qi (weakness, tiredness, poor digestion and other Deficiency signs), take Formula #44 (or 139).

Differentiation for Constipation:

(Be sure to see if other symptoms in this Pattern fit you.)

↪ Round, pebble-small and dry stools indicate Heat. Round, pebble-small but not dry stools indicate stagnant Liver Qi.

↪ Long and pencil-thick stools indicate Deficient Spleen Qi, or carcinoma of the bowel.

↪ Dry stools with strong thirst and the desire to drink cold fluids indicate Heat.

↪ Dry stools with dry mouth and desire to sip water indicate Deficient Blood or Yin.

↪ Loose stools that are hesitant and difficult to come out indicate Deficient Spleen Qi with stagnant Liver Qi.

↪ Watery, explosive stools that are yellow and frothy indicate Damp Heat.

↪ Watery, explosive stools with possible mucus and normal in color indicate Damp-Cold.

↪ Slight abdominal pain upon defecation with pro-

nounced abdominal distension indicates stagnant Liver Qi.

↪ Severe and spastic pain upon defecation indicates Cold.

↪ Difficult defecation with great effort and subsequent exhaustion indicates Deficient Qi or Yang.

↪ Cramping after defecation indicates stagnant Cold or stagnant Qi.

↪ Pale stools indicate Dampness, usually Damp Heat in the Gallbladder blocking secretion of bile.

↪ Dark stools indicate Heat.

↪ Green stools in children indicate Cold.

↪ Blood in stool (not on outside or on toilet paper) is a red flag for carcinoma—seek medical advice immediately.

↪ Blood on outside of stool or toilet paper can indicate an intestinal infection or irritation, or ailment such as a fistula, internal hemorrhoid, colitis, diverticulitis or Crohn's disease.

As well, try this soothing and astringent bolus for hemorrhoid relief (refer to *Herbal Preparations* to make): equal parts **bayberry** bark, **chestnut** bark, **comfrey** root, **slippery elm** and **witch hazel** bark.

Irritable Bowel Syndrome (IBS) is a more complicated condition with symptoms of abdominal bloating and pain (especially associated with bowel movements), mucus in the stools, a feeling of incomplete rectal evacuation, constipation, diarrhea, or alternating constipation and diarrhea. Several causes include stress, food intolerances (sugar or fiber), or being a "Type A" perfec-

tionist personality. IBS is generally due to stagnant Liver Qi and Deficient Spleen Qi. Caffeine (coffee, black tea, mate, colas, cocoa, chocolate), alcohol, nuts and nut butters, fried and greasy foods, avocados, chips, turkey, raw foods, cheese, soy products and iced drinks and foods should be eliminated from the diet. Use **peppermint**, **chamomile** and **licorice** tea, **deglycyrrhizinated licorice** and magnesium aspartate (800 mg daily), as these calm the GI tract. If a more complicated condition, see Patterns and combine applicable herbs. If diarrhea is a main symptom, see the section, Diarrhea.

CONSTIPATION—EXCESS PATTERNS:

INTERNAL HEAT	STAGNANT LIVER QI	EXTERNAL HEAT INVADING	EXTERNAL COLD INVADING
Dry stools with foul odor; infrequent bowel movements; possible blood from anus	Constipation with stools shaped like pebbles and not dry; desire to go but can't	Constipation with dry stools	Acute constipation with severe cramping during and after bowel movement

(continued on next page)

CONSTIPATION—EXCESS PATTERNS: *(continued)*

INTERNAL HEAT	STAGNANT LIVER QI	EXTERNAL HEAT INVADING	EXTERNAL COLD INVADING
Pain, burning, swelling of anus; scanty, dark urine	Desire to defecate but difficulty in doing so	High fever	Severe abdominal pain
Thirst	Abdominal distension	Profuse sweating	Possible shivering, chills
Feeling of heat	Irritability	Thirst	Feeling of cold
Aversion to heat	Chest and rib pain	Feeling of heat	Aversion to cold
Sweats easily	Abdominal pain comes and goes	Abdominal pain and fullness	No sweating
Foul breath	Swelling, congestion after eating	Dry mouth	Abdominal rumbling
Abdominal pain	Retention of urine	Red face	Dry mouth
Tongue: red, redder on sides, dry, yellow coat	**Tongue:** may be normal color or slightly red on sides	**Tongue:** red with dry, yellow coat	**Tongue:** pale and wet, thick, white coat on rear
Pulse: wiry and fast	**Pulse:** wiry on left side	**Pulse:** overflowing and Fast	**Pulse:** deep, slow, full and tight
Formulas: #13 or 175; tea or capsules of turmeric, cascara sagrada, yellow dock, dandelion, barberry, marshmallow, licorice and ½ part fresh ginger.	**Formulas:** #12 or 154; 1 capsule turmeric with tea of equal parts chamomile, lemon balm, marshmallow and ½ part each licorice and fresh ginger.	**Formulas:** tea of equal parts cascara sagrada, dandelion, chamomile, marshmallow and ½ part each licorice, ginger and rhubarb.	**Formulas:** #41; tea of equal parts fresh ginger, fennel and cascara sagrada with ½ part licorice.

CONSTIPATION—DEFICIENCY PATTERNS:

DEFICIENT QI	DEFICIENT BLOOD	DEFICIENT YANG/ INTERNAL COLD	DEFICIENT YIN
Desire to defecate but with difficulty and great effort	Difficult defecation; dry stools	Difficult defecation; stools not dry; abdominal rumbling	Difficult defecation; dry stools
Exhaustion afterwards	Dizziness	Exhaustion and sweating afterwards	Dizziness
Thin and long stools like a pencil; not dry	Blurred vision	Sore back and knees	Dry mouth and throat, especially in the evening
Pale complexion	Dull, pale complexion	Feeling cold	Tinnitus
Tiredness	Numbness of the limbs	Frequent, pale urination	Night sweats
		Possible cramping pain upon or after defecation	Thirst with desire to sip water

(continued on next page)

CONSTIPATION—DEFICIENCY PATTERNS: *(continued)*

DEFICIENT QI	DEFICIENT BLOOD	DEFICIENT YANG/ INTERNAL COLD	DEFICIENT YIN
Tongue: pale	**Tongue:** pale or normal	**Tongue:** pale and wet	**Tongue:** red without coat; cracks
Pulse: empty	**Pulse:** empty	**Pulse:** deep, slow and fine; slightly tight in rear position	**Pulse:** floating and empty
Formulas: #44; tea of equal parts licorice, codonopsis, cascara sagrada and dang gui.	**Formulas:** #106 or 175; tea, pills or syrup of dang gui.	**Formulas:** #75; eat walnuts and take 1 capsule/tablet dried ginger (#40) with tea of equal parts fennel cascara sagrada and 1/2 part licorice.	**Formulas:** #74 or 175; take aloe gel, psyllium seeds, castor, sesame and/or olive oils, or use cannabis seeds.

DIARRHEA

Diarrhea can manifest in various ways. While most think diarrhea is frequent passing of loose stools, it also encompasses loose, or poorly formed, stools that may be eliminated once a day as usual.

General Treatment for Diarrhea:

Acute diarrhea occurs when loose, watery stools pass several times daily with possible abdominal pain and bloody mucous feces. To treat, simplify the diet by eliminating sugar, caffeine, alcohol, raw foods, juices, iced drinks and foods, and fruit and eat a light diet of whole grains, legumes and cooked vegetables. Take **blackberry root** powder since its wonderful astringency binds loose stools (boil 1 oz./pint water for 20 minutes and drink 1 cup, three times daily). Other useful herbs for diarrhea (bleeding, too) include **agrimony**, **raspberry leaf**, **blackberry leaf**, **yarrow**, **oak bark** and **bayberry bark** (steep 1 tsp. each of above herbs; drink 1 cup, 3 times daily). Include 1/2 tsp. bifidus, 3x/day with meals.

Sudden diarrhea may be due to food poisoning or parasites, such as Giardia. If diarrhea occurs after eating spoiled food (there may also be a fever, stomach cramps and other flu-like symptoms), take 3 pellets of homeopathic *Nux Vomica*, 12C, 3 times daily. The diarrhea should clear up within a day or two. If diarrhea is due to parasites, see the section Candida.

Causes for Diarrhea:

- ↪ A chill (invasion of Heat or Cold from hot or cold weather. Heat can lock Coldness inside the body, especially in summer, leading to acute diarrhea; Cold invades when dressed inadequately for cool weather, directly penetrating intestines)

- ↪ Excessive consumption of Cold-energied foods (iced drinks and foods, raw foods, salads, soy milk, tofu, juices, fruit) or Dampening foods (same foods plus flour products, dairy, fatty, fried and greasy foods, melons, bananas; all injure Spleen Qi)

- ↪ Eating spoiled food

- ↪ Prolonged worry, brooding, stress, anger, frustration or irritability (injures Spleen and Liver Qi)

- ↪ Overworking or over-exercising along with irregular eating habits and/or insufficient rest (weakens Spleen and/or Kidneys)

- ↪ Chronic illness (weakens Spleen)

- ↪ Excessive sexual activity (injures Kidneys)

- ↪ Food poisoning or food allergies

Chronic watery, or loose stools are usually due to Deficient Spleen Qi—in which case there isn't enough Qi to hold stools together—or due to Deficient Kidney Yang—when there isn't enough metabolic fire to form stools (in this case, diarrhea may occur only at dawn, about 5 ᴀᴍ—called "daybreak diarrhea"). Spleen Qi tonics include **ginseng, codonopsis, white atractylodes** and **dioscorea** (Formula #44 or 139). Herbs sparking the Kidney fires include **evodia, cinnamon bark, cuscuta, schisandra, nutmeg** and **psoralea (dodder seeds**–Formula #75 or 194).

Add herbs to dry and form loose stools, such as **lotus seed, agastache, round cardamom, cinnamon bark, black atractylodes** and **magnolia bark. Pueraria (kudzu)** may also be used, particularly if flu-like symptoms are present, combined with **cinnamon, ginger** or **cardamom**. A folk cure for diarrhea, especially for the elderly, is boiling 2 cups milk in an iron pot down to half its volume, adding 1 tsp. **cinnamon** powder and/or three slices of **fresh ginger**, cooling and drinking 1 cup daily before each meal.

Abdominal pain frequently accompanies diarrhea (constipation, too), although it may appear with other symptoms of indigestion. Carminative herbs relieve abdominal pain by moving congestion, such as **cinnamon, ginger, fennel, chamomile, saussurea, dill, anise, fennel, citrus peel, cyperus**, and **cumin**, particularly if pain comes and goes or changes direction or location. Fixed abdominal pain that is stabbing in nature is due to stagnant Blood. **Corydalis** is the herb of choice, however **calendula, cayenne, tien qi ginseng, motherwort**, or **safflower** are also useful for this.

Abdominal distension or *bloatedness* is relieved by **cardamom, cinnamon, ginger, citrus peel** and/or **hawthorn** along with Spleen Qi tonics, such as **white atractylodes, dioscorea, ginseng**, and Dampness-removing herbs, such as **coix, fu ling** and **agastache**.

Dysentery, an acute condition caused by bacteria or amoebas, has symptoms of foul-smelling, yellowish and watery stools, possible abdominal pain and urgent diarrhea. In TCM, this is usually a condition of acute Damp Heat in the intestines. **Coptis** and **goldenseal** are two specific herbs, and may be taken alone or together. Another formula is one part each **scutellaria** and **mugwort** and $1/2$ part **rhubarb**. Alternatively, try two parts **goldenseal** with one part each **pueraria, black walnut, chaparral, garlic, bayberry bark** and **wormwood**. Other useful herbs for dysentery include **plantain, barberry, marshmallow, yarrow, mullein, blackberry root, Iceland moss, Irish moss** and **honeysuckle**. When there is Coldness (no odor, feelings of coldness, frequent and pale urination), use **cinnamon, cayenne, garlic, wild cherry** and **hawthorn**. If there's no improvement after taking herbs for 2 to 3 days, seek medical care.

Differentiation of Diarrhea:

- ↬ Acute diarrhea accompanied by fever is due to Exterior invasion of Damp Cold or Damp Heat (treat as Cold Dampness or Damp Heat)

- ↬ Foul-smelling diarrhea with abdominal pain and rumbling intestines is due to stagnant Food.

- ↬ Chronic diarrhea with abdominal distension, belching, gas and mood swings indicate stagnant Liver Qi invading the Spleen

- ↬ Diarrhea with frequent bowel movements and stools that are sometimes like water denote long-term Deficient Spleen Qi or Yang

- ↬ Early morning diarrhea is due to Deficient Kidney Yang (sometimes called "cock-crow diarrhea"). There may also be abdominal pain and intestinal rumbling during elimination and a feeling of coldness.

- ↬ Pale yellow stools indicate Damp Heat in the Liver and Gallbladder

- ↬ Very dark stools indicate Heat

- ↬ Foul-smelling stools indicate Heat

- ↬ Very watery stools indicate Cold

- ↬ Stools with no odor indicate Cold

- ↬ Burning sensations in the anus after bowel movements indicate Heat

- ↬ Abdominal pain worse after diarrhea indicates Deficiency

- ↬ Abdominal pain that is better after diarrhea indicates Excess

DIARRHEA—EXCESS PATTERNS:

COLD DAMPNESS	DAMP HEAT	STAGNANT FOOD	STAGNANT LIVER QI
Diarrhea; in severe cases, diarrhea is like water; little odor	Foul-smelling diarrhea, yellowish loose stools	Rotten-smelling stools; foul gas	Alternating diarrhea and constipation
Abdominal pain	Abdominal pain	Abdominal pain relieved by bowel movement	Abdominal distension
Rumbling intestines	Frequent bowel movements	Rumbling intestines	
Feeling of oppression in the chest	Burning sensation in the anus after bowel movement	No appetite	Poor appetite
No appetite	Feeling of heat	Feeling of fullness in the stomach region, diaphragm or abdomen	Moodiness
Possible fever	Thirst	Belching	Belching
Nasal obstruction	Scanty, dark urine	Sour regurgitation	Depression
Headache		Foul breath	Nervous tension
Feeling of heaviness		Bad digestion	Irritability
Possible mucus in the stools			
Tongue: thick, sticky, white coat	**Tongue:** thick, sticky, yellow coat	**Tongue:** thick coat	**Tongue:** possibly normal, or sides may be slightly red
Pulse: slippery and slow	**Pulse:** slippery and fast	**Pulse:** slippery	**Pulse:** wiry
Formulas: #41 or 236; tea of equal parts cranesbill, blackberry and/or raspberry leaves, agrimony and agastache with 1/2 part fresh ginger, cinnamon bark and licorice and 1/2 tsp. nutmeg.	**Formulas:** #266; 2 capsules of equal parts blackberry root and golden seal with tea of equal parts agrimony, mullein and plantain with 1/2 part fresh ginger and licorice.	**Formulas:** #25 or 146; tea of equal parts hawthorn berry, radish seeds, cyperus and green citrus peel.	**Formulas:** #12 or 239; tea of equal parts fennel, cumin, citrus peel, magnolia bark, fu ling and Chinese wild yam.

Colitis can be difficult to cure depending on its severity. For colitis with foul-smelling, frequent diarrhea and bleeding use equal parts **comfrey, marshmallow, plantain, slippery elm, scutellaria, pueraria (kudzu)** and **coptis.** Some benefit by squirting 4 oz. each **plantain juice** and water with a syringe into the colon twice daily for two weeks. If there are feelings of coldness, poor appetite, loose stools with no bleeding, gas and bloatedness, try 2 parts each **codonopsis, dioscorea, black**

atractylodes, agrimony and **coix** with 1 part each **saussurea, cinnamon bark** and **dry ginger** and 1/2 part each **fu ling** and **citrus.** Include 15-20 drops **horseradish juice** between meals. If intense pain occurs, add **corydalis, white peony** and **licorice,** and put six magnets negative pole down against skin over colon in line with navel, leaving in place until problem is healed.

Crohn's disease is a serious inflammatory ailment of the gastrointestinal tract with symptoms of diarrhea,

DIARRHEA—DEFICIENCY PATTERNS:

DEFICIENT SPLEEN QI	DEFICIENT KIDNEY YANG
Loose stools, sometimes like water	Early morning diarrhea
Thin stools like a pencil	Abdominal pain
Frequent bowel movements	Rumbling in intestines that stops after bowel movement
Poor appetite	Sore, weak lower back and knees
Slight abdominal distension	Nighttime urination or frequent, pale urination
Feeling of oppression in the chest	Low sex drive
Sallow complexion	Tiredness
Tongue: pale with teeth marks	**Tongue:** pale with teeth marks
Pulse: Weak	**Pulse:** Weak and Deep
Formulas: #44 or 184; 1 capsule of cardamom and nutmeg powders with a tea of equal parts jujube dates, astragalus, white atractylodes, Chinese wild yam, magnolia bark and black atractylodes and ½ part each fu ling and licorice.	**Formulas:** #75 or 194; 2 capsules of equal parts cardamom, nutmeg and ginger powders with tea of equal parts Chinese wild yam, white atractylodes, schisandra and psoralea.

crampy abdominal pain, fever, anal ulcers, fissures and/or fistulas and rectal bleeding with subsequent weight loss. Too complicated to deal with here, look at Patterns and try appropriate herbs, as they may bring relief and healing. For irritable bowel syndrome (IBS), refer to the section Constipation.

OTHER DIGESTIVE DISORDERS

Two other digestive disorders include gluten intolerance (celiac disease) and acid reflux (GERD).

Gluten intolerance (celiac disease) includes symptoms of: chronic fatigue, tiredness, weakness, headaches, feelings of having the flu, muscle and joint pains, allergies and food intolerance's, irritability, abdominal pain, constipation or diarrhea, anemia, cramps and muscles spasms, swollen glands, decreased concentration and focus, B12 deficiency, insomnia, vaginal burning and anxiety. A number of foods contain gluten: the grains rice, rye, oats and barley, imitation cheeses, malt extract, MSG, modified food starch, textured protein meat extenders, canned meat, binders, fillers, bulking agents, ice cream, catsup, mayonnaise, instant coffee, whiskey and more.

The best way to avoid these is to eat only whole foods and avoid processed foods. Also, eating a balanced diet for your body type, as described in *The Energy of Food*, and focusing more on protein, legumes, vegetables and fruits, helps avoid most glutinous foods. It may also be important to heal the intestines from leaky gut syndrome as well (see section Candida, for how to do this). Follow the Candida recommended herbs too.

Acid reflux or regurgitation (also called *GERD*) is due to stagnant Qi, food or Dampness (Phlegm) causing energy to flow in the opposite direction from normal, in this case, upwards. If due to stagnant Fluids, there may also be mucus in the chest or throat, or a need to clear the throat frequently, especially after eating. Symptoms of stagnant Qi and Food include acid reflux, belching, burping, bloatedness, heaviness, abdominal fullness, poor appetite and low energy.

The best treatment I have seen for this is a formula comprised of the following: 3 parts each *Melia toosendan* (Sichuan chinaberry—*chuan lian zi*) and **magnolia**

bark, 2 parts each **bupleurum**, **green citrus**, **citrus** (*chen pi*) and **evodia** and 1 part each **pinellia** and **hawthorn** (this formula is available in tablet form—see GERD in *Resources* to obtain). *Belching* is due to similar causes and patterns. **Ginger** and **cardamom** are also specific for belching.

Weight issues include both *underweight* and *overweight*. Covering these can encompass an entire book in itself, and so is only dealt with briefly here. In general, underweight and overweight are both caused by poor metabolism and dietary issues. In either case, eat a basic balanced diet of sufficient protein for your body's needs (see *The Energy of Food*), lots of mostly cooked vegetables and some whole grains and fruit. For both those who are underweight or overweight, use Qi tonification herbs, either as teas or cooked with foods. Choose **codonopsis**, **white atractylodes**, **astragalus**, **ginseng**, **fu ling** and **citrus** (Formula #44). Add **jujube dates** if underweight, and **black atractylodes** if overweight.

If underweight, also regularly incorporate figs, dates, milk, cheese, almonds, walnuts, nut butters, avocados, milk shakes and flour products into your diet. If overweight, be sure to avoid these foods along with alcohol, sugar (and other "white" foods) and high, glycemic foods and you'll be amazed at how quickly you lose weight. Perhaps even start with a 3-5 day kicharee fast (see *The Energy of Food*, for recipe).

If you are overweight and eat mostly salads and fruit juices, your digestion is now so Cold and Damp it can no longer properly metabolize these foods. To loose weight, eliminate all raw foods, fruit and juices and eat protein, cooked vegetables and dark leafy greens along with a little whole grains.

In general, weight loss is most easily accomplished by eating a balanced meal (in protein, carbohydrates and fats) three times a day, avoiding between meal snacking, cutting back on food intake overall and emphasizing protein and cooked vegetables, adding some whole grains and fruit in season as appropriate.

In terms of lifestyle issues affecting weight gain, be sure to exercise regularly, especially incorporating daily walks and stretching along with aerobic exercise and perhaps some weight lifting. Exercise is extremely important now to maintain or gain muscle mass rather than losing it while shedding weight. It's also vital to reduce stress, as chronic stress increases water retention and elevates blood sugar levels, leading to insulin resistance, blood sugar swings and weight gain. Lastly, get plenty of sleep since the body stores fat when sleep is inadequate.

GALLSTONES

Gallbladder stones, a mixture of cholesterol, bilirubin and protein, are formed when there is an excess of cholesterol in relation to bile acids. Stones may lay dormant and give little distress unless the gallbladder becomes inflamed and distended, or if the stones get stuck in bile ducts. Symptoms include cramping, aching or stabbing pain under the right ribs and/or in the right back and may extend to the right shoulder, particularly several hours after eating. In TCM, gallstones are formed when Damp Heat accumulates in the Gallbladder, arising from stagnant Liver Qi or Damp Heat in the Liver and Gallbladder.

Causes of Gallstones:

- Emotional strain, particularly anger, resentment and frustration (stagnates Liver Qi, which in time causes stagnant Liver Blood)

- Excessive consumption of dairy, fried, fatty and greasy foods, nuts and nut butters, avocados, cheese, alcohol, caffeine and chips (cause Damp Heat in Liver and Gallbladder)

- External invasion of Damp and Heat into the Liver channel, usually in tropical climates or summertime

- Overwork and excessive sexual activity (weaken Liver and Kidney Yin, leading to stagnant Liver Qi)

- Anemia, Deficient Blood from a poor diet, or excessive loss of blood from childbirth, heavy menses, hemorrhage or other factor (causes Deficient Liver Blood, leading to stagnant Liver Qi)

General Treatment for Gallstones:

Because gallstones can be very painful, surgical removal is quite seductive. Yet, this carries potential risks and doesn't treat the root cause underlying stone formation in the first place. Herbs and diet can be quite effective for helping dissolve or pass stones, especially if they aren't too large. Be sure to immediately eliminate all fried, fatty and greasy foods, caffeine (coffee, black tea, mate, cocoa, colas, chocolate), avocados, dairy, nuts and nut butters, chips and turkey from the diet (I have seen several people develop gallstones who ate turkey and drank coffee daily). Eat lots of cooked vegetables, artichokes (drink juice after steaming), beets, carrots, shiitake mushrooms, dark leafy greens, legumes, lean protein, grains and some fruit.

A specific formula for gallstones and gallbladder inflammation is 1 part each **Oregon grape** (or **barberry**), **gravel root**, **wild yam**, **turmeric**, **fennel** and **marshmallow** and 1/2 part **ginger**. Other useful herbs include **dandelion**, **artichoke** and **gentian**. Also try Formula #91. At the same time, use castor oil packs over the gallbladder and painful areas to relieve pain and help pass stones.

A liver flush that decongests and cleanses the liver and gallbladder, helping to pass gallstones, is 8 oz. water or grapefruit juice, 2 oz. olive oil and lemon juice and 2 cloves fresh garlic blended together. Drink 8 oz. first thing every morning for four days. Eat lightly during this time.

GALLSTONES—EXCESS PATTERNS:

STAGNANT LIVER QI	DAMP HEAT IN LIVER AND GALLBLADDER
Slight cramping pain in ribs	Dull pain in ribs
Pronounced distension in rib area	Feeling of fullness in rib and stomach areas
Feeling of oppression in chest	Bitter and sticky taste in mouth
Slight breathlessness	Nausea, vomiting
Poor appetite	Poor appetite
Frequent sighing	Dark urine
Belching	No jaundice
Moodiness, depression	Yellowish coloration in whites of eyes (sclera)
Tongue: may look normal	**Tongue:** sticky yellow coat
Pulse: wiry	**Pulse:** slippery
Formulas: #12 with 91, or #189; take 2 capsules turmeric with tea of two parts gravel root, 1 part each dandelion root and wild yam and 1/2 part each fennel, cyperus and lobelia.	**Formulas:** #13 with 91, or #173; take 2 capsules turmeric with tea of two parts gravel root, 1 part each dandelion root and wild yam & 1/2 part each barberry, rhubarb, fennel and lobelia.

❀ HEADACHES

In the West, we think headaches are a nuisance to be eliminated as quickly as possible by popping pills so we can continue with our current activities and habits. Only if headaches are recurring or debilitating do we pay them more attention and seek aid. If we use Western herbs, many of us look to **feverfew** or **rosemary** for the answer, yet since these herbs don't work for every headache, we may or may not receive relief. In TCM, there are more than five different types of headaches and each is treated differently. Further a headache is seen as a signal of an

Causes of Headaches:

↪ Inherited constitution (determined by parents' health at conception; older parents conceiving a child; mother's ill health during pregnancy; use of medications or recreational drugs during pregnancy)

↪ Childhood headaches that start between ages 7-10 are usually due to constitutional factors.

↪ Teenage headaches are often due to hormonal imbalances.

↪ Anger, frustration and resentment (stagnate Liver Qi, causing temple or vertex headaches)

↪ Excessive worrying (injures Spleen and Stomach, causing dull forehead or vertex headaches)

↪ Chronic anxiety or fear (depletes the Kidneys, causing headaches along back of head); shock (causes headaches affecting whole head)

↪ Excessive sexual activity (a common cause of headaches, especially in men—Kidney Qi lost during sex is replenished quickly, but when too frequent, Kidney Qi isn't restored and headaches result, especially if dizziness, mental tiredness and fatigue occur after sex)

↪ Birthing too many children (including miscarriages) too close together (depletes Kidney Qi and Liver Blood)

↪ Not eating enough (causes Deficient Qi and Blood and headaches along the top or back of the head—occiput)

↪ Overeating (leads to headaches on forehead)

↪ Excessive intake of Hot-energy or greasy foods and curries, spices, red meat and alcohol (cause sharp headaches along side of head or forehead)

↪ Excessive eating of Dampening foods, flour products, iced drinks and foods, dairy, raw foods, juices, soy milk, tofu and processed and refined foods (causes heaviness in head and dull frontal headaches)

↪ Eating too much salt (results in dull headaches throughout whole head, or along occiput)

↪ Overeating sugar (leads to frontal or occipital headaches)

↪ Excessive intake of sour foods (causes vertex or temple headaches)

↪ Excessive quantities of caffeine—coffee, black tea, cocoa, chocolate and colas (leads to many types of headaches)

↪ Trauma, such as accidents (stagnates Qi, Blood and Fluids, which causes chronic headaches)

↪ Colds and flu (caused by Wind invading body—particularly through the back of the neck—and creates headaches, stiff neck and shoulders and body aches—see the section Colds, Flu and Fevers, for treating these types of headaches)

underlying imbalance, a bank notice that something isn't right with our account. If we ignore it or mask it with drugs, the problem not only doesn't go away, but festers or moves deeper into the body. Thus, the underlying pattern needs be discovered and treated to prevent further health problems.

General Herbal Treatment for Headaches:

One of the best overall Chinese herbs for headaches is **ligusticum** (*chuan xiong*), or **Chinese lovage**, as it treats headaches in the occipital or temple regions and headaches due to stagnant Qi or Blood. A good general formula for treating headaches due to several causes is equal parts **feverfew**, **chamomile**, **willow bark** and Western **angelica** (or Formulas #37 and 105). Alternatively try equal parts **rosemary**, **poplar**, **willow**, **wintergreen** and Western **angelica**. Headaches normally are differentiated by their location, and these may alternate or co-exist at the same time. Since headaches tend to recur in specific locations, I have divided their treatments accordingly.

Temple region: Temple headaches may be located on both sides, though more frequently they are one-sided. Corresponding to the Gallbladder, temple headaches are due to Excess or Deficient Heat, or stagnant Liver Qi. A headache that arises mostly on the left side is usually due to Deficiency, while that which occurs mainly on the right side is usually due to Excess, though of course there may be exceptions to this rule.

Alcohol, caffeine, chocolate, fried and fatty foods, nuts and nut butters, turkey, cheese, chips, MSG, cured meats, pizza, red meat, tobacco, nitrates and sugar all lead to Liver and Gallbladder related headaches, including menstrual, PMS, peri/menopausal types and migraines. These headaches tend to be throbbing, intense and located in the temples, on the side of the head or behind the eyes. Eat lots of cooked vegetables, dark leafy greens, fruit, grains and legumes and some white meat. Herbs of choice include **ligusticum** (*chuan xiong*), **bupleurum**, **scute** and *Artemesia annua* (**sweet annie**). (Try Formulas #12, 37 or 105.)

Top of the head (vertex): Another type of Liver headache, if severe, it's due to Excess or Deficient Heat in Liver (see Migraines for more on this). If dull, it's due to Deficient Liver Blood or Yin, especially if dull and improves after rest. **Ligusticum** *gao ben* treats general vertex headaches while **ophiopogon, ghlenia,** and **raw rehmannia** treat vertex headaches due to Deficient Liver Yin (try Formula #74 or # 169). If the vertex headache is accompanied by nausea and vomiting and it's not a migraine, it may be due to Cold in the Middle Warmer transferring to the Liver. In this case, warming herbs are used, like dried and fresh **ginger**. See Patterns for more herbal specifics.

Sides of the head: These are due to the Gallbladder and Liver, usually from Heat, especially if sharp and throbbing. See Temple headaches for dietary and herbal specifics.

Behind the eyes: Dull pain is due to Deficient Liver Blood (try Formula #12); sharp pain is from Excess Heat with Liver rising (try Formula #192)—migraines frequently result in this type of headache. See Temple headaches for dietary guidelines. **Chrysanthemum** and **tribulus** are specific here, particularly if due to Heat. See Patterns for more herbal specifics.

Forehead (frontal): These are normally due to Stomach Deficiency or Heat. If pain is dull, it is from Deficiency—there may be accompanying poor appetite, low

energy, gas, bloatedness and possible loose stools. Use tonics such as **ginseng, codonopsis, astragalus, white atractylodes** and **dioscorea** (try Formula #43) and eat only cooked foods with plenty of protein. If pain is sharp, it is from Heat—there may be accompanying thirst with a desire to drink cold drinks (this only perpetuates headaches, by the way, since Coldness creates more Stomach Heat), pain in the stomach region, bad breath, bleeding gums and dry stools (maybe you have noticed headaches come on suddenly after consuming iced drinks or cold foods, like ice cream). Use **pueraria, chrysanthemum, cimicifuga (Chinese black cohosh)** and **angelica** *dahurica*.

Frontal headaches may also occur from Dampness or Phlegm retained in the head. If so, the head feels heavy and thinking is muddled or fuzzy. Be sure to eliminate all Dampening foods (flour products, dairy, iced drinks and foods, bananas and melons, fruit juices, raw foods, tofu and soymilk). Use **pinellia, coix, black atractylodes** and **agastache (**try Formula #240).

Back of the head (occiput): These are due to Deficient Kidneys (see Patterns), Deficient Blood (if occurring during the menstrual period), or acute invasion of Wind-Cold if a cold or flu is trying to occur. If pain extends up back to top of head and is sharp in nature, it is due to Damp Heat in Urinary Bladder (try Formula #99 with 105). If due to Deficient Kidneys, rest, stop excessive work, sex and mental activities and eliminate sugar, alcohol, caffeine, iced drinks and foods, fruit juices, soy milk and raw foods. Eat pork, legumes, grains and lots of cooked vegetables. Use herbs indicated in Patterns, adding a pinch of salt to the formula (this takes herbal energies to the Kidneys).

If due to Deficient Blood, it may arise during the menstrual cycle. Use **dang gui, cooked rehmannia, white peony** and **ligusticum,** or Formula #106 or 231. To build blood, eat more animal protein, and only cooked foods and use molasses. **Notopterigium** is the primary herb used for occipital headaches, particularly those due to Wind-Damp. Yet, **angelica** *du huo,* **ligusticum** and **ligusticum** *gao ben* (rhizome and radix) may also be used. Occipital headaches may be due to low blood sugar as well, in which case they will go away when you eat. If this occurs, regulate your blood sugar by balancing your diet with protein, carbohydrates and fats.

Whole head: Chronic dull headaches throughout the whole head are due to Deficient Kidney Essence (see Patterns for herbal specifics). Acute headaches throughout whole head that are severe and sharp in character are from invasion of External Wind (see section Colds, Flu and Fevers, for appropriate herbs).

Menstrual headaches: Hormonal headaches coming on during the menstrual cycle or PMS times respond best to **black cohosh** and **vitex**, since they regulate hormones, though **dandelion**, **chrysanthemum** and **feverfew** may also be used. If headaches occur during menses, they may be due to Deficient Blood (especially if there is dizziness and blurry vision). Use **dang gui**, **cooked rehmannia**, **white peony** and **ligusticum**, or Formula #106 or 231.

Sinus headaches: Sinus infection headaches go away when the infection is treated (see Sinus Infections in the section Cold, Flu and Fevers, for treatment). However, **Angelica *dahurica*** (*bai zhi*) is the herb of choice for relieving sinus headaches.

Migraine headaches: These are characterized by intense, severe, pounding, throbbing or pulsating pain. There may be visual disturbances, such as flashing lights or auras, with possible nausea, vomiting or diarrhea. There may also be a sensation of pressure behind the eyes, or hypertension. Pain may be on one or both sides of the head, eyes, temples, top of head or along eyebrows. Migraines are generally due to overworking, stress, insufficient rest and a diet rich in caffeine, alcohol, red meat, nuts and nut butters, cheese, turkey, chips and fried, greasy and fatty foods. These factors cause Excess or Deficient Heat in the Liver with possible Deficient Yin and uprising Liver Yang.

For best treatment, it's important to differentiate the cause, yet in general, **feverfew** and **siler** are both good herbs to use for migraines, although they may need to be combined with other herbs as appropriate for the underlying root cause (see Patterns). It's also important to follow dietary guidelines given for Temple headaches. As well, try Formula #37 or 192. Interestingly, some find immediate benefit from drinking a glass of tomato juice.

Hypertension headaches: These usually cause pressure behind the eyes and/or in the head, and feelings of energy being stuck in the head. Hypertension may manifest with vertex or occipital headaches accompanied by pronounced stiffness of neck muscles, tinnitus, irritability and, of course, elevated blood pressure. Hypertension can result from other issues, such as Deficient Kidney Yin or Yang (see Patterns to differentiate and determine herbs). Like migraines, overworking, stress, insufficient rest and aggravating foods are frequent causes for hypertension. Mung beans are a specific food for lowering

---

Types of Headache Pain:

The character of pain felt from headaches is a useful diagnostic tool:

- ↪ Dull—from Deficiency, usually of Blood, Yin, Qi or Kidneys
- ↪ Sharp—from Excess, usually of Heat or stagnation in Stomach or Liver
- ↪ Heaviness—due to Dampness or Phlegm obstructing head; there may also be difficulty thinking and concentrating, fuzziness, dizziness and/or blurred vision
- ↪ Stiff—stiffness along the occiput is usually due to invasion of Exterior Wind-Cold, although if chronic and in neck and shoulders, it is due to Excess or Deficient Heat in Liver
- ↪ Pulling—due to Internal Liver Wind
- ↪ Stabbing, boring, splitting, intense and fixed in one place—due to stagnant Blood (normally occurs in chronic headaches or migraines)
- ↪ Emptiness—due to Deficient Kidney Yin or Yang

blood pressure. Antihypertensive herbs that dilate the vessels include **pueraria**, **salvia** and **rhubarb**. A typical Chinese formula for hypertension is Formula #151. Also try equal parts **eucommia**, **motherwort**, **scutellaria**, **salvia** and **chrysanthemum**. A Chinese folk remedy is a daily tea of toasted **vacarria** seeds (*wang bu liu xing*).

If *high cholesterol* is a cause, use herbs to lower cholesterol such as **hawthorn leaf** and **berries** and **guggul** (refined **myrrh**)—alternatively, use Formula #18. **Garlic** has long been used to regulate blood pressure, and deodorized garlic in capsules seems to work well for this (Formula #39). Many find taking 1 Tblsp. of ground **flaxseeds** every morning valuable as well. Vegetarians can have high cholesterol as frequently as meat-eaters (stress is a contributing factor), so be sure to eat a balanced diet that is specific for your body's needs (see *The Energy of Food*). Include oatmeal or oat bran as it absorbs excess cholesterol in the intestinal tract and moves it out of the body. Exercise and take the supplement CoQ10. Check thyroid functioning as normalizing the thyroid lowers cholesterol levels (see section Tiredness, for thyroid information).

Qualities of Headaches:

- ↔ Worse in the daytime—due to Deficient Qi or Yang, or to Dampness.
- ↔ Worse in evening, or nighttime and is chronic—due to Deficient Blood or Yin
- ↔ Worse with activity—due to Deficient Qi or Blood
- ↔ Improves with light exercise—due to Phlegm, or Excess or Deficient Liver Heat or stagnant Liver Qi
- ↔ Improves with rest or lying down—due to Deficient Qi or Blood
- ↔ Worse with lying down—due to Dampness or Phlegm
- ↔ Worse with lying down but improved when sitting—due to Excess or Deficient Liver Heat
- ↔ Worse in heat—due to Excess or Deficient Liver Heat
- ↔ Worse in cold—due to Yang Deficiency
- ↔ Worse in damp weather—due to Dampness or Phlegm
- ↔ Improves with application of cold—due to Excess Liver Heat
- ↔ Worse when suddenly relaxes—due to Excess or Deficient Liver Heat (this frequently occurs on weekends or holidays)
- ↔ Improves after eating—due to Deficient Qi or Blood
- ↔ Worse before menses—due to Excess or Deficient Liver Heat
- ↔ Worse during menses—due to stagnant Blood, or Excess or Deficient Liver Heat
- ↔ Worse at end of menses—due to Deficient Blood
- ↔ Worse with pressure on the head—due to Excess or Deficient Liver Heat
- ↔ Improves with pressure—due to a Deficiency condition

HEADACHES—EXTERNAL PATTERNS:

EXTERNAL WIND-COLD	EXTERNAL WIND-HEAT	EXTERNAL DAMPNESS
Acute onset	Acute onset	Acute onset
Stiffness at the back of the neck	Distending sensation; headache felt inside the head	Heaviness in the head aggravated by damp weather
Can be severe, but of short duration	Can be severe, but of short duration	Can be severe, but of short duration
Body aches	Red eyes	Heaviness of the whole body
Aversion to cold	Aversion to heat	Aversion to cold
Shivering, chills	Slight chills and shivers, if any	Shivering, chills

(continued on next page)

HEADACHES—EXTERNAL PATTERNS: *(continued)*

EXTERNAL WIND—COLD	EXTERNAL WIND—HEAT	EXTERNAL DAMPNESS
Possible low fever	Higher fever	Possible low fever
No thirst	Thirst	No thirst
Achy shoulders	Sore throat; possible swollen tonsils	Heavy eyes
No sweating	Sweating	Possible light sweating
Runny nose with white discharge or blocked nose	Runny nose with yellow discharge	Runny nose with copious white discharge
Possible cough with white mucus	Possible cough with yellow mucus	Possible cough with copious white sputum; sensation of oppression in the chest and stomach region
Pale urine	Slightly dark urine	Possible cloudy urine
		Poor concentration
Tongue: normal or white coat	**Tongue:** slightly red sides or tip	**Tongue:** sticky coat
Pulse: floating and tight	**Pulse:** floating and fast	**Pulse:** floating and slippery
Formulas: #41 or 234; tea of equal parts fresh ginger and lovage with ½ part each sweet basil and lemon balm.	**Formulas:** #37 or 110; tea of equal parts lemon balm, feverfew and skullcap.	**Formulas:** #37 and 110; tea of equal parts willow bark and fresh ginger and ½ part licorice.

HEADACHES—INTERNAL EXCESS PATTERNS:

LIVER FIRE	LIVER WIND	STAGNANT LIVER QI	DAMPNESS	STOMACH HEAT	STAGNANT BLOOD	STAGNANT FOOD
Intense throbbing, distending, bursting or pulsating headache	Pulling sensation	Strong aching headache	Dull headache; heaviness in the head; worse in the morning	Acute or chronic headache; may be intense	Very severe and intense headache; stabbing and boring in character	Intense headache, usually acute
Headache fixed in one place	Affects whole head	Headache on forehead or temple and can move from side to side	Affects whole head, temples, sides of head or just the forehead	Headache affects forehead	Headache fixed in one place	Headache on forehead
Possible nausea, vomiting or thirst	Severe giddiness	Pain in the ribs	Possible nausea	Thirst with desire to drink cold water	Pain in ribs or abdomen	Aggravated by eating
Dizziness; insomnia; red eyes	Slight shaking of the head	Nervous tension	Difficulty thinking or concentrating	Dry stools	Dark complexion	Sour regurgitation

(continued on next page)

HEADACHES—INTERNAL EXCESS PATTERNS: *(continued)*

LIVER FIRE	LIVER WIND	STAGNANT LIVER QI	DAMPNESS	STOMACH HEAT	STAGNANT BLOOD	STAGNANT FOOD
Tinnitus; Deafness; Irritability	Numbness	Poor digestion	Lack of appetite	Possible pain in the stomach region	Painful periods with dark blood and clots	Belching
Bitter taste; dry throat	Tremor in a limb	Belching, sighing	Sinusitis			Foul breath
Constipation with dry stools; scanty dark urine		Flatulence; abdominal distension; small bits of stools	Feeling of fullness in chest and stomach region			Feeling of fullness In stomach region
Tongue: may be normal	**Tongue:** may be normal, or pale and thin	**Tongue:** may be normal	**Tongue:** thick, sticky coat	**Tongue:** thick, yellow coat	**Tongue:** purple	**Tongue:** thick, sticky coat
Pulse: wiry	**Pulse:** wiry, or fine/thin	**Pulse:** wiry	**Pulse:** slippery	**Pulse:** full and fast	**Pulse:** firm and wiry, or choppy	**Pulse:** slippery
Formulas: #37 or 170; 4 capsules of equal parts powdered dandelion, scullcap, goldenseal and feverfew with lemon balm tea.	**Formulas:** #192; tea of equal parts skullcap, lemon balm and chamomile with 5 drops lobelia tincture.	**Formulas:** #12, 63 or 154; 4 capsules equal parts powdered turmeric and cumin with fennel tea and 5 drops lobelia tincture.	**Formulas:** #150; tea of equal parts hawthorn berries, cumin, agastache and sassafras with 1/2 part fresh ginger and 5 drops lobelia tincture.	**Formulas:** #161; tea of equal parts cascara sagrada, barberry, dandelion and 1/2 part lobelia.	**Formulas:** #157; tea of equal parts corydalis, motherwort, salvia, cyperus and ligusticum.	**Formulas:** #25 or 146; tea of equal parts hawthorn berries, cardamom, cumin, dandelion, western angelica and radish seeds.

HEADACHES—EXCESS/DEFICIENCY PATTERNS:

This type of headache may be dull and aching, or resemble a migraine.

LIVER YANG RISING Due to DEFICIENT LIVER BLOOD	LIVER YANG RISING Due to DEFICIENT LIVER YIN	LIVER YANG RISING Due to DEFICIENT KIDNEY YIN	LIVER YANG RISING Due to DEFICIENT KIDNEY YIN and YANG
Dizziness	Dizziness	Pronounced dizziness	Dizziness
Blurred vision	Dry eyes	Dry eyes, skin, throat	Dry eyes, skin, throat
Possible palpitations	Irritability	Night sweats	Possible night sweats
	Possible pressure behind the eyes	Burning sensation in hands, soles and/or chest	Frequent, pale urination; nighttime urination
Wakes easily and can't go back to sleep	Insomnia (difficult to fall and stay asleep)	Insomnia (waking frequently)	

(continued on next page)

HEADACHES—EXCESS/DEFICIENCY PATTERNS: *(continued)*

LIVER YANG RISING Due to DEFICIENT LIVER BLOOD	LIVER YANG RISING Due to DEFICIENT LIVER YIN	LIVER YANG RISING Due to DEFICIENT KIDNEY YIN	LIVER YANG RISING Due to DEFICIENT KIDNEY YIN and YANG
	Possible hypertension	Possible hypertension	
Tongue: pale, thin	**Tongue:** red and peeled	**Tongue:** red and peeled	**Tongue:** pale and swollen
Pulse: floating and fine/thin	**Pulse:** floating and empty	**Pulse:** floating and empty	**Pulse:** deep and slow
Formulas: #51 with 106, or #192 with 231; tea of equal parts dang gui, white peony, ligusticum, lycii, cooked rehmannia, gastrodia and gambir.	**Formulas:** #51 with 74, or #163; tea of equal parts ophiopogon, lycii, raw and cooked rehmannia, gambir, epimedium (#51) and gastrodia.	**Formulas:** #51 with #74, or # 163; tea of equal parts cooked and raw rehmannia, epimedium (#51), lycii, dang gui, asparagus root, anemarrhena and phellodendron.	**Formulas:** #51 with 74 and 75; tea of equal parts epimedium (#51), eucommia, cooked and raw rehmannia, lycii, dang gui, asparagus root, anemarrhena and phellodendron

HEADACHES—DEFICIENCY PATTERNS:

DEFICIENT QI	DEFICIENT BLOOD	DEFICIENT KIDNEY YIN	DEFICIENT KIDNEY YANG
Dull headache that comes in bouts	Strong dull headache	More severe headache	Dull headache
Affects whole head or just the forehead	Affects top of head, back of head	Headache inside the head; may be on the vertex	Headache inside the head, may be on the back of the head
Aggravated by excessive work	Worse in afternoon or evening	Feeling of emptiness of the brain	Feeling of emptiness of the brain
Worse in the mornings	Worse at end of menses	Headache may occur after sexual activity	Headache may occur after sexual activity
Alleviated by rest, lying down	Better lying down	Feeling of heat in the evening	Feeling of cold
Poor appetite	Dizziness	Scanty urination	Abundant, pale urination
Tiredness	Blurred vision	Dizziness	Night time urination
Loose stools	Lack of concentration	Soreness of the lower back	Soreness of lower back and knees
Slight breathlessness	Poor memory	Slight constipation	
Possible palpitations	Possible palpitations	Tinnitus	
Tongue: pale	**Tongue:** pale and thin	**Tongue:** red without coat	**Tongue:** pale
Pulse: empty	**Pulse:** fine/thin	**Pulse:** floating and empty	**Pulse:** deep and weak

(continued on next page)

HEADACHES—DEFICIENCY PATTERNS: *(continued)*

DEFICIENT QI	DEFICIENT BLOOD	DEFICIENT KIDNEY YIN	DEFICIENT KIDNEY YANG
Formulas: #l06 or 198; tea of equal parts codonopsis, baked licorice, and white atractylodes with ½ part pinellia, citrus peel and fu ling.	**Formulas:** #106 or 198; tea of equal parts dang gui, cooked rehmannia, lycii, ligusticum, white peony, jujube dates and ½ part baked licorice (or powder the herbs and combine with blackstrap molasses).	**Formulas:** #74 or 166; tea of equal parts ophiopogon, raw and cooked rehmannia, lycii, epimedium (#51), and schisandra and ½ part white atractylodes.	**Formulas:** #75 or 180; 1 capsule equal parts powdered cinnamon bark and dried ginger with tea of equal parts epimedium (#51), eucommia, cooked rehmannia, Chinese wild yam and ½ part cornus.

❧ HEPATITIS

Hepatitis is an inflammation of the liver that blocks its ability to perform many functions: manufacture and store nutrients, purify blood, discharge bile for digestion and release glycogen for reserve energy. Not only are there hepatitis A, B and C, but also D, E and G and toxic hepatitis due to exposure from chemicals and toxins. (There are other viruses that affect the liver as well, such as herpes simplex, cytomegalovirus and Epstein-Barr virus.) Here, we'll only look at hepatitis A, B and C. In some cases a person may test for hepatitis antibodies, but not have any symptoms. Once hepatitis is chronic, it increases the risk of liver cancer. Each type of hepatitis is a contagious viral condition, but spreads in various ways. Herbs are very effective for hepatitis A, B and C.

Hepatitis A is an acute condition primarily spreading through fecal contamination. For example, if those who prepare food in kitchens, restaurants and other food services do not adequately wash their hands after using the bathroom, food can become contaminated. Hepatitis A takes two to six weeks to appear after exposure. It is contagious two to three weeks before, and one week after, jaundice appears.

Hepatitis B is primarily contracted through infected blood or blood products, saliva and sexual secretions. It can be acquired from blood transfusions, plasma therapy, contaminated blood entering a cut, or from needles used for drugs. It has an incubation time of

> ### *Causes of Hepatitis:*
>
> The virus may be contracted through:
>
> - ❧ contaminated blood or feces
> - ❧ contaminated drinking water or food
> - ❧ eating seafood harvested in polluted areas
> - ❧ injections with improperly sterilized hypodermic needles (including those used for recreational drugs)
> - ❧ infected blood passing through open cuts or sores

two weeks to four and a half months, but may go unrecognized.

Hepatitis C (HCV) is contacted through blood transfusions, infected needles (usually shared for drugs), sexual secretions and broken skin or mucous membranes. It may take six months to develop the antibodies. If left untreated, it can become serious, leading to cirrhosis of the liver and eventual liver failure. Today, the vast majority of those tested positive with hepatitis C antibodies have no symptoms at all, but are frightened out of their wits that they'll eventually develop fatal liver disease (because some do). Yet, hepatitis C is highly treatable and more often complicated by a congested liver from smoking, alcohol and other toxic substances rather than from a virus.

HEPATITIS SYMPTOMS:

HEPATITIS A	HEPATITIS B	HEPATITIS C
Acute condition	Slightly jaundiced (yellow cast to skin)	Chronic condition
Fever, chills	Dizziness	Possible mild fever
Exhaustion, drowsiness	Tiredness	Fatigue
Jaundiced (yellow cast to skin)	Indigestion	Hardening of the liver (under the right ribs)
Weakness	Weakness	Weakness
Vomiting, nausea	Nausea	Decreased appetite
Loss of appetite	Pain under the right ribs	Pain under the right ribs
Headache	Irritability, impatience and anger	Possible headache
Pale, almost white, stools	Pale, almost white, stools	Itching skin
Dark urine	Dark urine	Malaise
Elevated liver enzymes in the blood	Elevated liver enzymes in the blood	Elevated liver enzymes in the blood
Muscle aches and joint pains		There may be no symptoms at all and the person may feel fine but test positive for hepatitis C antibodies
Abdominal discomfort		

General Treatment for Hepatitis:

While herbs effectively clear acute hepatitis within several days, it may take up to three months to control hepatitis B and C, although they respond well to natural therapies (however, the antibodies may always remain present in the body). If there has been exposure to chemical toxicity, such as herbicides, pesticides, heavy metal poisoning (including metalworking, such as crafting jewelry), chlorinated hydrocarbons, arsenic and so on, the resulting liver toxicity and congestion can take much longer to clear. When treating hepatitis with herbs, it's important to note that you should *never give* **bupleurum** *to those on interferon* as they are incompatible, causing severe reactions.

Capillaris is one of the very best herbs to use as it treats all symptoms of *acute hepatitis*. **Dandelion, chicory** and **neem** are next best as they clear Damp Heat from the Liver (the major pattern characterized by acute hepatitis symptoms). Other useful herbs include **milk thistle, turmeric, barberry, Oregon grape, gardenia,** **rhubarb, isatis, baptisia, bupleurum, burdock, scutellaria, coptis, gentiana, artichoke leaves, shiitake, maitake, reishi** and **schisandra**. Alternatively, try Formula #162.

Vitamin C prevents and treats acute hepatitis (use 500-1000 mg/hour or to bowel tolerance). Eat very lightly, such as bean or vegetable soups with radish, fruit, juices, grains and **dandelion/chicory** tea. Avoid all fats, spicy, greasy foods, meats and most acidic foods. If nausea occurs, chew on a piece of lemon or orange peel (this gives relief within five minutes).

Effective formulas for *chronic hepatitis* (any type) include Formula #167 and 241. **Schisandra** and **calendula** lower liver enzyme levels (and schisandra increases immunity), so these are important herbs to take along with **milk thistle**, which regenerates the liver. A good formula includes 2 parts each **milk thistle, schisandra** and **calendula**, 1 part each **dandelion,** Oregon grape, **burdock root** and **isatis,** or **baptisia,** and $1/2$ part each **ginger, fu ling** and **licorice**. At the same time drink **roasted dandelion** and **chicory** tea and some sort of green drink daily, such as Green Magma, spirulina or blue-green algae.

Take 12 drops of grapefruit seed extract in water twice daily, include antiviral herbs such as **olive leaf extract**, **isatis** and **andrographis** (Formula #34), and antiviral immune tonics like **astragalus**, **shiitake** and **reishi** (Formula #77 or 82). (Keep in mind that it's a good idea to rotate antiviral herbs every week since the body gets smart and stops responding over time.) If you have poor digestion with symptoms of nausea, gas, bloatedness, poor appetite and loose stools, add herbs to strengthen Spleen Qi, such as one part each **ginseng**, **dioscorea**, **atractylodes** and **pinellia**, and 1/2 part each **fu ling**, **citrus** and **licorice** (Formula # 43 or 185).

It is extremely important to avoid all caffeine, alcohol, turkey, red meat, dairy, nuts and nut butters, fried and fatty foods, avocados, chips and fats (except ghee—clarified butter—or olive oil). Eat whole grains and legumes (especially aduki, black and mung), lots and lots of cooked vegetables, 1 cup daily dark leafy greens, carrots and carrot juice (room temperature and with ginger juice added to protect digestion), some fruits, fermented products, fish and chicken (avoid turkey and red meat). Take antioxidants and B Vitamins (try brewer's yeast). Regularly include **milk thistle** gomasio (see Recipes in *The Energy of Food*, substituting milk thistle seeds for sesame seeds).

As well, it's important to have your viral load tested regularly. Initially the antibody test will always be positive, since antibodies are produced as a defense response to the virus. From time to time, liver enzymes should be tested, especially the SGOT test, every three months until stabilized. If stable for a year, then test every six months. These tests, plus an overall feeling of well being, are generally a good sign that chronic hepatitis is at least controlled. Over time, it may be completely eradicated.

Meanwhile, maintain a calm and positive attitude. Emotional stress is a great way to help the hepatitis virus develop into a serious condition. Remember that herbs work exceedingly well for hepatitis and can completely reverse it, including type C, so maintain a peaceful state and let go. If you have any unresolved issues, then appropriately express and release your emotions, get therapy if needed, stay positive and laugh a lot. Release frustration, anger or irritability through exercise, creative expression or journal writing.

Liver cirrhosis occurs when liver cells lose function and are replaced by hard, connective fibrous tissues as the liver shrinks. To treat, eat lots of cooked vegetables and dark leafy greens, brewer's yeast (3-5 tablespoons daily), only organic vegetables, fats and protein, carrots, burdock root, beets and artichokes. Beneficial herbs are the same as for hepatitis—try two parts **capillaris**, one part each **safflower**, **dang gui**, **red peony**, **salvia**, **persica** and **ligusticum**, 1/2 part **green citrus** and 1/4 part **licorice**. A liver flush to decongest and cleanse the liver is 8 oz. water or grapefruit juice, 2 oz. olive oil, lemon juice and 2 cloves fresh garlic blended together. Drink 8 oz. first thing every morning for 4 days. Eat lightly during this time.

HEPATITIS PATTERN—DAMPNESS AND HEAT IN THE LIVER:

Jaundice; fever; loss of appetite; nausea; vomiting; bitter taste; fullness and pain of chest and ribs; abdominal distension; yellow sclera (whites of eyes); red face	
Tongue: red with sticky, yellow coat	**Pulse:** slippery, fast and wiry
Formula: # 13 or # 167; 1 capsule boldo with tea of equal parts dandelion, barberry, gentian, milk thistle, burdock root, capillaris, gardenia, neem and reishi. Eat shitake mushrooms.	

UNDERLYING HEPATITIS PATTERNS:

The main hepatitis pattern, Dampness and Heat in the Liver, may co-exist with one of the following underlying patterns. Treat together for best results.

STAGNANT LIVER QI	DEFICIENT LIVER YIN	DAMP SPLEEN
Feeling of distension or pain in ribs and chest	Dry eyes	Abdominal fullness
Frequent sighing	Dry throat	Loss of appetite, nausea
Mood swings, depression	Night sweats	Sensation of heaviness
Sour regurgitation	Scanty menses	Edema in face and eyes
Belching, hiccuping	Insomnia (wakes frequently, but can fall back asleep)	Thirst with desire to drink in small sips
Alternating constipation and diarrhea	Dull or throbbing headache at top of head or temples	Jaundice
Irregular menses	Dream-disturbed sleep	Watery diarrhea
PMS	Numbness of limbs	Pain in ribs
Abdominal distension	Propensity to outbursts of anger	Sallow complexion
Rumbling intestines	Blurred vision	Bitter taste
Tongue: may be normal	**Tongue:** red, especially on sides; peeled	**Tongue:** swollen and wet
Pulse: wiry	**Pulse:** wiry, fast and fine/thin, or floating and empty	**Pulse:** slippery and fast
Formulas: #12 or 189; 1 capsule boldo with tea of equal parts dandelion, bupleurum, white peony, milk thistle, lemon balm and ½ part tangerine peel.	**Formulas:** #74 or 166; tea of equal parts milk thistle, lycii, raw rehmannia, white peony, lycii, ophiopogon and ½ part each lemon balm and dandelion.	**Formulas:** #181; tea of equal parts dandelion, barberry, fennel, artichoke leaves, milk thistle, white and black atractylodes, magnolia bark and fu ling.

❦ INSOMNIA

There are many types of insomnia: inability to fall asleep, waking up during the night and not able to fall back asleep, waking up during the night but able to fall back asleep, restless sleep, dream-disturbed sleep and waking up too early in the morning. Most Western herbal approaches treat inability to fall asleep and stay asleep, but they don't always work for those who can't go back to sleep or who wake early in the morning. Insomnia is actually quite common and can be simple or

extremely difficult to treat, depending on the condition. Very difficult conditions—when insomnia doesn't respond to anything, even sleeping pills—need some form of therapy to clear deep emotional issues disturbing the Heart before regular sleep can be fully regained. Depression can also cause poor sleep (see Depression, for treatment strategies).

Simple factors that cause poor sleep, such as a cold or flu, aches and pains, sudden weather changes, full moon, bedroom too hot or cold, drinking caffeinated drinks, consuming too many fluids before bed, eating too late at night, sagging or lumpy bed, poor pillow, or itching skin diseases, are not classified as insomnia because when any of these causes are removed, sleep resumes.

In TCM, the ability to sleep well is generally connected to the Mind and Spirit (Shen), both of which are rooted in the Heart (especially Heart Blood and Heart Yin), and to the Hun (Ethereal Soul) in the Liver (again nourished by Blood and Yin). If Blood and Yin are abundant, then Shen and Hun are well rooted and can rest easily at night. If either are Deficient, or if Heat, Cold, or emotional factors or stress agitate the Heart or Liver, then sleep may be restless or difficult. Other factors may be involved, however, such as weak Lung Qi not able to descend at night, weak Kidney Qi not able to communicate with the Heart and/or weak Spleen Qi causing poor digestion and inability to form Blood.

General Treatments for Insomnia:

Thankfully, there are many wonderful herbs to support deep, restful sleep. However, it's important to know that herbs work best for sleep when they're taken throughout the day as well as before bedtime. This is because the conditions that create insomnia occur all day long so taking herbs regularly helps ameliorate these causes.

For some, a simple cup of warm milk or herbal tea 1/2 hour before bed works. Try **chamomile** or **skullcap** (good for insomnia from Heat), or **valerian** or **kava kava** tinctures in hot water (good for insomnia from Cold). For others, a formula of equal parts **passionflower**, **hops**, **kava kava**, **valerian**, California poppy and **skullcap** makes an effective combination (try Formulas #57, 92, 100 and/or 101). One of the most important herbs for sleep, **ashwagandha,** calms the nervous system and reduces stress (take in warm milk for best results, or try Formula #2). Simple calmatives that relax the body and induce sleep include **valerian**, **licorice**, **chamomile**, **skullcap**, **lemon balm**, **kava kava**, **schisandra**, **jujube dates** and **zizyphus**. Some find taking **St. John's wort** for several weeks is effective (For-

Causes for Insomnia:

- Emotional strain: long-term anger, frustration and resentment (lead to Heat in Liver); excessive worrying (injures Spleen, Lungs and Heart and weakens Heart Blood, or causes Heat in Heart)
- Constitutional weakness in the Gallbladder and Heart (may cause a timid character with shyness, indecisiveness and lack of self-assertiveness, leading to waking up early in morning)
- Physical or sexual overexertion, especially without adequate rest (depletes Spleen and Kidneys)
- Excessive mental activity, including over-studying and excessive concentration (injures Blood and over time, Yin)
- Poor, improper or irregular diet as well as overeating, eating too late at night and general improper nourishment (weakens Spleen and Blood)
- It is not unusual for women after childbirth to have insomnia (not just because of irregular sleeping hours of baby, but also because sudden loss of blood causes Blood Deficiency, which depletes Heart and Liver)
- Hormonal imbalances (see section Peri/menopause, to balance hormones)
- Excessive stress (weakens Kidneys and Spleen and stagnates Liver Qi)

mula #89). A calcium/ magnesium supplement also nourishes nerves and muscles, aiding sleep.

If insomnia becomes a routine problem, try one of the following:

- Unclutter and clear sleeping room of desks, computers and other work items.
- Change sleeping location or sleep away from electricity, lights, phones, and TVs for several days.
- Check for potential allergens such as molds, dust, pollens and mites.
- Ensure your bed gives proper support. Sagging, lumpy and overly soft or hard mattresses frequently

cause sleep issues. Uncomfortable pillows can also be irritants.

- Be sure to get sufficient exercise for your body's needs, at least twenty minutes, three to six hours before bedtime. Stretch before bed, as this moves stagnant Qi, allowing for deeper sleep.

- Journal writing at bedtime is a fabulous way to process emotions, thoughts and the day's events, which clears the Heart and Mind before sleep.

- Use relaxation and stress-reducing techniques before bed, such as yoga, meditation, contemplation and prayer, listening to soothing music, or tuning into the night sky and moon.

- Avoid excessive TV before bed, especially stimulating programs or movies (or any electronic stimulation for that matter). If you fit either of the Deficient Spleen and Heart Blood or Deficient Heart Yin Patterns, do not read before bed as this further depletes Blood and Yin (also avoid excessive reading, studying or computer work during the day).

- A head, neck, back or foot massage before bed can entice a good sleeping pattern again.

- A hot foot soak (add **ginger** tea if you are cold) can pull Excess Heat or energy down from the head, helping you to fall asleep.

- Moxibustion and a **ginger** fomentation over the Kidneys strengthen and warm, aiding sleep.

- Since irregular sleeping habits lead to sleep problems, create a regular bedtime and stick to it, preferably falling asleep between 9-11 PM for the best sleep quality.

- Examine your attitude about not sleeping, especially while lying awake. Anger or irritation can cause further restlessness and indicate Excess Heat in Liver and/or Heart. Sadness or crying usually signal underlying emotional issues that need attention before sleep will return.

- If you can't sleep, get up and do a few things, then lie down again (rather than just toss and turn) or listen to music or a book on tape.

- The best position for good sleep is on the right side, with legs slightly bent, right arm bent and resting in front of pillow, and left arm resting on left thigh. In this position the heart is up high so Blood can circulate freely, while the liver is low, allowing blood to collect and root the Ethereal Soul.

- Sleeping on a magnetic mattress can promote more restful sleep.

- Sun yourself daily, especially in the afternoon, to keep your body clock regulated.

If insomnia doesn't respond to any of the above, there is a deeper underlying imbalance to identify (there may also be hyper- or hypothyroidism—see Tiredness, for more details). I have divided sleep issues into the various timeframes during which insomnia patterns tend to occur. It is common for people to wake up, or stay awake, during the same hours every night, but be able to sleep at other times. If true, check the following, or refer to insomnia Patterns. As insomnia can become a long-term issue, it may need several simultaneous approaches. Don't get discouraged, but try combinations of the listed methods. There are, however, a few simple tricks that have helped many to break insomnia patterns:

Nutmeg technique: take 1 capsule of *freshly* ground **nutmeg** (it doesn't work with dried) four to five hours before bedtime. Increase dose as needed by 1 capsule/day, until sleep regulates. Nutmeg is usually more powerful and longer lasting and helps you stay asleep more than **valerian**.[1]

Body temperature regulation technique: get in mildly hot water (that doesn't cause a sweat) five hours before you plan to sleep. Stay in twenty minutes, dry off, dress and complete your day. Be sure to get in bed five hours later.

Herbal technique: Rather than using herbs only before sleep, take throughout the day (3-4 times) as well as 1/2 hour before bed. If you wake and can't go back to sleep, take another dose (keep herbs and water by bed). Combine several herbs or formulas for best results.

Hard to Fall Asleep Any Time of Night: Not able to fall

---

[1] Karta Purkh Singh Khalsa, *Herbal Defense: Positioning Yourself to Triumph Over Illness and Aging,* Warner Books, 1997.

asleep is commonly due to emotional disturbances, such as anxiety or depression, or to pain, a variable sleep schedule or a stimulant, like caffeine. If none of these is an issue and you have difficulty falling asleep any time of night, it's generally due to Deficient Blood, low blood sugar or Heat in the Liver. Build Blood with **dang gui**, or Formula #231 (suck on 8 pills or dissolve in warm water and drink as tea), or try Formula #106 with 57 or 100. Alternatively, use an iron supplement, preferably one derived from herbs and blackstrap molasses (such as *Floridex*) as this won't cause constipation as do most iron supplements. As well, eat more animal protein along with mostly cooked foods.

If not able to fall asleep from low blood sugar, eat a protein snack before bed to elevate blood sugar levels and keep a snack by the bed if you wake up. If you are not able to fall asleep due to Heat in the Liver, see Awake 11 PM–3 AM. You may also be too tired to fall asleep (as strange as this may sound). Overworking with insufficient rest sets the body on overdrive, overstimulating adrenals and keeping the body awake, no matter how tired you are. If this fits you, stop overworking (of course!), get more rest during the day, exercise more and eat well. Take **ginseng** to strengthen Qi and aid sleep (while ginseng can stimulate some to stay awake, it aids sleep in Deficient types). Formula #54 and 159 help regulate blood sugar (but don't substitute for proper diet).

Sometimes the body gets stuck in the sympathetic nervous system, unable to switch to parasympathetic and go to sleep. People often experience this just as they're falling asleep by body jerks or being easily startled awake. The best ways to deal with this include foot massage, head massage, hot foot soaks and/or journal writing before bed and daily exercise. Also try **ashwagandha** (Formula #2, or 192).

Restless sleep is generally due to Heat, either Excess or Deficient. Look at one of the Fire, Heat or Deficient Blood or Yin Patterns. Sweating a lot during the day, particularly in hot, humid climates, can cause itchy skin resulting in restless sleep. Vigorously dry brush the skin over your entire body before bed to improve sleep.

Awake on and off during the night, yet able to go back to sleep: If you wake frequently at various hours but are able to go back to sleep fairly quickly, this is usually due to Deficient Kidney Yin or Yang. If Deficient Yin, there may also be restlessness, frequent dreaming, dizziness, irritability, a dry throat, feelings of heat, sore and dry eyes, night sweats and a possible burning sensation in the palms, soles and/or chest. Use the herbs listed under Deficient Yin Patterns. If due to Deficient Yang, there is usually nighttime urination, sore low back and knees, lowered sex drive and feelings of coldness. Use herbs listed under Coldness in category, Awake 5-7 AM.

Awake 11 PM–3 AM: If you are unable to fall asleep during this time, or wake up now and can't fall back asleep, it's due to one of the following: Liver or Heart Fire, Deficient Heart Blood or Yin, or Deficient Liver Blood or Yin. Check the Patterns to see which is applicable and use the indicated herbs. Heat in the Liver is a common cause and has additional symptoms of restlessness, irritability, anger and frustration. Be sure to eliminate all Liver-congesting foods, such as caffeine, alcohol, dairy, turkey, nuts and nut butters, cheese, chips, fried and fatty foods and avocados. Formula #13 with 100 may be useful here.

Also, follow good sleep habits by getting in bed and being asleep by 11 PM, as those who go to bed after that time often get a second wind and can't fall asleep until between 1–3 AM or after 3 AM. This is because Liver/Gallbladder time is between 11 PM to 3 AM, and once awake into that time it may be difficult to fall asleep until energies pass into the next Organ complex. (Going to bed earlier, around 9 PM, is even better as it replenishes the Kidneys.) *Restless legs* frequently occur at this time and can be alleviated by clearing Excess Liver Heat or Deficient Liver Yin (if from Deficient Yin, take Formula #149 or 169, or Formula #74 with 57).

Awake 3–5 AM: Lung time during the 24-hour cycle, Lung Qi flourishes now. If awake only during these hours, Lung Qi is unable to descend. Often coughing, bronchitis, asthma, wheezing and other breathing problems are worse at this time (see section Coughs, for treating these). For some, taking Formula #202 helps Lung Qi descend and sleep return. Those with Deficient

Qi often benefit from taking **astragalus**. Take Formula #44 (or #139) with #77, during the day since they tonify Lung Qi, helping it properly descend at night.

Sleeplessness from indigestion can occur at this time. Often Lung Qi is burdened by stagnation in the Large Intestines, it's paired partner, resulting in nocturnal gas, restless sleep and insomnia. Improve digestion, check for leaky gut syndrome or Candida (see Candida) and take digestive tonics during the day. A good formula to strengthen digestion and clear intestinal stagnation includes 2 parts each **ginseng** or **codonopsis**, **atractylodes**, **dill** and **hawthorn berries**, 1 part each **fu ling** and **sprouted rice** and $1/2$ part each **ginger** and **coptis**. Alternatively, take Formula #25 or 146, as needed.

Being awake at this time may also be due to Deficient Spleen Qi, especially if there is worry, or constant mental thoughts. If Spleen Qi is weak, Blood becomes Deficient and is unable to nourish the Heart. Other symptoms may include poor concentration, gas, bloatedness, sleepiness after meals, heaviness in the arms and legs, fatigue and weakness. Use Spleen Qi tonics during the day, such as **ginseng** or **codonopsis**, **white atractylodes**, **fu ling** and **citrus**. At night, take Formula #43, both before bed and if you wake during these hours. Also try Formula #50.

If Spleen Qi is weak, low blood sugar may be an issue. Be sure to eat meals balanced in protein, carbohydrates and fats during the day and include a balanced snack with protein before bed. If need be, get up and eat a similar snack when you wake in the night, then go back to bed. Take **longan berries**, **ginseng**, **hawthorn**, **pinellia** and **sausurrea**, or Formula #50 or 159, throughout the day. If Coldness is an issue at this time of night, follow directions for Coldness under Awake 5-7 AM timeframe.

Awake 5–7 AM: The Large Intestine time of the 24-hour cycle, it is also the opposite of Kidney time. Thus, Deficient Kidneys usually cause waking at this time with inability to fall asleep. Kidney Qi is supposed to rise and meet the Heart to communicate harmoniously. If this doesn't occur wakefulness results, particularly at this time (although it can happen any time of night—see

Pattern, Heart and Kidneys not Harmonized). If due to Deficient Kidney Yin, night sweats, frequent waking and nocturnal emissions may occur (try Formula #74, 166 or 169, or see Deficient Yin Patterns). Formula #230 works quite well for this, especially if taken throughout the day and before bed. If you wake at 5 AM and can't go back to sleep, then take an extra dose.

If wakefulness is due to Deficient Yang, feelings of coldness, possible nighttime urination, low back pain, knee weakness and/or lowered sex drive may arise. Put more covers on your bed or use a duvet or other warm comforter. Make a formula of 1 part each **fenugreek**, **cinnamon bark**, **ginseng**, **eucommia**, **dioscorea**, **cooked rehmannia** and **dried ginger** and drink three times daily. Also try **dried ginger**, **valerian**, **prickly ash**, **fennel**, **angelica** or **cloves** (or Formula #75 or 180). Eat a warming diet, increase protein and include **ginger**, **garlic**, **black pepper** and **walnuts** with food. Check your thyroid as well (see section Tiredness, for directions).

As well, put a hot water bottle against your lower back or other cold body part (go to sleep with it, too). I don't recommend heating pads or electric blankets because electricity disrupts the body's electrical pattern and may actually cause insomnia. Avoid cold and raw foods, salads, juices, alcohol, sugar, soymilk and iced drinks and foods, as these create Coldness in the body.

Waking up at this time may also be due to Gallbladder insufficiency. If so, there may be timidity, shyness, indecisiveness and lack of self-assertiveness. Take Formula #181 3 times daily. Lastly, waking now may arise from the Kidneys and Heart not communicating.

Snoring: Snoring can cause restlessness and insomnia, and may be the main cause for sleep difficulties without you even knowing it. Snoring is most always due to Dampness collecting in the head and sinuses. This may arise out of Dampness in the Lungs or in the Spleen/Stomach. If in Lungs, there may be cough, mucus in the chest and possible shortness of breath (see section Cough, for herbs to clear Dampness from Lungs). If in Spleen/Stomach, there may be excessive saliva, drooling at night, clearing of throat after eating, possible mucus in lungs after eating, stuffiness in stomach and diaphragm regions and a feeling of heaviness.

For either, use herbs to metabolize Dampness, such as **pinellia** (an herb that also helps Qi descend for better sleep), **black atractylodes**, **agastache**, **cardamom**, **coix**, **grindelia**, **fuling** and **citrus**. Take Spleen Qi tonics as well, such as **ginseng** or **codonopsis** and **white atractylodes**. At the same time, use specific herbs to clear Dampness from head and sinuses, such as Formulas #25, 84, 94, or 237. Also try: 5 parts **coix**, 3 parts **black atractylodes**, 2$^{1}/_{2}$ parts **agastache**, **fennel** and **grindelia** and 2 parts each **citrus**, **magnolia bark**, **baked licorice**, **fresh ginger** and **jujube dates**.

If sinus congestion is predominant, use Formula #84 or 94. Don't eat heavy meals in the evening or before bedtime, and get more rest during the day, as exhaustion leads to snoring. Nasal wash is excellent for clearing Dampness from the head, preventing snoring. (Also, refer to Colds, Flu and Fevers, for more ideas.)

Anxiety can accompany insomnia or cause it, and is due to Excess Heat in the Liver and/or Heart, or due to Deficient Blood, Yin or Kidney/Heart Qi. If due to Excess Heat, try **black cohosh**, **skullcap**, **chamomile**, **kava**, **California poppy**, **wood betony**, **passionflower**, **lady's slipper**, **white peony**, **coptis** and/or **scutellaria** (Formulas #57 & 89). If due to Deficient Blood or Yin, take Blood or Yin tonics (see those Patterns). Other useful herbs include **valerian**, **motherwort**, **sarsaparilla**, **cactus grandiflorus**, **longan berries**, **ginseng**, **schisandra**, **jujube dates**, **dioscorea**, **fu ling**, **zizyphus** and the Formula #50. **Albizzia** is particularly good for anxiety with depression and/or anger.

Formula #131 is a useful general formula in reducing anxiety. Further, anxiety may be a signal that some emerging possibility or potential is too scary to face because doing so involves losing one's present security. Journal write about emotional issues, worries and fears before bed to empty Mind and Heart.

Palpitations may also accompany insomnia. Beneficial herbs reducing palpitations include **arjuna**, **cactus grandiflorus**, **black haw**, **hawthorn**, **licorice**, **motherwort**, **lady's slipper**, **cayenne**, **valerian**, **lotus seeds**, **fu ling**, **zizyphus**, **dang gui**, **cooked rehmannia**, **ginseng** and **longan** (alternatively, try Formula #112). As with anxiety, journal write about emotional issues or worries to clear and settle the Heart.

Differentiation of Insomnia:

- ↝ Difficulty falling asleep is due to Deficient Blood, or Heat in Liver or Heart.

- ↝ Falling asleep easily but waking up frequently during the night is due to Deficient Yin.

- ↝ Excessive dreaming causing restless sleep or nightmares is due to Deficient Blood or Yin, or Heat (Fire) in Liver or Heart. Frightening dreams that awaken you are due to Deficient Gallbladder and Heart. Restless dreams are due to Phlegm-Heat affecting Stomach and Heart.

- ↝ If you must sleep on your back with arms outstretched, this indicates Excess Heat.

- ↝ Inability to sleep on your back indicates Excess of Lungs and/or Heart.

- ↝ If you must sleep in a prone position, this indicates Deficiency, usually of Stomach.

- ↝ If you must sleep on your right side, this indicates Deficient Liver Blood, or Excess Lungs or Heart.

- ↝ If you must sleep on left side, this indicates Deficiency of Lungs or Heart, and Excess Liver.

- ↝ Snoring is usually due to Phlegm affecting Stomach, causing congestion in head.

- ↝ Body jerks or spasms when falling asleep indicates Deficient Kidney and Liver Yin.

- ↝ Sleepwalking is due to Deficient Liver Yin.

- ↝ Talking in sleep is due to Deficient Liver Yin.

- ↝ Restless legs at night indicate Excess or Deficient Heat.

- ↝ Feeling cold at night indicates Deficient Kidney Yang.

Hyperthyroidism, a condition caused by excessive secretion of the thyroid gland, increases basal metabolic rate and possibly causes insomnia. Symptoms include goiter, fine tremor of extended fingers and tongue, increased nervousness, weight loss, altered bowel activity, heat intolerance, excessive sweating and increased heart rate.

Bugleweed (*Lycopus virginicus/europaeus*) blocks conversion of thyroxin to T3 in the liver, interferes with iodine metabolism and inhibits thyroid stimulating hormone. Thus, it is the herb of choice for hyperthyroidism. As well, it is beneficial for tachycardia and arrhythmias in conjunction with insomnia. Combine with **lemon balm** and **motherwort**. In TCM this condition is generally one of Deficient Yin, thus Yin tonics are given, such as Formula #149.

INSOMNIA—EXCESS PATTERNS:

LIVER FIRE	HEART FIRE	PHLEGM HEAT
Restless sleep; possibly very difficult to fall asleep	Waking up in night; possibly very difficult to fall asleep	Restless sleep, tossing and turning
Nightmares, unpleasant dreams, possibly dreaming of fires	Nightmares, possibly dreaming of flying	Unpleasant dreams
Dizziness	Palpitations	Dizziness
Irritability	Mental restlessness	Mental restlessness
Bitter taste in the mouth	Bitter taste in the mouth in the mornings only	Sticky taste in the mouth
Headaches	Tongue ulcers	Feeling of heaviness
Thirst	Thirst	Feeling of oppression in the chest
Dark urine		Nausea
Dry stools		No appetite
		Palpitations
Tongue: red, redder on sides; dry, yellow coat	**Tongue:** red, redder tip with red points; yellow coat	**Tongue:** red with sticky, yellow coat; sticky, rough, yellow coat inside crack in Stomach area
Pulse: wiry and fast	**Pulse:** fast and full on left front position	**Pulse:** slippery and fast
Formulas: #13, 57 or # 170, 1 capsule goldenseal with tea of equal parts St. John's wort, hops, California poppy, chamomile, skullcap, passionflower, lemon balm and ½ part licorice.	**Formulas:** #57; 1 capsule goldenseal with tea of equal parts skullcap, chamomile and hops.	**Formulas:** #13 with 57, or #230; 1 capsule goldenseal with tea of equal parts albizzia bark, schisandra, pinellia, zizyphus and ½ part each green citrus, fresh ginger and licorice.

INSOMNIA—DEFICIENCY PATTERNS:

DEFICIENT HEART BLOOD	DEFICIENT HEART YIN	DEFICIENT LIVER YIN	HEART and KIDNEYS NOT HARMONIZED	DEFICIENT HEART AND GALLBLADDER
Difficulty falling asleep, but once asleep, sleeps soundly	Waking up frequently at night, and difficulty falling back asleep	Waking up during the night; possibly very difficult falling back asleep	Waking up frequently during the night, difficulty falling back asleep	Waking up early in the morning and unable to fall asleep again
Palpitations	Palpitations; anxiety	Talking in one's sleep	Palpitations; anxiety	Palpitations
Tiredness	Mental restlessness	Possible sleepwalking	Mental restlessness	Tiredness
Poor appetite	Sensation of heat in the palms, soles and/or chest	Dreaming a lot; sore, dry eyes	Sensation of heat in the palms, soles and/or chest	Dreaming a lot
Slight anxiety	Night sweats	Feeling of heat, especially in the evening	Night sweats	Lack of initiative and assertiveness
Pale face	Dry throat	Dry throat	Dry throat	Easily startled
Poor memory	Poor memory	Irritability	Poor memory	Breathlessness
Dizziness		Dizziness	Dizziness	Timidity
Blurred vision		Blurred vision	Backache	
		Dry skin and hair	Tinnitus	
Tongue: pale	**Tongue:** red without coat, tip redder; crack in Heart area	**Tongue:** red without coat	**Tongue:** red without coat; tip redder; dry crack in Heart area	**Tongue:** pale, crack in Heart area
Pulse: choppy	**Pulse:** floating and empty, especially on left front position	**Pulse:** floating and empty, especially on left side	**Pulse:** floating, empty and slightly fast	**Pulse:** empty
Formulas: #50 or 132; tea of equal parts dang gui, longan, polygala, zizyphus, schisandra, reishi and 1/2 part licorice.	**Formulas:** #57 or 149; 1 tablet #51 (epimedium) with tea of equal parts ophiopogon, lycii, schisandra, albizzia, dang gui and zizyphus with 1/2 part licorice.	**Formulas:** #169 or 190; tea of equal parts ophiopogon, lycii, dang gui, zizyphus, white peony, raw rehmannia, albizzia, anemarrhena he shou wu vine and 1/2 part green citrus peel.	**Formulas** #51 with 57 and 74, or # 230; 1 tablet #51 (epimedium) with tea of equal parts reishi, raw and cooked rehmannia, asparagus root, dang gui, ophiopogon, polygala, albizzia and reishi.	**Formulas:** #13 with 57, or #230; tea of equal parts albizzia bark, fu ling, zizyphus, reishi, cooked rehmannia and schisandra.

 MENSTRUAL ISSUES

Gynecology is a very broad topic encompassing menarche through pregnancy to menopause. For that reason, I have separated out the most common menstrual issues affecting the majority of women in these age groups and only dealt with them here. There are several excellent books on treating women's ailments, including pregnancy, and some of these are listed in the *Bibliography*.

Some important notes should first be mentioned here about *vaginal health*.[2] Most commercial tampons and sanitary napkins contain anti-clotting chemicals, which cause more bleeding and cramping. Since they are also bleached (to turn them white), they contain harmful dioxins (a by-product released during the bleaching process of sanitary napkins, tampons and toilet paper). Interestingly, women with endometriosis have been found to have higher levels of dioxins in their bloodstreams.[3]

Further, it is not unusual for tiny fibers to rub off tampons and interweave with vaginal tissues (this happens with sea sponges, too, which by the way, are endangered live animals). Over time, these minuscule fibers harbor bacteria, causing vaginal infections, yeast and discharge. As well, the absorbency of tampons also soaks up vaginal secretions, leading to microulceration, peeling and Toxic Shock Syndrome. Thus, I do not recommend women use tampons, or if they absolutely must, only those made of untreated cotton. Menstrual pads should also be made of untreated cotton to prevent infections.

Kegel exercises are important for maintaining vaginal tone and health and preventing urinary incontinence, dry vagina and a prolapsed uterus. To do kegels, contract and release the PC muscle—this is the same muscle stopping urination and contracting the anus—working up to 200 a day of alternating rapid and slow contractions. This can be done any place, any time, with no one ever being aware of it. Lastly, while douches can be beneficial, avoid excessive use as this throws off the important vaginal pH balance, causing vaginal dryness.

Since menstrual issues revolve around blood, it is good to review the TCM definition of Blood. Blood in Western medicine is just that, blood circulating in veins. In TCM, Blood has broader characteristics and functions: it is a very dense and material form of Qi, and, as such, is inseparable from it. In fact, a person may experience Deficient Blood (dizziness, blurry vision, floaters or spots in the visual field, numb limbs, scanty menses or amenorrhea and dry skin and hair) and still not be anemic. Thus, TCM Blood must be considered as different from blood in gynecological conditions.

In general, there are three major causes for women's health issues: emotional stress, diet and External Pathogenic Influences (particularly Damp and Cold). Emotional stress has many origins beyond the obvious, such as cultural influences and societal expectations. To keep emotions from festering and causing gynecological complaints, journal write, talk with a friend or counselor, appropriately express and release pent-up emotions, go on retreats or vision quests, work with dreams, do rituals, or find productive or creative outlets directly working with blocked emotions. External Damp and Cold can be prevented from invading the body by dressing appropriately (keep midriff and lower back covered) and avoiding sitting on concrete and other cold, damp areas, wearing wet bathing suits for extended periods and exposure to cold drafts after sex. Helpful diets are also discussed under each of the following topics.

SCANTY BLEEDING

Scanty bleeding occurs when the period is so light that few changes of tampons or pads are needed, or when bleeding lasts only 2-3 days and is extremely sparse.

General Treatment for Scanty Bleeding:

There are several general approaches to induce a regular blood flow. First of all, build Blood in the body by boosting iron levels (take an iron supplement, such as

---

[2] For a wonderful, provacative poem about vaginal health, read "Tampons" by Ellen Bass.

---

[3] Dioxins are inescapable in our environment. They are legally released as a manufacturing by-product of certain plastics, waste incineration, diesel fuel burning, the bleaching of many paper products and in animals eating foods exposed to dioxin in the air and water. "The Dioxin-Endometriosis Link", Ms., Volume VI, Number 1.

Floridex or blackstrap molasses), increasing vitamin B12 and/or taking a B vitamin complex, or taking Blood tonic herbs, especially **dang gui,** since it increases red blood cells, but also **white peony, cooked rehmannia, jujube dates,** and **lycii berries.**

Western herbs that build blood through increasing iron include **yellow dock, nettles, alfalfa, burdock, dandelion, red clover, sarsaparilla, kelp** and **chickweed** (note that these herbs high in iron are also drying, which depletes Blood; therefore, it's necessary to combine them with blackstrap molasses for best results). **Mulberry fruit, blackberries, raspberries, huckleber-**

ries, and **black currants** also build the Blood, but you must eat a lot of them frequently. Alternatively, take Formulas #106 or 231, as these are quite useful for *anemia* as well.

If blood flow is impeded, emmenagogues are indicated, as they move blood circulation, bringing on menstrual flow. Try **dang gui, mugwort, motherwort, salvia, ginger, chamomile, angelica root, white peony, ligusticum** or **lovage.** If Coldness blocks blood flow (feelings of being cold, pale face, nighttime urination, no thirst), use moxibustion over abdomen and sacrum and take Internally warming herbs, such as **dried ginger, garlic, cinnamon bark, cayenne, prickly ash, anise, star anise, cloves, bayberry** or **galangal** (Formula #41). If there is Yin Deficiency, rest, do gentle exercises that don't cause excessive sweating, avoid hot tubs (injures Yin, Blood and Yang) and take Yin tonics, such as **American ginseng, marshmallow root, ophiopogon** and **asparagus root** (try Formula #74 or 166).

Next, moonbathe, especially under the full moon, as this helps regulate and bring on the cycle, and surround yourself with menstruating women at work, school and home (when women menstruate, they secrete a chemical, called a pheromone, that triggers a hormonal reaction in other women and brings on menstrual flow).

Be sure to balance body weight by eating a balanced diet for your body type (see *The Energy of Food*). If you have just stopped using the birth control pill and your period hasn't begun again, use **vitex** for a minimum of three months to re-regulate your cycle.

It is normal before puberty, during pregnancy and breast-feeding, and after menopause to not bleed. Abnormal lack of menstrual bleeding (*amenorrhea*) occurs when a period stops three months or more in a row and is not due to pregnancy. The longer amenorrhea continues, the more difficult to treat and the more possibility of untreatable infertility. Those women who exclusively eat raw foods often experience stopped periods. This is not from a renewed state of "cleanliness", as some believe, but from insufficient Blood to even bleed.

Amenorrhea is almost always due to extreme Blood Deficiency, stagnant Blood, or from hypothyroidism

SCANTY BLEEDING PATTERNS:

EXCESS PATTERNS;		DEFICIENCY PATTERNS:		
STAGNANT BLOOD	**PHLEGM OBSTRUCT-ING THE UTERUS**	**DEFICIENT BLOOD**	**DEFICIENT KIDNEY YIN**	**DEFICIENT KIDNEY YANG**
Scanty periods	Scanty period	Scanty periods	Scanty periods	Scanty periods
Dark blood	Brownish discharge	Pale, dilute blood	Normal color	Pale blood
Blood clots	Obesity	Dizziness	Dizziness	Dizziness
Painful periods	Tiredness	Blurred vision	Tinnitus	Tinnitus
Abdominal pain that is better after passing clots	Feeling of oppression in the chest	Tingling in limbs; poor memory	Feeling of heat; hot flashes	Backache; knee pain
	Period stops and starts	Insomnia	Dry throat	Night time urination
	Excessive vaginal discharge	Palpitations	Night sweats	Coldness
	Feeling of heaviness	Dull, pale complexion	Malar flush	Frequent, pale urination
Tongue: purple	**Tongue:** swollen	**Tongue:** swollen	**Tongue:** red without coat	**Tongue:** pale and swollen
Pulse: wiry	**Pulse:** slippery	**Pulse:** choppy or fine/thin	**Pulse:** floating and empty, or fine/thin and fast	**Pulse:** deep and weak
Formulas: #107 or 157; tea of equal parts blue cohosh, Western angelica, dang gui, lovage, corydalis and ½ part turmeric.	**Formula:** tea of equal parts cyperus, fu ling, citrus peel, agastache and fresh ginger.	**Formulas:** #106 or 231; tea of equal parts dang gui, white peony, cooked rehmannia, lovage and jujube dates with ½ part citrus peel.	**Formulas:** #74 or 166; tea of equal parts raw and cooked rehmannia, Chinese wild yam, salvia, lycii, cornus and epimedium (#51).	**Formulas:** #75 or 180; 1 capsule powdered ginger & cinnamon bark with tea of equal parts lovage, lycii, cooked rehmannia, false unicorn and ½ part licorice.

(see Tiredness, for more on this), and must be treated immediately, or run the risk of later infertility. **Dang gui** is the best herb for building blood and bringing on menses. As well, the following formula works well for amenorrhea by regulating hormonal balance: equal parts **vitex**, **black cohosh**, **licorice**, **sarsaparilla** and **false unicorn**, or Formula #104.

It is also extremely important to increase protein in your diet, eating it 3 times/day, including animal sources, for at least 3-6 months or more.

HEAVY BLEEDING (MENORRHAGIA)

Heavy menstrual bleeding is excessive menstrual flow during the proper period time. **Flooding** occurs when a period starts suddenly with a flood, or spotting of blood, often before the proper time, while **trickling** is a period continuing with a trickle after proper time. Flooding is different than a heavy period—it is heavier bleeding and a more serious condition. Flooding and trickling are treated the same way as heavy bleeding.

Causes for Heavy Bleeding:

- Emotional stress or shock, such as repressed anger, resentment and frustration (leads to stagnant Qi and then to Fire, which causes Heat in Blood, pushing it out of vessels—this is one of most common causes)

- Mental overwork and excessive sex (weakens Liver and Kidney Yin, causing Deficient Heat in Blood, pushing Blood out of vessels)

- Physical overwork and chronic illness (weaken Spleen Qi, which then fails to hold Blood in vessels and it leaks out)

- Fibroids (block blood flow)

- Missing a period (can cause excessive bleeding during the next cycle)

- Hypothyroidism (see Tiredness, for further details)

- Adrenal or pituitary dysfunction

- Uterine inflammation such as endometriosis or PID

- Estrogen imbalance (too high or too low)

- Excessive eating of cold, raw foods, salads, soy milk, tofu, fruit, juices, iced drinks and foods and melons (weaken Spleen Qi, which then fails to hold Blood in vessels and it leaks out)

- Excessive intake of alcohol, caffeine (chocolate, coffee, black tea, colas, maté, cocoa), cheese, nuts and nut butters, avocados, turkey and fried, fatty and greasy foods (create Heat and stagnation, causing Heat in Blood and pushing it out of vessels)

- Overexposure to environmental toxins (congest the Liver, affecting blood flow)

General Treatment for Heavy Bleeding:

Heavy bleeding is a relative term loosely defined as an increase from what is normal for each woman. However, if blood soaks one tampon or pad per hour for more than three hours in a row, bleeding is considered heavy. Unfortunately, the typical Western treatments for repetitive heavy bleeding is to either give the birth control pill, or a hysterectomy. For most women, neither option is good, nor need they be as many wonderful herbs exist for regulating excessive menstrual bleeding.

To stop excessive bleeding, combine herbs that stop bleeding (**shepherd's purse** tincture, 3-6 drops every 2 hours, or **cattail pollen**, **agrimony**, **mugwort**, **yarrow**, **shepherd's purse**, **raspberry** and **blackberry leaves**, taking 1 dropperful of the tinctures every two hours) with those that eliminate stagnant Blood (**tien qi ginseng**, **cattail pollen**—these herbs also eliminate *blood clots* and stop bleeding), herbs that calm the Blood (**white peony**, **cooked rehmannia**, **moutan pi**) and those that nourish the Blood (**dang gui**, **cooked rehmannia**). Putting it all together, a possible formula is two parts each **mugwort**, **yarrow**, **cattail pollen** and the herbs specific to your condition (according to heavy bleeding Patterns) and 1 part each **tien qi** (Formula #201), **cooked rehmannia** and **astragalus**.

A useful home remedy to stop any type of bleeding (including *hemorrhage*) is to place 1/2 tsp. of ashes (they are quite astringent) in water and drink every hour or two until bleeding slows. Use ashes left over from moxibustion (**mugwort**), burn an herb to ash, such as **mugwort**, **agrimony** or **yarrow**, or in a pinch, burn enough strands of human hair to create 1/4 tsp. of ash. Tonifying and raising Qi holds Blood in vessels so it doesn't leak out (**astragalus** is the best herb for this). Lastly, if anemia results from heaving bleeding, build Blood with iron supplementation (Floridex or blackstrap molasses are good) and Blood-building herbs, such as **dang gui**, **lycii**, **cooked rehmannia** and **white peony**.

To correct the root cause for heavy bleeding, balance hormones with a daily tea of equal parts **vitex**, **wild yam**, **dang gui**, **false unicorn**, **cramp bark** and **black haw**. Include seaweeds in the diet to nourish endocrine glands and increase minerals. Next, see which heavy bleeding Pattern(s) fits and take indicated herbs. It is not unusual to find Heat in the Blood with stagnant Blood, Deficient Qi and Yin appearing together, or Deficient Qi and Kidney Yang with stagnant Blood co-existing. To treat, combine herbs for co-existing patterns.

At the same time, it is extremely important to alter the diet, as this has tremendous impact on heavy bleeding. For those who bleed heavily from Excess Patterns, eliminate alcohol, caffeine (chocolate, coffee, black tea, maté, cocoa), cheese, nuts and nut butters, diary, turkey and fried, fatty and greasy foods. Eat lots of vegetables, fruits, dark leafy greens, grains and legumes. For those who bleed heavily from Deficiency patterns, eliminate cold, raw foods, salads, soy milk, fruit, juices, iced drinks and foods, and eat all cooked foods and vegetables, animal protein, dark leafy greens and some grains and legumes.

Fibroids, a type of benign tumor made of hardened nodules from muscular tissue encapsulated in connective tissue, can also cause heavy bleeding (and menstrual pain and leukorrhea). Abdominal masses are too complex to deal with here, however, one of the best treatments I've seen for fibroids (and *cysts*) is **partridgeberry** tea 2-3 times daily along with high doses of **vitex** tincture (1 tsp., 3 times daily), a dropperful of **cotton root** tincture 3 times daily and Formula #107. A kicharee fast for 5-10 days also shrinks fibroids and cysts along with increasing vitamins E and C, magnesium and selenium supplementation.

All forms of caffeine and dairy (especially cheese— I've seen fibroids increase in size just from cheese alone) along with nuts, turkey, popcorn, avocados, alcohol and fried and fatty foods must be stopped for any results (A good caffeine substitute is 1 part **dandelion root** and $1/2$ part **chicory root**.) Journal write about what wants "birthing" or letting go in your life or any underlying stuck emotional issues. Lastly, the underlying Pattern(s) must be treated as well, such as stagnant Qi and Blood, and/or Deficient Spleen Qi and Dampness.

Spotting throughout the cycle may be due to deficient estrogen and/or excess progesterone (use phytoestrogen herbs—see Peri/Menopause, or see which heavy bleeding Pattern (especially Deficiency) fits and use indicated herbs. **Raspberry** and **wild yam** are specific for *mid-cycle spotting*.

Trickling occurs when the period continues beyond its normal flow with spotting or a slight trickling of blood. See Patterns to treat.

HEAVY BLEEDING (FLOODING/TRICKLING)—EXCESS PATTERNS:

EXCESS HEAT IN THE BLOOD	DEFICIENT HEAT IN THE BLOOD	STAGNANT LIVER QI TURNING TO HEAT	STAGNANT BLOOD	DAMP HEAT IN THE UTERUS
Flooding suddenly, often before proper period time	Flooding suddenly outside of proper period time	Profuse bleeding with sudden flood	Period is hesitant, starting and stopping and then starting again with a flood	Bleeding which could be be either scanty or abundant
Trickling of blood for a long time after the end of the proper period time	Trickling for many days after proper period		Trickling for a long time after the period	Bleeding on mid-cycle
Blood is bright-red or dark-red	Blood fresh-red and watery	Possibly very small blood clots	Dark blood with larger clots	Blood sticky; no clots
Thirst	Malar flush	Thirst	Dark complexion	Vaginal discharge
Red face		Depression	Pain before the period	Yellowish-brown discharge appearing before period starts

(continued on next page)

HEAVY BLEEDING (FLOODING/TRICKLING)—EXCESS PATTERNS: *(continued)*

EXCESS HEAT IN THE BLOOD	DEFICIENT HEAT IN THE BLOOD	STAGNANT LIVER QI TURNING TO HEAT	STAGNANT BLOOD	DAMP HEAT IN THE UTERUS
Agitation	Mental restlessness	Irritability	Abdominal distension	Irritability
Feeling of heat	Feeling of heat in the evening	Moodiness		Burning pain in the lower abdomen
Dark urine	Dark scanty urine	Nausea		Scanty dark urine, pain on urination
Constipation	Dry stools	Acid regurgitation		Feeling of heaviness
		Pain, distension under the ribs		Pain in the joints
				Dragging sensation in the lower abdomen
				Feeling of oppression of the chest
Tongue: red with yellow coat	**Tongue:** red without coat	**Tongue:** redder on sides	**Tongue:** bluish-purple or reddish-purple	**Tongue:** sticky, yellow coat
Pulse: fast and full	**Pulse:** floating and empty	**Pulse:** wiry	**Pulse:** choppy	**Pulse:** slippery
Formulas: #73 or 170 with 201; shepherd's purse tincture (60 drops, 3-5x/day with tea of raspberry leaves, partridgeberry and tree peony.	**Formula** #147 or 153; shepherd's purse tincture (60 drops, 3-5x/day) with tea of equal parts partridgeberry, raspberry leaves, raw rehmannia and American ginseng.	**Formulas:** #12 with dandelion, or #154; shepherd's purse tincture (60 drops, 3-5x/day) with tea of equal parts vitex, white peony, moutan peony, raw rehmannia, bupleurum and cyperus.	**Formulas:** #107 and 113, or 201; shepherd's purse tincture (60 drops, 3-5x/day) with tea of equal parts safflower, motherwort, mugwort, corydalis and salvia.	**Formulas:** #13 or 170; shepherd's purse tincture (60 drops, 3-5x/day) and 1 capsule goldenseal with tea of equal parts raspberry leaves, plantain and partridgeberry.

HEAVY BLEEDING (FLOODING/TRICKLING)—DEFICIENCY PATTERNS:

DEFICIENT SPLEEN QI NOT HOLDING THE BLOOD	DEFICIENT KIDNEY YANG	DEFICIENT KIDNEY YIN
Flooding at the beginning of the period	Periods coming late with prolonged bleeding	Late cycle
Trickling for a long time after proper period	Trickling for a long time after proper period	Trickling of blood after proper period
Pale and watery blood	Pale blood	Fresh-red and watery blood
Pale face	Pale complexion	Malar flush

(continued on next page)

HEAVY BLEEDING (FLOODING/TRICKLING)—DEFICIENCY PATTERNS: *(continued)*

DEFICIENT SPLEEN QI NOT HOLDING THE BLOOD	DEFICIENT KIDNEY YANG	DEFICIENT KIDNEY YIN
Tiredness	Feeling cold	Feeling of heat in the evening
Slight dizziness	Sore back	Dizziness
No appetite	Cold limbs	Tinnitus
Loose stools	Pale urine	Night sweats
Weak limbs and muscles	Weak knees	Weak knees
Gas, bloatedness	Nighttime urination	Hot flushes
Hemorrhoids; prolapsed organs	Feelings of coldness	Mental restlessness
Tongue: pale with teeth marks	**Tongue:** pale and swollen	**Tongue:** red without coat
Pulse: weak	**Pulse:** deep and weak	**Pulse:** floating and empty
Formulas: #159; shepherd's purse tincture (60 drops, 3-5x/day) and rice congee with astragalus, jujube dates and codonopsis, eaten 2 times/day.	**Formulas:** #75 or 180; shepherd's purse tincture (60 drops, 3-5x/day) with 1 capsule dry ginger, cinnamon bark and tea of equal parts eleuthro, mugwort and licorice.	**Formulas:** #74 or 166; tea of equal parts asparagus root, lycii, anemarrhena, cornus, cooked rehmannia, nettle and shatavari.

MENSTRUAL PAIN (DYSMENORRHEA)

Painful periods can range from dull aching cramps in lower abdomen or sacral region to such excruciating pain that a woman passes out. I have seen women who took massive doses of painkillers and still passed out every month from debilitating menstrual pain. Herbs are very effective in treating menstrual pain, alleviating it tremendously, or eliminating it altogether.

General Treatment for Menstrual Pain:

Menstrual pain varies tremendously—there may be pain immediately before, during, or near the end of menses—while quality of pain may be dull, aching, sharp, stabbing or come and go. Each characterizes a different cause for the pain and, therefore, a different approach. Accompanying symptoms may include bloating, gas, abdominal distension, headaches, water retention, achiness, depression, insomnia, diarrhea, constipation or low back pain (to treat related symptoms, see sections by those names).

Causes for Menstrual Pain:

- ↬ Emotional strain, such as anger, frustration, resentment and hatred (cause stagnant Liver Qi, leading to stagnant Blood in uterus, or Liver Fire turning to Heat in Blood)

- ↬ Excessive exposure to cold and dampness, especially during puberty (causes Cold to invade uterus, leading to stagnant Blood—this is frequently seen in young girls who bare their midriffs, especially in cold and/or damp weather, or in women who excessively eat diets high in cold, dampening foods, such as raw foods, salads and fruit juices)

- ↬ Physical overwork or chronic illness (cause Deficient Qi and Blood, leading to stagnant Blood and pain)

- ↬ Excessive sexual activity and too many childbirths too close together (cause Deficient Liver and Kidneys, leading to stagnant Qi and Blood)

- ↬ Imbalance between estrogen and progesterone

Differentiation of Menstrual Pain:

The various characteristics of pain give clues as to its cause:

- ↩ Pain before and during the period is usually due to Excess (especially stagnant Qi or Heat).

- ↩ Pain after the period is due to Deficiency (especially Blood).

- ↩ Pain worsened from pressure ("don't touch my belly!") is due to Excess.

- ↩ Pain improved by pressure (holding the abdomen feels good) is due to Deficiency.

- ↩ Pain aggravated by heat is due to Heat in Blood.

- ↩ Pain relieved by heat (such as that from a hot water bottle) is either a Cold condition or stagnant Blood from Cold.

- ↩ Pain better after passing clots is due to stagnant Blood:

- ↩ Pain with pronounced feeling of distension is due to stagnant Qi.

- ↩ Burning pain is due to Heat in Blood.

- ↩ Cramping pain is due to Cold in Uterus.

- ↩ Fixed, stabbing pain is due to stagnant Blood.

- ↩ Pulling pain is due to stagnant Blood.

- ↩ Bearing-down pain before period is due to stagnant Blood.

- ↩ Bearing-down pain after period is due to Deficient Kidneys.

- ↩ Pain on both sides of lower abdomen is due to Liver.

- ↩ Pain in the lower abdomen is due to Kidneys.

- ↩ Pain on the sacrum (lower back) is due to Deficient Kidneys.

To treat menstrual pain, begin with prevention measures by first increasing intake of calcium/magnesium (eat calcium-rich foods such as sesame seeds, dark leafy greens—kale and collards, yogurt, sardines, seaweeds) and iron (take a supplement if needed, such as Floridex or blackstrap molasses) and taking an herbal formula to regulate hormones 2-3 times/day for 10-14 days before period is due—try equal parts **vitex**, **wild yam**, **black cohosh**, **dang gui**, **sassafras** and **licorice** with 1/2 part **ginger**. Be sure to avoid using tampons as they can cause menstrual pain. Alternatively, try Formula #107 for the first two weeks after menses and Formula #22 from ovulation until menses.

Next, take herbs most appropriate for your type of menstrual pain (see Patterns) 2-3 times daily for a week or more before onset of menses. Take during menstrual pain as well, increasing dose to 1/4 to 1/2 cup tea (or 4-6 "00" capsules) every 15 to 30 minutes. Mix combinations of herbs as appropriate. To best create a formula, use 1 part each of main herbs with 1/2 part each **ginger** and **licorice**. Remember, it takes about three months to change anything related to the menstrual cycle, so be patient for lasting results. An overall formula might be: tea or powder of 1 part each **cramp bark** or **black haw**, **salvia**, **safflower**, **chamomile** and **false unicorn** and 1/2 part each **licorice** and **ginger** (or try Formula #22).

Dull, aching pain: tea or powder of **cramp bark** or **black haw**, **wild yam**, **vitex**, **cyperus**, **fu ling**, and **dang gui** (or Formula #22); eliminate caffeine, alcohol, fried, fatty and greasy foods, avocados, cheese, turkey, nuts and nut butters, chips and vinegars.

Fixed, stabbing pain: tea or powder of **salvia**, **ginger**, **safflower**, **motherwort**, **mugwort**, **dang gui**, **tien qi ginseng**, **corydalis**, **turmeric rhizome**, **white peony**, **angelica**, tinctures or tablets of **frankincense** and **myrrh** (or Formula #107 or 157); get plenty of daily exercise (belly dancing and yoga are especially good here); eat eggplant (moves Blood) and build Blood if Deficient (use **dang gui**, **white peony**, **cooked rehmannia** and **licusticum** (Formula #106 or 231); or take an iron supplement, such as Floridex or blackstrap molasses; avoid cold, raw foods, juices, iced drinks and foods and soy milk; use moxibustion over lower abdomen during pain and throughout month (see *Home Therapies*).

Cramping pain: tea or powder of **wild yam**, **black haw** or **cramp bark**, **blue cohosh**, **black cohosh**, **false uni-**

corn, ginger (Formula #22); eat calcium-rich foods, take calcium and magnesium supplements, get plenty of exercise; use moxibustion and a **ginger** fomentation over lower abdomen; drink hot ginger-lemonade.

Pain with Cold signs (relieved by application of heat): tea or powder of **ginger, mugwort, Western angelica, corydalis, safflower, blue cohosh, cinnamon branch, dang gui, sassafras** (Formula #41); use a hot water bottle, moxibustion, or ginger fomentation over lower abdomen and back; take sitz baths; eat animal protein and all cooked foods; eliminate cold, raw foods, salads, soy products (soy milk, tofu), juices and fruit, iced drinks and foods.

Pain with Heat signs: tea or powder of **motherwort, vervain, salvia, coptis** or **goldenseal**; eliminate caffeine,

alcohol, fried, fatty and greasy foods, avocados, cheese, vinegar and red meat; eat lots of dark leafy greens, vegetables, fruits, beans and grains.

Mid-cycle pain: drink 1 cup **raspberry, wild yam** and **partridgeberry** leaf tea 2-3 times daily for several months.

Endometriosis, a more complicated condition, occurs when endometrial cells usually lining the uterus grow elsewhere, such as on ovaries, fallopian tubes, vagina, bladder, intestines, pelvic ligaments, ureters or other areas in body. Over time, these cells grow into a mass that can scar and form adhesions. Most endometriosis symptoms correspond to the Patterns Damp Heat or Blood stagnation (see those for appropriate herbal choices). Be sure to avoid tampons. If excessive bleeding occurs, see

MENSTRUAL PAIN—EXCESS PATTERNS:

STAGNANT QI	STAGNANT BLOOD	STAGNANT COLD	DAMP HEAT	STAGNANT QI TURNING TO FIRE
Lower abdominal pain during the period or one or two days before the period	Intense, stabbing pain before or during the period	Lower abdominal pain before or after the period	Hypogastric pain before the period and sometimes on mid-cycle	Abdominal pain before or during the period
Pain relieved after movement	Pain relieved after passing clots	Pain relieved by application of heat	Burning sensation extending to the sacrum	Pain not relieved by heat
Dark blood; no clots	Dark blood with clots	Blood scanty and bright red with small, dark clots	Red blood with small clots	Dark blood; heavy period; dry stools
PMS and irritability	Mental restlessness	Sore back	Mental restlessness	Irritability
Pronounced breast and abdominal distension		Feelings of cold	Feelings of heat; thirst	Feelings of heat; thirst
Period starts hesitantly			Vaginal discharge; scanty dark urine	Propensity to outbursts of anger
Tongue: may be normal, or with raised edges	**Tongue:** purple	**Tongue:** pale-bluish, or bluish-purple	**Tongue:** red with sticky, yellow coat	**Tongue:** red with redder sides
Pulse: wiry	**Pulse:** choppy	**Pulse:** deep and choppy, or deep and wiry	**Pulse:** slippery	**Pulse:** wiry and possibly fast

(continued on next page)

MENSTRUAL PAIN—EXCESS PATTERNS: *(continued)*

STAGNANT QI	STAGNANT BLOOD	STAGNANT COLD	DAMP HEAT	STAGNANT QI TURNING TO FIRE
Formulas: #12 or 153; 1 capsule turmeric with tea of equal parts cyperus, dang gui, white peony, corydalis & ligusticum. Eat rose petal paste.	**Formulas:** #107, 113 or 157; tea of equal parts turmeric, motherwort, tien qi ginseng, dang gui, lovage, salvia, corydalis, cyperus and cinnamon branches.	**Formulas:** #41 or 137; equal parts angelica, ginger, caraway, dang gui, lovage, corydalis and cinnamon branches.	**Formulas:** #13 or 170; 1 capsule goldenseal with tea of equal parts dandelion, barberry, turmeric tuber, salvia, and fennel with ½ part wild yam.	**Formulas:** #12 with dandelion, or #154; 2 capsules powdered goldenseal and turmeric tuber with tea of equal parts dandelion, barberry salvia, motherwort and fennel with ½ part wild yam.

MENSTRUAL PAIN—DEFICIENCY PATTERNS:

DEFICIENT QI AND BLOOD	DEFICIENT BLOOD AND YANG	DEFICIENT KIDNEY AND LIVER YIN
Dull hypogastric pain towards the end of or after the period	Dull abdominal pain after the period	Dull hypogastric pain towards the end of or after the period
Pain relieved by pressure and massage	Pain relieved by pressure and application of heat	Pain relieved by pressure and massage
Scanty bleeding	Scanty pale blood with no clots	Scanty bleeding
Dragging sensation in the lower abdomen	Dull headache	Sore back
Pale complexion	Blurred vision	Blurred vision
Tiredness	Feeling of coldness	Exhaustion
Slight dizziness	Dizziness	Dizziness
Loose stools	Depression	Tinnitus
Tongue: pale and possibly thin	**Tongue:** pale, swollen and wet	**Tongue:** red without coat
Pulse: choppy	**Pulse:** fine/thin, slow and empty	**Pulse:** floating and empty
Formulas: #106 or 198; tea of equal parts astragalus, dang gui, jujube dates, codonopsis, salvia, motherwort and corydalis.	**Formulas:** #107 or 113; 1 capsule cinnamon bark and dried ginger with tea of equal parts dang gui, white peony, lycii and corydalis.	**Formulas:** #74 or 166; tea of equal parts asparagus root, dang gui, white peony, salvia, raw rehmannia and corydalis.

Heavy Bleeding in this section.

IRREGULAR MENSTRUAL CYCLES

The average cycle length is 28 days, meaning a normal cycle can vary from 25-32 days. Irregular cycles are unpredictable: sometimes coming early and sometimes coming late (those that come consistently early or late are not

General Treatment for Irregular Menstrual Cycles:

The very best herb to regulate the menstrual cycle is **vitex**, although **black cohosh**, **dang gui** and **false unicorn root** (only use cultivated) are also quite useful. Start with just one dropperful vitex every morning, or take equal parts of all four herbs in a tea, 2-3 times daily. This protocol must be followed daily throughout the month for at least 3-6 months to see results. Alternatively, try Formula #12.

At the same time, "moonbathe" every night, since regularly exposing yourself to the moon normalizes menstrual flow, and surround yourself at home, school and work with menstruating women. If after trying everything your cycle is still irregular and you are in your late thirties or in forties, it is likely you have entered the peri-

irregular). An irregular cycle that occurs for only a few months may be due to one ovary not functioning properly, although this is normal during peri/menopausal years.

IRREGULAR CYCLES PATTERNS:

EXCESS PATTERN:	DEFICIENCY PATTERNS:	
STAGNANT LIVER QI	**DEFICIENT KIDNEY YANG**	**DEFICIENT KIDNEY YIN**
Irregular periods	Irregular periods	Irregular periods
Possible early or late periods	Possible late periods	Possible early periods
Usually with scanty bleeding	Scanty and pale blood	Scanty bleeding
Some small clots	No clots	No clots
Abdominal & breast distension	Backache	Night sweats
PMS	Frequent, copious urination	Blurred vision
Depression	Feeling cold, cold knees	Feeling of heat in the evening
Irritability	Night time urination	Tinnitus
Sighing	Low sex drive	Dizziness
Tongue: normal or possibly red sides	**Tongue:** pale and swollen	**Tongue:** red without coat
Pulse: wiry	**Pulse:** weak and deep	**Pulse:** floating and empty, or fine/thin and fast
Formulas: #12 or 153; 1 capsule turmeric with tea of equal parts bupleurum, cyperus, dang gui, white peony and lemon balm. Eat rose petal paste.	**Formulas:** #75 or 180; 1 capsule cinnamon bark and ginger powders with tea of equal parts false unicorn, epimedium (#51); saw palmetto and lycii.	**Formulas:** #74 or 166; rice congee with equal parts lycii, asparagus root, epimedium (#51) and American ginseng, eaten twice daily.

menopausal phase of life (see section Peri/Menopause for more details). Be sure to avoid using tampons, as they can negatively affect the menstrual cycle (see Vaginal Health at the beginning of Menstrual Issues).

PRE-MENSTRUAL SYNDROME (PMS)

PMS broadly describes the emotional and physical symptoms occurring anywhere from one to three days before the period, or as early as ovulation, fourteen days before the period. I have seen all sorts of PMS cases. Some women feel extremely crabby or can easily burst into tears. Others complain about uncomfortable breast distension or lack of sex drive. A few have experienced tremendous food cravings, swinging between eating everything in sight to not wanting food at all. Yet, the most common symptom I see among those who experience PMS is moodiness and depression (see section Depression).

General Treatment for PMS:

While Western medicine sees PMS as a hormonal swing (caused by dropping progesterone levels leaving estrogen unopposed, also called estrogen dominance), wholistic medicine sees PMS as an important signal that something is not right with our bodies and/or psyches that needs attention. Just like the effects of lunar tides upon people, the ten to fourteen day phase before bleeding may be an extra sensitive time.

In fact, it is during this phase when women become barometers for their environments—their personal, family and community lives. In the past, women retreated to "moon lodges" where, being fed and cared for, they envisioned, dreamed and received inner guidance. When the bleeding phase ended, they brought visions back to the tribe and shared them for the good of all people.

Women not only don't do this today, many try to ignore and mask their cycles as best possible. This is quite unfortunate because emotional issues arising at this time are valuable red flags signaling what's off and needs correction. When focus is placed on enhanced emotionality, we can contact its causes and plan for the

PMS Symptoms:

These may occur in combination and range in severity from mild to serious: depression, mood swings, breast distension and tenderness, cramps, menstrual pain, acne, irritability, sadness, anxiety, lethargy, tension, water retention, loss of concentration, appetite swings, food cravings, crying, outbursts of anger, clumsiness, nervousness, insomnia, lowered pain threshold, aggressiveness, changes in libido, intense food/sweet cravings and abdominal distension.

Causes for PMS:

- Emotional strain from long-term unexpressed or repressed emotions, especially anger, frustration and resentment (one of the most common cause of PMS, this leads to stagnant Qi, particularly in the Liver)
- Excessive intake of dairy, alcohol, caffeine, nuts and nut butters, avocados, chips, fried, fatty and greasy foods, turkey and recreational drugs (causes stagnant Liver Qi)
- Excessive intake of flour products, dairy and fried, fatty and greasy foods (cause Phlegm to accumulate in breasts, leading to breast tenderness)
- Overwork with inadequate rest and excessive sexual activity (causes stagnant Qi and weakens Liver and Kidneys)
- Hormonal imbalance (occurs from any of the above, inherited factors, excessive exposure to environmental toxins, or from some drugs, such as the woman's mom taking DES while pregnant)

indicated changes. Thus, concentrate on your feelings and intuition during this phase, for in doing so, not only may your health improve, but also that of your family and community. While herbs relieve PMS symptoms, they don't take away these red flags, or the need for retreat or reflection.

That said, there are several approaches for treating these monthly symptoms. First, PMS responds very well to the same treatment used for depression: get lots of exercise, focus on creative projects, appropriately express and release emotional issues and eat a balanced diet. (For more details on these, or to treat depression and moodiness, see section Depression.) If you experience extreme PMS, try not to use oral contraceptives because in disrupting the natural hormonal cycle, they can cause menstrual issues, such as amenorrhea and infertility, and proliferate yeast in the body, possibly leading to Candida.

PMS-causing foods include dairy, alcohol, caffeine (coffee, black tea, colas, chocolate, cocoa, maté), nuts and nut butters, avocados, chips, flour products, fried, fatty and greasy foods, sugar, refined and processed foods, red meat and turkey. Beneficial foods encompass dark leafy greens (kale, collards, etc.), lots of cooked vegetables, grains, legumes, protein as appropriate for your body's needs, and some fruit.

Be sure to include seaweeds for their high mineral content, calcium-rich foods to nourish nerves and muscles, and 500 mg two times daily of essential fatty acids, such as **evening primrose, borage (**Formula #11), or **black current seed oils,** as these aid proper liver functioning. Some women benefit by taking B vitamins, especially B6, as these calm PMS tension and irritability. General food cravings respond well to **evening primrose oil** and **vitex.** Control sugar cravings by eating something bitter (believe it or not, this really works)

and premenstrual chocolate cravings (a signal of magnesium deficiency) by taking magnesium supplementation for seven days before the cycle (or throughout the whole month for intense, or constant, cravings).

One of the best overall herbs for PMS is **vitex** (Formula #102), since it regulates hormonal balance. I have seen it clear up the worst imaginable cases of PMS when a woman claims she is a living Jeckyll and Hyde. In general, vitex needs to be taken for three months up to a year or more for lasting results in severe cases. For minor cases, take one dropperful vitex tincture every morning; or 1 tsp. vitex tincture, one to three times daily for severe cases, tapering dosage as symptoms improve.

Gentle diuretic herbs are useful in eliminating excess water weight, relieving emotional tension, breast tenderness and abdominal bloatedness. Try equal parts **nettles, parsley** and **dandelion,** or Formula #99. Since the liver is responsible for breaking down hormones and cleansing the blood of toxins, include detoxifying and decongesting Liver herbs. **Dandelion, Oregon grape, barberry, milk thistle** and **burdock** clear Heat from the Liver. **Vitex, cyperus, green citrus** and **bupleurum** move stagnant Liver Qi. **Dang gui, lycii** and **white peony** tonify Blood, easing Liver functioning. Diminish stress and PMS through nervines such as **skullcap** and **valerian,** calmatives like **chamomile** and **hops,** calcium supplementation, rest, meditation and regular exercise.

One of the very best formulas for most all PMS symptoms is the Chinese Formula #12 (or #153), also

PMS—EXCESS PATTERNS:

STAGNANT LIVER QI	PHLEGM-FIRE HARASSING UPWARDS
Abdominal and breast distension before the period	Feeling of oppression in the chest
Irritability	Slightly manic behavior
Mood swings, depression	Depression, agitation
Under the ribs pain and distension	Red face; bloodshot eyes
Clumsiness	Possible phlegm, nausea, vomiting, dizziness, palpitations and/or insomnia

(continued on next page)

PMS—EXCESS PATTERNS: *(continued)*

STAGNANT LIVER QI	PHLEGM-FIRE HARASSING UPWARDS
Tongue: may be normal, or with raised sides, or red sides	**Tongue:** red with sticky, yellow coat
Pulse: wiry	**Pulse:** full, slippery and fast
Formulas: #12 or 153; tea of equal parts St. John's wort, black cohosh, black haw, lemon balm, vitex and ½ part fresh ginger. Eat rose petal paste.	**Formulas:** #13 with 64, or #181; 4 capsules, 2-3 x/day of powdered barberry, dandelion, cyperus, goldenseal and ½ part fu ling and fresh ginger.

PMS—DEFICIENCY PATTERNS:

DEFICIENT LIVER BLOOD	DEFICIENT LIVER AND KIDNEY YIN	DEFICIENT SPLEEN AND KIDNEY YANG
Depression and weepiness before the period	Irritability before the period and sometimes after it	Slight PMS with depression and weeping
Slight abdominal and breast distension	Slight breast distension before period and sometimes after it	Slight abdominal and breast distension
Scanty periods	Scanty periods	Low sex drive
Tiredness	Poor memory	Tiredness
Poor memory	Sore back and knees	Sore back
Poor sleep	Insomnia	Feelings of cold
Slight dizziness	Dizziness	Frequent and pale urination
Dull-pale complexion	Dry eyes and throat	Poor digestion
Floaters or black spots before the eyes	Burning sensation in palms, soles and/or chest	Gas, bloatedness; loose stools
Tongue: pale, possibly only on sides	**Tongue:** red without coat	**Tongue:** pale and swollen
Pulse: choppy, fine/thin and wiry	**Pulse:** floating and empty	**Pulse:** deep and weak
Formulas: #12 or 153; tea of equal parts dang gui, white peony, lycii, lovage and cooked rehmannia. Eat mulberries, blackberries, raspberries, huckleberries and black currants.	**Formulas:** #74 or 166; tea of equal parts lycii, dang gui, ophiopogon, raw rehmannia, epimedium (#51) and asparagus root (also cook with rice and chicken to make soup).	**Formulas:** #75 or 180; 1 capsule cinnamon bark and dried ginger powders with tea of equal parts epimedium (#51), Chinese wild yam, cuscuta, cooked rehmannia and lycii.

known as *Free and Easy Wanderer*, an apt name for what it does. If there are additional symptoms of irritability, frustration and anger, add dandelion tea or take its modified version, Formula #154. Alternatively, try Formula #63. If none of these fully relieve your symptoms, look to one of the PMS Patterns and try the listed herbs.

Menstrual Acne: Usually due to hormonal fluctuation, *vitex* is the herb of choice for menstrual acne. Try for at least three months, and if desired results do not occur,

Causes for Vaginal Infections and Discharge:

- ✦ Emotional strain or any long-term unexpressed or repressed emotion (lead to stagnant Qi invading Spleen, impairing its transformation and transportation functions and resulting in Dampness pouring downwards to genital system.)

- ✦ Excessive intake of dairy, greasy foods, sugar, raw foods, juices, flour products (lead to formation of Dampness that pours downwards to genital system)

- ✦ Irregular eating habits (leads to formation of Dampness that pours downwards to genital system)

- ✦ Excessive physical work (weakens Spleen, impairing its transformation and transportation functions, leading to Dampness collecting and pouring downwards to genital system)

- ✦ Overwork for a long time (leads to Kidney Yang Deficiency, impairing Kidneys from storing and holding fluids so they leak out in vaginal discharge). Overwork with inadequate rest (depletes Liver and Kidney Yin, causing excessive vaginal discharge)

- ✦ External Dampness directly invading the body and settling in the genital system can occur at vulnerable times, such as after childbirth, after each period, or from prolonged sitting/standing in wet bathing suits, cold environments such as basements and concrete areas, or wearing clothes that don't cover midriff and lower back regions.

- ✦ Stress

- ✦ Leaving a tampon, sponge, diaphragm or other foreign object in the vagina too long

- ✦ Synthetic underwear, pantyhose and pants (trap moisture and heat since these fabrics don't breathe)

- ✦ Lice, crabs, wounds, reactions to feminine sprays, hot tub chemicals or bacteria, reactions to detergents and/or scented/colored toilet tissue, talcum powder, bubble baths (possible irritants).

see section Skin Conditions.

Types of Vaginal Infections and Discharge:

- ✦ Bacterial infections generally have white, watery or creamy discharge with foul or fishy odor and itchiness.

- ✦ Yeast infections are normally itchy and have thick-white discharge (it can be like cottage cheese) with a possible yeasty smell.

- ✦ Trichomonas, a one-celled parasitic microorganism that is spread during intercourse or bathing, causes intense symptoms of vaginal itching, irritation and yellow to green discharge that may also be frothy with a foul odor. Both discharge and urine burn genital area while the vaginal opening itself is very red with severe burning and itching. There may also be other signs of infection, such as a fever, chills, nausea, irritability or tiredness. It occurs through contact from sexual intercourse with an infected partner. (Since it is possible to re-infect your sexual partner, sexual abstinence is important during its treatment.)

- ✦ Gardnerella vaginalis is a bacterial infection with fishy smell and thin grayish discharge that may have tiny bubbles.

- ✦ Chlamydia trachomatis, generally classified as a bacterium, is actually a type of intracellular parasite with symptoms of vaginal discharge, painful urination and low abdominal pain.

VAGINAL INFECTIONS AND DISCHARGE

Vaginal infections can manifest in a variety of ways, from no symptoms at all, to burning and itching pain of the vagina and external genitalia, or pain during intercourse. Vaginal infections include monilia, gardnerella, trichomonas, Candida and nonspecific vaginitis. Normal vaginal discharge has a clear color, is stretchy or rubbery in consistency and has no odor. It is normal for vaginal discharge to increase during ovulation and sexual stimulation. Pathological discharge is different than this—it may be excessive, have color or odor, or be thick and copious.

General Treatment for Vaginal Infections and Discharge:

One of the best ways to treat **most vaginal infections**, including *cervical dysplasia*, is with a bolus (see *Herbal Preparations*), such as 2 parts each **echinacea**, **chaparral** and **partridgeberry**, one part each **marshmallow** and **goldenseal** and $^1/_2$ part **bayberry bark**. At the same time take 10-15 drops grapefruit seed extract in water, 3 times/day and douche with tea of equal parts **comfrey**, **raspberry**, **lady's mantle** and **partridgeberry**. Use bolus nightly and douche daily until 3-5 days after infection or discharge is gone. A sitz bath of **raspberry** or **daikon radish leaves**, or **rose petals**, is also helpful.

Be sure to avoid caffeine, alcohol, fried, fatty and greasy foods, nuts and nut butters, dairy, cheese, chips, turkey, sugar and raw and cold foods. Eat lots of cooked vegetables and dark leafy greens. If Damp Heat is present (see Patterns), cleanse liver with herbs such as **dandelion**, **burdock root**, **barberry** and **milk thistle** (or take Formula #13 or 170).

Chronic vaginal infections and discharge are frequently caused by a Deficiency condition. Be sure to tonify Kidneys, Spleen, Qi, Blood and/or Yang while clearing Damp Heat at the same time. To do so, combine herbs from applicable Patterns, or try Formula #140.

Bacterial infections respond especially well to the following douche: one cup each 3% hydrogen peroxide and water (distilled is best). Douche with this twice daily for three days. A bolus and douche of **echinacea**, **goldenseal** and **raspberry** also works well. If the infection does not clear up with these, it is probably not from bacterial causes.

For *yeast infections*, try Formula #17, 140 or 242, plus 10-15 drops grapefruit seed extract internally 3 times daily for 3-7 days (slowly work up to this dose). The very best douche I have used for yeast infections is this

Chinese formula: $^1/_2$ oz. **cnidium** (*Semen Cnidii monnieri—she chuang zi*), $^1/_3$ oz. each **lycii bark** (substitute **phellodendron** if needed), **stemonia**, **lithospermum** and **sophora** and $^1/_4$ oz. **prickly ash**. Simmer all herbs except prickly ash and lithospermum in 6 cups water down to 4 cups. Add prickly ash and lithospermum, cover and steep 15 minutes. Cool and add 2 tablespoons baking soda. Douche with 2 cups in the morning and 2 cups in the evening for three days. If using Western herbs, try a bolus of equal **parts pau d'arco**, **black walnut hull**, **echinacea**, **goldenseal**, **slippery elm**, **gentian** and **calendula** powders. Alternatively, use **garlic** bolus, or 2 "00" capsules boric acid powder for a week (know that boric acid may burn for a few days, but is very effective). If none of the above work, see associated Patterns and try indicated herbs. Also refer to Candida, for other treatment approaches.

Trichomonas requires at least two months of treatment since it is a more difficult condition. A garlic bolus (be sure to wrap in cheese cloth and soak in olive oil before inserting) is specific for Trichomonas. Also, follow herbal directions and Patterns for treating Candida (see

---

Differentiation of Vaginal Infections and Discharge:

- ↬ Consistency: Profuse discharge is typically due to Deficient Kidneys; a white-sticky discharge usually reflects a Deficient Spleen.

- ↬ Color: White, clear discharges indicate Cold and may be from Deficient Spleen and Kidney Qi; yellow, red or green discharges indicate Heat; a profuse red discharge (whether dilute or sticky) indicates Yin Deficiency with Damp Heat (this must be distinguished from mid-cycle bleeding).

- ↬ Thickness: Dilute, watery discharges indicate Cold or Deficiency; thick, sticky discharges indicate Heat or Dampness.

- ↬ Odor: Strong odors indicate Heat; fishy odors indicate Cold.

VAGINAL INFECTIONS AND DISCHARGE—EXCESS PATTERNS:

DAMP HEAT	TOXIC HEAT	STAGNANT LIVER QI
Profuse vaginal discharge that has odor	Profuse vaginal discharge that has odor	Profuse vaginal discharge without odor
Yellow or brown discharge	Blood-stained discharge	White or yellow discharge
Sticky consistency	Sticky consistency	Sticky consistency
Loose stools	Dark urine	Pain in the ribs
	Thirst	Irritability
	Feelings of heat	Depression
Tongue: sticky, yellow coat on root with red spots	**Tongue:** red with sticky, yellow or brown coat with red spots	**Tongue:** slightly red on sides
Pulse: slippery	**Pulse:** slippery and fast	**Pulse:** wiry
Formulas: #13 or 170, or # 242; 1 capsule goldenseal with tea of equal parts barberry, partridgeberry and raspberry leaves.	**Formula:** 4 capsules, 3x/day of equal parts powdered goldenseal, chaparral, yellow dock, baptisia, echinacea, dandelion and sarsaparilla.	**Formulas:** #12 or 153; tea of equal parts lemon balm, chamomile, dandelion and fennel.

VAGINAL INFECTIONS AND DISCHARGE—DEFICIENCY PATTERNS:

DEFICIENT SPLEEN QI	DEFICIENT KIDNEY YANG	DEFICIENT KIDNEY YIN
Excessive vaginal discharge	Profuse and dilute vaginal discharge	Lighter discharge flow
White or slightly yellow discharge	White or clear discharge	White discharge
Sticky discharge, persistent	Discharge resembles water or egg whites	Diluted discharge
No smell	No smell	No smell
Dull complexion	Pale complexion	Malar flush
Tiredness	Tiredness	Tiredness
Depression	Dizziness	Dizziness
Cold limbs	Feelings of cold overall	Feeling of heat in the evening
Loose stools	Backache	Tinnitus
	Frequent, pale to clear urination	Burning sensation in palms, soles and/or chest
Tongue: pale with sticky, white coat	**Tongue:** pale and wet	**Tongue:** red without coat
Pulse: weak and slightly slippery	**Pulse:** deep and weak	**Pulse:** floating and empty

(continued on next page)

VAGINAL INFECTIONS AND DISCHARGE—DEFICIENCY PATTERNS: *(continued)*

DEFICIENT SPLEEN QI	DEFICIENT KIDNEY YANG	DEFICIENT KIDNEY YIN
Formulas: #140; tea of equal parts eleuthro, Chinese wild yam, white peony, black and white atractylodis, phellodendron, astragalus and fu ling.	**Formulas:** #75 with 80, or #194; take 1 capsule cinnamon bark and dried ginger powders with tea of equal parts schisandra, cuscuta, lycii, epimedium (#51), cooked rehmannia, Chinese wild yam and fu ling.	**Formulas:** #74 with 80, or #166; tea of equal parts Chinese wild yam, schisandra, raw rehmannia, anemarrhena, phellodendron and asparagus root.

section Candida), and use an external wash made of 3 oz. **cnidium**, 1 oz. **sophora** and $1/2$ oz. each **dang gui** and **clematis**. Simmer herbs in 6-8 cups water for 30 minutes and divide into three equal doses. Dilute each dose with cold water and use as a sitz bath for external genitalia, or an herb wash that air dries. Alternatively, use external wash made of **agrimony** (*Agrimonia pilosa*). Also take Formula #242.

PERI/MENOPAUSE

Over the years I have clinically treated many women for the wide range of symptoms bundled together under the terms, perimenopause and menopause. I have found herbs to be amazingly effective in alleviating symptoms that arise during this phase, especially when combined with an alteration of diet, exercise and lifestyle activities. While some women seemingly breeze through this life passage, most experience anywhere between a few to a large array of symptoms, some of which can have tremendous impact on a woman's quality of life. While peri/menopause is not a disease but a normal life phase, it is included here because its many symptoms may be alleviated with natural treatments.

By definition, the perimenopausal phase begins when hormone-related changes kick in and continues until hormones stabilize a few years after menopause has occurred. Thus, the perimenopausal stage encompasses the years before menopause itself (called climacteric), whereas actual menopause begins twelve months after the menses has ceased. So when most people talk about menopausal symptoms, they usually refer to those of the perimenopausal period, which can last up to ten, or even fifteen, years before the period stops. Because perimenopause and menopause symptoms are virtually the same, I use the combined term, peri/menopause, to mean both.

The mean age of menopause is just over 50. Menopause is classified as premature if the period stops earlier than age 35. Interestingly, ovarian follicles slowly decline over time, starting in the fetus and continuing through menopause. As follicle activity declines, estrogen drops. This means your lifestyle and dietary habits from childhood on determine what kind of menopause you're going to experience. If you overwork, bear too many children too close together, overindulge in sex or eat a poor diet, the peri/menopausal period reflects this accordingly. In fact, how you treat your body in your teens and twenties usually determines the ease or difficulty of the peri/menopause phase you'll experience.

Peri/menopause symptoms include headaches, tiredness, lethargy, irritability, anxiety, nervousness, depression, mood swings, insomnia, heart palpitations, inability to concentrate, memory lapses, hot flashes, vaginal dryness, dry skin, bone loss, lowered libido, erratic menstrual cycles, urinary incontinence, weight gain and night sweats. Western medicine states only hot flashes and vaginal dryness are estrogen-deficiency related, while other symptoms are due to increased stress at this time of life. However, the Chinese perspective sees these symptoms as related to an underlying pattern, most usually Kidney Deficiency, although this can be complicated by other patterns.

In Western terms, the body's response during peri/menopause is as follows: when estrogen drops, the hypothalamus secretes gonadotropin-releasing hormone (gnRH) to the pituitary gland, which in turn sends follicle-stimulating hormone (FSH) to signal the ovaries, asking them to please produce more estrogen. As ovaries age, they become less responsive, causing the hypothalamus and pituitary to send out even more signals to crank them up. When the ovaries don't release estrogen, the various functions of the hypothalamus are disrupted, affecting many aspects of the body: temperature regulation, perspiration, metabolism and emotional states. At the same time, if an egg doesn't ripen, ovulation doesn't occur and progesterone isn't secreted. This lack of progesterone accompanied by relatively higher levels of estrogen result in peri/menopausal symptoms (and together this is sometimes called estrogen dominance).

Many hormonal issues actually occur from excessive xenoestrogens found in plastics (plastic wrapping, water jugs and baby bottles, for instance) in sprayed fruits and vegetables, herbicides (DDT, DDE, etc.), processed foods, petrochemicals and DES (the morning sickness drug given to pregnant women in the 1950s). Xenoestrogens mimic natural estrogen in the body by sitting on estrogen receptor sites. Highly fat soluble and non-biodegradable, they accumulate in fat tissues and affect hormonal glands as well. (It is the presence of these, plus hormones in foods, that are contributing to young girls menstruating so early in life.) Excessive collection of xenoestrogens in fat cells leads to cancer, particularly breast cancer, because of the high number of fat cells there, although prostate cancer can occur, too.

At the same time, the liver has to process these wild hormonal fluctuations. If congested from stress or an inappropriate diet (now is when a woman can really feel the adverse effects of such aggravating foods as caffeine and alcohol), symptoms can soar or plummet on a roller-coaster ride that may last for years. This causes not only physical symptoms, but emotional and mental ones as well. Most people are familiar with the typical symptoms of hot flashes and night sweats, but it is not unusual for women during these years to also cry easily, have poor memory or concentration gaps, and feel undecided about what to do with the rest of their lives. While traditionally there has been a strong place in many cultures for a menopausal woman as the wise woman, shaman, healer, or spiritual or political leader, she has been considered old (hags, shrews, old bags), sick, used up, and even hysterical in the West until only recently. With so many baby boomers passing into menopause today, it is finally receiving the recognition it deserves as a time of normal change.

However, Western treatment still gives hormone replacement therapy (HRT) as a quick bullet cure, causing more estrogen dominance and resulting in a severity of already existing symptoms and, of course, a possibility of the known side effect of excessive estrogen, cancer. However, because symptoms are still present and perhaps worse, the estrogen dose is increased. Now signs of hypothyroidism may occur because estrogen interferes with how the thyroid hormone works. Thus, there can be apparent hypothyroidism but with blood tests showing normal thyroid levels. Yet, thyroid is commonly given anyway to make up for thyroid sluggishness, forcing out more thyroid hormone than the cells really need. This sets up the possibility of Hashimoto's thyroiditis in the future.[4]

Rather than using HRT, many women are considering taking progesterone alone, or along with synthetic

---

4 For further in-depth information on this hormonal cascade see the book, *What Your Doctor May Not Tell You About Menopause* by Dr. John R. Lee. If you must use synthetic estrogen, choose the more natural estrogen patch, as less estrogen is needed with a patch than through oral pills since estrogen passes directly through the skin into the bloodstream, bypassing the liver.

---

5 Know that "natural" progesterone creams, such as wild yam cremes, all contain synthetic progesterone because the wild yam molecule is too large to pass through the skin.

---

6 I should also mention here that oral estrogen and progesterone create a further burden on the liver, as it has to break them down to make thems available to the body. From a Chi-

estrogen, since this hormone usually alleviates peri/menopausal symptoms. One of the most common methods is using one of the many progesterone creams available on the market today.[5] Of course, it is possible to take too much progesterone, and women with a history of Candida often find those symptoms aggravated. Either way, undergoing HRT is definitely a personal decision, which hopefully, is only chosen after careful consideration, or if alternative therapies do not help.[6]

In TCM, menopause is considered the completion of a thread of life when the "Dew of Heaven", or life Essence, dries up and the "Heavenly Waters", or menstrual blood, is circulated within rather than shed monthly. Essence provides the ability to grow, mature, reproduce, generate Blood and marrow, adapt to stress, repair body tissue and maintain stability. The Chinese Kidneys preserve Essence in the body and govern all these functions. Further, Essence is the origin of Yin (Blood and Moisture) and Yang (Qi and Warmth) in the body, both of which are rooted in the Kidneys.

When Essence is plentiful, we easily adapt to change and resist illness, yet as we age, or if we unwittingly use up our reserve Essence through hard living and poor diet, these resources ebb. Essence can be likened to a trust fund we inherit at birth and which we maintain through the air we breathe and food we eat. We each inherit larger or smaller trust funds to begin with, then some of us relentlessly spend whatever we have through inadequate rest, excessive intake of alcohol, caffeine and/or sugar, inappropriate diet (excessive or insufficient protein, for example), recreational drugs, smoking, excessive sex and stress.

---

nese point of view, if the Liver is already congested from dietary indiscretions or drug use (medications included), then it reacts accordingly. Because the Liver rules the breasts, it is not uncommon for women to develop tender breasts and eventually, breast cancer, particularly on the left side, since the Liver rules the left side of the body. The Liver also rules the groin, and so fibroids and cysts, or uterine cancer, may also develop. Further, it can cause more emotional swings, depression, tight neck and shoulders and headaches. Thus, if you absolutely need to use HRT, I highly recommend during so only through the skin (patches and creams).

The list goes on, but results are the same—depletion of: Kidney Yin (night sweats, insomnia, five palm heat, hot flashes, dry vagina), Kidney Yang (nighttime urination, lowered sex drive, frequent urination), Blood (insomnia, dry skin and eyes, blurred or weak vision, dizziness, muscle cramps), and/or Qi (fatigue, weakness, dull thinking and decreased motivation). Any of these may lead to stagnant Liver Qi (depression, mood swings, irregular menstrual cycle, tight neck and shoulders, irregular menstrual flow), Excess Heat in the Liver from Deficient Blood and Yin (irritability, frustration, anger, more frequent hot flashes), or a combination of Deficient Yin and Excess Liver Heat resulting in Liver Fire rising (dizziness, pronounced insomnia and hot flashes, migraines, hypertension). Other patterns may be present, but these are the most common.

General Treatment of Peri/Menopause:

Thankfully, there are many useful herbs to help women comfortably transition through this life passage. As well, they offer the potential of self-regulation rather than direct substitution, thus alleviating side effects from taking synthetic hormones. Interestingly, there are many herbs available, both Western and Chinese, which mimic the hormonal effects of estrogen and progesterone in the body. Called phytohormones, these plants do not actually contain hormones, but substances that either bind with cell estrogen or progesterone receptor sites, or promote progesterone, making the body think it's getting the hormones.

There are literally hundreds of plants (both herbs and foods) that contain substances which bind on estrogen receptor sites, such as **black cohosh**, **red clover**, **pomegranate**, **dates**, **hops**, **motherwort**, flax seeds, green beans and **licorice**. **Vitex** and **wild yam** promote progesterone as well as relieve PMS, depression and bone loss. Many other herbs are beneficial in menopause (see chart), especially those that boost and regulate hormones in general, such as **black cohosh**, **vitex**, **wild yam**, **false unicorn**, kelp and **licorice** (or Formula #104).

In TCM, menopause arises from a Deficiency of Essence that normally occurs around age 49, with signs of hot flashes, night sweats, graying hair, wrinkles, loose teeth, brittle and thinning bones, memory loss, low back pain, vaginal dryness and atrophy, deterioration of teeth and gums, diminished hearing and eyesight, sore hips or knees, loss of stamina, apathy, despair and dull mindedness. Deficient Essence leads to Deficient Blood and Yin, causing poor sleep, blurred or weak vision, dry skin and eyes, dizziness, hot flashes, night sweats and muscle cramps, and Deficient Qi with signs of fatigue, weakness, dull thinking, decreased motivation and hypo-functioning of Organs.

By combining herbs that regulate Qi with herbs that tonify Yin, support Yang and clear uprising Heat, many of these symptoms can be alleviated. Possible herbs include **anemarrhena**, **phellodendron** (both clear uprising Heat and nourish the Yin), **epimedium** (nourishes Yin and Yang) and **ophiopogon**, **marshmallow**, **asparagus root**, and **eclipta** (all Yin tonics). Alternatively, take 2-6 tablets of Formula #63, 3 times/day (I specifically created this formula to help most women I see with peri/menopausal issues).

Along with taking herbs, it is important to watch certain dietary guidelines and follow particular lifestyle habits to alleviate peri/menopausal symptoms naturally. First, eat an appropriate amount of protein for your body's needs, whole grains and legumes, lots of cooked vegetables, dark leafy greens and some fruit in season. Add in seaweeds, **flaxseeds** and other phytoestrogen foods and calcium-rich foods and herbs. Avoid crash dieting as this only further weakens Essence. Regulating blood sugar is important as it stabilizes the body, reducing hot flashes and other symptoms.

Although it has been found that high-protein diets cause bones to loose calcium, certain blood types (especially Os) and those with northern European and northern climate ancestries need more protein than others. These same types also need more exercise, which helps metabolize calcium into the bones. Thus, if you physically need a higher protein intake, drink plenty of water, choose more neutral sources such as fish, chicken, pork and eggs, be sure to exercise regularly and drink plenty

Beneficial Herbs for Peri/Menopause

Black cohosh—hot flashes, insomnia, irritability, vaginal dryness, prolapsed uterus and bladder, vaginal and uterine atrophy, phytoestrogen effects

Motherwort—palpitations, hot flashes, sloughing of the lining, phytoestrogen effects

False unicorn—vaginal and uterine atrophy, menstrual irregularities

Wild yam—muscle and menstrual cramps, prevents bone loss, regulates moods (PMS, depression)

Vitex—water retention, depression, uterine fibroids, breast lumps, menstrual flooding, skin breakouts

Dang gui—nourishes and builds Blood, hot flashes, irregular cycle, dry vagina

Nettles—water retention, weight gain; strengthens bones (high in calcium and other minerals)

Oatstraw—tension, nervousness, insomnia; builds bones (calcium content)

Cramp/black haw—menstrual cramps and pain, flooding or excessive bleeding

Kava kava—tension, anxiety, insomnia

Ginseng—tiredness, poor memory and concentration, anxiety, insomnia (from Deficiency), low libido

Asparagus root—strengthens female hormones, tonifies Yin

Solomon's seal—builds reproduction secretions; vaginal dryness

Deer antler—hormonal deficiencies, night sweats, hot flashes

Epimedium—hot flashes, night sweats, headaches, dizziness, light headedness; tonifies Yin and Yang

of water. Keep in mind that those eating high levels of protein who lose bone mass are also usually consuming high levels of sugar, alcohol and caffeine, all of which either directly or indirectly affect bone loss.

I purposely haven't listed seeds and nuts here as protein or essential fatty acid choices because, with the exception of walnuts (which tonify Kidney Yang), nuts congest the Liver, leading to an aggravation of peri/menopausal symptoms (women are always amazed at the positive results they experience simply by eliminating their handfuls of daily seeds and nuts). I also don't recommend eating lots of fruit, juices, raw foods and cooling foods like cucumbers, bananas, melons and soy milk, because their cool and damp natures contribute to symptoms of diarrhea, low energy, frequent urination, low sex drive, memory issues, lowered libido and weight gain.

Because Japanese women eating their traditional diet including soy have a low incidence of breast cancer, research has focused on the use of soy for supplying needed estrogen to the body. While soy is a phytoestrogen, it can be difficult to digest for many (the Japanese use small amounts of tofu and supplement with fish) and further, it creates a Cold, Damp Spleen with resulting Deficient Spleen Qi and symptoms such as gas, bloatedness, water retention, edema, coldness, frequent urination, nighttime urination, lowered sex drive, feelings of heaviness, diarrhea and poor memory.

Actually, all legumes contain gestein, a constituent that prevents cancer (Formula #85). As tempeh and miso are fermented and so pre-digested, they are the best soy choices. Tofu should be eaten sparingly and never raw, but cooked with a spice such as **cumin** (**ginger**, **turmeric** or **garlic** may cause more hot flashes because they are so heating or drying to Blood). Alternatively, eat other legumes as they are equivalent in phytoestrogens, particularly black beans.

In general, avoid spicy foods—chilis, curries and hot spices—red meat, refined flour, junk food, additives, salt, iced drinks and foods that deplete Essence—alcohol, caffeine in all its forms, sugar, fruit juices, excessive intake of raw foods and fruit, soy milk, iced drinks and foods and marijuana. Other foods which cause peri/menopausal symptoms are those congesting to the Liver—alcohol, caffeine (coffee, chocolate, black tea, colas, maté, cocoa), nuts and nut butters, avocados, dairy, chips of all types, fried, greasy and fatty foods, turkey, vinegar, excessive intake of red meats, cheese (except cottage cheese) and recreational drugs.

In terms of lifestyle habits, it is well known that smoking aggravates hot flashes, increases calcium loss, causes abnormal vaginal bleeding, increases heart disease risk, respiratory problems, and cancer and osteoporosis risk. Alcohol decreases hormonal production in the ovaries, leads to irregular bleeding, increases calcium loss and the risk of osteoporosis, induces hot flashes and congests Liver Qi (increasing moodiness and depression). Caffeine (coffee, black tea, chocolate, colas, maté, cocoa) causes irritability, tension, heart palpitations, hot flashes, insomnia, elevated blood pressure, fibrocystic breasts, fibroids, ovarian cysts, moodiness and depression, since it congests Liver Qi and depletes Essence.

Recreational drugs, stress, excessive sexual activity and overworking deplete Essence and congest the Liver. Instead, get extra rest at this time of life, particularly going to bed by 10 or 11 PM at the latest (9 PM is even better to replenish the Kidneys), take a nap around 3 or 4 PM, and exercise daily in gentle forms that don't cause excessive sweating (which depletes Yin and Blood)—walking, yoga, Tai Chi, swimming and so on. Sleep in cool environments and limit time under the hot sun. Avoid hot tubs and saunas, not just because you sweat more, but also because in excess they cause Kidney Yang Deficiency by dissipating inner body heat through sweating (unless you get in a cold shower or plunge immediately afterward, which pushes body heat back to the Interior) and Deficient Blood and Yin (by losing their fluid component). Manage stress through exercise, yoga, gardening, creative projects, baths, listening to music, or meditating, as stress over-stimulates adrenals, weakening Kidney Qi and throwing off blood sugar levels.

Many supplements can be helpful at this time. Vitamin E (300-600 I.U. daily) reduces hot flashes, vaginal dryness, breast tenderness and the risk of heart disease. Calcium and magnesium supplementation is a good idea since calcium loss is greatest during the first five years of menopause (see Osteoporosis for details). B vitamins may help with energy, mood swings and irritability (try the food source, brewer's yeast). Vitamin B6 helps clear estrogen through the liver, making it more available to the body. Vitamin A can decrease heavy menstrual bleeding (carrots, yams, dark leafy greens and red, yellow and orange vegetables and fruits are food sources). My only caution is to not take too many synthetic supplements, as over time they build up toxic Heat in the body, taxing digestion.

Mental attitude has a lot to do with how well peri/menopause is experienced. In many cultures, women earn more respect as they age. Take time to reflect on your own beliefs and perhaps choose a new view of your body and maturation process. It's also important to acknowledge that peri/menopause is a time of great inner change, giving an opportunity to partially withdraw from active, outer life and replenish within. Doing so allows you to dive deeply into your psyche where you can meet your shadow and transform its "dross" into gold. Through this you may discover new potentials and spiritual power. Thus, this life passage can be an alchemical journey, should you so choose that to happen.

A note should be mentioned here about *hysterec-*

PERI/MENOPAUSE—EXCESS PATTERNS:

STAGNANT QI AND ACCUMULATION OF PHLEGM	STAGNANT BLOOD
Obesity	Hot flashes
Feeling of oppression in chest	Mental restlessness
Sputum in chest	Irregular menses, stopping for a long time, then starting again
Feeling of fullness in epigastrium	Possible fixed, stabbing or boring menstrual pain
Feeling of distension of the breasts	Insomnia
Irritability	High blood pressure
Belching; nausea	Abdominal pain
Irregular menses; possible small blood clots	Large blood clots in menses
No appetite	Dark menstrual blood
Moodiness, depression	
Tongue: slightly red sides, sticky coat	**Tongue:** purple
Pulse: wiry	**Pulse:** choppy or wiry
Formulas: #12 or 154; 2 capsules, 2-3 times/day for 3-6 months, of equal parts powdered sarsaparilla, angelica, false unicorn, cramp bark, black cohosh, blue cohosh, vitex and ½ part ginger. Eat rose petal paste.	**Formulas:** #113 or 143; 2 capsules, 2-3 times/day, of equal parts powdered dang gui, turmeric, motherwort, safflower, angelica, salvia and red peony.

PERI/MENOPAUSE—DEFICIENCY PATTERNS:

DEFICIENT KIDNEY YIN	DEFICIENT KIDNEY YANG	DEFICIENT KIDNEY YIN and YANG	DEFICIENT KIDNEY and LIVER YIN with LIVER YANG RISING	KIDNEYS and HEART not HARMONIZED
Hot flashes	Hot flashes	Hot flashes	Hot flashes	Hot flashes
Tinnitus	Swelling of ankles	Tinnitus	Tinnitus	Tinnitus
Malar flush	Pale face	Pale face, periodic malar flush	Malar flush	Malar flush
Night sweats	Night sweats in early morning	Chilliness	Night sweats	Night sweats
Irritability	Depression	Slightly agitated	Irritability	Anxiety, mental restlessness
Heat in the palms, soles and/or chest	Cold hands and feet	Cold hands and feet	Heat in the palms, soles and/or chest	Feelings of heat in the evenings
Dizziness	Dislike of cold	Dizziness	Dizziness	Dizziness
Sore back	Backache	Backache	Sore back	Backache
Dry mouth	Chilliness	Dry throat	Dry eyes	Dry mouth and throat
Constipation	Frequent pale urination	Frequent pale urination	Ache in joints	Dry stools
Dry hair			Blurred vision	Blurred vision
Dry skin, itching			Dry skin, headaches	Palpitations, insomnia, poor memory
Tongue: red without coat	**Tongue:** pale	**Tongue:** mainly Deficient Yin: red; mainly Deficient Yang: pale	**Tongue:** red without coat	**Tongue:** red without coat and redder tip
Pulse: floating and empty, or fine/thin and fast	**Pulse:** deep and fine/thin	**Pulse:** mainly Deficient Yin: floating and empty, or fine and fast; mainly Deficient Yang; weak and deep	**Pulse:** floating and empty, wiry on left middle position	**Pulse:** fast and fine/thin, or floating and empty
Formulas: # 63; 1 tablet #51 (epimedium) with tea of equal parts asparagus root, American ginseng, dang gui, lycii, cooked rehmannia, schisandra and anemarrhean.	**Formulas:** #63 and 51; (epimidium);1 tablet #1 (deer antler) with tea of equal parts ashwagandha, cornus, lycii cooked rehmannia.	**Formulas:** #63; 1 tablet #51 (epimedium) with tea of equal parts cooked rehmannia, lycii, Chinese wild yam, cornus, American ginseng and eucommia.	**Formulas:** #51 with (epimedium) 166; tea of equal parts ophiopogon, asparagus root, dang gui, lycii, schisandra, anemarrhena.	**Formulas:** #51 and 149; tea of equal parts zizyphus, cooked rehmannia, asparagus root, schisandra, dang gui, eucommia, phellodendron and anemarrhena.

tomies. Women who experience complete hysterectomies are dependent on using HRT, yet it is possible to keep the dose extremely low by using herbs. The information given here on diet, lifestyle and herbs is still applicable and very effective in reducing symptoms and using a minimum of HRT, even taking it only every other day (for instance, try Formulas #147 and 154 together for the herbal part.).

DRY SKIN

General treatment includes taking oils high in essential fatty acids, such as **flaxseed**, **borage** and **evening primrose oils**, tonifying Kidneys and Lungs with herbs such as **asparagus root**, **coix** and **ophiopogon**, and moistening skin with herbs like **ghlenia** and **coix**. As well, check thyroid levels to be sure the thyroid is properly functioning (see section Tiredness).

HEART PALPITATIONS AND THE CARDIOVASCULAR SYSTEM (CVS)

The cardiovascular system (CVS) is at risk as we age, and usually women rely on HRT estrogen for prevention. However, there are many wonderful herbs that effectively strengthen the heart, averting heart problems. **Motherwort** is terrific for alleviating heart palpitations and tachycardia. Not only is it a phytoestrogen, but it moves blood circulation and is cooling, both qualities beneficial to the peri/menopausal body. However, as it is very bitter tasting, take in powdered form. **Arjuna** also relieves palpitations and arrhythmias and tones the heart.

Hawthorn treats palpitations while **garlic** lowers cholesterol and blood fats, normalizes blood pressure and lessens arteriosclerosis (Formula #50). **Salvia** (red sage root) lowers cholesterol, disperses stagnant Blood, dilates vessels, treats angina, dysmenorrhea and abdominal masses and cools Heat, treating restlessness, irritability, palpitations and insomnia (Formula #113). Palpitations frequently occur with hot flashes and night sweats, so using herbs to treat the latter conditions usually helps the former (also see section Insomnia).

There are many causes for heart palpitations, but in peri/menopause they are usually due to either Excess Heat in the Liver and/or Heart, or Deficient Heart Blood. Following the general peri/menopausal guidelines usually alleviates these. If not, try one of the following:

Heat in Liver and/or Heart: gardenia, scute, coptis, motherwort, salvia, kava kava (Formula #13)

Deficient Heart Blood: longan berries, cooked rehmannia and biota seeds (Formula #50 or 231)

Dampness: fu ling

Stagnant Blood: salvia (Formula #113 or 182)

HOT FLASHES
(Is it Hot in Here? Or Is it Me?)

Hot flashes, one of the most common signs of impending menopause, usually last several minutes and may occur any time of the day or night. The milder type leads to a general heating of the body or a light sweat (termed hot flush by some women), whereas the more severe type can cause such intense sweating that clothes and bedsheets need be frequently changed. I once had a patient who experienced a hot flash every hour for 10 years. Within two weeks of taking herbs, these reduced by half.

I've found two approaches to be effective in alleviating hot flashes: "Excess treatment" or "Deficient treatment". Excess types have good energy regardless of the number or severity of hot flashes, more Excess and Heat symptoms (see Excess Peri/Menopause Patterns) and usually have a history of eating meat. These women need Kidney-supporting herbs (**rehmannia, dioscorea, cornus** and **epimedium**) along with Excess Heat-clearing herbs (**coptis, scute, gardenia, moutan**) and some Blood tonics (**dang gui, white peony**). Try a formula of 2 parts each **bupleurum, raw rehmannia,** and **dang gui**, 1 part each **alisma, scute, forsythia, gardenia, coptis, phellodendron, anemavrhena,** $1/2$ part **licorice** and $1/4$ part **ginger** (or take Formula #195 with 262).

Eat lighter proteins, such as chicken, fish and grains with legumes, plus lots of vegetables and some fruit. Avoid Liver-congesting foods, such as alcohol, caffeine (coffee, chocolate, black tea, colas, maté, cocoa), sugar, red meats, nuts and nut butters, avocados, chips, fried, fatty and greasy foods, vinegar, turkey and dairy.

Those with Deficiency have symptoms of low energy, fatigue, lowered immunity, weakness, other Deficiency symptoms (see Deficient Peri/Menopause Patterns) and usually eat little to no meat. These women do best with a combination of Yin tonics (**ophiopogon, asparagus root, American ginseng**), gentle herbs to clear Deficient Heat (Deficient Yin) and support Yin (**anemarrhena**), herbs to regulate Liver Qi (**bupleurum** and **white peony**), Blood tonics (**cooked rehmannia, dang gui** and **lycii**) and mild Kidney Yang tonics (**epimedium** and **cuscuta**). Try equal parts each **American ginseng, asparagus root, anemarrhena, phellodendron, dang gui, cooked rehmannia, epimedium** and **cuscuta**, or Formula #63. Alternatively, take Formula #147 with 154. Eat protein three times daily—fish, chicken, pork, eggs, a little beef—lots of cooked vegetables and some whole grains. Avoid raw foods, salads, juices, iced drinks and foods, soy milk, fruit and Liver-congesting foods (listed under Excess type above).

A Western herbal formula may be made of **black cohosh** (Europeans have long used it to treat hot flashes), **red clover, dang gui, licorice** and **motherwort** as useful phytoestrogens, **eleuthro** for adrenal

support and antistress herb) and **skullcap, hops** and **chamomile** to clear Heat and lower hot flashes (because these are drying to the Blood, also include **dang gui** or **lycii berries**). See general Peri/Menopause Patterns for other herbal possibilities. As well, rub essential fatty acid oils (**borage, flaxseed, evening primrose**) over ovaries (right and left sides of lower abdomen), as these are precursors to prostaglandin hormones. Also take 600-800 I.U. vitamin E and 6-10 caps of evening primrose oil daily.

INSUFFICIENT SLOUGHING OF UTERINE LINING

When progesterone levels drop through the peri/menopausal phase, the uterine lining may not fully slough during menses, leaving toxic blood in the uterus that can turn cancerous over time. To prevent, take **vitex** and **wild yam daily** (stopping during menses) to boost effects of progesterone in the body, along with Blood-moving herbs, such as **mugwort, dang gui, safflower, motherwort** or **salvia** (Formula #113), near the end of menses to help the uterus fully empty. If you bleed excessively, only take these herbs when bleeding has slowed and add hemostatics such as **shepherd's purse, yarrow** or **cattail pollen**. If the problem is chronic, take Blood-moving herbs throughout the entire month. As well, do deep abdominal massage with ginger/sesame or other stimulating oils and/or ginger fomentations over lower the abdomen.

LOWERED LIBIDO

One of the best herbs to increase sexual drive is **epimedium**, also known as "horny goat weed" (Formula #51). Other useful herbs include **damiana, saw palmetto, cuscuta, ashwagandha, ginseng** and **deer antler** (Formulas #1 & 51). Also, follow general treatment section under Peri/Menopause, balancing hormones, and try Formulas #1, 6 or 51 (men, try Formulas #1, 5 or 51).

MEMORY ISSUES

For details, see Poor Memory. Generally, estrogen is needed for synapses in the brain to work smoothly. Thus, as estrogen dips, poor memory results and it's not unusual until hormones level off after menopause. In general, **bacopa** and **gotu kola** are very useful (alternatively, use Formula #7).

NIGHT SWEATS

Night sweats may be considered a nocturnal hot flash, although it is possible for anyone to have them even if not peri/menopausal. Follow the herbs given for hot flashes, or try Formula #130. Other possible herbs include **American ginseng**, **schisandra**, **zizyphus**, **oyster shell** and **biota** for night sweats due to Yin Deficiency, and **dioscorea** with **cooked rehmannia** and **cornus** for night sweats due to Kidney Deficiency (or Formula #63). See general Peri/Menopause Patterns for other herbal possibilities.

OSTEOPOROSIS

A crippling, degenerative disease marked by gradual loss of bone mass, osteoporosis can lead to height loss, a stooped appearance, back pain and skeletal deformities or fractures, especially of hips (the latter is often the beginning path to death since it is slow to heal, with much ground lost in exercise and activity). Bone loss occurs at different locations depending on the woman, the most common being the spine and hips. Those with highest risk have Caucasian or Asian ancestry, a family history of osteoporosis, take excessive amounts of thyroid or cortisone-like drugs, are physically inactive, have early or surgically induced menopause, a diet low in calcium sources and smoke or drink alcohol.

Although bone mass starts declining around ages 30-35, the first five years *after* menopause is the major time of bone loss for most women. The following are various ways bone mass and density can be built and maintained. If none works, check vitamin B levels and thyroid function, as these influence bones as well. While estrogen slows bone loss, it does not contribute to bone formation. On the other hand, progesterone quickly promotes bone building and density by stimulating osteoblasts (cells building bone mass). **Vitex** and **wild yam** are good herbal progesterone promoters, and many women benefit from a progesterone cream.

Hands down the best prevention and treatment for osteoporosis is weight-bearing exercise. A friend once told me about her 101-year-old small-boned grandmother who, after starting to lift some light weights, didn't have a single bone break or fracture when she fell over a grocery cart six months later. Other benefits of weight-bearing exercise include diminished risk of heart disease, better sleep, fewer mood swings and decreased pain. Be sure to choose exercise that is fun and doesn't cause excessive sweating or depletion. The old adage, "Use it or lose it" is particularly apt here. Sun yourself 15 minutes daily, as this helps production of vitamin D, improving calcium absorption.

In Chinese medicine, the Kidneys rule bones and bone marrow through Essence, so weak Kidneys means bones don't hold alignment well and/or become deformed. Thus, herbs nourishing Kidney Yin and Yang also help bones, such as **deer antler** (Formula #1), **eucommia**, **dipsacus (teasel)**, **drynaria** and **loranthus (Chinese mistletoe)**. Also eat bone marrow soup regularly to build bones (see Recipes in *The Energy of Food*).

Of course it is extremely important to take some form of calcium (from 1000-1500 mg/day), magnesium and vitamin D during the peri/menopausal years, as the body doesn't absorb calcium at this time, but only circulates it in the blood. Calcium-rich herbs and foods include: sesame seeds, seaweeds, parsley, chickpeas, broccoli, sardines, salmon, shrimp, dark leafy greens (**dandelion**, bok choy, kale, collards, amaranth—be cautious with spinach and chard as they are high in oxalic acid, which binds with calcium, making it unavailable to the body), **flaxseed** oil, bone marrow soup (see Recipes in *The Energy of Food*), dairy (although most dairy congests the Liver or causes Dampness and impairs digestion, cottage cheese and yogurt are fine choices since they are cultured, just don't eat them cold or if you have Dampness) and herbs such as **oatstraw**, **alfalfa**, **nettle**, **horsetail**, **rosemary**, kelp and **chickweed**.

Some women make herbal vinegars with these herbs, including eggshells, and sprinkle on daily dark leafy greens (vinegar pulls calcium out of food, shells and bones). Be sure to avoid alcohol, caffeine, smoking, salt and excessive phosphorous (all carbonated drinks), as these cause bone loss. Extreme dieting depletes estrogen, adversely affecting bones as well. For more dietary factors concerning osteoporosis, review the General Treatment section under Peri/Menopause.

THINNING HAIR

Common at times of hormonal changes (including after childbirth), thinning hair is usually due to Deficient Blood and Kidney Qi. Avoid crash dieting, caffeine, alcohol, sugar, iced drinks and foods, excessive raw foods, and marijuana, as all deplete Blood and/or Kidney Qi. Get plenty of rest and sleep. Regularly massage the scalp with essential oils of **lavender** and **rosemary** mixed with sesame oil and leave on several hours before washing the hair. Alternatively add $1/2$ ounce cayenne tincture and 2 tsp. each **rosemary** and **lavender** oils to 1 pint sesame oil and massage into scalp regu-

larly. Also, tap entire scalp with a dermal hammer for 20-30 minutes daily to stimulate hair growth. Beneficial herbs include *Polygonum multiflorum* (**he shou wu**), **lycii**, **cooked rehmannia**, **dioscorea** and Formula #183.

URINARY INCONTINENCE

Urinary incontinence includes urgent urination, frequent urination, enuresis (when bladder isn't able to

---

Causes for Urinary Incontinence:

- ↪ Inherited weak constitution (particularly nighttime urinary problems)

- ↪ Shock, fright or prolonged fear (injure Kidneys, resulting in lack of urinary control)

- ↪ Aging (Qi becomes Deficient, making it unable to hold urine in)

- ↪ Excessive sexual activity (weakens Kidneys, leading to slight incontinence)

- ↪ Chronic cough (puts strain on Bladder and weakens the Lung Qi's ability to control the Bladder)

- ↪ Childbirth (weakens Kidney Qi, causing slight incontinence during postpartum months)

URINARY INCONTINENCE—EXCESS PATTERN:

LIVER FIRE POURING DOWNWARDS	
Bed-wetting or nighttime urination	
Grinding of teeth at night	
Restless sleep; nightmares; waking up crying	
Thirst	
Bitter taste in mouth	
Pain in ribs	
Tongue: red with redder sides, yellow coat	**Pulse:** wiry and fast
Formulas: #13 or 170; take 1 capsule goldenseal with a tea of equal parts dandelion root, burdock root, barberry, wild yam and fennel.	

hold urine and it leaks out) and incontinence (inability to control voiding of urine). Urge incontinence occurs with an overpowering need to urinate followed by leakage of a large amount of urine. Stress incontinence occurs when laughing, coughing, running, jumping or lifting pressures the bladder, causing urine to leak.

Western medicine sees these conditions as caused by a weakening of the pelvic floor as women age, or a malfunctioning of one of the two bladder sphincters. The bladder may also weaken and become mis-shapened, causing it to not fully empty and creating a frequent desire to pee. Kegel exercises are useful here, preventing urinary incontinence (for how to do, see Menstrual Is-

General Treatment for Urinary Incontinence:

URINARY INCONTINENCE—DEFICIENCY PATTERNS:

DEFICIENT LUNG QI	DEFICIENT SPLEEN QI	DEFICIENT KIDNEY QI AND YANG	DEFICIENT KIDNEY YIN
Frequent urge to urinate with inability to contain it	Slight incontinence	Frequent urination	Incontinence of urine but in scanty amounts
Slight incontinence, often on coughing or sneezing	Urinary urgency	Nighttime urination	Dribbling after urination
Dribbling urine	Frequent desire to go with inability to contain it	Slight dribbling	Dark urine
Weak voice	Loose stools	Bedwetting	Dry throat
Tiredness	Tiredness	Incontinence in elderly	Night sweats
Slight sweating or spontaneous sweating	Poor appetite	Pale to clear urine with no odor	Sensation of heat in palms, soles and chest
Shortness of breath	Bloatedness	Exhaustion	Tinnitus
Chronic cough	Poor digestion	Dizziness	Dizziness
		Tinnitus	Insomnia
		Weak and sore back and knees	
		Feeling cold	
Tongue: pale	**Tongue:** pale	**Tongue:** pale, wet and swollen	**Tongue:** red without coat
Pulse: weak	**Pulse:** weak	**Pulse:** Weak, empty and deep	**Pulse:** floating and empty
Formulas: #44 with 80, or #118; tea of equal parts astragalus, schisandra, white atractylodes and licorice.	**Formulas:** #44 with 80, or #139; tea of equal parts codonopsis or ginseng, astragalus, jujube dates, white atractylodes, Chinese wild yam, fu ling and 1/2 part citrus and licorice.	**Formulas:** #80; tea of equal parts eleuthro, epimedium (#51), cornus, Chinese wild yam and schisandra. Eat green raspberries and drink diluted, room temperature black cherry juice.	**Formulas:** #74 with 80, or #147; tea of equal parts asparagus root, alisma, euryales (fox nut), fu ling, cornus, Chinese wild yam and cinnamon twig.

sues). In terms of TCM, there are many possible causes for this condition (see associated Patterns and take indicated herbs). As well, do moxa on the top of head for 15 minutes, once or twice daily, as this is a major point for lifting up prolapsed organs.

Frequent urination is due to Deficient Kidney Qi. Avoid Kidney-depleting substances, such as caffeine, alcohol, sugar, raw foods, juices, iced drinks and foods and marijuana. Eat pork, legumes and dark leafy greens along with a balanced diet. Add a pinch of salt to herbal formulas, as salt carries herbal energies to the Kidneys.

VAGINAL DRYNESS

Because drying of Essence during peri/menopause causes vaginal dryness and the Kidneys rule the reproductive organs, Kidney Yin tonics are sometimes helpful for this—try Formula #74 or 166. Phytoestrogens treat vaginal dryness and thinning of vaginal lining. **Black cohosh** is one of the best choices since it also tones uterine muscles, preventing against prolapse and atrophy. Also try wild yam cream to lubricate a dry vagina. Avoid unnecessary douching, as this can dry the vagina over time. Take essential fatty acids, such as **evening primrose**, **borage** seed or **flaxseed oils**, as they can enhance vaginal lubrication

The Ayurvedic herb **shatavari** is the most esteemed herb for toning the female reproductive organs. It is very effective for hormonal deficiencies that result in vaginal dryness. In addition, Ayurveda recommends a preparation called *Kumari*, meaning Goddess. Derived from **aloe vera gel**, a known uterine rejuvenative, it also prevents wrinkling of skin at the same time it builds reproductive secretions (as does **Solomon's seal**).

One of the best and easiest treatments I have seen work for vaginal dryness is vitamin E vaginal suppositories. Every night for a month, prick a vitamin E capsule (I.U. doesn't matter) with a pin and insert vaginally (you may need to wear a light pad to catch leakage). Repeat the next month every other night. Do every third night the third month and gradually taper down to whatever minimal dosage is needed for desired results.

It's also useful to regularly exercise the PC muscle through **kegel** exercises (for instructions, refer to Menstrual Issues).

WEIGHT GAIN

Believe it or not, it's normal to gain 5-10 pounds through peri/menopause. First of all, estrogen fluctuations cause elevation of sodium levels, while progesterone, the body's natural diuretic, declines, meaning the body carries more water weight through this phase. Secondly, as the ovaries stop producing hormones, adrenal glands and fat cells take up their production. Thus, fat cells are necessary and needed to continue producing diminishing hormones.

Do not limit water intake during this time, as it builds Blood and nourishes cells. Instead, decrease salt intake, use herbs such as **vitex**, which works as a gentle diuretic through its indirect hormonal-balancing effects, include diuretic foods, such as asparagus, parsley and carrots and take gentle diuretic herbs, such as **cornsilk**, **parsley**, **chickweed**, **nettle** and **coix**, or Formula #99 (but be cautious about overusing, as diruretics can further dry Yin and Blood, aggravating the very peri/menopausal symptoms you are trying to eliminate.). See Weight Issues under section Digestive Disorders, for further details and information, including helpful dietary guideline.

❦ POOR MEMORY

Poor memory can range anywhere from frequent forgetfulness to dementia and even Alzheimer's disease. While poor memory is common, it signals an imbalance that can worsen if left untreated. Simply put, memory is a refection of your health. In TCM memory depends on the condition of three different Organs: the Heart, Spleen and Kidneys. The Heart houses Mind, that part which thinks coherently and remembers long term events. Spleen houses Intellect and holds the ability to concentrate, study and memorize. Kidneys house Will Power and influence the brain, since they produce bone

Causes for Poor Memory:

- ↭ Overwork with insufficient rest (weakens Kidneys)
- ↭ Excessive sexual activity (weakens Kidneys)
- ↭ Birthing too many children too close together (weakens Kidneys); excessive bleeding at childbirth (weakens Blood, making the Heart unable to nourish the brain and Mind)
- ↭ Prolonged worry and pensiveness (weaken Lungs, Spleen and Heart); prolonged sadness (depletes Heart Qi so it cannot brighten the Mind)
- ↭ Prolonged use of marijuana (injures Kidneys, Spleen and Liver, and causes loss of brain substance)
- ↭ Lack of sleep and sleep deprivation (interrupted sleep is so common in the elderly that people accept it as normal—see section Insomnia, for treating this)
- ↭ Not drinking enough water (causes dehydration, resulting in Deficient Blood and poor memory—people frequently confuse hunger with thirst and so eat instead)
- ↭ Low blood sugar (depletes Spleen)
- ↭ Hormonal imbalance, such as decreased estrogen and low thyroid function (see sections Peri/Menopause for decreased estrogen, and Tiredness for hypothyroidism)
- ↭ Excessive caffeine and alcohol (weaken Kidneys)
- ↭ Mental laziness (weakens memory—the brain is like a muscle that needs exercising—"if you don't use it, you lose it" is especially true here)
- ↭ Strokes, alcoholism, Parkinson's, drugs and hypothyroidism (causes of dementia and Alzheimer's)

The best and first approach for maintaining good memory is prevention, since cerebral nerve cell loss starts around age forty, but doesn't show up until the sixties or seventies. Get plenty of rest and balance work with rest, play, exercise and creative activities. Regularly challenge your mind, especially as you age. Learn and memorize new things, read more and watch less TV, take on new activities or hobbies, vary routines, stay active and interested in life, exercise daily and keep circulation and your heart healthy and strong. Exercise your mind through challenging pursuits such as crossword puzzles, chess, or learning a musical instrument or foreign language.

The Western cultural myth states we should expect to decline as we age. Other cultures hold different beliefs, such as the South American tribe that believes its best runners are men in their sixties (when examined in a Harvard study, this was found to be true). Prevention also encompasses avoiding alcohol, caffeine (coffee, black tea, cocoa, colas, maté, chocolate), stress, physical and mental overwork, marijuana, iced drinks and foods, excessive intake of raw foods and soy products (in excess, soy causes learning disabilities in children, hypothyroidism and poor memory). As well, be sure to eat sufficient protein for your body's needs and drink plenty of water to keep the brain hydrated (there are lots of fluids in the brain).

At the first signs of poor memory, immediately start taking herbs, as there are several commonly available ones that are wonderful for improving memory. Most people have heard of **ginkgo** (50:1 extract), which stimulates blood circulation to the brain and eyes (and is at least as good as the commonly used medications for Alzheimer's (but do not take if you are on blood-thinners, as it thins blood). However, **bacopa** is probably one of the greatest herbs known for improving mental function, and **gotu kola** is quite good as well.

Try this memory formula: 2 parts each **bacopa** and **ginkgo**, 1 part each **gotu kola**, **schisandra**, **polygala**, **lemon balm**, **ashwagandha**, **ginseng**, **jujube dates** and **longan berries**, and ¹/₂ part each **fu ling**, **citrus** and **licorice**. For poor memory due to Deficient Yin (night

marrow, which nourishes the brain. As well, the Kidneys are responsible for short-term memory, that ability to remember such things as what you just walked into the next room to get, people's names, faces and dates. It is Deficient Kidneys that most often cause dementia or Alzheimer's.

General Treatment for Poor Memory:

sweats, malar flush, dizziness, burning sensation in palms, soles and/or chest), add 1 part **loranthus (Chinese mistletoe)**. For poor memory due to constrained emotions, add 1 part **albizzia (mimosa tree bark)**. Royal bee jelly is also a useful tonic for brain energy. Alternatively, try Formulas #7 and 42.

In the meantime, stimulate blood circulation to the brain through exercise, Qi Gong, yoga postures (especially inverted postures like the shoulder and head stands, as they circulate blood to the brain) and other therapies (such as therapeutic massage) and make sure arteries are cleared of cholesterol (use purified **myrrh**, called **Guggul**, or Formula #47, and eat oats; also check this topic in the section Headaches). Use moxibustion over the waist of the lower back in a line extending about 3″ on either side of the spine (this strengthens the Kidneys). Definitely stop all caffeine, alcohol, excessive sex and overwork, and change eating and resting habits accordingly.

Eventually, cognitive decline results in *senility* (senile dementia) if occurring in old age, or *Alzheimer's* (presenile dementia) if before old age (as early as the fifties), a progressive process that kills brain cells and destroys synaptic connections between nerve cells in the brain. More serious symptoms arise now, such as feeble-mindedness, impaired memory, deranged speech and withdrawn or aggressive behavior. In advanced stages, memory and recognition of people, things and places may be lost. Early onset Alzheimer's is usually genetically linked whereas late onset is mostly due to lifestyle and environmental factors, such as clogged or hardened arteries, aluminum toxicity, smoking, low educational attainment, hypertension, head injuries, stress, solvent exposure, thiamine deficiency and/or a history of depression along with the causes listed in the chart below.

To prevent Alzheimer's or senility, wear protective

POOR MEMORY PATTERNS:

DEFICIENT HEART QI	DEFICIENT SPLEEN QI	DEFICIENT KIDNEY ESSENCE
Poor memory, especially long-term	Poor memory	Poor memory, especially short-term
Forgetfulness; forgetting names	Inability to concentrate, memorize and study	Forgetfulness
Absent-mindedness	Poor appetite	Tinnitus
Palpitations	Loose stools	Weak knees and lower back
Slight breathlessness on exertion	Poor digestion	Dizziness
Tiredness	Tiredness	Tiredness
Possible anxiety	Gas and bloating	
Tongue: crack in Heart area; with Deficient Yang: pale; with Deficient Yin: red	**Tongue:** pale	**Tongue:** Deficient Kidney Yang: pale; Deficient Kidney Yin: red without coat in rear
Pulse: weak	**Pulse:** weak	**Pulse:** deep and fine
Formulas: #7 and 42, or #136; take ginkgo 50:1 extract with tea of equal parts longan, reishi, zizyphus, dang gui, lycii, schisandra, polygala, codonopsis and ½ part each cinnamon branches, fu ling and licorice.	**Formulas:** #7, 42 and 43; tea of equal parts reishi, codonopsis, astragalus, baked licorice, dang gui, polygala, zizyphus and white atractylodes with ½ part fu ling and citrus.	**Formulas:** #7, 42 and 51; tea of equal parts cooked rehmannia, lycii, Chinese wild yam, he shou wu, polygala, asparagus root, alisma, American ginseng, epimedium (#51) and ½ part cornus.

head gear as appropriate, avoid hypertension, alcohol and stress, exercise, take antioxidants (such as vitamins C, E and selenium), use monounsaturated fats (like olive oil), eat less meat and more vegetables and fruits, take calcium and silicon (the latter protects against aluminum absorption), eliminate all sources of aluminum from your diet (cook in stainless steel pots and pans instead), eat two tablespoons of lecithin, three times daily (or take four 500 mg capsules of **evening primrose oil**), maintain thyroid function (see the sections Insomnia or Tiredness), treat depression (see Depression), get sufficient rest and sound sleep at night (see Insomnia), drink plenty of water, stay interested in life, visit with your family and other people, laugh a lot and *be mentally active.*

Herbally, follow the given suggestions, or see Patterns for more herbal choices. Many know of **ginkgo**, which is neuro-protective, and taking 120-240 mg of its standardized 50:1 extract is as strong as the drugs tacrine and donepezil (note that only the 50:1 ginkgo extract works this way). Further, it can stop the progression of Alzheimer's whereas drugs don't (note that ginkgo tinctures or teas do not work for this; only the standardized extract is effective).

A general formula can be made of equal parts **bacopa**, **dang gui**, **polygala**, **gotu kola**, **ginseng**, **deer antler** (Formula #1), **corydalis** and **loranthus**. (Alternatively, take Formula #7.) At the same time, take a dropperful of ginkgo leaf (50:1 extract) three times daily (if you are not on blood thinners). Useful supplements to include are *Hyperzine*, which increases mental alertness and improves memory, and L-carnitine, which helps transport nutrients to brain cells. Of course, resting, eating a balanced diet, exercising and stimulating your mind are also important at this time. Do all of this at least three months to see good results.

Several Chinese patents particularly useful for poor memory and other ailments of the elderly include Cerebral Tonic Pills (Formula #136) for aging, hardening of arteries, insomnia and restlessness and Recovery of Youth Tablet (Formula #260) for senility, fatigue and lowered resistance.

Causes for Skin Conditions:

↬ Irregular diet, excessive consumption of hot and spicy foods, alcohol, caffeine, acidic foods and red meat.

↬ Poor digestion, assimilation and elimination

↬ Candida

↬ Hormonal imbalance, particularly during adolescence in teens and peri/menopause in women

↬ Overwork, chronic illness and hemorrhaging after childbirth (all lead to Deficient Blood, which can stir up Wind, causing skin eruptions)

❦ SKIN CONDITIONS

The skin is the largest elimination organ in the body, so what you see on your skin is a reflection of your body's internal condition. Skin outbreaks and diseases are a direct message to you that something is off. The more serious the skin condition, the greater the internal imbalance. Quite often skin problems are due to Heat toxins and a congested colon that cannot fully eliminate (leaky gut syndrome), so they pass through to the skin instead (refer to section Candida, for how to treat).

General Treatment for Skin Conditions:

Skin problems are a warning signal that your body needs cleansing, and doing so brings renewed health to your entire being. There are three general approaches for this and they should be followed before turning to more specific treatments. First, check to see if there's any constipation for it there is, then the skin automatically breaks out to release trapped toxins in the colon. Treating constipation then clears the skin (see the topic, *Constipation*, under the Section, *Digestive Disorders*). Secondly, if you're a meat-eater, skin eruptions frequently occur if meat toxins aren't properly neutralized through a balance of water, alkalinizing foods and exercise. Thus, it's important to do the following while eating meat: increase water intake to at least 8 glasses/day, eat at least five or more vegetables and fruits daily and exercise so you sweat 3-4 times/week.

Thirdly, if skin conditions still persist, then its time for a kicharee fast, the best and quickest cure I've seen for most skin problems (see Recipes in *The Energy of Food*). Eat only kicharee for 5–10 days, adding cooked vegetables (especially **burdock root**, a great blood purifier and skin cleanser) and dark leafy greens, such as kale, collards or bok choy, after 3–5 days. For people who need less protein, kicharee itself suffices; for those who need more, add yogurt or whey protein powder into mix, and/or cook kicharee in chicken stock. To break the fast, stick mainly to an alkaline diet (acidity causes skin problems) and combine lots of other grains and legumes, cooked vegetables and dark leafy greens. After a few more days, add in some animal protein, if appropriate.

In general, eating alkaline foods heals and prevents skin problems—these include lemons, limes, millet, amaranth, quinoa, umeboshi paste, vegetables (except tomatoes, peppers, eggplants and potatoes) and fruit (except most citrus). Further, quickly alkalinize the body by taking 1 tsp. baking soda in 1 glass water, 1-2 times daily for a week. Since skin ailments may also improve by taking essential fatty acids (especially if the skin is dry), try including a capsule or teaspoon of **evening primrose**, **borage seed** (Formula #11) or **flaxseed oil** in your daily diet (be sure to purchase these oils in small amounts and refrigerate in dark bottles, as they go rancid very quickly). Alternatively, eat fish high in fat.

At the same time, take a blood-purifying formula, such as equal parts **burdock root** and **seeds** (burdock seeds are specific for clearing skin), **yellow dock**, **dandelion**, **red clover**, **milk thistle**, **lycii**, **neem**, **sassafras**, **sarsaparilla**, **forsythia** and **honeysuckle** with ½ parts each **licorice** and **ginger**. Formula #109, while normally used for colds and flu, opens the skin surface, releasing Heat causing red skin eruptions. Formulas #73 and 108 also effectively treat skin eruptions, especially for those from Damp Heat (red, itchy and oozing skin eruptions). As well, take **red marine algae** and essentail fatty acids.

If skin conditions are due to hormonal imbalances,

take 1 tsp. **vitex**, three times daily, tapering to 1 dropperful, once a day in the morning when skin is clear. Vitex wonderfully regulates hormones and clears related skin eruptions, even *acne* (in adolescent males, too)—try Formula #102. I've seen the worst imaginable cases of acne quickly resolve when all fats (pizza, french fries, chips, etc), salt, processed foods, sugars and acidic foods and drinks are eliminated from the diet (particularly fats and sugars if you "just can't leave it *all* out"). Add in a blood-purifying formula and kiss your acne goodbye. If skin conditions are due to candida, see section Candida, for treatment.

Poultices are quite valuable for treating skin conditions, and many herbs may be used either in powder, tincture, or freshly bruised, herb form. If a skin condition blisters, it has moved deeper into the body, and herbs that cleanse blood as well as release the surface need be used together. Try 1 part each **forsythia**, **honeysuckle**, **mint**, **yellow dock**, **burdock seed** and **root**, **dandelion**, **red clover** and ½ part each **ginger** and **licorice**, or use Formulas #73 and 109. As well, a few products are valuable for skin conditions: beta glucan creams boost local skin immunity and heal skin problems, alpha-lipoic acid is anti-inflammatory, and zinc pyrithone (only get it without chemicals added) very effectively clears certain difficult skin conditions, such as psoriasis and eczema (see *Resources*).

Usually the kicharee fast and herbs clear most skin problems, but sometimes other therapies are needed as well. Soak the affected skin area in saltwater and let it air dry, and/or journal write about any underlying emotional issues, such as any repressed or suppressed emotions (erupting as skin conditions), boundary issues (difficulty claiming your space at home or work, inability to say "no" when appropriate, and so forth, and so your body's boundary, the skin, reflects this) and/or being out of integrity with one's self.

Edgar Cayce is responsible for popularizing **castor oil** packs for all sorts of ailments. Because this oil is so healing and clears toxins from blood, it is quite effective for many skin ailments (see *Herbal Preparations*, for making and using castor oil packs). Finally, manage stress through relaxation techniques, exercise, meditation, contemplation, rest and massage and herbs, as this is a frequent causative factor for many skin outbreaks.

Psoriasis responds particularly well to natural therapies. Regularly apply **castor oil** packs to area and follow dietary and herbal guidelines given above. Those who are easily tired need to tonify Spleen Qi with **ginseng, white atractylodes** and **dioscorea**. There is also a product, zinc pyrithione, that many find very effective for psoriasis (see *Resources* to obtain).

Eczema, a dry or weeping skin condition characterized by severe itching and possible burning, frequently arises in children who have childhood asthma, or in those who have Deficient Lung Qi (shortness of breath, coughing, low resistance to colds or flu, weak voice, pale face). In babies, eczema is due to the surfacing of toxic Heat from the mother's uterus. Because eczema is very close to asthma and is due to the same root causes, see Asthma and Wheezing in section Cough, for further information.

I have seen eczema clear in children just by eliminating soap for washing body and clothes, as a soap allergy often causes this condition. As well, chlorinated water can worsen many eczema cases—put water filter on shower. For others, following a kicharee fast for 5-10 days works wonders. Also take 2 parts each **yellow dock** and **burdock seed** along with 1 part each **dandelion, red clover, sassafras, sarsaparilla, forsythia** and **honeysuckle** and ¹/₂ part each **licorice** and **ginger**. Include **neem** internally and topically. A Chinese patent specific for eczema is Formula #158. Otherwise, it is necessary to treat the root cause by determining which Patterns best fit your symptoms and taking the indicated herbs.

Topically, many herbs heal the surface manifestation of weeping eczema. An herb paste can be made out of **aloe vera gel** alone or with **chickweed, calendula** and **phellodendron**. Because chronic recurring eczema weakens the local skin immunity. Thus, it may also be necessary to boost skin immunity in that area. The best

substance I have found for this is beta glucan, a powerful immune stimulant that may be taken internally in capsule form, but is most valuable when applied topically as a cream (see *Resources*). Be sure to include 500 mg daily of essential fatty acids in the diet, such as **evening primrose, flaxseed** or **borage seed oils** (or Formula #11). There is also a product using zinc pyrithione many find very effective for eczema (see *Resources* to obtain).

Shingles (post-hepatic neuralgia), caused by a virus attacking the nerves, usually runs its course and goes away, but can be quite painful during the wait. **Cayenne oil** applied topically to the area eliminates pain, quickly healing shingles. **Calendula** cream is soothing and healing, particularly if mixed in equal parts with black tea. As well, a **burdock leaf** poultice pulls out inflammation. While I don't have experience with this, it seems to me an antiviral herb should be useful here as well, such as **St. John's wort**, both as an internal tincture and a topical oil (which also treats the nerves), and perhaps **olive leaf extract, lemon balm oil, isatis** or **andrographis** internally.

Manage stress through relaxation techniques, exercise, meditation, contemplation, rest and massage, and follow a cleansing diet, such as the kicharee fast given earlier. Vigorously tap a dermal hammer around affected area to cause bleeding, as this clears underlying stagnant Blood causing this condition, helping to reduce pain and heal the condition. Lastly, try placing magnets (negative pole down) on skin area to reduce pain. Also try Formula #92.

Rosacea is a skin condition with varying degrees of papules, pustules and hyperplasia of the sebaceous glands. It predominantly appears on the nose, face and chin. In TCM, this is usually due to Stomach Heat (from Excess or Deficient Heat). Generally, Formula #197 works well for this as does cutting out all acidic foods and eating an alkaline diet (emphasizing millet, legumes, quinoa, vegetables and lemons/limes). If you are vegetarian, add some animal protein (even if acidic,

Simple Skin Conditions:

In the following, the most specific herb(s) are in *italics*. The best salve I've ever used for many of these simple skin conditions is made of equal parts **comfrey**, **echinacea**, **plantain**, **yarrow**, **calendula** and **chickweed** (see *Herbal Preparations*, for making salves).

BURNS: *aloe gel*, St. John's wort, plantain, comfrey, marshmallow, slippery elm, calendula and yarrow

SUNBURN: pat vinegar over burned area and air dry; topically apply aloe gel; take antioxidants (vitamins A, C, E) to neutralize free radicals caused by excessive sun exposure

ITCHING: *chickweed*

WOUNDS: *comfrey*, calendula, slippery elm, plantain, elder, aloe, marshmallow, tien qi ginseng, St. John's wort, yarrow; also, soak area in water 15 minutes and let air dry, repeating several times daily

CUTS: *comfrey poultice or salve*, echinacea, plantain, calendula, yarrow and elder

BLEEDING: *cayenne* powder or *moxibustion ashes* (the latter stops continuous bleeding from deep cuts, but also "tattoos" the skin for several months)

INSECT BITES AND STINGS: *mud*, clay, aloe, comfrey or plantain poultice or *echinacea* drops (put echinacea tincture on cotton ball and tape over area)

BEDSORES: *slippery elm*, *marshmallow*, *comfrey* and *echinacea* poultice

NON-HEALING SORES: *astragalus*, codonopsis (when unhealed sores linger for a long time, there is Deficient Qi)

BOILS: *echinacea*, *goldenseal*, *plantain*, dandelion, chickweed, comfrey, marshmallow, slippery elm poultices externally; *burdock seeds* and root, dandelion, honeysuckle, turmeric internally

RASHES: *calendula*, *slippery elm*, *marshmallow*, elder, echinacea, chamomile, powders or salves; plantain wash; internally, take isatis, dandelion, burdock, red clover, calendula and/or chamomile

CHICKENPOX: *calendula* tincture externally; calendula, yarrow, dandelion, echinacea internally

MEASLES: *calendula* tincture externally; calendula, yarrow, dandelion, mint, gotu kola, pueraria internally

CANKER SORES: *calendula* tincture externally; *burdock seeds* and root, calendula, red marine algae, alkalinizing foods internally; *lemon balm tea extract in a salve*

---

it helps in this case).

Lupus is a chronic, progressive, usually ulcerating, skin disease causing lesions of the face, neck and upper extremities. When systemic, a characteristic butterfly rash appears across malar areas (cheeks and nose). While too complex a condition to discuss here, the same treatment for rosacea is useful for some stages of lupus. Also see the Skin Conditions Patterns.

Herpes is a chronic viral infection of nerve tissues producing small blisters on the skin. Transmitted sexually, it tends to manifest under high stress or lowered immunity. When flaring up, painful open sores manifest, usually on genitalia, anal region or mouth, with possible accompanying muscle aches and pains. Some people carry the virus but don't know it because they never have

an outbreak. If you have herpes, be sure to inform potential sexual partners, and if a herpes outbreak occurs, stop sex until healed, as these open sores are contagious.

As genital herpes is generally a condition of Damp Heat in the Liver (acidity, too), and oral herpes is usually due to Stomach Heat, either must cleared for the herpes to resolve. The best herb I have seen for either type of herpes is **red marine algae** (I think it works well because it quickly alkalinizes the body). Take 2-4 tablets every 3 hours at the beginning signs of an outbreak, as this usually prevents its full manifestation (continue this dose if outbreak occurs). At same time, or alternately, take Formula #13 with 108, or Formula #170 for genital herpes, and Formula #170 or 197 for oral herpes.

Externally **lemon balm salve** works especially well by itself, yet also try **calendula, St. John's wort, licorice,**

Simple Skin Conditions: *(continued)*

MOUTH SORES: *echinacea, goldenseal* tinctures externally; echinacea, goldenseal, gardenia, *chrysanthemum* internally

TONGUE SORES: *echinacea, goldenseal,* coptis

SCABIES: *blood root ointment; lemon balm salve, neem,* cnidium, isatis, turmeric, chaparral internally and externally

IMPETIGO: *echinacea,* goldenseal, isatis, usnea externally and internally; regularly scrub area well with antibacterial soap

SEBOREA: *chickweed, burdock*

POISON OAK AND IVY: *plantain,* burdock seed, clay poultices, *jewelweed lotion, grindelia, echinacea*

WARTS: apply drynaria tincture directly on wart; homeopathic Antimonium tartarum 30C, 3 pellets, 3 times daily for two weeks; then homeopathic Thuja 30C, 3 pellets, 3 times daily for two weeks; repeating this cycle three times total. (Warts will slowly disappear within three to six months.)

GUM SORES OR GUM DISEASE: brush with cayenne and prickly ash powders 2 times daily for 3-6 weeks (beware—this is quite stimulating, but very effective and may even prevent gum surgery); topical vitamin E oil (very effective and anti-inflammatory); gargle 2-3 times daily with mouthwash made from equal parts echinacea, goldenseal, myrrh, bayberry and blood root; squirt echinacea tincture on sores or inflamed areas every hour or two.

An effective general treatment is to make a tincture of equal parts neem and prickly ash and 1/4 part cloves and licorice. Squirt on gums, or mix with toothpaste, and brush upwards and downwards into gums. Be sure to also floss and use a Proxy brush twice daily. Have dental hygienic cleaning every three months. Continue procedure for 1-2 years (although results will be seen within two weeks).

LIVER "SPOTS": take antioxidants, alpha lipoic acid (see *Resources* for an effective product) and vitamins A, C, E, as these are usually due to excessive amounts of free radicals in body.

VARICOSE VIENS: externally, use horse chestnut salve, hyssop poultice; witch hazel wash; internally, take tien qi ginseng, and/or horse chestnut; dermal hammer over the affected area(s); Formulas # 52 and 53.

neem, **tienqi ginseng** tincture, or baking soda compress. Also take antiviral herbs, such as **St. John's wort, isatis, lemon balm** and/or **andrographis**, stress-relieving herbs, such as **chamomile, oatstraw, skullcap, passionflower** or **kava kava**, and immune-boosting herbs such as **astragalus, eleuthro** or **reishi**. (Whenever you are under high stress, *rest* and take immune tonics and stress herbs to prevent outbreaks.)

SKIN CONDITIONS—EXCESS PATTERNS:

WIND-HEAT INVADING THE BLOOD	WIND AND DAMP HEAT	TOXIC HEAT IN BLOOD	STAGNANT QI AND BLOOD
Itchy skin eruptions	Weeping skin eruptions; dry, scaly skin	Toxic skin eruptions or with oozing fluid	Skin problems worsen with stress or emotional issues
Irritability	Itchiness worse in heat or sun	Pus	Pain
Dry mouth	Possible ulcers of mouth and tongue	Inflamed and infected skin lesions	Restlessness

(continued on next page)

SKIN CONDITIONS—EXCESS PATTERNS: *(continued)*

WIND-HEAT INVADING THE BLOOD	WIND AND DAMP HEAT	TOXIC HEAT IN BLOOD	STAGNANT QI AND BLOOD
Red skin eruptions	Thirst	Ulcerated skin lesions	Dark red or purple skin lesions
Thirst	Restlessness	Itching, redness and pain	Thirst
Tongue: red; possible strawberry and/or crooked	**Tongue:** swollen, red, sticky yellow coat	**Tongue:** red with yellow coat	**Tongue:** bluish-purple, or reddish-purple
Pulse: fast	**Pulse:** floating and slippery	**Pulse:** rapid and overflowing	**Pulse:** choppy
Formulas: #110 with 73; 5 drops lobelia tincture and 1 capsule chaparral with tea of equal parts red clover, yellow dock, sarsaparilla, burdock seeds and ½ part each barberry and fresh ginger.	**Formulas:** #108 or 152; 5 drops lobelia tincture and 1 capsule chaparral with tea of equal parts yellow dock, sarsaparilla, burdock seed, barberry and ½ part fresh ginger.	**Formulas:** #73 or 142; 1 capsule chaparral with tea of equal parts yellow dock, burdock seed, sarsaparilla, barberry, honeysuckle, forsythia, red peony and ½ part fresh ginger.	**Formulas:** #12 with 73; 1 capsule equal parts powdered turmeric and gardenia with tea of equal parts redclover, calendula, barberry and burdock seeds.

SKIN CONDITIONS—DEFICIENCY PATTERNS:

DEFICIENT QI AND BLOOD	DEFICIENT BLOOD	DEFICIENT YIN
Pale skin	Itchy, papular skin eruptions	Red skin conditions
Non-eruptive skin conditions	Worse at night	Dry, scaly skin
Slow healing	Insomnia	Possible afternoon fever
Little or no pain	Dizziness	No pain
Fatigue	Scanty periods	Night sweats
		Fatigue
Tongue: pale, thin, wet	**Tongue:** pale, thin	**Tongue:** red without coat
Pulse: Thin and Empty	**Pulse:** Thin	**Pulse:** Floating and Empty
Formulas: 1 tablet #106 with 1 tablet 73; or #198; tea of equal parts astragalus, codonopsis, jujube dates, dang gui, white peony and red peony.	**Formulas:** 2 tablets #106 with 1 tablet 73; tea of equal parts dang gui, lycii (bark if possible), red peony, cooked rehmannia, ligusticum, astragalus, schizonepeta and burdock seeds.	**Formulas:** 1 tablet #73 with 2 tablets #74; tea of raw and cooked rehmannia, ophiopogon, red peony, moutan peony, burdock seeds, anemarrhena and sarsaparilla.

It is also extremely important to avoid foods creating Damp Heat in the Liver and/or promoting herpes—alcohol, turkey, fried, greasy and fatty foods, avocados, spicy foods, nuts and nut butters, caffeine (coffee, black tea, cocoa, maté, colas, chocolate), cheese, dairy, vinegar, sugar, chips of all kinds, all acidic foods and foods high in the amino acid arginine, such as nuts, seeds, oatmeal, wheat, raisins and rice as well as recreational drugs. Using lysine relieves herpes (fish, chicken and

Causes for Tiredness:

- ⊷ Overworking, mental or physical, and without adequate rest (depletes Spleen and Kidney Qi)

- ⊷ Mental, physical or emotional stress (depletes Kidney Qi and stagnates Liver Qi)

- ⊷ Excessive standing, especially if combined with irregular eating habits (depletes Kidney Qi)

- ⊷ Straining the eyes (such as computer work, reading or studying)

- ⊷ Inadequate diet for the body's needs, including improper dieting—particularly over many years, or simply not eating enough for the body's needs (depletes Spleen Qi)

- ⊷ Excessive eating (burdens Stomach and Spleen Qi)

- ⊷ Excessive intake of cold, raw foods, smoothies, juices, fruit, soy milk, iced drinks and foods, sugar, flour products (weakens the Spleen)

- ⊷ Excessive intake of meat, spicy foods, alcohol and fried, fatty and greasy foods (create Heat and stagnation of Liver Qi)

- ⊷ Excessive intake of caffeine—coffee, black tea, cocoa, colas, maté, chocolate (injures Kidney Qi and Liver)

- ⊷ Insufficient food and/or protein for the body's needs depletes blood

- ⊷ Excessive physical exertion without adequate rest (weakens muscles and Spleen Qi)

- ⊷ Prolonged illness (injures Spleen Qi)

- ⊷ Excessive sexual activity (injures Kidney Qi—if there is dizziness, lower backache, or frequent urination, that amount of sex is definitely excessive)

- ⊷ Chronic bacterial or viral infections

- ⊷ After childbirth (including miscarriages), it is common for mothers to be tired (sudden loss of blood coupled with demands of newborn lead to Deficient Blood, especially if mother doesn't rest adequately and quickly returns to work). It is also common for nursing mothers to be tired until they stop nursing (mother's milk is partially made from Blood, thus potentially causing Deficient Blood).

- ⊷ Prolonged use of recreational drugs, such as marijuana, cocaine or heroine (injures Kidneys and Liver)

- ⊷ Excessive time spent at computers (depletes Kidney Qi and causes not only tiredness, but also thinning hair, night sweats and dizziness)

- ⊷ Inherited weak constitution (creates tendency toward chronic low energy)

- ⊷ Candida, gluten intolerance, food allergies and/or heavy metal poisoning (can cause tiredness to the point of chronic fatigue)

- ⊷ Stress, stress, stress (weakens Kidney Qi and stagnates Liver Qi)

- ⊷ Exposure to drugs, chemicals and environmental pollutants

- ⊷ Sometimes low energy results after invasion of a cold or flu (see Cold, Flu and Fevers)

most beans contain lysine) along with B vitamin–rich foods (nutritional yeast, bee pollen, spirulina, blue green algae, seaweeds, and peas).

❧ TIREDNESS/LOW ENERGY

A major complaint in the West, tiredness can occur periodically, chronically or as extreme exhaustion that even rest doesn't alleviate. Those who experience chronic fatigue syndrome (CFS) not only find it difficult to get out of bed, but live with limitations around where they can go and what they can do. While some may be diagnosed as depressed, far more are excited about life but just do not have the energy to do what they want (if you suspect depression is involved, refer to section Depression).

General Treatment for Tiredness:

No matter the cause for tiredness, the two best approaches for regaining energy are to rest and eat an appropriate diet. Resting is difficult for many people because it isn't considered productive. Yet, allowing the body to rest replenishes energy and refreshes the mind, increasing mental abilities and immunity. Only 10–20 minutes are needed, although the siesta so prevalent in other cultures is a wonderful concept to adopt. Ideally, after every meal one walks ¹/4 mile and then rests 15 minutes (this supports good digestion). Then in the mid-afternoon, rest for 15–60 minutes as needed. Lastly, go to bed by 9 or 10 PM at the latest, and you'll be amazed at how quickly your energy is restored (if you also follow the dietary guidelines given and take the suggested herbs!).

An overly acidic body causes tiredness, particularly in those who eat meat—eat alkaline foods for awhile, such as vegetables and fruits. In general, however, an appropriate diet varies according to the cause of low energy. As well, be sure to quit all caffeine—see Tiredness Due to Other Causes below. Usually tiredness arises either from some type of stagnation, making energy unavailable for use (an Excess condition), a Deficiency of Qi, Blood, Yin and/or Yang, or a combination of the two.

Tiredness Due to stagnation: Stagnation of Qi or Fluids (Dampness) is an Excess condition that makes energy unavailable. It usually occurs in those who excessively eat animal protein, dairy, dampening foods, sugar and processed foods. Accompanying symptoms include headaches, heaviness, irritability, sluggishness, thirst, digestive upset, constipation, easy sweating, yellow urine and feelings of being stuck. By all respects, these folks eat and look as if they should have energy, but don't. Rather than eating more concentrated sources of protein, like meat, those with A or B blood types mainly need plant sources such as grains and legumes, along with some fish, lots of vegetables and some fruit.

To treat, reduce meat, dairy, sugar, processed foods, flour products, iced drinks and foods, potatoes. As well, take herbs that clear Excess and move stagnation. One famous Chinese practitioner always first gave (usually for three days) the Chinese formula #265 before giving any other herbs. It is comprised of equal parts of five herbs, each of which clears a different type of stagnation: **cyperus** (Qi), **black atractylodes** (Damp), **ligusticum** (Blood), **gardenia** (Heat), and *Massa fermentata*, or *shen qu* (food). A Western herbal variation can be made with equal parts: **green citrus peel**, **agastache (patouchli)** or **asafoetida**, *Angelica archangelica*, **turmeric** and **hawthorn berries**, **radish seeds** and **sprouted barley or rice**.

Tiredness may also be due to chronic infections, and people don't always know this until they feel better and their energy increases after taking antibiotics. Thus, treat possible infections first by taking **echinacea, goldenseal, red clover** and **dandelion** for a week. Add **isatis** and **andrographis** for possible viral infections. Alternatively, take 2-4 tablets of Formula #33 or 34 for one week. Be sure to eat a simple diet during this time. If energy doesn't increase after one week, try other herbs given and/or look to the Patterns.

Tiredness Due to Deficiency: Those who are tired from Deficiency have different symptoms: weakness, lowered immunity, dizziness, anemia, blurred vision, loose stools or diarrhea, coldness, breathlessness, weak voice, exhaustion, pale urine, spontaneous sweating and no thirst. These people need to build (Qi, Yang, Blood and/or Yin), both with herbs and foods.

Those who eat mentally rather than according to their bodies' needs frequently experience tiredness from Deficiency (by eating mentally, I mean the person thinks this is what is best and right to eat without paying attention to what it does to his/her body). I've had young women come to me complaining of tiredness and upon examining their diets found they were eating bagels for breakfast, skipping lunch and having a light dinner. Many young women do this not just because of busy lifestyles, but to maintain slim figures. (Believe it or not, young men do this, too.)

Not eating enough food is similar to not putting oil in the car, or asking a business to run short-handedly. The body has to work extra hard while it gets weaker and weaker, eventually reaching burnout and then stopping altogether. Ultimately, not eating enough actually leads to an overweight condition, as the resulting weakened Spleen Qi can no longer transform food and fluids, causing them to collect as edema, cellulite and excess weight instead.

Others desire to be vegetarian or vegans for spiritual

reasons, but their body types need animal protein. Not eating sufficient amounts of concentrated animal protein is depleting to Blood and Qi and, eventually, poor energy results. In this case, it is necessary to increase quality and quantity of protein, switching to animal products and having a serving of protein at every meal (include fermented products for live enzymes). At the same time, cold-energied and dampening foods need be eliminated, such as soy milk, tofu, fruit juices, raw foods, iced drinks and foods, excessive fruit, smoothies, flour products and processed foods (even though they may be organic and "healthy").

To alleviate tiredness from Deficiency, incorporate herbs to tonify Qi, Blood, Yin or Yang as appropriate. Unfortunately, there are few Western tonifying herbs, which is one reason Chinese herbal tonics have become so well known in the West. To choose which are most applicable for your condition, see Deficiency Patterns. When using tonic herbs to treat tiredness, it is best to cook in soups, teas and stocks. **Astragalus**, **reishi**, **jujube**, **lycii**, **ginseng**, **dang gui**, **dioscorea**, **atractylodes**, **fu ling** and **citrus** make a great combination for building Qi and Blood from Deficiency. Alternatively, take Formulas #45 and 77 daily, and/or dissolve 4–6 tablets each in grains, hot cereals, soup stocks, or tea water. If tiredness is due to Deficient Blood, use Blood tonics, such as **dang gui**, **white peony**, **cooked rehmannia**, **blackberries**, **raspberries** and blackstrap molasses, or some other iron supplement (or Formula #106).

Therapies that alleviate tiredness from Deficiency include moxibustion: on lower abdomen between navel and pubic bone (this enhances Qi); over lower back, level with waist, covering a line that includes area between three inches on either side of spine; and on a point below width of the hand on outside of the knee, about 1-1^1/2 inches from bone (find tender spot there—called "beside three mile", when stimulated this point gives enough energy to walk another 3 miles). As well, wear a harimake to maintain the body's energy and improve immunity. Lastly, bear in mind it can take from a few days up to a year or so to regain good energy, de-

pending on your condition and how long you have had it.

Tiredness Due to Other Causes: There are many other causes and remedies for tiredness. While it may seem the only crutch helping you get through the day, **caffeine** weakens the Kidneys, robbing energy and perpetuating the cycle. Those who use caffeine for their daily energy boost are only hastening the ultimate: ***adrenal exhaustion***. Caffeine (coffee, colas, black tea, cocoa, chocolate, maté) spends your inherited Qi trust fund rather than saves it to collect interest (so does keeping on the go, day and night, without getting sufficient rest and food). Eventually the bank sends out overdraft notices and symptoms such as low energy, weakness, lowered immunity, poor digestion, low back pain, nighttime urination, lowered libido and knee weakness result. If you don't stop, rest and eat adequately, but continue to use caffeine—or other stimulants (sugar)—as your energy source, then your constitutional trust fund goes bankrupt and adrenal exhaustion results. (Try Formulas # 51 and 80 to improve adrenal function)

Although it can take up to one month for your true energy to return after quitting coffee, its higher quality and quantity make it well worth doing. The best way to stop caffeine is drink a caffeine substitute. 1) **Roasted dandelion** and **chicory**, a traditional blend that works for many, is dark, full-bodied, bitter tasting and you can grind the beans and use a filter, just as for coffee. Because it clears Heat in the body, it eliminates those headaches so many experience when going off caffeine. 2) Grain blends, such as roasted barley, beet root, chicory and rye (there are many brands available at health food stores). 3) Herb teas (those that don't have black tea in them!). 4) Green tea—while this has caffeine, it has a very small amount, and is cooling and drying in energy versus the dampening and heating effects of most caffeine. 5) Chew on several slices of honeyed **ginseng**—a Qi tonic, this gives a gentle lift that doesn't swing to a low, as do caffeine and sugar (to make: peel and slice ginseng root thinly, place in jar and pour over just enough honey to lightly coat each piece; let soak until softened; store in jar).

Likewise, using **sugar** to increase energy sends blood sugar levels on a roller-coaster ride. It also creates acidity and Heat in the body, weakens Spleen Qi, lowers immunity and depletes Kidney/Adrenals. The result is indigestion, poor energy, lowered immunity, frequent urination, decreased sex drive, hearing and memory problems and premature aging symptoms, for example. Ultimately, this creates cravings for more sugar and the cycle repeats itself. Those who have sugar (especially chocolate) cravings before menses, usually have magnesium deficiency—thus, take a magnesium supplement one week before menses.

There are several ways to break the sugar cycle: eat or drink something bitter instead (believe it or not, this really works!), increase whole grains and legumes in diet (if you are a meat-eater), or increase protein in diet (if you eat little meat, or are vegetarian). Rarely do I tell someone to stop sugar, because if they do any of the above, sugar cravings stop.

Candida yeast overgrowth causes low energy, and is discussed as the topic Candida, under the section Digestive Disorders.

Gluten intolerance (celiac disease) can also cause low energy (see section Digestive Disorders).

Chronic fatigue syndrome (CFS) is a far more complicated condition because it is a combined condition of Excess with Deficiency. Not only is digestion usually impaired and thus, Qi and Blood weak, but also Liver Qi is stagnant and generally toxic. At this point, tonics alone don't work because they can actually aggravate stagnant Liver Qi, like adding more cars to a traffic jam. Rather, herbs that detoxify, clear Heat and regulate Liver Qi are needed as well. A good combination is **milk thistle**, **dandelion**, **bupleurum**, **green citrus**, **lycii** and **gardenia** (**red marine algae** is good here, too, especially if there is Epstein Barr). These may be added to Liver immune tonics, such as **shiitake** and **schisandra**, and Qi tonics such as **dioscorea**, **ginseng** or **codonopsis** and **white atractylodes**. It may take one to two years to heal

CFS, but if after six months you don't feel better, it's possible hypothyroidism is causing fatigue and should be addressed.

Hypothyroidism also causes tiredness and is a common undiagnosed ailment in the West. Prolonged Deficiencies or Excesses affect the hormonal system, including the thyroid. Further, it's not unusual for women to experience low thyroid symptoms after childbirth or during peri/menopausal years. Women on estrogen replacement without progesterone may also experience hypothyroidism symptoms because estrogen dominance can slow the thyroid, whereas progesterone is supportive. Stress, environmental pollutants (including fluoride in toothpaste and water and mercury in amalgam dental fillings), yeast infections (Candida), certain drugs, hormones in food, excessive iodine, soy products, lack of sunshine, lack of sleep and insufficient essential fatty acids in the diet can all cause hypothyroidism. Further, fungal infection symptoms mimic those of hypothyroidism, so clear any fungal infections first.

The easiest way to test for hypothyroidism is the basal thermometer test. To do, first put thermometer by bed before sleep (if using a mercury thermometer, shake it down then, too). When waking in morning and *before doing anything else*, put thermometer under armpit and wait ten minutes. Be sure to lie still and relax during this time. Remove and record temperature. Do three consecutive days, then average temperatures. (For women, it is best to do on the 2nd, 3rd and 4th days of menstrual cycle.) If average basal temperature is consistently below 97.6 degrees F, thyroid may be underactive. Oral temperatures may be taken, instead (follow same procedures)—if below 98 degrees F, hypothyroidism is possible.

Many with low thyroid respond well to taking glandular products along with the amino acid, L-tyrosine. Usually these products include bovine sources of thyroid, adrenal and other glands, kelp, L-tyrosine, B12 and substances boosting the thyroid. At the same time, eliminate thyroid-inhibiting foods, such as all soy products (isoflavones suppress thyroid function), Brassica family

Low Thyroid Symptoms:

Primary Symptoms: General tiredness, fatigue, exhaustion; feeling of being overwhelmed, rundown, sluggish; lethargic; family history of thyroid disease; weight gain and unable to lose weight with diet/exercise; constipation, sometimes severe; very dry skin, coarse and pale skin or thickened, scaly skin; low body temperature; feeling cold even in warm temperatures; Low basal temperature (below 97.6); **Other symptoms:** Mental sluggishness; decreased ability to focus and concentrate; brain fog; poor memory; aches and pains in joints, muscles, hands and feet; yellowish complexion; edema; hypoglycemia; skin problems; chronic infections (yeast, viral, or bacterial); poor vision; hearing impairment; heart disease; muscle cramps; high cholesterol; muscle weakness; brittle, dry, coarse hair; hair loss, including loss of eyebrow hair; dry and gritty eyes; eyes sensitive to light; eyes get jumpy/tics in eyes; dizziness/vertigo; tinnitus; lightheadedness; milky discharge from the breast; voice hoarse, deep, husky and slow; speech thick; facial puffiness; puffiness and swelling around the eyes; palms of hands yellowish; swollen feet; swollen ankles; shortness of breath even with minimal exercise; heart rate decreases; high or low blood pressure; fungal infections (Candida); numbness and a sensation of pins and needles in the hands or feet; myopathy; seizures; excessive muscle bulk in children; muscle coordination problems with loss of equilibrium, unsteadiness on the feet and trembling; sleep apnea; pleural effusion; depression, mood swings; Increased sleepiness; restlessness; forgetfulness; anxiety; paranoia; inappropriate crying; slow reaction time; ADHD; excessive worrying; panic attacks; emotional instability; sadness; loss of ambition; loss of interest in normal daily activities; feelings of worthlessness; slowing of thought and speech; irritability; fear of open or public spaces; audiovisual hallucinations and paranoid delusions; dementia; manic behavior; history of miscarriage; infertility; menstrual irregularities—cycle longer, more frequent, or heavier; menstrual cramps severe; loss of sex drive; shortness of breath and tightness in the chest; yawning a lot to get oxygen; frequent infections that last lon ger.

vegetables (mustard greens, kale, cabbage, spinach, Brussels sprouts, cauliflower, broccoli and turnips), as well as almonds, peanuts, soy flour, millet and apples (thyroid-suppressing foods). Instead, eat thyroid-stimulating foods: seaweeds, garlic, radishes, shrimp, egg yolks, wheat germ, brewer's yeast, mushrooms, oats, parsley, apricots and yams.

Take 800-1,200 IU of vitamin E daily, 10,000 IU of vitamin A, a multivitamin with zinc, copper, selenium and iron, use natural sources of iodine, such as kelp, cod liver oil, lobster, shrimp and saltwater fish like cod, halibut, haddock and herring, and take essential fatty acids such as **evening primrose**, **borage seed** (Formula #11) or **flaxseed oil**. Get plenty of sleep and sunshine exposure and reduce stress. Some use iodine therapy to boost the thyroid, but this is only indicated for poor T4 function (take 4-6 drops/day then). If hypothyroidism isn't caused by poor T4 function, iodine supplementation can actually contribute to cancer formation.

In terms of Western herbs, many find **royal bee jelly** and **rosemary** very helpful in improving thyroid function. A Chinese thyroid-boosting herbal formula is equal parts **ginseng** and **lycii**, 3/4 parts, **deer antler** (Formula #1) and 1/2 part **tortoise shell** along with 10 tablets daily of kelp. In TCM, low thyroid is very similar to the Pattern Deficient Yang, so taking Yang and Qi tonics frequently stabilizes low thyroid symptoms, including tiredness. (try Formulas #77 with 74 and 75).

If after taking these and following a diet change (see treating Deficiency tiredness earlier) your energy isn't

TIREDNESS—EXCESS PATTERNS:

LIVER QI STAGNATION	LIVER YANG RISING	LIVER FIRE BLAZING	PHLEGM	DAMPNESS
Tiredness that Is worse in the afternoon: 3-5 PM	Throbbing headaches	Tiredness	Tiredness	Tiredness and sleepiness
Tiredness	Dizziness	Dizziness	Slight dizziness	Lack of concentration
Depression	Tinnitus	Tinnitus	Lethargy	Lethargy
Moodiness	Dry mouth and throat	Deafness	Feeling of heaviness in the body	Feeling of heaviness in the body or head
Irritability	Irritability	Headache on the temples	Numbness	Dull headache
Feeling of distension or pain under the ribcage or chest	Short temper	Red face and eyes	Cloudy or foggy mind	Feeling of oppression in the chest or stomach region
Sighing	Insomnia	Nosebleeds	Possible mucus	A foggy feeling in the head
Nausea		Bitter taste in the mouth; thirst		Cloudy urine; urinary difficulty
Poor appetite		Dream disturbed sleep		No appetite; a sticky taste
PMS		Constipation with dry stools		Mucus in the stools
		Dark yellow urine		Excessive vaginal discharge
Tongue: may be normal, or slightly red on sides, or with raised sides	**Tongue:** red sides	**Tongue:** red, redder on sides, yellow coat, dry	**Tongue:** swollen, sticky coat	**Tongue:** sticky coat
Pulse: wiry, especially on left side; in women may be choppy or fine/thin	**Pulse:** wiry, often only on left side	**Pulse:** full, wiry and fast	**Pulse:** slippery	**Pulse:** slippery
Formulas: #12 or 153; tea of equal parts bupleurum, dang gui, white peony, cyperus, Chinese wild yam, ligusticum and 1/2 part fennel and licorice. Eat rose petal paste.	**Formulas:** #192; tea of mung beans, burdock root, dandelion, raw rehmannia, gambir and gastrodia.	**Formulas:** #13 or 170; 1 capsule goldenseal with tea of burdock root, yellow dock, isatis, gentian, lycii, bupleurum and raw rehmannia.	**Formulas:** #181; tea of one part each codonopsis, pinellia, fu ling, bamboo leaves and 1/2 part each citrus, ginger and licorice.	**Formulas:** #236; tea of one part each dandelion, buchu, parsley, coix, cardamom, nettle and 1/2 part each licorice and dried ginger.

improved within three to six months, it may be neces- sary to see a thyroid specialist. If you do this, be sure to

TIREDNESS—DEFICIENT QI AND YANG PATTERNS:

DEFICIENT LUNG QI	DEFICIENT SPLEEN QI	DEFICIENT HEART QI	DEFICIENT HEART YANG	DEFICIENT SPLEEN YANG	DEFICIENT KIDNEY YANG
Tiredness	Tiredness	Tiredness	Tiredness, weariness	Tiredness	Extremely tired, exhaustion
Slight breathlessness	Poor appetite	Shortness of breath on exertion	Shortness of breath on exertion	Poor appetite	Frequent, pale urination; night-time urination
Low voice	Weak muscles	Palpitations	Palpitations	Weak muscles	Listlessness
Pale, white complexion	Weakness in arms and legs	Depression	Cold limbs, especially hands	Weakness in the arms and legs	Mental depression
Slight spontaneous sweating	Loose stools	Slight spontaneous sweating	Slight sweating	Loose stools; undigested food in the stools	Diarrhea, especially early morning
Timidity	Sallow complexion	Pale complexion	Bright pale face	Sallow complexion	Bright white complexion
Propensity to catching colds and flu	Uncomfortable feeling in the abdomen after eating	Dislike of talking	Slight feeling of discomfort in the heart region	Slight abdominal pain	Soreness of the lower back and knees; weak knees
	Poor digestion		Palpitations	Feeling of cold; Cold limbs	Feeling of cold; Cold limbs, Especially legs
	Prolapsed organs		Feeling cold	Dislike of speaking	Edema of the ankles
	Gas and bloatedness			No appetite	Impotence; Infertility
				Edema	No sexual desire
Tongue: slightly pale	**Tongue:** pale with teeth marks	**Tongue:** pale, midline crack reaching the tip	**Tongue:** pale, wet, swollen	**Tongue:** pale, swollen, teeth marks	**Tongue:** pale, swollen
Pulse: weak or empty, especially left Front position	**Pulse:** empty, especially right Middle position	**Pulse:** empty, especially left Front position	**Pulse:** weak and deep; knotted in severe cases	**Pulse:** weak, especially in right Middle position	**Pulse:** deep, slow and weak
Formulas: #44 with 77; tea of equal parts jujube dates, codonopsis or ginseng, astragalus, and dang gui (best cooked as congee or in beef soup).	**Formulas:** #44 and 77; tea of equal parts jujube dates, Chinese wild yam, ginseng or codonopsis, astragalus, jujube dates and dang gui with ½ part baked licorice and ½ part dried ginger (best cooked as congee or in beef soup).	**Formulas:** #50 and 77; tea of reishi, astragalus, ginseng, longan and jujube dates with royal bee jelly.	**Formulas:** #50 with 75; 1 tablet of deer antler (#1) with tea of astragalus, reishi, ginseng, longan, dang gui and cinnamon branches.	**Formulas:** #43 with 75; 1 capsule ginger powder and tea of equal parts ginseng, baked licorice, jujube dates, astragalus, fennel, Chinese wild yam, cardamom, white atractylodes and ½ part fu ling and citrus.	**Formulas:** #75 or 156; 1 tablet deer antler (Formula #1) with tea of epimedium (#51), fenugreek, ashwagandha, cooked rehmannia, Chinese wild yam, lycii and ½ part each alisma and cornus.

TIREDNESS—DEFICIENT BLOOD PATTERNS:

HEART BLOOD DEFICIENCY	LIVER BLOOD DEFICIENCY	SPLEEN BLOOD DEFICIENCY
Tiredness which is worse at midday	Tiredness (11AM-1PM)	Tiredness
Palpitations	Feeling of weakness	Slight palpitations
Poor memory, forgetfulness	Cramps	Poor appetite
Insomnia or dream disturbed sleep	Blurred vision; Dizziness	Pale lips
Dull pale complexion	Dull pale complexion	Dull pale complexion
Dizziness	Propensity to being easily startled	Desire to lie down
Pale lips	Slight constipation	Loose stools
Anxiety	Scanty periods or no period	
Easily startled	Brittle nails	
	Dry skin and hair	
	Numbness or tingling of limbs	
Tongue: pale and thin, may have midline crack reaching the tip	**Tongue:** pale and thin, especially sides; dry	**Tongue:** pale, slightly thin with teeth marks
Pulse: choppy or fine/thin	**Pulse:** choppy or fine/thin	**Pulse:** weak or fine/thin
Formulas: #50 or 231; tea of equal parts longan, dang gui, lycii, jujube dates, codonopsis and tien qi ginseng with royal bee jelly.	**Formulas:** #12 or 231; tea of equal parts dang gui, lycii, white peony, ligusticum, cooked rehmannia and jujube dates with blackstrap molasses.	**Formulas:** #50 or 159; tea of equal parts dang gui, longan, white peony, codonopsis, astragalus and jujube dates with blackstrap molasses.

TIREDNESS—DEFICIENT YIN PATTERNS:

DEFICIENT LUNG YIN	DEFICIENT HEART YIN	DEFICIENT STOMACH YIN	DEFICIENT LIVER YIN	DEFICIENT KIDNEY YIN
Exhaustion	Exhaustion	Tiredness	Tiredness that is worse in the afternoon: 3-5 PM	Exhaustion; worse in late afternoon: 5-7 PM
Dry cough; unproductive	Mental restlessness	Dry mouth, lips and throat	Headaches at the top of the head	Depression
Dry throat	Palpitations	No appetite	Dizziness	Dizziness
Breathlessness	Poor memory	Dry stools	Dry eyes	Weak legs and knees
Hoarse voice	Anxiety	Thirst with no desire to drink or only drink in small sips	Irritability	Dry mouth and throat that are worse at night

(continued on next page)

TIREDNESS—DEFICIENT YIN PATTERNS: *(continued)*

DEFICIENT LUNG YIN	DEFICIENT HEART YIN	DEFICIENT STOMACH YIN	DEFICIENT LIVER YIN	DEFICIENT KIDNEY YIN
Feeling of heat in the afternoon	Feeling of heat in the afternoon	Slight pain in the stomach region or diaphragm	Restlessness	Soreness of the lower back
Malar flush	Malar flush	Malar flush	Malar flush	Malar flush
Burning sensation in palms, soles and/or chest	Burning sensation in palms, soles and/or chest	Fever or feeling of heat in the afternoon	Tinnitus	Tinnitus, deafness
Night sweats	Night sweats	Feeling of fullness after eating	Numbness of the limbs	Night sweats; thin body
Emaciated appearance	Dream-disturbed sleep	Constipation with dry stools	Cramps	Disturbed sleep (waking frequently at night)
Insomnia	Propensity to be easily startled		Blurred vision	Lack of drive and will-power
Tongue: red without coat, especially in front part; possible cracks in Lung area	**Tongue:** red without coat, especially in front part; deep midline crack reaching to the edge of the tip	**Tongue:** midline crack in center with rootless coat, or no coat	**Tongue:** red without coat; dry	**Tongue:** red without coat
Pulse: fine and fast, or floating and empty	**Pulse:** fine and fast, or floating and empty	**Pulse:** fine and fast, or floating and empty on right Middle position	**Pulse:** fine and fast, or floating and empty	**Pulse:** fine and fast, or floating and empty
Formulas: #168; tea of equal parts ophiopogon, schisandra, American ginseng and astragalus.	**Formulas:** #149; tea of equal parts ophiopogon, raw rehmannia, asparagus root, dang gui, salvia, schisandra and reishi.	**Formulas:** #169; tea of equal parts ophiopogon, glehnia, raw rehmannia, chrysanthemum and ½ part licorice.	**Formulas:** #74 or 169; tea of equal parts raw rehmannia, ophiopogon, dang gui, lycii, white peony, zizyphus and epimedium (#51).	**Formulas:** #74, or 166, and 51; tea of equal parts asparagus root, American ginseng, cooked rehmannia, lycii, phellodendron, Chinese wild yam, epimedium (#51), white atractylodes and anemarrhena.

get a *complete* thyroid panel (TSH, T3, T4, free T3, free T4, reverse T3, thyroid antibodies and TRH), as it is not unusual for TSH to be within "range" because it's circulating in the blood while the thyroid is actually deteriorating (this is subclinical hypothyroidism). If left undiscovered until too late, ***Hashimoto's autoimmune thyroiditis (HAIT)*** can occur. Since hypothyroidism and HAIT are extensive and complicated topics, they aren't dealt with any further here.

❧URINARY BLADDER INFECTIONS (Cystitis)

Urinary frequency, urgency, pain, difficulty and scantiness characterize bladder infections (cystitis). They can be very painful, not to say extremely disruptive to one's life. Unfortunately, women experience bladder infections more than men because of the proximity of their urethra to vaginal and anal bacteria. In fact, cystitis is often called the "honeymoon disease" because so many new brides get bladder infections then. Some doctors recommend women get up and pee right after having sex to prevent infections from occurring. While this may help, there are far more causes for bladder infections than bacterial transmission.

I've seen all types of bladder infections: acute with blood, recurring, and chronic painful ones that women live with daily. The easiest to treat, of course, are the acute ones, and typical Western herbs given for bladder infections usually work especially well here. Chronic ones can be tricky to heal, while long-term daily bladder infections are the most difficult to treat, although I have seen eventual results.

General Treatment for Urinary Bladder Infections:

Ideally, stop a bladder infection at onset of the first symptoms. For those who have had them before, these are quite recognizable: slight burning sensation upon urination and slight fullness or distension in the lower abdomen (the urinary bladder region). Immediately use the baking soda trick I learned from a doctor: take 1 teaspoon baking soda in one glass water morning and again in evening for five days. Taper dose to one teaspoon daily for the next five days. Baking soda affects the acid/alkaline balance between the urethra and bladder walls, eliminating oncoming bladder infections. In the meantime, eat simply and rest. If Coldness is present (lower abdomen feels better with application of heat), take hot sitz bath, or use a **ginger** fomentation or moxibustion over lower belly (these may be done in appropriate acute conditions, too).

If the bladder infection progresses, or comes on full-blown, immediately cut back all protein, sugar, fruit, juices and other aggravating foods (see list of causes) and eat a very simple diet of soups, hot cereals, grains, legumes and cooked vegetables (especially asparagus). Next, take two "00"-sized capsules of **goldenseal** powder every 2-3 hours along with one cup of a diuretic herbal tea at room temperature (this temperature enhances its diuretic action)—try equal parts **uva ursi**, **cornsilk**, **parsley**, **cleavers**, **dandelion** and **marshmallow. Buchu, usnea, nettle, horsetail** and **plantain** are other possible diuretics to include (alternatively take 4 tablets of Formula #99). If you have pH strips, use them (they are easily purchased from pharmacies)—if urine pH is above 6.0, drink **cranberry** juice; if below 6.0, take vitamin C (or Formula #23).

Extreme burning on urination with scanty, dark urination indicates Heat. Include more cooling herbs in your herbal formula, such as **goldenseal** and/or **chaparral**, **gentian**, **gardenia** and **scutellaria**, or the Chinese Formulas #142 or 170. If blood is present in urine, include **shepherd's purse**, **yarrow**, **cattail pollen** or **dianthus** (pinks). Chronic, recurring bladder infections are due to Deficient Qi, Yin or Yang, so include herbs to tonify as appropriate (see Patterns). At the same time, do regular **castor** oil packs over the bladder and/or kidneys. If there is cramping pain or muscle spasms with the infection, include **cramp bark** with your other herbs.

Kidney infections have similar symptoms, but may include pain over kidney region (around and above waist on either side of spine). Follow same procedure for acute bladder infections, but be sure to rest a great deal. A castor oil pack over the kidneys wonderfully reduces pain, while drinking **dandelion leaf** tea is specific for kidney infections. If pain is excruciating, or fever high, seek medical attention.

Kidney stones can cause the worst pain there is, I'm told.

Differentiation of Urinary Bladder Infections:

- ↜ Frequent, pale urination indicates Deficient Kidney Yang, or Deficient Spleen Qi.

- ↜ Frequent, dark, painful urination is due to Damp Heat, or Deficient Kidney Yin.

- ↜ Frequent, dark, scanty urine is due to Deficient Kidney Yin.

- ↜ Frequent, cloudy urine indicates Dampness.

- ↜ Rust or blood-tinged urine indicates presence of blood (blood in urine is due to Heat in the Blood, or to Deficient Qi). Dark blood with small clots indicates stagnant Blood.

- ↜ Difficult urination where flow is hesitant or fitful indicates Dampness obstructing Water passages.

- ↜ Weak-stream urination is due either to Dampness obstructing Water passages or to Deficient Kidney Yang unable to push urine along.

- ↜ Burning pain during urination is due to Heat or Damp Heat.

- ↜ Pain before urination indicates stagnant Qi.

- ↜ Pain after urination indicates Deficient Qi.

- ↜ Pain over the hypogastrium indicates stagnant Liver Qi or Liver Fire.

- ↜ Pain over the sacrum indicates Deficient Kidneys.

- ↜ A feeling of distension in lower abdomen area indicates stagnant Liver Qi.

- ↜ Intense pain is due to either stagnant Liver Blood or to Liver Fire.

- ↜ A feeling of fullness over the hypogastrium indicates Dampness.

- ↜ A dragging, bearing-down feeling in lower abdomen area indicates sinking of Spleen Qi.

- ↜ If lower abdomen feels hard and distended to touch, it indicates stagnant Qi or Dampness. If soft and flaccid, it indicates Deficient Kidney Qi.

Usually blood is present in the urine with possible burning pain and slight difficulty in urination. There may also be cloudy or turbid urine, lower backache, tiredness and dizziness. Take herbs that dissolve stones (lithotriptics such as **gravel root**, **cleavers**, **parsley**, **dandelion**, **nettle**, **uva ursi** and **horsetail**) along with diuretic herbs—try 2 parts each **gravel root**, **parsley root** and **uva ursi** and 1 part each **cleavers**, **dandelion**, **nettle**, **buchu**, **marshmallow** and **horsetail**. Drink 1/2 cup every 2-3 hours. Other useful herbs include **corn silk**, **shepherd's purse**, **agrimony**, **fennel**, **huckleberry leaves**, **alisma**, **fu ling**, **oyster shell**, **white peony**, **codonopsis**, **dioscorea**, **saussurea**, **corydalis** and **dipsacus**. Alternatively, try Formula #91. Do castor oil packs over the kidneys, as they not only reduce pain, but also dissolve stones. It can take weeks to months to naturally dissolve stones, so be patient. If pain is extreme, seek appropriate medical attention. Avoid extra calcium supplementation, vitamin C, spinach, and chard, as these are stone forming.

Frequent urination and nighttime urination with-

URINARY BLADDER INFECTIONS—EXCESS PATTERNS:

DAMP-HEAT	HEART FIRE	STAGNANT QI	HEAT IN THE BLOOD	DAMPNESS OBSTRUCTING
Frequent, scanty, and difficult urination	Difficult urination	Difficult and painful urination	Difficult urination with burning pain on urination	Difficult turbid or cloudy urine (it looks like it has patches of oil floating on the surface)
Dark urine with a strong odor;	Reddish or yellowish urine	Irritability	Blood in the urine, which could take the form of small clots	Possible blood or sediment in the urine
Constipation	Insomnia			
Hypogastric pain, nausea	Mouth and/or tongue sores; bleeding gums	Hypogastric pain and distension	Fullness and pain In hypogastrium	
Bitter taste; thirst	Palpitations		Mental restlessness	
Tongue: yellow, sticky coat on root with red spots	**Tongue:** red with redder tip	**Tongue:** may be normal, or raised on the sides	**Tongue:** red	**Tongue:** sticky coat
Pulse: slippery in left Rear position and slightly fast	**Pulse:** fast and full on left Front position	**Pulse:** wiry	**Pulse:** full and fast	**Pulse:** full and slippery
Formulas: #13 with 23 or 99, or #170: 2 capsules goldenseal with tea of equal parts uva ursi, plantain, cleavers, dandelion root and leaves, and burdock root.	**Formulas:** #148; 2 capsules goldenseal with tea of dandelion root, uva ursi, cleavers, buchu, parsley, marshmallow root, and 1/2 part ginger.	**Formulas:** #12 and 99, or #153; tea of equal parts uva ursi, plantain, cleavers, dandelion root and leaves, burdock root, cyperus, green citrus, and white peony.	**Formulas:** #73 and 99; 2 capsules goldenseal with tea of equal parts uva ursi, plantain, dandelion root and leaves, burdock root, agrimony, nettle, and marshmallow.	**Formulas:** #23 and 99; 2 capsules goldenseal with tea of equal parts uva ursi, plantain, dandelion leaves, burdock, parsley, and buchu.

URINARY BLADDER INFECTIONS—DEFICIENCY PATTERNS:

DEFICIENT QI	DEFICIENT QI WITH DAMPNESS OBSTRUCTING	DEFICIENT YIN CAUSING EMPTY HEAT IN THE BLOOD	DEFICIENT KIDNEY YANG
Difficult urination	Slight difficulty in urination	Slight discomfort on urination with little pain	Difficult urination; coming in bouts with no burning
Weak stream urination	Cloudy or turbid urine	Pale blood in urine	Dribbling after urination
Slight hypogastric distension	Lower backache	Sore back	Sore back
Tiredness	Tiredness	Depression	Exhaustion
	Dizziness	Feeling of heat in the evening	Depression
			Feeling cold
			Dragging feeling in hypogastrium
Tongue: pale	**Tongue:** pale with sticky coat	**Tongue:** red and peeled	**Tongue:** pale
Pulse: weak	**Pulse:** weak and floating	**Pulse:** fast, floating and empty	**Pulse:** weak
Formulas: #44 & 99; tea of equal parts American ginseng, plantain, nettles, parsley root, uva ursi and ½ part marshmallow root and fresh ginger.	**Formulas:** #23 & 99; tea of equal parts American ginseng, plantain, nettles, parsley root, uva ursi, corn silk and ½ part marshmallow root and fresh ginger.	**Formulas:** #74 & 99, or #147; tea of equal parts American ginseng, nettle, marshmallow root, alisma, fu ling, anemarrhena and phellodendron.	**Formulas:** #75 & 99, or #180; 1 capsule cinnamon bark with tea of equal parts saw palmetto, parsley and black cherry stems.

PART III

Regaining and ❧ *Maintaining Health* ❧

CHAPTER 9

The Energy of Food

Most people are disconnected from the food they eat—they don't plant it, grow it, harvest it, or even cook it. In fact, many young children don't understand that the milk bought at a store actually comes from the cows they see in fields! The first medicine is always food; only after proper nutrition is established do herbs come next. If you want to heal, particularly from a complicated condition, it is necessary to treat your entire life, not just take a magic herbal bullet, and this starts with nutrition and diet.

In *The Energy of Herbs*, we learned that all herbs have a warm, neutral or cool energy. Like herbs, every type of food has an inherent cool or warm energy. The cooling or warming energy of food affects the body by cooling it down, or heating it up. While in the West we create food groups, those in the East recognize the energy of food regardless of the group it is in.

Learning the energy of food is important in order to regain and maintain health. If you have Excess Heat, as described in *The Energy of Illness*, and continue to eat warming and heating foods, then your body only becomes warmer inside, eventually creating disease. The same is true if you have Coldness: eating a lot of cooling foods causes your body to get colder.

As a result, it is very important to choose foods according to their heating or cooling energies. If you are taking the right herbs to heal your condition but are eating foods with the wrong energy, then you will receive little or no benefit from the herbs: The herbal treatment will either be less effective, will take longer to heal, or will have no effect at all. For this reason, it is extremely important to learn about and understand the energy of food. Furthermore, eating appropriately for your body's energy helps prevent illness.

For example, Neil came to me with low energy and frequent colds. I gave him warming and building herbs and a balanced diet to eat, but he made little progress in two weeks time. When discussing his diet, Neil admitted he drank fruit juices, believing them healthy and important foods. Yet, these same foods continually caused his poor digestion, mucus, lowered immunity and tiredness. When Neil eliminated the fruit juices, within a week he felt stronger and had better digestion and more energy.

Rose had skin problems, frequently breaking out on her face, back and shoulders. Again I gave her an appropriate energetic diet along with Heat-clearing and detoxifying herbs. Within a few weeks, Rose felt better and her face cleared, but skin eruptions continued to appear on her back and shoulders. When questioned further I learned that she still ate a weekly dose of chocolate chip cookies, white sugar included. When she stopped these, Rose's skin fully cleared.

Every food we eat affects our bodies in some way. Food can add Warmth, Coldness, Dampness, Dryness, strength, weakness, maintain balance, create disease and so forth. Because most people eat two to three times a day, then two to three times a day the body's energy is affected by the energy of the food ingested. "You are what you eat" is not such a strange adage from this perspective.

THE ENERGY OF FOOD

A balanced diet is one that uses foods energetically, incorporating more foods with a neutral to cool and neutral to warm energy, less food with warm or cool energies and sparing use of hot and cold energy foods.

Consider this continuum as a child's seesaw and imagine a person sitting at each of the hot and cold ends, one in the air and the other on the ground. Now if the person on the ground suddenly gets off, the one in the air quickly slams to the ground. Likewise, if eating hot and cold foods at the extreme ends, the disease 'crash' is likely to be sudden, more intense and harder to cure.

Now imagine both people sitting a little distance away from the center point. If one gets off, the other only lightly taps the ground. Thus, eating closer to the balanced energy point creates less disease potential and only slight ailments may occur and are more easily healed. When eating according to the energy of foods, include more foods close to the balance point and fewer foods away from it.

The more warm or hot foods you eat, the more potential there is for an Excess Heat illness to manifest (such as high fever, thirst, constipation, craving for cold, blood in the nose, stool or urine, yellow mucus, stools or urine, red tongue body and rapid pulse). Likewise, the more cool to cold foods you eat, the more likely an Excess Cold illness can manifest (such as feelings of coldness, diarrhea or loose stools, poor appetite, clear discharges, urine or mucus, no thirst, no sweating, a pale frigid appearance, frequent and copious urination pale tongue body, and slow, deep pulse).

You can determine yourself how food makes you feel by noticing how it affects you after eating it. Some effects are evident immediately, such as those from spicy hot peppers, or it may take three days or more for you to experience it, such as the effects of cold energy ice cream. Most foods affect you within three days. An excess amount of one type of food builds over time and within a month you can feel its effects.

Another way of looking at the warm-cool energy of food is in terms of acid-alkaline. The acid-alkaline determination is not the pH of food itself, but the residue ash that forms when food is oxidized. In general, foods that are cool or cold tend to make the body more alkaline. Foods that are warm or hot tend to make the body more acidic (of course there are exceptions). Most people eat too many acidic foods and not enough alkaline ones. Being either too acidic or too alkaline can imbalance your health (see page 332 for specific acid and alkaline foods).

Sometimes just cutting back on acidic or alkaline foods quickly alters the body's condition. In fact, I know of one woman who healed herself of multiple illnesses simply by testing her pH balance frequently throughout the day and then altering her diet accordingly (you can purchase pH strips at your local drugstore and do this yourself).

The taste of each food also indicates its warming, cooling or neutral energy. Bitter foods, like endive or spinach, cool and eliminate toxins. Sour foods refresh and cool, like lemons, while small amounts aid digestion. Spicy foods stimulate and heat metabolism and move Blood and Qi. Salty foods, like seaweed and miso, cool and soften because they retain Fluids in the body. Full sweet foods, like protein and complex carbohydrates, are hot to cool in energy and nourish bones, muscles, Qi and Blood.

| Hot | Warm | Neutral-Warm | Neutral-Cool | Cool | Cold |

The energy of a food is inherent to it regardless of how the food is eaten or prepared, though the energy can be modified somewhat. Overall, adding heat, pressure, cooking time and spices makes a food less cooling and more warming. Adding water, refrigeration or freezing, eating raw and unspiced makes food less warming and more cooling. Yet, despite preparations, a cool food can never be warm and vice versa. For example, an apple, with a cool energy, can be baked with **walnuts** and **cinnamon** to make it less cool in energy instead. Likewise, eating warm shrimp in a raw state gives it a less warm energy since the shrimp isn't cooked.

EMPTY-FULL

Along with warming and cooling energies, foods are either empty or full. Empty and full refer to a food's building or eliminating effects on the body and not its nutritional contents. Like energy, empty-full is on a continuum; each food is not absolutely empty or full. Full foods are highly concentrated nutritionally, like animal protein. Empty foods lack protein, such as fruits and vegetables. Solid foods are building while simple foods are eliminating. Relative to each other, fruit and juices are empty, vegetables are neutral to somewhat empty, meat and dairy are full, grains and legumes are neutral, protein-rich foods are full and more water-containing foods are empty.

For instance, fruit and juices are empty foods, although they range from warm to cold in energy. They generally lower body temperature and metabolism by creating elimination. A little periodically eliminates toxins and moistens Dryness. Yet, if eaten too frequently or predominantly, they cause Coldness, poor digestion, gas, possible low-back pain. Dampness, lowered immunity and resistance and feelings of being ungrounded and unfocused.

On the other hand, prolonged eating of mostly full foods stagnate Energy, Blood, Fluids, Food or Heat, ultimately resulting in Excess conditions. Those who predominantly eat full foods often feel congested, stuck, explosive and hypertensive. For example, red meat and dairy are full foods, although they are neutral to warming in energy. They strengthen Blood and Qi, building strength and endurance. Yet, excess red meat or dairy ultimately creates too much congestion, resulting in a red neck and face, irritability, a loud voice, aggressive behavior, constipation and toxicity.

Putting empty-full together with warming and cooling energies helps us look at food in a different way. For instance, some foods may be warm in energy but also empty. The spice cayenne is hot, but it doesn't build or strengthen. Instead, it stimulates and disperses and, in excess, causes elimination. On the other hand, some foods may be cool in energy but also full, such as barley. It expands the intestines and eliminates Dampness, helping stop diarrhea. It also strengthens digestion.

Thus, along with the energy of a food, it is important to look at its empty-full effects. Overall, a balanced diet is comprised predominantly of foods with a neutral-warm and neutral-cool energy that are neutral-full to neutral-empty in quality. Eating large amounts of the more extreme foods, those that are hot, cold, full and/or empty, creates imbalance and disease.

DETERMINING THE RIGHT DIET FOR YOU

I frequently hear this comment: "I've looked at every diet out there and they all say I should eat something different. I'm confused and don't know what to do. Which one is right?" Always I answer in return: *there is no one specific diet for all people*. This cannot be overstated. Because all people's bodies are different, everyone requires

meat & eggs	dairy	grains & legumes	vegetables	fruit
Full	**Neutral-Full**		**Neutral-Empty**	**Empty**

different types of foods to stay in balance, and even this may vary from season to season and year to year. Each person should learn what his/her current body's needs are and eat the right foods for those personal conditions.

Eating raw foods makes Karen feel so fantastic, she tells you (and everyone else) that this is the best diet to follow. Yet, when Suzie ate the same, she got diarrhea, gas and lowered immunity. Eating frequent amounts of animal protein healed Ken of prolonged weakness and tiredness, and he scoffed at vegetarians. But it caused headaches, constipation and high blood pressure when Steve followed this diet. Thus, what benefits one person won't necessarily be healthy for your body, and could even make you sick over time.

Every one of us is born with unique traits based on ancestral heritage, blood type and inherited constitution. Further, your childhood dietary and lifestyle habits strongly influence your body type and food needs. The speed of your metabolism plus what you currently experience in life—stress, giving birth or having a specific ailment, for instance—also indicates what is best for you to eat. Therefore, diet must be individually tailored to your unique body needs. This is an extremely important point: never blindly follow a mass diet, no matter how good it sounds, or how much it has helped someone you know.

Most of us eat according to our minds or emotions, such as following a specific dietary regime for spiritual, cultural or peer group reasons, long-standing habits, according to ongoing emotional issues, or how we feel about food. Eating according to your mind or emotions rarely serves your body. Instead, choose to eat according to your individual body needs.

The following keys can help determine the appropriate diet for your individual needs.

Constitution: Each of us is born with a different constitution determined by the health of our parents at the time of conception, and inherited weaknesses and strengths. These help determine our immune strength, susceptibility to disease and, consequently, our food needs. Those with weaker constitutions must be much more careful with their diets, ensuring sufficient build-ing foods are incorporated. Those with stronger constitutions do not need to be as strict.

Body Type: TCM categorizes body types according to the Five Phases—Fire, Earth, Metal, Water or Wood (refer to *The Energy of Illness*). Ayurvedic medicine recognizes the body types Vata (Air), Pitta (Fire) or Kapha (Earth). Other cultures identify further body types. For example, Western medicine used to categorize people according to sanguine, phlegmatic, choleric and melancholic. Each body type has its own dietary and lifestyle needs to stay in balance and eating accordingly maintains strength and immunity (see The Five Phases, in *The Energy of Illness*).

Metabolic Power: This is the ability to digest food normally. If metabolism is too slow, lethargy, sluggishness and easy weight gain result; if metabolism is faster than normal, foods burn too quickly, causing constant hunger, irritability and drastic energy drops (see table, Slow Burner or Fast Burner? to determine which you are). People with slow metabolisms do better with lean proteins, little fat and some complex carbohydrates. Those with fast metabolisms need more concentrated proteins and healthy fats, both of which take much longer to metabolize than carbohydrates. Both types should avoid processed carbohydrates, the former because they'll experience severe blood sugar swings, the latter because they'll experience congestion and weight gain.

Ancestry and Genetic Heritage: People with unmixed heritages, like pure Japanese, Chinese, Indonesian, African, Indian, German, Italian, French, or Middle Eastern constitutions, for example, do better eating as their ancestors did and usually have stronger and healthier bodies. Most of us, however, have mixed heritages. To help determine your ancestral needs, consider whether most of your ancestors came from northern areas (cold climates) or southern areas (warm climates). Those from colder climates need concentrated diets with more protein and less carbohydrates. Those from warmer climates need lighter diets with less protein and more carbohydrates. If you are half-northern and half-southern, see which feels best and eat accordingly.

SLOW BURNER OR FAST BURNER?

Answer questions that apply to you most of the time with a check. Add up every checked question. The column with the most checks determines which type you are.

SLOW BURNER	FAST BURNER
Can you skip breakfast without losing energy or getting hungry?	Do you enjoy a hearty breakfast high in protein?
Do you prefer a "light" meal of salad to a "heavy" one of steak and potato?	Do you feel better eating steak and potatoes rather than leaner foods like chicken and vegetables?
Are you somewhat "laid back" and even-tempered?	Are you Type A, high strung or hyperactive?
Do foods like cheese, butter and avocados seem to make you sluggish?	Are cheese, butter, avocados and full-fat dairy products satisfying to you?
Do you approach problems one at a time, rather than juggling many things at once?	Do you like to juggle several problems at a time?
Do sweets give you quick energy?	When you eat sweets, do you burn out quickly after a short energy burst?
Does red meat feel heavy in your body?	Do you reach for salty snacks when stressed?
Do spices and condiments give an energy lift?	Do you have a hearty appetite?
Are you more satisfied by jam on toast than butter?	Are you more satisfied by butter on toast than jam?
Do you feel better eating two meals daily?	Do you feel better eating full meals every three to four hours?

Blood Types: Much study has been done on how blood types affect us, not only on our nutritional needs, but also our personalities.

Blood type O is the oldest and most common blood type on the planet, derived from the original hunter-gatherer population. These people survived by eating lots of animal protein with some vegetables, fruits and wild grain supplementation (along with enormous amounts of exercise). Thus, O blood types need higher amounts of full proteins in their diets, especially from animal sources such as wild game. To offset the potential stagnating effects of this full diet, be sure to eat copious amounts of vegetables (part raw and part cooked), some fruit, plenty of water and get lots of exercise. Blood type O should especially avoid pork products and refined grains and flour products, since they don't as easily assimilate these domesticated products.

Blood type A, generally does well with a vegetarian diet, needing protein from lean and carbohydrate sources. They tolerate more grains, legumes and vegetables and should limit intake of red meat and dairy.

Blood type B appeared less than 10,000 years ago, after the introduction of grains into the diet. Thus, B blood types can handle a wide range of animal products, dairy and complex carbohydrates. This blood type should avoid chicken and sesame seeds/oil as they cause clumping in B type blood.

The most recent blood type on the planet and thus the rarest, **AB blood types** do very well on a vegetarian diet. They can easily digest dairy, grains and domesticated meat.

Environment/Climate Influences: This refers to the influences of where you live. Regardless of your heritage and blood type, for instance, if you live in a cold, northern climate, your body generally needs more protein and fewer carbohydrates. If you live in a warm, southern climate, your body needs a lighter diet of less protein and more complex carbohydrates.

Inherited Influences: What health issues exist in your family also determines your body needs or intolerances. If there's diabetes, it's generally safe to assume you may be sugar sensitive and thus need to ingest simple sugars (fruit, honey, etc.) and complex sugars (grains) in moderation. If there's asthma or allergies, dairy products should be limited. If there's alcoholism, there's generally a greater sensitivity to Liver heating and congesting foods such as nuts, nut butters, avocados, cheese, caffeine, alcohol, turkey, chocolate and fried and fatty foods.

Putting it all together: Taking all these keys into account, if you look at the current dietetic food pyramid guide you will be shocked to see that it is beneficial for only certain types of people (fast-burners, and A, AB and some B blood types living in warmer, southern climates). This guide is devastating for slow burners, O blood types and those living in colder, northern climates, and helps account for the rampant obesity, hypothyroidism, Syndrome X, diabetes and other health issues we see today. Thus, be sure to use these keys as clues so that when put together, they determine the right diet for you personally. The importance of one key over another varies individually. Experiment with these keys to help determine which are most important and influential for your unique dietary needs.

THE PROCESS OF DIGESTION

Your digestion can be likened to a pot of soup bubbling at about 98-99 degrees F on the stove. In TCM, the pot of soup is the Spleen, the burner under the pot is the Stomach, and the pilot light of the stove is the Kidneys. Foods that digest easily in this soup pot are thoroughly cooked and warm in temperature.

When added to the soup pot, raw foods, cold foods eaten directly out of the refrigerator or freezer and cold energy foods all stop the soup from bubbling and slow the digestive process until they are heated up to match the body's temperature. If digestion is strong, this occurs fairly quickly, but over time the body has to turn up the burner underneath the pot to counteract the coolness obstructing digestion.

When the metabolic Stomach burner suddenly "turns up" symptoms often arise, such as forehead headaches, gum infections, bleeding gums, increased appetite, dry lips, mouth sores and/or bad breath. If the intake of cold foods continues, it also dampens the pilot light in the Kidneys, making it difficult to stay lit. This is similar to putting wet wood on the fire—it creates smoke (Stomach Heat) and burns low, providing little heat (Deficient Spleen Qi and Yang).

Eventually, the burner cannot be turned up any further. Digestion becomes sluggish until, ultimately, food is not fully broken down and passes through the stools undigested, like wet wood dampening the fire so in time it goes out altogether (Deficient Kidney Yang). When digestion gets this Cold, other symptoms manifest, such as gas, bloating, sleepiness after eating, anemia, fatigue, weakness, lowered immunity, poor appetite, amenorrhea (lack of menstrual bleeding), loose stools or diarrhea, frequent copious urination, lowered sex drive, achy lower back and knees and a variety of other complaints. Although these symptoms can occur at any time of year, they are generally aggravated in late summer (due to the excessive intake of cooling summer foods) or winter (the coldest season and Kidney time of year).

On the other hand, excessive amounts of hot foods, either from a high temperature or heating Energy, such as greasy or oily foods, excessive intake of hot spices or lamb, cause the soup pot to suddenly boil and splatter. This causes too much Heat in the body, leading to headaches, hypertension, irritability, restlessness, difficulty falling asleep, hyperacidity, hyperactivity and thirst, among numerous other symptoms. Thus, you need the correct energied fuel to maintain healthy digestion and stoked fires.

COOKED VERSUS RAW FOODS

Easily digested and assimilated foods build Blood and supplement your Essence trust fund with usable energy. When digestion is poor or sluggish, the body withdraws Essence in order to meet its daily demands. Ultimately, this causes Deficient Qi and Blood, aches and pains, anemia, gas, bloatedness, lethargy, weakness, lowered immunity, recurring infections and chronic ailments. This is why it is better to eat cooked foods rather than raw ones: they digest better and protect the digestive soup pot, thus providing more assimilated nutrients even if they do not contain live enzymes. Of course, healthy cooked food does not mean burnt or over-cooked. It means properly soaked and cooked grains and legumes, slightly crunchy vegetables and just-cooked meats.

At this point I am frequently told: "But raw foods are loaded with enzymes while cooked foods are dead! I need them to stay vital and well." Frankly, I have seen just as many sick raw vegetarians as I have meat eaters, and generally it is more difficult to bring them to health. While it is true raw foods have many "live" enzymes necessary for good digestion and health, if your digestion is sluggish, you won't fully metabolize or assimilate them and then the vitality of raw foods is totally lost. It is not only what you eat that is important, but also what you assimilate.

In addition, vegetable digestion takes little hydrochloric acid so that over time, your body produces a smaller amount. As digestive ability decreases, it becomes more difficult to digest other foods since they need more hydrochloric acid to metabolize. It is then that I hear, "I can't handle anything other than vegetables, fruit and juices. Everything else is too heavy too digest." This is always a sign of impaired digestion. Now it takes time and focus, along with eating only cooked foods, slowly introducing more concentrated protein and taking digestive tonic herbs to restore good digestion.

This is why fermented foods and cultured products are so important throughout all cultures: they provide the valuable "live" enzymes so important for good digestion. As predigested foods, they are not only easily assimilated, but also provide the valuable nutrients and live enzymes our bodies need. Thus, fermented and cultured foods are the best substitutes for raw vegetables. Most traditional cultures have a native fermented or cultured food with every meal. Choose the ones that most closely match your ancestral heritage.

A BALANCED DIET

The following basic balanced diet serves as a guideline for most people. It is broken into the Western categories, protein, carbohydrates and fats, with a look at specific food energies in each of them. To create your own personal dietary plan, vary the ratio of proteins, carbohydrates and fats according to the keys given earlier in the section Determining the Right Diet for You. Then choose the appropriate energy foods within each category to match your body's needs.

PROTEIN
- Animal protein in amounts personally needed; eggs, grains and legumes together; cultured dairy in moderation; protein powders only as necessary; some fermented soy

CARBOHYDRATES
- Whole grains and legumes properly soaked and cooked
- Mostly cooked vegetables (still slightly crisp)—5 different ones per day of varying colors
- Dark leafy greens (collard, kale, mustard, bok choy, **dandelion**, chard, spinach)
- Fruit in season—mostly cooked and with spices (**cinnamon, ginger, cardamom**)
- Some salads in warmer seasons
- Fermented and cultured foods

FATS
- Small amounts of essential fatty acids, ghee, olive oil, sesame oil; small amounts of nuts and seeds as appropriate for your body's balance

PROTEIN

Protein, the body's building block of life, creates Qi and Blood and from there, muscles, tissues and so on. It also gives strength, endurance, immunity, resistance and Heat. Excessive protein intake, however, taxes the kidneys and creates toxins, congestion, irritability and Excess Heat. Bear in mind that some proteins, such as red meat, are highly concentrated and only small amounts are needed, while other proteins, such as combined grains and beans, are less concentrated and so not as readily accessible to the body as are animal proteins.

Each person needs to determine his/her own protein level and needs. Don't go by an intellectual idea or theory but experiment with how you feel when you don't eat enough, or eat too much. Find what amount helps you feel good, strong, energetic and flexible. Bear in mind that your protein needs change from day to day and week to week according to what is going on in your life. In general, physical work requires more carbohydrates to sustain, while mental work demands more protein.

To determine how much and what type of protein you require refer to the keys under the section Determining the Right Diet for You. In general, those with O blood types, northern European or Northern Hemisphere ancestries and living in cold climates need substantial amounts of concentrated protein in their daily diets. Those with A or AB blood types, living in southern or hot climates and having Mediterranean, East Indian or tropical ancestries need less protein. B Blood types vary in protein needs; experimentation helps determine what is needed for each individual. Regardless of the quantity or type of protein eaten, everyone needs to include a complete protein with every meal, three times a day. It is the proper combination of protein, carbohydrates and fats that forms a complete nutritional meal.

Meat

Meat ranges from neutral-hot to neutral-cold in energy, yet it is full in quality. Meat, particularly red meat, is a very concentrated protein. If you have Excess Heat and need to eliminate, meat should be limited to white meats 2-3 times a week. If you need to build a Deficient condition, eat meat 1-2 times/day. In general, limit red meat and turkey to 1-2 servings per week (because they are quite congesting) and emphasize neutral-warm meats, such as fish and chicken.

A danger of eating meat is ingesting the drugs and chemicals injected into those animals. Thus, try to eat only organic meat because it is relatively pure and the animals are usually treated better. Avoid eating processed meats as they generally contain preservatives and carcinogens. Further, cook meat with spices, such as **ginger**, to help neutralize toxicity and aid quick metabolism and assimilation (see Recipes at the end of this chapter for how to detoxify meat).

The issue of whether to eat meat or not is a personal one. All foods are neither inherently "good" nor "bad" but subject to each individual's needs and preferences. I

ENERGY OF MEAT

HOT	WARM	NEUTRAL		COOL	COLD
Lamb	Chicken	Herring	Pork	Mussel	Clam
Trout	Fresh ham	Oyster	Beef		Crab
	Anchovy	Sardine	Eggs		
	Shrimp	Duck	Carp		
	Turkey	Goose	Tuna		
		Whitefish	Oyster		

have seen people eliminate meat from their diets and feel much better. I have also seen ten-year vegetarians begin to eat a little meat and become healthier and stronger than ever before.

Excessive meat eating causes Heat, stagnation, toxicity and acidity, resulting in symptoms such as constipation, abdominal stuffiness, headaches, restless sleep, headaches, hypertension, heart attacks, arthritis, strokes, aggressiveness, irritability, red face and neck, rheumatism, stiff neck and shoulders and gout. Also, as a food dense in protein and fat, excess amounts set up cravings for sugar (and vice versa), a substance high in carbohydrates and devoid of protein, minerals and fat.

On the other hand, vegetarians must eat more strictly to maintain health, eating only cooked food and a balanced protein at every meal. This does not allow for inclusion of many empty foods in the diet, such as fruit, salads, juices and other raw uncooked foods. Be sure to include warming and building herbs to provide warmth, resistance and immunity. Ideally include some fish for a concentrated protein source.

In traditional medicine, meat is classified according to its therapeutic value (along with herbs and other foods): beef is neutral, sweet in taste and nourishes Qi and Blood and the Spleen-pancreas and Intestines, but its full energy easily leads to stagnation; lamb is hot in energy and nourishes Blood, the Heart, Spleen and Kidneys; pork is neutral, moistening and nourishes the Kidneys and Liver Yin; chicken is warming and tonifies Spleen, Stomach and Liver Qi; and duck is neutral, moistening and nourishing to the Lungs and Kidneys. Although a lean meat, keep turkey to a minimum because it is too Heating, Drying and stagnating to Liver Qi.

Consider adding small amounts of organ meats (liver, heart, kidney, gizzards, etc.) back into your weekly diet. Historically, organ meats have been an important part of most all culture's diets. They strengthen their associated organs and glands (heart strengthens the Heart, liver the Liver and so on). The rampant hypothyroidism found today is often due to insufficient nutrition and poor glandular function, which organ meats support. Sausage was one of the best forms for eating organ meats as all edible parts of the animal were ground together to create this food. If you don't like organ meats, locate organic sausage made this old-fashioned way.

Dairy

The basic energy of dairy is neutral to warm and full/building. It adds valuable protein to the diet, especially for vegetarians, and moistens and builds, particularly for those who are underweight or have Dryness. In India, diary is widely used as a major source of protein. Yet, dairy is also Dampening and in excess, quite stagnating to Energy, creating mucus, cysts, fibroids, mood swings, cough, tight neck and shoulders, lung ailments, allergies and other conditions. Often children's asthma, coughs, runny noses, diarrhea or constipation disappear when diary and juices are eliminated from the diet. This is even truer if the dairy is eaten cold directly out of the refrigerator.

Curtail dairy's dampening energy by drinking milk warm and eating yogurt or cottage cheese with cooked foods. Thus, be sure to heat dairy or bring it to room temperature before eating. Further, add a little **cinnamon, cardamom** or **ginger**, plus take with some honey to counteract its mucus-producing effects.

ENERGY OF DAIRY

HOT	WARM	NEUTRAL	COOL	COLD
	Goat's milk	Cow's milk		
	Goat's cheese	Cow's cheese		
	Butter	Cottage cheese		
	Ghee	Yogurt		

Milk has different properties according to the animal from which it is taken. The cow has more fat content and its milk induces more mucus in the system. Yet, because the cow has a more peaceful disposition, its milk is "calmer." Goat's milk, on the other hand, is more alkaline and has a composition similar to that of human milk. Yet, goats tend to be more restless and aggressive, and this more "heating" characteristic of the goat makes its milk less mucus forming. Therefore, goat's milk is a better choice for people who can't tolerate cow's milk, get mucus easily, or have Coldness.

The best ways to ingest dairy products are in cultured forms (yogurt, cheese, clabber, curds, whey, kefir, koumiss, longfil, crème fraiche, sour cream, cottage cheese, yogurt cheese, kefir cheese and buttermilk). This is because the fermentation (souring) process breaks down casein (milk protein), a very difficult protein to digest. Further, culturing restores many of the enzymes destroyed during pasteurization. Finally, cultured dairy products are much easier to digest and provide important friendly bacteria and lactic acid to the digestive tract. Often people who have dairy allergies do fine with cultured dairy.

Ideally, dairy products should be whole rather than low fat. Fats are needed with protein intake for mineral absorption and adequate protein utilization. Also, a lack of fat causes blood sugar dips, ultimately resulting in hunger and snacking (and weight gain rather than loss). Dairy should also ideally be purchased raw, non-homogenized and non-pasteurized. Homogenization makes fat more susceptible to rancidity and oxidation, while pasteurization destroys vital enzymes, making it less digestible and dairy allergies more likely. As well, be sure to eat only organic dairy to avoid drugs, hormones and antibiotics injected into cows (these substances concentrate in animal fat).

Eggs

Eggs, like meat, contain all amino acids and are high in protein and fat-soluble vitamins. They are neutral, full in energy and moistening. The idea that eggs increase cholesterol is a controversial one. In fact, eggs are high in lecithin, a cholesterol-lowering agent that also keeps cholesterol moving in the bloodstream. Eggs are best eaten in their whole, complete form, which contains both protein and fat together, an essential combination for protein metabolism and mineral assimilation. It is also best to purchase eggs from free-range chickens not given hormones or antibiotics.

Soy

When vegetarianism became popular in the late 1960s and 70s, many turned to tofu as their main source of protein. Fifteen to twenty years later, numerous of these same folks complained of fatigue, poor digestion, poor memory and hypothyroidism among many other symptoms. While several factors contributed to this, such as "poor vegetarianism" (i.e., insufficient protein and poor food combining), a main culprit was the heavy use of soy products. Children fed soy in school lunches react with vomiting, diarrhea, upper respiratory infections, rashes, fevers, extreme emotional behavior, immune problems, thyroid disorders and pituitary insufficiency. Infants fed soy-based formula have a higher incidence of learning disabilities and early-onset puberty.[1]

Clinically I have seen such issues over and over and experienced them personally with family and friends. Since then, much important research brings the true nature of soy to light, despite the explosion of soy protein sources over the last decade from intense marketing strategies promoting its apparent health benefits.

Traditionally, the soy legume was used to fix nitrogen in the soil. Only when fermentation processes were applied around 2500 years ago was soy eaten as food—tempeh, miso, natto and soy sauce. In recent times, it was processed into the common forms used today—soymilk, tofu, soy protein powders, texturized

---

[1] For further information and scientific studies, refer to the article "Newest Research On Why You Should Avoid Soy", by Sally Fallon and Dr. Mary G. Enig, extracted from Nexus Magazine, Volume 7, Number 3 (April-May 2000).

vegetable protein, soy protein isolate and soy infant formulas.

In actuality, soy contains many anti-nutrients, or natural toxins. It is rich in potent enzyme inhibitors that block the action of trypsin and other enzymes needed for protein digestion, resulting in reduced protein digestion and amino acid deficiencies. Soy also contains hemagglutinin, a clot-promoting substance that causes red blood cells to clump. As well, both trypsin and hemagglutinin are growth inhibitors. Fortunately, these components are deactivated during the process of fermentation.

Soy also contains goitrogens—substances that depress thyroid function (babies fed soymilk formula have a higher incidence of thyroid issues). Hypothyroidism is now a rampant problem in the West, and excess intake of soy products is certainly a contributor. As well, soy is very high in phytic acid, a substance that interferes with protein absorption and blocks the uptake of essential minerals in the intestinal tract, particularly calcium, magnesium, copper, iron, iodine and especially zinc. Such mineral deficiencies can lead to problems involving the bones, blood sugar, nerves, memory and brain. Further, soy notably lacks important vitamins such as A, D and B12.

Energetically, soy is cold and dampening, depleting digestive fires (Spleen Yang) and slowing metabolism (Kidney Yang), setting the stage for hypothyroidism, Candida, chronic fatigue, cold hands and feet, gas, bloatedness, coldness, lowered immunity, anemia and scanty menstruation, among many other conditions.

By now many of you are wondering about all the touted soy health benefits, such as lowering cholesterol, aiding menopause with estrogen-like compounds and preventing cancer. Yet, how can soy help alleviate osteoporosis if it blocks calcium absorption? And all beans contain genistein, the cancer-reducing component of soy. Further, while Asians do have a lower incidence of breast, uterine and prostate cancer, they have much higher rates of other types of cancer, especially of the esophagus, stomach, pancreas and liver.

Thus, many of these health claims are premature and biased. While the Japanese do consume soy daily, it's mainly in fermented form and only as much as 1-2 tsp./day. Further, a mineral-rich fish broth and serving of fish or meat generally follow it.

Thus, if you eat soy, only eat fermented soy products, such as tempeh and miso. Limit intake of soymilk, tofu, soy isolate protein powders and all other soy forms if you are concerned about their cold, dampening energies, mineral-blocking effects, enzyme inhibitors, goitrogenicity, endocrine disruption and increased allergic reaction results.

Protein Powders

Protein powders, mostly made from whey or soy, are now readily available in pure form, or mixed with sugar (usually fructose) and vitamins/minerals. Like all supplements, these are concentrated substances separated from their whole food source. It is always better to eat a whole food rather than its parts, because the whole food contains added components that metabolize and balance its other elements. However, for those with Deficiency, or vegetarians who won't eat meat but need higher levels of protein than a typical vegetarian diet provides, protein powders can be useful, even essential.

I generally recommend undenatured whey protein powder rather than soy because it metabolizes better, doesn't have any added sugar and boosts immunity (some are even lactose free). Soy protein powders tend to be genetically manufactured, have added sugar, are difficult to digest and their processing leaches high levels of aluminum into the final product, not to mention the other negative effects of soy (read about soy above).

Because protein powders are mostly predigested, they quickly metabolize. Yet, a small part generally remains in the stomach unless the protein powder is taken with carbohydrates, such as whole grains, vegetables or fruit. The bulk and fiber of carbohydrates help metabolize the residue protein, moving it through the stomach and intestines. If protein powders are taken alone, the undigested portion remaining in the stomach blocks digestion in time, causing food stagnation, stuffiness in the abdomen, constipation and headaches. Further, if the protein powder isn't natural, but partly artificial, the artificial part causes toxicity, as seen in resulting skin outbreaks.

Other Protein Sources

The combination of grains with legumes/seeds/nuts provides all the amino acids necessary to form a complete protein. For many people, particularly blood types A, AB, and some B's, this less-concentrated protein is adequate, especially if living in hot, southern climates. For blood type O and some B's, and for those living in cold, northern climates, grains and beans alone usually do not provide sufficient protein for all meals, and so some animal protein usually needs be included to maintain a healthy body. This is because grains and legumes are carbohydrates high in fiber, which must first be broken down in order to get to the protein. Thus, grains and beans are considered a "weak" or less concentrated protein.

CARBOHYDRATES

Carbohydrates are comprised of starch and sugar. When broken down in the body, they form the primary sugar in the blood. There are three types of carbohydrates: complex, simple and processed. *Complex carbs* include whole grains, legumes and starchy vegetables, such as potatoes, broccoli and asparagus. They digest slowly in the body.

Simple carbs include all sugars and sweeteners, such as sugar, honey, molasses and the fructose found in fruit and fruit juices. Simple carbs enter the blood at various rates, though much more quickly than complex carbohydrates, raising blood sugar levels and increasing fat storage (fructose and agave are the slowest metabolizing of the sugars).

Processed carbs act just like simple carbs in their effect, whether from whole sources or not. They include all flour products, such as pasta, breads, pastries, pie crust, cakes, crackers, cookies, bagels, muffins, cold cereals, rice cakes, quick oats, pre-prepared and packaged foods, many desserts, pancakes, waffles, flour-coated fried foods, donuts and all types of chips. Often people

gasp when they see this list, for these foods usually comprise 70% or more of their diets! Further, junk food is generally made from vegetable oils, white flour and sugar. While it quickly satisfies taste buds and hunger, it just as quickly stores as fat and drops blood sugar levels.

Flour products acidify and strongly imbalance blood chemistry. Even those from recently ground, whole grain, organic flour are made from flour and water which together form—does this sound familiar?—glue, or paste. This is exactly what these foods turn into inside our intestines. In excess, they cause tremendous congestion, particularly if coupled with insufficient protein.

I frequently see people develop carbohydrate sensitivity leading to food allergies, hypoglycemia, Candida, leaky gut syndrome, Syndrome X, hypothyroidism, weakness, gas, bloatedness, anemia, diabetes, lowered immunity, food allergies and/or chronic fatigue as a result. Folks usually eating diets high in carbohydrates and low in protein for ten to twenty years and developing these health issues are generally O blood types with northern European ancestries. When eating flour products in excess, even those made of organic whole grains, coupled with insufficient protein intake, these ailments (and many others) ultimately arise.

Grains and Legumes

Grains and legumes are predominantly neutral-warm and neutral-cool in energy and neutral in quality. A complex carbohydrate, grains are broken down slowly by the body, giving long-lasting energy and strength, particularly to AB, A and some B blood types. Adding beans to grains provides a complete protein that should be regularly eaten by those who don't include meat, or as a periodic protein substitute for meat eaters. Further, beans are high in genistine, an anticancer agent. Bread and pasta are not substitutes for grains, even if organically grown and made from whole grains. Once ground into flour and mixed with water, you get a glue-like flour product that is dampening and congesting to digestion.

It is extremely important that all grains and legumes be soaked before they are eaten. As complex carbohy-

ENERGY OF GRAINS AND LEGUMES

HOT	WARM	NEUTRAL	COOL	COLD
	Sweet rice	Adzuki (azuki) bean	Barley	Soymilk
		Kidney bean	Wheat	
		String bean	Tofu	
		Rice	Mung bean	
		Yellow soybean	Soybean	
		Black soybean	Millet	
		Peas	Buckwheat	
		Corn	Wheat gluten	
		Rye		

drates, their protein content is not readily available, but obtained only after the fiber is broken down. Soaking grains 12-24 hours and beans 12-36 hours catalyzes this process and, more importantly, neutralizes the phytic acid content. If not soaked, phytic acid actually interferes with protein absorption. When grains and beans are properly soaked, phytic acid is neutralized and protein availability shoots up sixfold. Fermented foods with phytic acid, like tempeh, are fine as the fermentation process neutralizes this acid.

After eating a high-grain diet for ten to twenty years, many Westerners today are experiencing low energy, depressed immunity, Candida and hypoglycemia (among other problems), especially those of O blood type and northern European ancestry. This occurred because the grains and legumes generally weren't soaked and were also used as the primary source of protein along with soy products. While eating lots of grain usually works fine for AB, A and some B blood types, over time it causes a myriad of problems for O blood types. Thus, the proper quantity of grains to include in your diet varies according to your blood type, ancestry, climate and digestive strength.

In general, those with blood types AB and A, living in southern climates, or with strong digestions tolerate grains well and can incorporate a larger percentage into the diet, from $1/2$–1 cup per meal. O blood types, those living in colder climates and people with weakened digestions should decrease this amount to $1/4$–$1/3$ cup per meal. B blood types may or may not tolerate high quantities of grains; determine your needs through experimentation.

For soy products, see the section Soy in this chapter.

Vegetables

While vegetables range from slightly neutral-warming and neutral-cooling in energy, they are neutral to empty in quality. An important addition to any type of diet, most people don't eat enough vegetables and they should comprise about 30-40% of each entire meal. Ideally, eat a minimum of five different vegetables a day and from all color groups (green, white, yellow, orange and red), as the various colors supply the different nutrients our bodies need. Dark leafy greens, such as kale, collards, **dandelion**, mustard and bok choy, are one of the most important groups as they clear Heat, toxins and acidity from the Blood, decongest Liver Qi, aid in grain digestion and supply important vitamins and minerals. Their tremendous value cannot be overstated.

Most vegetables alkalinize the body, creating balance to acidifying meat, grains and flour products. They also supply nutrients and are a primary help in waste

ENERGY OF VEGETABLES

HOT	WARM	NEUTRAL	COOL	COLD
	Onion	Carrot	Cucumber	Tomato
	Garlic	Shiitake mushroom	Eggplant	Seaweed
	Winter squash	Beet	Lettuce	
	Mustard leaf	Potato	Swiss chard	
	Kale	Sweet potato	Button mushroom	
	Chestnut	Yam	Watercress	
		Cabbage	Asparagus	
		Pumpkin	Summer squash	
		String bean	Celery	
			Lotus root	
			Spinach	
			Cauliflower	
			Broccoli	

elimination. Since a wall of cellulose that is difficult to break down surrounds vegetables, cook them to facilitate assimilation of their vital nutrients. While raw vegetables supply vital "live" enzymes, they are extremely difficult to digest, so less nutrition is metabolized from them than from cooked vegetables (use fermented and cultured foods for the "live" enzymes). However, never overcook vegetables so they are mushy, as this destroys important nutrients. Cooked and still slightly crunchy, vegetables are less cold and digest and assimilate well. A little bit of raw food is beneficial for meat eaters, who can healthily include some salads, fruits and juices to help counteract their warmer diet.

Unfortunately, most vegetables today (even organic) are grown in soil depleted of nutrients, particularly minerals. Thus, it is extremely important to include sea vegetables in the daily diet, as they provide the essential minerals our bodies need. Some, such as arame and hiziki, are bland and make colorful additions to vegetable dishes. Others are stronger in taste, such as the more detoxifying kelps, and cooked best with legumes.

All sea vegetables are very cooling and Dampening in nature, particularly the kelps, yet therapeutically they soften lumps and masses in the body.

Nuts and Seeds

When combined with grains, nuts and seeds provide all needed amino acids to form a complete protein. However, and this is a BIG however, nuts and seeds are highly concentrated foods high in fat, which in excess easily stagnate Liver Qi, causing PMS, tight neck and shoulders, depression, moodiness, anger, irritability, stress, headaches and gallbladder pains, just for starters. Because they are so rich, most should be eaten infrequently and even then in moderation, like a condiment.

The only exception I've seen is walnuts, since they tonify Kidney Yang, thus supporting Liver Qi. Walnuts, (and almonds), are also roborants (thus building the body and increasing weight). A couple tablespoons of walnuts each day can treat chronic weakness of the lower back and joints and lung weakness. Peanuts make

ENERGY OF NUTS AND SEEDS

HOT	WARM	NEUTRAL	COOL	COLD
	Walnut	Almond		
	Pinenut	Sesame seed		
	Chestnut	Peanut		
		Sunflower seed		

delicious stir-fries and sauces, and help circulate Blood. In general, you can consume more seeds, such as sesame or sunflower, than nuts. Sesame seeds are a great tonic food that can be added to dishes as gomasio, a Japanese condiment (see Recipes later in this chapter).

Fruit

Rich in vitamins and minerals, but lacking in protein, fruit has a neutral-warm, neutral-cool or cold energy and an empty quality. Fruit is best eaten locally grown and in season, and better digested and assimilated when eaten baked, stewed, sauced, or cooked, with **cinnamon**, **ginger** and/or **cardamom** and **walnuts** added to make it less cooling. Additionally, include a little pro-

tein on the side to balance its higher glycemic (blood sugar raising) effects.

Meat eaters should regularly include fruit (of different colors) in their diets to eliminate Heat toxins, acidity and Excess. Young children (who naturally have more Internal Heat) also benefit from moderate fruit intake on a daily basis with occasional use of juices (be sure to add a dash of **ginger**, **cinnamon** or **cardamom** and dilute it by half with water to lower its concentrated fruit sugar). Excessive intake of fruit juices, however, contributes to children's runny noses, coughs and diarrhea.

Vegetarians should moderate fruit intake and only eat it cooked and with spices and protein. Excess fruit

ENERGY OF FRUIT

HOT	WARM	NEUTRAL	COOL	COLD
	Cherry	Fig	Apple	Banana
	Date	Grape	Lemon	Mango
	Peach	Loquat	Lime	Watermelon
	Coconut milk	Papaya	Pear	Cantaloupe
	Guava	Plum	Strawberry	Grapefruit
	Kumquat	Raspberry/blackberry	Tangerine	Star fruit
		Blueberry	Orange	Melons
		Olive	Mandarin orange	Persimmon
		Coconut meat		Mulberry
		Pineapple		
		Apricot		

thins the Blood and creates Dampness, causing anemia, weakness, scanty menses, fatigue, poor digestion, weakness, lowered immunity, diarrhea, frequent and recurring colds and flu, mucus, chronic asthma and other lung problems, low back pain, sciatica, impotence, infertility, nasal drip or runny noses and many other ailments. This is especially true of fruit juices, which are highly concentrated. Few people could eat the eight or more carrots or apples it takes to make a glass of juice, plus the important fiber is lost, which aids in the fruit's digestion. Thus, keep juices to a minimum, dilute them and add spices to aid in their digestion.

While eating fruit and protein together is generally considered poor food combining, many who experience gas, bloatedness, runny nose, diarrhea and abdominal cramps after eating fruit alone do not experience these symptoms when intaking fruit with a protein (try cottage cheese). Further, these folks feel more satisfied, don't get blood sugar peaks and drops, or hypoglycemia, and their energy is sustained longer.

FATS

Perhaps the most misunderstood food group is fats. Many people run from fats, fearing they cause weight gain, high cholesterol and heart disease. Yet fats are not only unharmful to the body, they are essential to protein metabolism and mineral absorption, and are the primary fuel warming your body and providing energy to your muscles. They also slow carbohydrate release and keep your appetite satisfied for hours.

What is most important about fat is *quantity* and *quality*. Slow-burners, A, AB and some B blood types, and those living in warmer climates need less fat. Fast-burners, O blood types and those living in colder climates need more fat. In terms of fat quality, be sure to consume only organic fats, as chemicals and pesticides are concentrated in fats. Further, there are three types of fats: saturated, unsaturated and transfats and not all of these act the same in the body.

Saturated fats, solid at room temperature, are found in meat, dairy, lard, beef tallow, and coconut and palm kernel oils. They provide good sources of stored energy for the body, insulate vital tissues against the cold, provide fat-soluble vitamins and enhance immunity. The problem related to saturated fats has more to do with their excess consumption rather than the fats themselves. Many saturated fats are hidden in restaurant foods, fast foods and highly processed and frozen foods.

There are two types of *unsaturated fats*: monounsaturated and polyunsaturated. *Monounsaturated fats*, solid at cold temperatures, include canola oil, olive oil, peanuts, almonds, cashews and avocados. They metabolize quickly and can increase weight gain because the body mostly uses saturated fats for energy. (Olive oil, ghee, or clarified butter, and sesame oil are monounsaturated fats that don't go rancid.)

Polyunsaturated fats are found in fish (salmon, mackerel, halibut), vegetable oils (sunflower, safflower, sesame) and botanicals (**borage**, **evening primrose**). These fats rapidly go rancid from heat and light, and should be used quickly, or refrigerated in dark containers.

It is from the polyunsaturated fats that we obtain *essential fatty acids* (**EFAs**)—once known as vitamin F. There are two types of EFAs: omega 3's and omega 6's. *Omega 3 oils* come from flax, chia and pumpkin seeds, **walnuts**, canola oil, seaweeds and cold-water fatty fish such as salmon, sardines, butterfish, tuna and anchovies. *Omega 6 oils* come from plant sources such as unprocessed, unheated vegetable oils (safflower, sunflower, corn and sesame), botanicals (**borage**, **evening primrose**), and saturated animal fat (choose free-range organic meats because drugs concentrate in animal fat). While omega 3's and 6's each have individual functions, both are necessary for health and should be taken in equal amounts rather than one over the other.

Transfats, "modern" manufactured oils, are hands down the most harmful fats for your body. They include hydrogenated and partially hydrogenated vegetable oils shortening, margarine and soybean oil. The manufacturing process of transfats strips the original oils of their EFAs, creating a chemical makeup closer to plastic. Subsequently, these fats cannot be broken down in the body, but are stored in fat tissues (like the breasts), eventually leading to such diseases as cancer, obesity, diabetes, heart disease, depressed immunity and the formation of free radicals (causing wrinkles, age spots and tumors for starters). Transfats are commonly found in commercial as well as health foods, such as breads, crackers, chips, cookies, rolls, muffins, cakes, pies, donuts, pre-prepared packaged foods and most restaurant foods. Read labels for hydrogenated oils and avoid margarine, whether from butter, vegetable or soy sources.

In excess, most fats create Heat in the body, particularly in the Liver and Gallbladder, causing hypertension, PMS, depression, headaches, insomnia and a propensity toward anger and irritability. Those with Liver Heat or stagnant Liver Qi should only use small amounts of saturated fats. Nuts, nut butters, avocados and tahini all have a very high fat content and should be eaten infrequently and in small amounts. The best fats include olive oil, sesame oil and ghee (clarified butter). These are natural sources of important vitamins and minerals. Not only do olive oil and ghee not go rancid, ghee has the added energetic quality of sparking metabolic fires without adding unwanted Heat.

Now before you shy away from fats altogether, remember the problem is not with fats themselves, but with the quantity and type. We do need fat with every meal, but most of us don't need more than $1/4$–$1/2$ teaspoon, depending on our dietary needs. In fact, fat is needed to lose fat! Those who lose body fat from reducing food fats in their diet usually do so because they were eating excess fats to begin with.

However, those who don't eat fat, or only low fat, may ultimately gain weight. If there is not enough fat in the diet, then protein can't be properly metabolized and the unsatisfied body tells the brain to keep eating. This is the reason most people cannot stay on low-fat diets and eventually develop other health problems, such as mineral deficiencies. Fat is essential for mobilizing stored fat out of the body; thus, some fat in the diet is necessary for reducing stored body fat.

FERMENTED AND CULTURED FOODS

Fermented and cultured foods are extremely important, not only for digestion, but also for health and well-being. These foods are partially predigested, making them easily digested and assimilated. The fermentation or culturing process further adds invaluable enzymes back into the food, which provide nutrients and assist digestion. These foods also supply friendly bacteria to the digestive tract. Thus, fermented, cultured, pickled, leavened and sprouted foods are the best substitutes for raw, "live" vegetables and juices.

Most traditional cultures have a fermented or cultured food with every meal. For example, yogurt is traditionally eaten in India, sauerkraut in Germany, kimchi in Korea, cultured dairy products in Scandinavia, miso and umeboshi plums in Japan, and pickled fruits and vegetables in many countries. Choose the fermented or cultured products that most closely match your ancestral heritage.

An easy recipe is to chop enough vegetables to fill a mason jar $3/4$ full. Place cut vegetables in a bowl and mix with 3 tsp. salt and 2 Tblsp. whey (make yourself by

FERMENTED AND CULTURED PRODUCTS

Fermented		Cultured		
Umeboshi plum	Sauerkraut	Yogurt	Sour cream	Cheese
Pickles	Kimchi	Cottage cheese	Clabber	Curds
Pickled vegetables	Pickled rinds	Yogurt cheese	Kefir cheese	Kefir
Chutney	Pickled fruit	Crème fraiche	Cream cheese	Whey
Pickled grape leaves	Relishes	Koumiss	Longfil	Buttermilk

straining yogurt through cheesecloth overnight, catching the liquid—this is the whey—if you don't add whey, add 4 tsp. salt). Toss mixture well, stuff into mason jar and pack down. Screw on lid and let sit unrefrigerated for 3 days, turning once a day. Then refrigerate and eat small amounts with every meal.

EXTREME FOODS

There are several other foods worth discussing here since they frequently comprise a large percentage of most diets: sugar, salt, alcohol and caffeine. Tobacco, although smoked and not eaten, is still ingested and, since its effects are severe and serious, it's also included here. Ingesting any of these extreme foods usually sets up a craving for the other and creates an endless cycle. For example, after eating sugar for awhile, the body craves salt and vice versa. Yet this type of "balance" is extreme, like the seesaw described in *The Energy of Food*.

Processed **sugar** causes Stomach Heat with accompanying forehead headaches, gum problems, dry lips, mouth sores and bad breath, among other health issues. As well, sugar over-tonifies the Spleen, eventually leading to digestive problems, poor energy and a big stomach (sugar expands the abdomen).

Refined white sugar is an empty food that leaches important vitamins and minerals (such as calcium) from the body, depletes the immune system by half and feeds infections. As well, white sugar causes muscle cramps and spasms and makes it difficult for the body to hold alignment (because it weakens the Kidneys). If that were not enough, it also gives an energy boost so you skip eating when food is actually what your body needs. Excessive sugar intake also causes salt cravings.

Many people are amazed at how good they feel simply by eliminating sugar from their diets. Those with strong sugar cravings generally eat insufficient amounts of protein. Rarely do I tell someone to stop eating sugar. Rather, when people increase protein, grains and legumes in their diets, their sugar cravings quickly disappear.

Whole sugars, such as maple sugar, honey, barley and rice malts and raw unrefined sugar cane, are healthier choices, though they should be used sparingly since they are empty foods. Fructose metabolizes more slowly than other sugars and so is frequently used in health foods. Yet, fructose is bleached and so should be eaten more sparingly. Agave metabolizes slowly, too, perhaps even more so than fructose (Native Americans traditionally use cactus sweeteners like

ENERGY OF EXTREME FOODS

HOT	WARM	NEUTRAL	COOL	COLD
	Coffee	Honey	Green tea	Salt
	Tobacco	White sugar		Sugar cane
	Vinegar			
	Wine/alcohol			
	Brown sugar			
	Malt/maltose			
	Molasses			
	Chocolate/cocoa			
	Black tea			

agave with no problems, but quickly develop diabetes on refined white sugar). Thus, agave is one of the best sweeteners to use.

Salt is cooling and softening in nature. A little salt tonifies the Kidneys, but in excess it causes water retention and subsequent edema, high blood pressure and other problems. Ideally, use unrefined sea or earth salts because they are high in minerals. Alternatively, use gomasio, a combination of sesame seeds and salt (see Recipes at the end of this chapter). When the seeds are ground, their oil coats the salt particles, thus metabolizing the salt directly into the cells and preventing water retention. Excessive eating of salty foods causes sugar cravings.

Alcohol, **caffeine** and **tobacco** all cause Heat and irritation, particularly in meat eaters. In vegetarians, alcohol, caffeine and tobacco can provide the Heat the body craves since it is usually fed a very cooling diet. This quite often makes it much more difficult, if not impossible, for vegetarians to quit smoking tobacco and drinking coffee without a diet change, even more so than meat eaters. In addition, because of its sugar content, alcohol creates the same sugar swings and addictions as sugar does (this is why it goes so well with a meat diet), and it is quite Heating to the Liver and depleting to the Kidneys. As well, alcoholic beverages cause stagnant Blood, which can be seen as a purplish discoloration on the nose and cheeks of alcoholics or heavy alcohol drinkers.

Caffeine drains energy reserves from the adrenals to create a temporary sense of well-being. Drinking coffee to push through tiredness ultimately leads to adrenal exhaustion, which is very difficult to replenish (bags under the eyes are one impending sign of this). It may take years for adrenal exhaustion to show up, and then suddenly take you by "surprise." Coffee is especially harmful this way and becomes a "catch-22" of needing coffee to wake up while at the same time it makes you tired (the adrenal exhaustion). If you can drink coffee after 5 PM and it doesn't affect your sleep, worry about it! This means your adrenals aren't responding and well on their way to exhaustion. (See the chart, Caffeine Contents, for specific foods and how much caffeine they contain.)

While not containing caffeine, **chocolate** contains theobromine and **maté** contains mateine, both of which energetically act like caffeine by creating Liver Heat and depleting Kidney Qi, Yin and Yang. Further, when eaten excessively, chocolate causes toxins in the Liver, which generally show up as skin outbreaks. Perhaps the only caffeine exception is green tea, which is Cooling and Drying in energy rather than Heating and Dampening. It clears Heat from the Liver, is anti-tumor and anticancer and has the lowest caffeine content of all caffeinated substances.

To get off caffeine, drink a beneficial coffee substitute, such as **dandelion/chicory** "coffee" made from 1

CAFFEINE CONTENTS[2]

SUBSTANCE	CAFFEINE IN MG.
Drip coffee (7 oz.)	115-175
Jolt (12 oz.)	100
Espresso (7 oz.)	100
Iced tea (12 oz.)	70
Instant coffee (7 oz.)	65-100
Tea, brewed, imported (7 oz.)	60
Mountain Dew (12 oz.)	58.8
Coca-Cola (12 oz.)	45.6
Tea, brewed, U.S. (7 oz.)	40
Diet Pepsi (12 oz.)	36
Cadbury Chocolate Bar (1 oz.)	15
Hot cocoa mix (one envelope)	5
Decaf coffee, brewed (7 oz.)	3-4
Jello Pudding Pop (47 g.)	2

[2] From seas.upenn.ed/~epage/caffeine/FAQmain, copyright 1994 by Alex Lopez-Ortiz.

part dandelion root with 1/2 part roasted chicory root (to prevent caffeine withdrawal headaches, slowly reduce the caffeine while proportionately increasing the dandelion/chicory coffee). Grind the herbs like coffee beans and put in a filter or percolator. The resulting tea is dark, full bodied and bitter in flavor, satisfying all coffee needs but the taste. Yet, it does exactly the opposite of coffee: it clears Heat, Dampness and toxins from the Liver and helps the Kidneys to filter fluids.

Alternatively, try drinking grain drinks, green tea or herb teas to eliminate coffee. The longest I've seen it take people to regain their true energy after quitting coffee is about a month. Until that time, you may experience more tiredness than before, but keep going, for the results are well worth it. Once caffeine is eliminated from the diet, you'll not only feel more energy, but also notice that it is of better quality and clarity than you ever felt while on caffeine.

Tobacco injures the circulation because it constricts blood vessels. It also robs the cells of their much-needed oxygen supply, causing a weakening of cell functions throughout the body and injuring the Blood. Further, it causes wrinkles, lung mucus and a husky voice, not to mention all sorts of cancers. To get off tobacco, smoke herbal cigarettes, gradually reducing the amount over time. As well, take 2-3 drops of **lobelia** tincture when cravings arise, ingest 2-4 caps 3 times daily of a lung decongesting formula (such as equal parts **mullein**, **coltsfoot**, **chickweed**, **horehound**, **loquat** and **grindelia** or **yerba santa**) and eat a piece of honey-soaked **ginseng** (slice ginseng root very thinly and "marinate" in honey) periodically throughout the day.

Water is worth mentioning here because it, too, can cause disease when taken improperly. Often the brain is unable to distinguish between the need for water and the need for food. Most people are under-hydrated rather than over-hydrated and so need to drink more water. Most meat eaters crave iced water because it seemingly offsets their thirst, which is caused by the Internal Heat and acids created by excessive red meat eating. Yet iced water is one of the largest contributors to weakened digestion.

Imagine throwing iced water on a fire and the resulting steam and eventual extinguished fire. The same occurs in the stomach where digestive fires must be kept continually burning. If doused by iced water, the results are gas, bloatedness, lethargy, forehead headaches, drippy and stuffy nose, postnasal drip, ulcers and poor digestion among other ailments. Thus, drink water warm, or at room temperature.

The average meat eater should have a minimum of 6-8 glasses of pure water daily to dilute and flush meat toxins from the body and uric acid from the blood (it also relieves chronic pains in the joints and lower back). For those who eat little or no meat, less water is needed, from 4-6 glasses a day, because vegetable foods have higher water content. Excessive drinking of water causes frequent urination, while too much carbonated water creates gas, bloatedness, hiccuping, poor digestion, dizziness, spaciness, lethargy and poor bone formation. Further, excess water intake in vegetarians can cause Dampness and overwork the Kidneys, thus weakening them.

SUPPLEMENTS

While herbs are whole food-like substances, supplements are concentrated components extracted from whole foods and synthesized in laboratories. Taking extensive amounts of vitamins, minerals, body-building substances, energy boosters and other similar products have strong actions that over time, can imbalance the body. While many people are familiar with excess vitamin C intake causing diarrhea, most do not know that prolonged excessive intake of supplements creates toxic Heat and stagnation in the body, in time causing many health issues. In fact, minerals are best absorbed by the body in their whole organic form, i.e., in food.

Taking a multivitamin or mineral supplement can be useful over a short period of time (several months), yet prolonged intake of these and/or other supplements is not a substitute for good food and proper nutrition. In time, health issues arise, not to mention digestive problems, such as gas, bloatedness, diarrhea or constipation, headaches, poor appetite and low energy.

Supplements create a false environment—they are not the body's true energy. Only use them short term as an aid and support while getting your diet, rest, sleep and general life back on track (unless, of course, you are dealing with serious health issues that need such supplementation). Using herbs to obtain your desired vitamins and minerals can also cause problems because herbs have many other uses that may not be appropriate for you. For instance, while **nettle** is high in iron, it's a diuretic and while **goldenseal** contains vitamin C, it's drying to the Blood and very cooling, all of which actions may not be suitable for your particular body.

FOOD THERAPY

Food can be used therapeutically to heal disease by following its inner warming or cooling nature. A body with Excess Heat can be balanced by eating more cooling foods and less heating ones. A body with Excess Coldness can be balanced by eating more warming foods and less cooling ones. Thus, it's important to tailor your diet according to any disease or imbalance you're experiencing, along with taking the proper herbs. Known as food therapy, this not only enhances the healing process, but usually speeds it up as well. In contrast, eating improper foods can actually drain your healing energies and prolong illness.

To use food therapeutically, first determine if your condition is one of Coldness, Heat, Dampness, Dryness, Excess, or Deficiency as outlined in *The Energy of Illness*. Then create your food plan accordingly. If the plan is to maintain existing good health, then follow the balanced diet outlined under the section A Balanced Diet, earlier in this chapter.

More specifically, when treating an illness of Heat (feeling irritable, thirsty, always hungry, sweating easily and always feeling warm), it's important to eliminate foods with a hot energy, eat only a few with a warm energy and focus more on neutral, cool and a small amount of cold energy foods. Eat mostly cooling foods until the illness is healed and the body is brought back to balance. Then a balanced diet should be adapted, for otherwise, the continued eating of cooling foods (salads, raw foods, fruit juices, etc.) over time creates the opposite energy in the body: Coldness.

It is not uncommon for someone with too much Heat from excessive meat eating to adapt a vegetarian or raw foods diet and feel great for awhile. Yet, upon continued eating of these foods, Coldness is created several years later, eventually causing emaciation, lowered immunity, fatigue and a feeling of coldness. Thus, it is very important to always come back to a balanced diet once the illness has healed.

When treating an illness of Coldness (frequent colds and flu, lowered immunity, runny nose, tiredness, weakness, diarrhea, poor appetite and/or feelings of chill and cold), eliminate all cold foods, eat some cool foods, but only in cooked form, and focus more on balanced, warm and some hot energy foods. This means eating only cooked foods and eliminating all raw foods, salads, fruit and vegetable juices and anything directly out of the refrigerator or freezer. Along with the cooked foods, more concentrated protein and warm-natured foods should be ingested with every meal three times a day, including animal protein such as beef, fish, pork or chicken. In time, adding more warming foods and meat into the diet makes vegetarians feel great again. When the illness is healed and the body brought back to balance, adapt a balanced diet, for if these foods are eaten to excess over a few years, then problems of Excess Heat and stagnation can eventually arise.

In general, vegetarians must eat much more strictly to regain and maintain balance in the body. This means ingesting only cooked foods, including sufficient protein with every meal, and cooking food with spices such as cumin, coriander, **garlic** and onions to warm and spark digestion. Further, vegetarians with O type blood and/or northern European ancestry have even less leeway and absolutely need adequate protein 3 times/day to maintain health.

The following categorizes foods according to their energies and effects in the body.

DIGESTION-IMPAIRING FOODS

- Sugar
- Refrigerated/frozen foods and drinks (iced drinks, frozen yogurt, ice cream, popsicles)
- Excessive intake of raw foods, including salads
- Excessive intake of flour products (breads, pasta, chips, cookies, crackers, pastries, etc.)
- Fruit; fruit and vegetable juices
- Potatoes (in excess)
- Excessive and prolonged intake of supplements
- Insufficient protein and nutrition

OVERLY HEATING FOODS

- Turkey
- Lamb
- Nuts and nut butters
- Alcohol
- Caffeine (coffee, black tea, cocoa, colas, maté, chocolate)
- Fried, fatty and greasy foods
- Hard cheeses
- Vinegar
- (Plus: tobacco smoking)

OVERLY-COOLING FOODS

- Refrigerated/frozen foods and drinks (iced drinks, frozen yogurt, ice cream, popsicles, etc.)
- Raw foods, including salads
- Most fruit and vegetable juices
- Melons
- Bananas
- Crabmeat and shellfish
- Soymilk, tofu

ACIDIC FOODS

- Flour products (breads, pasta, chips, cookies, crackers, pastries, etc.)
- Red meats
- Grains (except millet, barley, amaranth and quinoa)
- Citrus (except lemons and limes)
- Tomatoes
- Green bell peppers
- Sugar

ALKALINIZING FOODS

- Umeboshi plums
- Lemons, limes, grapefruit, cranberries, blueberries
- Millet, quinoa, amaranth, barley, white rice

DAMPENING FOODS

- Flour products (breads, pasta, chips, cookies, crackers, pastries, etc.)
- Bananas, citrus, persimmon
- Cucumber, plantain, olives, seaweed
- Raw foods, including salads
- Wheat, wheat gluten, oats, potato
- Refrigerated or iced foods and drinks
- Dairy (cheese, milk, sour cream, cottage cheese, etc.)
- Honey
- Frozen foods, such as yogurt, ice cream, popsicles
- Salt
- Potatoes
- Fruit and vegetable juices
- Excessive intake of fruit
- Soymilk, tofu and other soy products
- Goose, oyster, clam, pork, duck

DRYING FOODS

- Adzuki, kidney and mung beans
- Asparagus, celery, carrots, cabbage, lettuce, dark leafy greens
- Barley, rye, millet, quinoa, rice
- Tuna, chicken, lamb
- Berries

WIND AGGRAVATING FOODS

Avoid if there's arthritis, rheumatism, asthma, or any other patterns with Wind:

- Shrimp
- Prawns
- Crab

- Lobster
- Spinach
- Rhubarb
- Mushrooms
- Caffeine
- Alcohol

FOODS THAT STRENGTHEN OR WEAKEN EACH ORGAN

Each food has a special affinity for a specific Organ. When eaten in moderation, it strengthens that Organ, but weakens it when eaten to excess. The following lists foods according to the Organs it strengthens or weakens.

SPLEEN STRENGTHENING FOODS	SPLEEN WEAKENING FOODS
Protein (all proteins, especially beef)	Insufficient protein and nutrition
Cooked foods	Excessive intake of raw foods, including salads
Warm/room temperature drinks	Refrigerated foods and drinks
Root vegetables	Iced drinks
Winter squash	Frozen yogurt, ice cream, popsicles
Rice, quinoa, barley, amaranth, buckwheat, millet; peanuts; tofu	Excessive intake of flour products (breads, pasta, chips, cookies, crackers, pastries, etc.)
Spices (garlic, cumin, ginger, black pepper, etc.)	Excessive hot, spicy foods (ex. salsa)
Soups	Excessive intake of vegetable juices
Congees	Excessive intake of potatoes
Peach, apple, mango, papaya, loquat; cook fruit with spices	Excessive intake of fruit and fruit juices
Beets, cabbage, carrot, yam, sweet potato, potato, string beans, peas, winter squash, lotus root	Excessive intake of supplements
Small amounts of whole sugar, especially malt	Excessive intake of sugar, especially white, refined
LUNG STRENGTHENING FOODS	**LUNG WEAKENING FOODS**
Black beans, tofu	Dampening foods
Rice	Digestion-impairing foods

(continued on next page)

LUNG STRENGTHENING FOODS *(continued)*	LUNG WEAKENING FOODS *(continued)*
Almonds, walnuts, peanuts	Citrus
Pear, loquat, tangerine, olive	Dairy
Garlic, onions, black pepper	Flour products
Duck, chicken	Raw foods
Warm foods and drinks	Cold refrigerated and/or iced foods and drinks
Water chestnuts, mustard greens, carrot, lotus root, asparagus, radish	Cigarette smoking
KIDNEY STRENGTHENING FOODS	**KIDNEY WEAKENING FOODS**
Adzuki beans, kidney beans	Raw foods
Pork, duck, lamb, oyster	Alcohol
Asparagus, celery, sweet potato, string beans, parsley	Caffeine (coffee, black tea, cocoa, colas, chocolate)
Black sesame seeds	Refrigerated foods and drinks
Grapes, plums, raspberry, strawberry, black cherry, blueberry, tangerine	Excessive intake of fruit and fruit juices; sugar and sweets
Millet, wheat	Insufficient protein and nutrition
Seaweeds; salt	Excessive protein intake (prolonged high-protein diets)
Walnuts	Marijuana and similar recreational drugs
Sufficient protein	Iced drinks
	Frozen yogurt, ice cream, popsicles
LIVER STRENGTHENING FOODS	**LIVER WEAKENING FOODS**
Mung beans, garbanzo beans	Alcohol
Beef liver, oysters, pork	Turkey
Vegetable juices	Fried, greasy and fatty foods
Carrots, beets, celery, tomato, seaweed	Avocados; nuts and nut butters
Dark leafy greens (collards, kale, bok choy, **dandelion**, chard, spinach), **burdock root**	Caffeine and caffeine-like substances: coffee, black tea, cocoa, colas, chocolate, maté)
Lemons, loquat, plum, raspberry, strawberry, mulberry, watermelon	Cheese
Oats; black sesame seeds	Chips of all kinds

(continued on next page)

LIVER STRENGTHENING FOODS *(continued)*	LIVER WEAKENING FOODS *(continued)*
Shiitake mushrooms	Excessive intake of vinegar
Vinegar in small amounts	Excessive intake of oils
Essential fatty acids	Recreational drugs
	Cigarettes
	Mega doses of vitamins
	Environmental chemicals
	Synthetic drugs
HEART STRENGTHENING FOODS	**HEART WEAKENING FOODS**
Mung beans, adzuki beans	Fried, greasy and fatty foods
Lamb	Excessive red meat intake
Amaranth, rye, wheat	Alcohol
Cherry, papaya, watermelon	Hard cheeses
Burdock root, lotus root, eggplant	Insufficient protein and nutrition
Dark leafy greens (collards, kale, bok choy, **dandelion**, chard, spinach)	Caffeine (coffee, black tea, cocoa, colas, chocolate)

FASTING

Fasting is a good way to rapidly change the body by voluntarily throwing it into imbalance so it can reintegrate at a higher level. However, to be effective and strengthening, it must be tailored to your body's unique constitution and current imbalance for, like diet, there is no one fast best for everyone. In general, those with Excess benefit most from fruit juice fasts and can fast longer, while those with Deficiency benefit from a kicharee fast (see Recipes at the end of this chapter), and should fast for short periods only.

Know that fasting is not necessarily a comfortable process. It is not unusual to experience irritability, headaches, dizziness and lack of focus. Yet, after a day or so when the body becomes accustomed to the fast, these symptoms disappear and, in its place, a new inner calm and evenness occurs, signifying that the body is healing. In time, depending on the length and frequency of a fast, deeper levels heal, and past acute and chronic diseases resolve (see Healing Crisis in *The Process of Healing*).

In many cases, no other therapy works as well to overcome disease as an organized fast. Yet, like anything, one can become addicted to fasting and actually feel a certain high from metabolic excretions called ketones. Therefore, one must practice moderation. Fasting to excess can also damage the body's ability to properly digest solid food.

Coming off a fast is as important as the fast itself. It should be ended gradually, taking an equal amount of time to end the fast as was spent on it. For example, after a three-day fast it should take three days to build to a regular diet. During this time, eat easy to digest foods, such as warm vegetable broth, watery grains, soups, oatmeal or rice cream, and then slowly add steamed vegetables and more grains. Lastly, add in animal protein, if ingested, and return to a balanced diet.

Nervous or unfocused people may have more trouble fasting because food is grounding. These folks should incorporate meat broth or a little fish in their fasts. Others who have a fast metabolism may experience excess stomach acids. Take herbs to neutralize the acids (and digestive enzymes) by drinking this fasting tea: steep equal parts **violet** leaves (**gotu kola** or **chickweed** may be substituted), **chicory** or **dandelion** and $1/4$ part each **black peppercorns**, **anise seed** and **rose petals**. Strain and mix with equal parts milk. Add honey to taste.

Fast for those with Excess conditions: Drink only fruit or vegetable juices for 3-10 days, choosing according to your needs. For example, apple juice opens the channels, cherry juice eases arthritic, rheumatic complaints and gout and a combination of carrot, celery, beet and **parsley** juices detoxifies the Liver.

Here is a sample four-day fast: Every day for the first three days drink three 8-ounce glasses of fresh-squeezed apple or vegetable juice mixed with 1 tsp. agar seaweed flakes (agar replaces the loss of important minerals and binds with toxins to efficiently remove them from the body). Include $1/2$–1 tsp. **cayenne** pepper with 1 Tblsp. olive oil, three times daily. Also take 2 tablets or 1 tsp. **Triphala** powder (Formula #95 or 97) three times daily to cleanse and regulate the bowels. On the fourth day, continue with the olive oil, cayenne and Triphala, but eat a light vegetable broth. On the fifth and sixth days, eat steamed vegetables and a light soup or rice porridge. On the seventh day, return to a balanced diet.

Fast for those with Deficient conditions: Individuals who are thin or malnourished should generally not fast, but build their bodies with solid nutrition. However, upon occasion it can be beneficial for those with Deficiency to fast, although never on just water or juices. Instead, fast on kicharee (see Recipes at end of this chapter) for 3-4 days to promote detoxification without overly depleting the body. Be sure to soak rice and mung beans for 12 hours and (ideally) cook in organic chicken stock. To come off the fast, gradually add in vegetables and dark leafy greens, then vary the beans and grains. Lastly, add in some animal protein and return to a balanced diet.

WHOLE FOODS

Regardless of the energies of food, there is a big difference between whole (healthy) foods and disease-causing foods. Whole foods are those that come directly from nature with the least possible interference. This means they are unrefined and preferably organic (and ideally from animals given free-range and humane treatment). As well, we should ideally consume foods that are locally grown, limiting those that come from far away. Brown rice, maple syrup, earth salt and organic vegetables and meats are examples of whole foods.

On the other hand, disease-causing foods are highly refined with additives, preservatives, hormones, chemicals and/or colorings added. Refined white rice, white sugar, table salt, flour products and prepared packaged foods are examples of processed, disease causing foods. The chart Whole Foods, suggests healthy foods to eat and unhealthy foods to avoid.

Unfortunately, many chemicals, additives and preservatives are hidden in food. For instance, MSG is a known irritant that causes skin rashes, headaches, nausea, palpitations, insomnia, hyperactivity, depression, panic attacks, migraines and asthma for starters. Yet, MSG is hidden in many forms, such as hydrolyzed vegetable protein, natural flavors and natural flavorings, autolyzed yeast, sodium or calcium Caseinate and more. Thus, get in the habit of reading labels and researching "foreign" names.

In today's mass-produced food market, most every stage of development is negatively affected in some way. Fruits and vegetables are hybridized to grow bigger and faster and are subjected to plant hormones, insecticides and chemical fertilizers to increase production. Unfortunately, this sacrifices flavor and enhances the potential of disease. Animals are force-fed, given massive amounts of antibiotics, and subjected to extremely inhumane treatment, all to increase production. The result is toxicity and lowered immunity in those who eat these foods. Thus, get in the habit of reading labels and shopping selectively. There are plenty of healthy alternatives available. Eating whole foods according to a balanced energetic diet is eating to maintain strength, health and disease prevention.

Further, more and more foods are genetically manufactured organism (GMO), completely mixing different food chemistries together in order to prolong shelf life, resist pests and enhance other commercial purposes. European countries, such as the U.K., strictly forbid all GMO foods while in the U.S. these foods are slipped past an unsuspecting public because no legal requirements exist for their labeling. In fact, most soy is now genetically manufactured, including that widely used in health foods.

How foods are cooked affects their quality as well. Never use aluminum pots and pans as aluminum is toxic, contaminates food and causes disease, such as Alzheimer's. Glass, stainless steel and ceramic containers are best for cooking food. As well, use gas or wood heat, as electric heat is fine for strong bodies, but for those with lowered immunity and severe or degenerative disease, it can alter the food enough to interfere with the healing process. Microwaves should ideally never be used. They rearrange the molecular structure of the food, altering the electromagnetic field of its atoms and making the food something different than nature created. Microwaved food doesn't cook evenly and even tastes strange to some.

WHOLE FOODS

HEALTHY FOODS	UNHEALTHY FOODS
Whole, organic grains	White sugar
Organic legumes	White flour
Vegetables, especially organic	White bread and other flour products
Sea vegetables	"Junk foods"
Sea or earth salts	Refined (table) salt
Fermented foods	Additives; preservatives; artificial colorings
Organic fruit in season and cooked (if needed)	Chemicals in foods (MSG, etc.)
Small amounts of whole, organic dairy	Soda pop
Sufficient organic protein for your body's needs	White sugar
A little sea or earth salt	Tobacco
A little honey, maple or grain syrups, or whole unrefined sugar cane	Caffeine (coffee, black tea, maté, cocoa, chocolate)
Very small amounts of red wine or beer	Larger amounts of alcohol
	Genetically manufactured food (GMOs); irradiated food

Ideally, eat foods within two days after being prepared. After 24 hours food quickly looses energy and nutrients, while molds start growing, even though they can't be seen. Thus, prepare food as freshly as possible. The best methods for food preservation include cold storage (refrigeration), drying, salting, fermenting, pickling and smoking. Only freeze foods with low water content to prevent cellular deterioration caused by water turning to ice. Eat canned foods only sparingly, as many nutrients are lost in the canning process (foods must be cooked at very high temperatures to create a vacuum and resulting hermetic seal, killing important nutrients).

HEALTHFUL EATING ROUTINES

How food is eaten and prepared also contributes to health or disease. These and other cooking/eating routines are discussed at length in the section Health and Healing Routines, in *The Process of Healing*. However, the most important thing to remember is no matter what or how you eat, be *fully* present with your food and give thanks for it. When you do this, you'll digest it better and become more aware of *what* and *how* you're eating.

KITCHEN TIPS

Those with busy lifestyles (probably most of you!) may feel overwhelmed at first with this diet change. To heal disease, regain health and maintain wellness, however, an appropriate energetic diet is absolutely essential. Old habits die hard, yet new ones can actually be formed fairly quickly with attention and intention. Give yourself two to four weeks of focused energy on your dietary changes and needs. Afterward, it'll be much easier and slip into your lifestyle as new habits. Following are several tips to aid this process.

Plan Ahead

Always think of what must be done for the next three meals. For instance, put grains and legumes on to soak and marinate meats a day in advance. Prepare your evening meal in the morning (try a Crock-Pot) so it's ready after a busy afternoon. Plan meals several days ahead so you can shop for what you need only once or twice a week.

Crock-Pots

Although cooking with electricity is not ideal, Crock-Pots are so convenient and useful, I recommend them. It's an easy way to prepare meals, soups, stocks, beans, breakfast and dinner with little time and effort. Ingredients are put into the pot at night for the next morning, or in the morning to be ready for dinner. Turn pot on high, medium or low, depending on length of time available/needed to cook its contents.

Meal Ideas

Breakfast: Throw away all your whole-grain boxed cereals even if organic and start your day with oatmeal, multi-grain cereal, soup, congee, kicharee (see Recipes at end of this chapter), or even leftover dinner. Side proteins can include eggs, sausage, Canadian bacon, tempeh or cottage cheese, or if necessary, whey protein powder, for instance.

Lunch: Heat up leftover dinner, kicharee (see Recipes at end of this chapter) or soups. If traveling away from home, put in wide-mouthed thermos or warmth-holding food containers (pickled and fermented foods do not need refrigeration and can be kept in a drawer at work). Sandwiches also travel well.

Eating out: Ethnic restaurants usually offer the most nutritional and balanced meal choices, such as Chinese, Indian, Japanese, Korean, Indonesian, Middle Eastern and Malaysian. Avoid fast-food restaurants.

Condiments

Add condiments to every meal to aid digestion and impart flavor and color. This is very important, not only to the taste of food, but its desirability. Try **garlic** powder, kelp powder or dulse flakes, miso paste, umeboshi plum paste (instead of salt), **ginger** powder, tamari, Bragg Liquid amino acids, yeast flakes and varied spices.

Enzymes

Include a little fermented, cultured or sprouted food with every meal. These aid digestion and provide invaluable nutrients, especially when eating mostly cooked foods. See Fermented and Cultured Foods listed earlier in this chapter. To make your own, refer to the *Bibliography* for a book with recipes.

Meat

Many cookbooks teach how to cook meat (see *Bibliography*). Roasting is also an excellent and simple method. Cook all meat with **ginger** to aid digestion of meat and prevent toxin buildup.

To detoxify chicken and other poultry before cooking: remove skin, rub salt (rock salt is best) over chicken for one minute, rinse, then cook with ginger.

To detoxify red meat before cooking: rub with salt (rock salt is best) one minute, then soak in water for ten minutes to remove the blood. Cook with ginger.

RECIPES

Kicharee

This wonderfully balancing food detoxifies, yet supports. It makes a good fast for all body types, though it may be eaten as a meal any time. Vegetables may be added or eaten on the side. Vegetarians and O blood types benefit from cooking the rice and mung beans in meat stock, or adding meat on the side.

To make: soak and cook 1 cup rice and $1/3$ cup mung beans separately. Brown 1 tsp. **turmeric** powder, 1 tsp. **cumin** seed and $1/2$ tsp. **coriander** powder in 2 Tbsp. ghee (or sesame oil). Mix all together. Add water to make soupier, if desired.

Congee

Congee, called *jook*, is a well-cooked soupy grain or for-tified porridge. A very therapeutic food, it's perfect during convalescence from sickness, for treating acute diseases, strengthening digestion and assimilation and alleviating general debility and low vitality. Congee gives strength and energy to the whole body and helps those who can't digest carbohydrates or keep food down. Traditional Chinese families serve congee to the whole family on a weekly basis, varying herbs according to weather and health needs to enhance immunity, strengthen digestion and prevent illness.

Congee is made with a grain, usually rice (or $1/2$ part rice and $1/2$ part barley or **coix**), water and your chosen herbs. It is then cooked a long time over low heat, which slowly and thoroughly breaks down the grain so it's extremely easy to digest and assimilate. Thus, the body gets the most nutrients possible, perfect for weak digestion, those who are ill, convalescing, or needing strength and vitality. Ideally enamel, clay, glass or good quality stainless steel pots are used in making congee. Don't use aluminum, iron or water-soluble metal pots. A Crock-Pot may also be used. Vary herbs to satisfy your current health and healing needs. In a pinch you can use herbal tablets instead of fresh herbs.

Basic Morning Congee Recipe

(Four servings)

6 cups water
1 ounce herbs
1 cup rice, or $1/2$ cup rice and $1/2$ cup coix
    or pearled barley

Combine all ingredients and cook in Crock-Pot for 8-10 hours, or in glass-covered dish in 250 degree oven for 4-6 hours. If congee consistency is too thick, add water to thin. Include honey, as desired.

Gomasio

Gomasio, or sesame salt, is a great way to include small amounts of salt in the diet. When made, the salt crystals are coated with sesame oil, aiding its quick assimilation into the body's cells while preventing water retention. Gomasio also provides a good source of calcium to the diet and is beneficial to the heart.

To make: separately, dry toast sesame seeds and sea salt in pans. Then grind 20 parts sesame seeds with 1 part sea salt in a surabachi, nut and seed grinder, food processor, or blender. Bottle a small amount and leave on table; refrigerate the rest. Yellow sesame seeds are typically used; **black sesame seeds** are best for tonifying Yin.

Ghee

Ghee, or clarified butter, is the oil *par excellence* because it sparks digestive fires without creating Heat, as do most other oils. Further, it doesn't go rancid and so needn't be refrigerated.

To make: melt 1 lb. *unsalted* butter in a pan over low heat. Periodically scrape foam off surface. When golden and clear, pour through sieve into container.

Dark, Leafy Greens

Include $1/2$–1 cup of dark, leafy greens (collards, kale, bok choy, mustard, **dandelion**) per day in your diet.

To cook: wash, chop and blanch (boil) greens in 1-2″ water for 5 minutes. Drain, set aside and add miso to greens' water to create an additional nutritious drink or broth. Add lemon juice to greens to make the iron more available, top with a little olive oil or salad dressing, if desired, and make these vibrant greens your daily "salad" rather than raw foods.

Stocks

Stocks have been used worldwide for a very long time. They are extremely nutritious and easily assimilated. Use them for soups, grains, beans, stir-fries, and cereals and to flavor other meals. Stocks are excellent for vegetarians. They supply highly assimilated nutrients and protein not found in vegetarian food. Cook all beans and grains in stocks to increase flavor and nutrition. Stocks can be made in bulk (easily done in a Crock-Pot) and stored until needed. They keep several months in the freezer (pour into ice cube trays).

To make: prepare stock by stuffing a large pot full of bones. Add any vegetable peelings and eggshells (saved in freezer). Add water, covering bones by 2-3 inches, and $1/4$ cup vinegar to pull minerals out of bones. Add whole cut vegetables (such as onions, carrots and celery) and herbs (if desired). Cook in a Crock-Pot, or simmer on stove, for 12-72 hours, removing dirty foam for first two hours or so. Strain, then cool soup overnight. Skin off fat the next morning, then pour resulting stock into pint-sized mason jars or ice cube trays. Refrigerate and/or freeze.

Bones to use: ribs, knuckle, meaty shanks, oxtail, lamb, beef, pork and/or chicken bones, wings, backs, breastbones, necks, whole fish carcasses and heads.

Cooking Beans

All beans need picking through for stones and washing before soaked and cooked. At cooking, add a strip of kombu or other seaweed for minerals and to aid digestion.

Hard beans, such as adzuki (adzuki), black and garbanzo beans, must be soaked 12-36 hours to neutralize phytic acid (and other antinutrients) and increase protein content substantially (or otherwise it prevents protein absorption). Beans also cook more evenly and prevent gas formation. Cook 2 hours.

Softer beans, such as lentils, split peas and dahls, should be soaked 3 hours, then cooked 30-60 minutes.

Cooking Grains

Pre-soaking grains 12-48 hours increases protein content six-fold (a USDA-published fact). It also neutralizes their phytic acid content (and other antinutrients), which otherwise inhibits protein absorption, and they become more digestible and increase in protein content substantially. Try mixing various grains together. The following is a table of grains and their cooking specifics.

GRAINS

1 CUP GRAIN	CUPS WATER	COOKING TIME	YIELD
Amaranth	3	45 min.	2½ cups
Barley, hulled	2½	1 hr.	3½ cups
Barley, pearled	2	30 min.	3 cups
Buckwheat groats	2	20 min.	2½ cups
Couscous	1	20 min.	1½ cups
Millet	2½	30 min.	2 cups
Oat groats	2	1-2 hr.	2½ cups
Polenta	4	20-25 min.	3½ cups
Quinoa	2	15 min.	2½ cups
Basmati white rice	2	15 min.	3 cups
Basmati brown rice	2	45 min.	3 cups
White rice	1	15 min.	3 cups
Brown rice	2	45 min.	3 cups
Wild rice	3	1 hr.	4 cups
Rye berries	2	45 min.	3 cups
Teff	4	15 min.	2½ cups
Wheatberries	2	1½ hr.	2 cup
Bulgur wheat	2	20 min.	2½ cups
Kamut and Spelt: follow directions on package			

CHAPTER 10
Living with the Seasons

Without fail, when a season changes, I frequently see people present with similar symptoms. While fall and winter are obvious times for these to appear, the seasons and their changes constantly affect us, no matter the season nor where we live. Even in extreme hot or cold climates there are seasonal differences with distinct qualities and traits. Coping with these changes can be difficult for some of us. Not adjusting well to each season's differences lowers resistance, creating sickness. The ancient Chinese have long acknowledged how seasons affect health. In fact, each season is associated with particular aspects of nature, climate, Organs, emotions, foods, activities, energies and ways to dress. By knowing these, we can learn their unique opportunities and discover how to balance the extremes of each season's energy.

Our well-being is connected with nature. The seasons' energies, qualities and traits affect all our eating, dressing and lifestyle habits. When we adjust our life patterns to match these seasonal influences, we promote health and enhance our quality of life. For instance, herbs that cool and eliminate toxicity from Blood and Organs are most appropriate to use during the spring and summer; others that warm and build strength and energy specifically support the body through fall and winter. Living according to the seasons in this way is an ancient wisdom still alive in the Orient.

In China, traditional people cook weekly soup, differing herbs according to the current weekly weather patterns. They do this in part based on the Chinese theoretical system called the Five Phases (refer to *The Energy of Illness*), a type of "user's guide" for living in balance through the seasons. The elements and Organs describe not only the ailments most likely to arise in each season, but also give clues as to what foods, herbs and lifestyle habits support health at those times. When we follow the "way" of each season, we maintain balance and protect our inherited constitutional energy, or Essence.

The TCM concept of Essence is extremely important here as it determines our constitutional strength and thus our individual potential for withstanding disease. Constitutional Essence can be likened to an inherited trust fund. The trust fund can be supplemented with deposits of good food and healthful lifestyle activities. On the other hand, eating poorly, skipping meals, staying up late, or overdoing it physically, mentally or sexually withdraws from our trust funds.

Eventually, the bank sends us overdraft notices in the form of frequent colds and flu, headaches, menstrual problems or other health issues. If we don't focus and take care of ourselves, we ultimately bankrupt our trust funds and experience chronic degenerative disorders, immune system diseases or adrenal exhaustion, for instance. Unfortunately for many, this is the only way the body can get our attention so we start caring for ourselves. Because some of us receive large trust funds of Essence and others smaller ones, how quickly an overdraft occurs differs for each of us.

THE SEASONS AND THEIR CORRESPONDENCES

Element	WOOD	FIRE	EARTH	METAL	WATER
Yin Organs	Liver	Heart	Spleen	Lung	Kidney
Yang Organs	Gallbladder	Small Intestine	Stomach	Large Intestine	Urinary Bladder
Season	Spring	Summer	Indian Summer	Autumn	Winter
Opens To	Eyes	Tongue	Mouth	Nose	Ears
Sense	Sight	Speech	Taste	Smell	Hearing
Fluid	Tears/bile	Sweat/blood	Lymph/saliva	Mucus	Cerebral spinal fluid/sexual secretions
Body Part	Tendons	Pulse	Muscles	Skin/body hair	Bones
Emotion	Anger	Overexcitement	Melancholy, worry	Grief	Fear
Sound	Shouting	Laughter	Singing	Sobbing	Groaning
Color	Green	Red	Yellow	White	Black/dark blue
Taste	Sour	Bitter	Sweet	Pungent	Salty
Activity	Looking	Walking	Sitting	Reclining	Standing
Climate	Wind	Heat	Damp	Dryness	Cold
Manifestation	Nails	Complexion	Lips	Body hair	Head hair
Time of Day	11 PM to 3 AM	11 AM to 3 PM; 7 AM to 11 AM	7 AM to 11 AM	3 AM to 7 AM	3 PM to 7 PM

Diet and herbs are the most important supplements to our trust funds. Remember that your digestion can be likened to a pot of soup bubbling about 98-99 degrees on the stove (refer to *The Energy of Food*). Food digesting easily in this soup pot is cooked and warm in temperature. Excessive amounts of hot foods, either from a high temperature, or a heating energy (such as greasy or oily foods, hot spices or lamb) cause the soup pot to suddenly boil and splatter. On the other hand, surplus intake of cooling foods, such as iced drinks, frozen treats (ice cream, frozen yogurt, popsicles), iced drinks and foods with a cooling energy (melons, bananas, soymilk, seafood and salads) stops the soup pot from bubbling.

Thus, you need the right fuel to keep the soup pot bubbling and the fires stoked. When the body easily digests and assimilates foods, it supplements your trust fund with beneficial energy. When digestion is poor or sluggish, the body withdraws Essence in order to meet its daily demands. All the methods used for living harmoniously with the seasons focus on maintaining effective digestion and a strong trust fund of Essence.

Tips for staying healthy through the seasons:

↪ Take your environment into account. Use foods and herbs following the different seasonal lengths and influences where you live. For instance, if you reside in New York, continue using winter herbs until the weather warms your area, even though summer temperatures heat Florida.

(continued on next page)

❧ Consider your unique needs. Pay attention to your body's needs regardless of the season. If you feel cold in summer, for example, avoid cooling summer foods such as cucumbers, watermelon and raw foods, since these weaken digestive energy and cool metabolic fires.

❧ Keep moderation in mind no matter the time of year. Although activity in summer and rest in winter are best at these times, too much of either can respectively cause burn-out or stagnation.

❧ Prepare one to two seasons ahead to get results in the next. If you tend to get sick in fall, drink a fall immune tonic tea during late summer. If you fall prey to spring illnesses, exercise more in winter and start spring cleansing teas during late winter.

❧ How well you take care of yourself in one season influences how you feel the rest of the year. For instance, if you tend to get ill in winter, you may have over-indulged in cooling foods the prior summer, or been excessively active. It is possible to improve your health that winter by following a winter diet and using building winter herbs, yet to prevent the same winter illnesses recurring again, it's necessary to take care of yourself in summer and fall to plan for the coming winter.

❧ Avoid sudden changes in temperature. In winter use clothing and exercise to stay warm rather than indoor heat. In summer, wear a sweater or vest in air-conditioned rooms. The more extreme temperature differences between outdoors and indoors, the more it stresses your immune system, making you susceptible to colds and flu.

❧ Eat what is locally grown as much as possible. This assures your diet is seasonally appropriate and adjusts your body chemistry to the climatic conditions where you live. Doing so adapts your body to local pollens and grasses better, helping prevent seasonal allergies.

❧ Although ailments may occur any time of year, they're aggravated during particular seasons.

SPRING

Spring is the beginning of the year, when the earth awakens and new life bursts forth. It's a time of planting seeds, physically and mentally. This season stirs the uprising of vital energy; just as sap begins to rise in trees, so our inner fire stirs and ascends in spring. The hint of new growth surges through us, moving us out of winter's cocoon with renewed vitality. It's time now to shake off any excess or sluggishness developed during winter. This is the key to spring: cleansing.

The Chinese associate spring with the Wood Element and its Organs, the Liver and Gallbladder. A healthy Liver is like a young sapling growing strong, yet flexible, flowing and rooted. Thus, the Liver controls the smooth and even flow of Energy and Blood. This is nurtured by the trust fund energies in the Kidneys, just as a tree (the Wood Element and Liver) is nourished by water (the Water Element and Kidneys). The Liver also stores and replenishes Blood, a function similar to a Western understanding of the Liver. Spring is the time to cleanse the Blood and Liver, and to regulate our habits and activities.

Spring Ailments: If spring winds invade, or stir Internal Wind, they cause tension, stiffness, spasms, tics, clumsiness, numbness, headaches, allergies, convulsions, itching, skin conditions and pains which change severity and location. The Liver then becomes congested, resulting in anger, frustration, irritability, stiff neck and shoulders, hypertension, PMS, depression, mood swings and irregular menstruation. People who feel worse in spring often have congested livers.

Those who experience red face and eyes, irritability, propensity to outbursts of anger, dizziness, dry mouth, splitting headaches or migraines, insomnia, thirst and constipation at this time of year have Excess Heat in the Liver, or Deficient Liver Yin. Prolonged ingestion of caffeine (including coffee, black tea, cocoa, colas and chocolate), alcohol, sugar, fried, fatty and greasy foods, dairy, nuts and nut butters, turkey, avocados, chips, cheese and spicy foods causes this condition. It is further aggravated when the Kidney's trust fund is depleted from prolonged over-activity (mental, physical or sexual) and insufficient food or protein to sustain that activity.

To balance Spring's energy, eat plenty of dark leafy greens, such as collards, kale, mustard, and chard, as these cleanse the Blood and Liver. Include other greens naturally growing at this time, such as watercress, lamb's quarters, **malvae**, **chickweed**, **nettle**, purslane and **dandelion**. Add lemon juice (to make iron more available from the greens and clear Liver Heat) and an oil high in GLAs, such as flaxseed oil (which supports normal liver function). Ingest white meats (except turkey, which "Heats" the Liver) instead of red, legumes, a large variety of cooked vegetables, some fresh fruit and whole grains. Use grain drinks, green tea or **dandelion** tea instead of coffee for energy, and **chamomile** tea in place of alcohol to relax.

Others may experience Dampness and Heat in the Liver this time of year, with symptoms of nausea, jaundice, vaginal discharge and itching, migraines, headaches, redness and swelling of the scrotum and frequent urinary infections. Dampening and Heating foods help cause these conditions, such as caffeine (including coffee, black tea, cocoa, colas and chocolate), alcohol, sugar, fried, fatty and greasy foods, dairy, nuts and nut butters, turkey, avocados, chips, cheese and spicy foods. Further, if the digestive soup pot is injured from prolonged intake of Cold and Damp foods (iced foods and drinks, juices, raw foods, salads, soymilk and flour products) then Dampness accumulates and impairs the Liver function.

These folks should eat plenty of protein from white meats (except turkey) and legumes, a large variety of cooked vegetables and dark leafy greens (collards, kale, mustard, **dandelion** and chard) and a small amount of whole grains. Avoid all cold, raw, greasy, damp foods and iced drinks and foods. Drink herb teas or green tea, and eliminate caffeinated substances and alcohol.

Many may experience symptoms of pain in the sides and chest, depression, moodiness, frustration, anger, PMS, swollen breasts before periods, irregular menses, nausea, belching, poor appetite, alternating diarrhea and constipation, abdominal distension and lumps in the neck, breast, groin or sides this time of year. Due to stagnant Liver Energy, these are caused by a sedentary lifestyle and lack of exercise, long-term stuffed or repressed emotions, unexpressed creativity and/or weakened Kidneys and/or excessive intake of Liver-congesting foods.

Physical movement and exercise are extremely important to moving stagnant Energy. Moderate your habits and balance your focus between inward and outward activities. Set routines for eating, sleeping and exercising and keep them with regularity. Alternate work with rest and play. Discover creative outlets and actively pursue them, yet pace yourself. Use appropriate channels to express pent-up emotions.

Go to sleep by 11 PM, as the Liver peaks between 11 PM and 3 AM (you'll actually feel more rested than if you went to bed later and got the same hours of sleep). Directing the Liver's energy into other activities during these hours diverts it from cleansing and renewing the Blood, causing tiredness, toxicity and stagnation. Following the dietary guidelines for a Damp and Heated Liver above, as these protect the digestive soup pot and nourish the Kidney's trust fund, both of which support the Liver.

If you start dressing and eating as if it were summer instead of spring, or inadequately exercised during winter, then you'll more easily experience colds and flu now. Although your internal body heat is moving toward the surface, there is still sensitivity to cool air, so remain wrapped up outdoors. This is the windy season, and External Wind blows colds and flu into the body at the back of the neck. Wear a scarf until it warms up. Likewise, refrain from eating cold foods and drinks (iced drinks and foods, juices, raw foods, salads, soymilk). Continue eating cooked foods, including beef, pork, chicken and eggs, to help your body adjust to temperature changes. Add in a large variety of cooked vegetables, dark leafy greens, some whole grains and cooked fruit with spices.

Spring Herbs for Balance: Gently stimulating herbs with pungent, bitter or sour tastes are particularly good for spring. Sorrel, **dandelion**, **nettles**, watercress and other young green leaves provided by nature now are perfect balancing foods for the liver as they cleanse the blood and release toxins. Dandelion, **gentian**, **barberry**, **sarsaparilla, turmeric, chamomile, isatis, burdock, yellow dock** and **gardenia** cleanse the liver and bowels and strengthen digestion. **Bupleurum**, **fennel** and **green tangerine peel** regulate Liver energy, as **lycii** and **dang gui** build Liver Blood. **Milk thistle** is particularly good for spring allergies, while an antiviral tea of 1 part each **dandelion root**, **forsythia** fruit and **isatis** leaf quickly clears spring colds and flu.

Fasting, the traditional ritual of spring, cleanses the Blood and assists the Liver in releasing stored toxins and winter's accumulated fat (see section Fasting, in *The Energy of Food*). A good liver fast combines 8 ounces each water and apple juice with 1-4 cloves **garlic** and 1-4 Tblsp. olive oil. Take each morning on an empty stomach for four days. Follow with tea decoction of equal parts **fennel** seeds and **dandelion** root. If appropriate for your body, also fast on warm apple juice and green vegetable juice, and take 1-2 "00" capsules **cayenne** powder 1-3 times daily. Alternatively, eat spring kicharee for four days (or add into your regular diet): make kicharee (see section Recipes, in *The Energy of Food*), adding shiitake mushrooms, burdock root, carrots and dark leafy greens. Season with lemon juice.

SUMMER

Summer is the essence of life, growth, heat and activity. Not surprisingly, the Fire Element and its Organs, Heart and Small Intestine, correlate with summer. With the sun at its zenith, nights are short and days are long. Our energy is expansive now, flowing outward to act on the plans and seeds sowed in spring. Similarly, the body's heat, or "inner fire," starts rising close to the surface, cooling us inside. We are motivated now to pursue sports, gardening, yard work, hiking or other outdoor activities. We feel compelled to get things done, work and socialize. With increased heat, circulation and joy (the Heart's emotion), we generally feel more optimistic, find it easier to work on relationship issues, and experience increased sex drive.

Because our fires are closer to the surface, we can easily overheat through overexposure to the sun, heated environments, or hot-natured foods. Lighter, easier to digest foods are appropriate now, such as fruit, salads, grains and legumes. Red meat should be kept at a minimum, if eaten at all.

Summer Ailments: People with Excess Heat often feel worse in summer and are generally tired, sluggish and easily overexcited or impatient in hot environments. Many are easily prone to heat exhaustion, headaches, arthritis, colds, allergies, hypertension, chest pains and palpitations. Eating too many hot, spicy, greasy, fried foods, red meats, alcohol, sugar, or caffeine, or smoking tobacco, aggravates these symptoms. Instead, eat fresh vegetables, salads, fruits, legumes, white meats, mung beans, watermelon, soybean sprouts and room temperature herbal teas.

Drinking excessive amounts of cold and iced drinks causes Stomach Heat (any season) with headaches across the forehead, bad breath, bleeding gums, ravenous hunger, extreme thirst (especially for cold drinks), constipation, nausea, vomiting, sour regurgitation or mouth ulcers. In fact, iced drinks taken with fatty or fried foods causes cholesterol, according to the Chinese, because cold drinks "encapsulate" fat, making it indigestible and turning it into fatty deposits in the blood vessels. Although we like iced drinks in the West, they also ultimately create this Heat because the body has to increase metabolic warmth in order to digest them. People who live in hot climates mostly drink hot teas and eat spicy foods since these make the body sweat, ultimately cooling it.

Other people eat excessive amounts of cooling foods in summer, such as salads, raw foods, iced drinks/foods, juices, smoothies, melons, soymilk and excessive fruit. Since these cool the digestive soup pot, in excess they cause poor digestion and assimilation, resulting in undigested food in the stools, gas, bloatedness, sleepiness after meals, low immunity, weakness, tiredness, nausea, loose stools, or diarrhea. Thus, if you tend to feel cold, even in summer, limit intake of cold foods, eat all cooked foods, add spices (such as **ginger** and **cardamom**), increase protein (such as red and white meats) and drink warm herbal teas. Balance fruit intake by eating its seeds (like watermelon) or a piece of its peel (these are ancient Asian secrets to "keep the doctor away").

While the fiery energy of summer pulls us into activity, we need to guard against overactivity and over-excitement, as these injure the Heart, deplete our trust fund's energy reserves and rob our bodies of their vital Essence needed the rest of the year. If we experience low energy now, it's often because we didn't rest sufficiently during winter, or were overly active. Tiredness, exhaustion and "burn-out" result, particularly if we go from dawn to midnight, accomplishing many different tasks, socializing more, working out a lot, skipping meals and snacking instead, having more sex and fitting in vacations, house repairs and yard work with everything else.

Summer is actually the time to protect your energy, especially for those who already have low energy. Thus, rest during the hotter hours of the day (this is siesta time in many countries), pace yourself, delegate, prioritize, moderate activities and exercise, and eat three regular meals daily. Take **eleuthro** to enhance endurance and immunity.

Dressing in summer seems easy—the fewer the clothes the better. Yet, regularly baring midriffs exposes the Kidneys and abdomen to Coldness, ultimately depleting Essence and metabolism, respectively. Those who frequently feel cold should maintain body heat by covering up on cooler summer days. Air conditioning can lower immunity and cause colds or chills, especially if kept too high, or if indoor/outdoor temperatures differ extremely. If air conditioning is a must, keep at a higher temperature to more closely match that of the outdoors, and wear a sweater.

Summer Herbs for Balance: The cooling and drying qualities of the bitter taste strengthen the Heart and Small Intestines and eliminate excess fluid and cholesterol from the blood. Spicy herbs, such as chilies and curries, open the pores and create perspiration to cool the body. Herbs such as **mint, lemon balm, chrysanthemum, hibiscus, red clover, violet** leaves, **honeysuckle,**

borage, rosehips and **green tea** also cool the body and make refreshing summer drinks. **Hawthorn** and **longan,** because they nourish the Heart, are good now as well. Don't take **ginseng** or other strong warming tonics during summer (unless you're weak) because they're too heating and stagnating now, potentially causing headaches, chest pains, stomachaches, or excessive thirst and sweating.

LATE SUMMER

Many climates throughout the world have five seasons— late summer, or Indian Summer, is usually the fifth. Associated with the Earth Element, it's a time of stability and rootedness, qualities that nourish and balance so we withstand the changes of upcoming fall. At this time, we are fully assimilating our year's experience from the initial planting to its full growth, associated with the Spleen and Stomach, which rule digestion and assimilation. The quality of late summer is transformation, symbolic of digestive functions and our shift from warming spring and summer into cooling fall and winter.

Late Summer Ailments: Dampness easily occurs now (as seen externally in monsoons or heavy, late summer rains), causing digestive problems, diarrhea, fluid retention, lethargy, gas, bloatedness, cough, allergies, poor appetite, malnutrition or weight gain in late summer and mucus in fall. Use general tonic herbs now to strengthen and improve digestion and follow diet, herbs and lifestyle activities for fall. The sweet taste (Earth Element) strengthens digestion and includes complex carbohydrates and protein. Add more of these foods along with plenty of vegetables into the diet now. As fall is around the corner, it is best to limit intake of juices, salads, fruit and raw foods.

Late Summer Herbs for Balance: Herbs that are sweet and strengthen the Spleen's digestive functions include **ginseng, codonopsis, dioscorea** and **fu ling.** Other beneficial herbs at this time are **hawthorn, licorice** and carminatives such as **citrus peel, cardamom** and **ginger.**

FALL

In the fall, we harvest the fruits and labors of spring's planting and planning. Shorter days and cooler nights send the surface fires into the body. Just as many people harvest bounty from their gardens to stock up for coming winter, it's time now to pull back from multiple summer activities and store energy in your trust fund reserves. Similarly, change the diet to warming foods to protect strong digestive fires for the cold winter to come.

This is the time to discriminate and separate out what is needed from what isn't. The ability to receive, or take in, and to release the unnecessary is attributed to the Metal Element ruling the fall, with its corresponding Organs, the Lungs and Large Intestine. Change and old age represent this, and when we don't release the old or accept changes, we experience grief and sadness. The Lungs open to the nose and control breathing and the skin, including the opening and closing of pores, while the Large Intestine rules elimination.

If Lungs are weak, or you overindulged in cooling summer foods or overactivity, then excessive mucus now builds in the Lungs, impairing their breathing function. Asthma, bronchitis, allergies and other lung ailments also result and often kick up at this time of year. Since the Large Intestine and skin eliminate what is unnecessary, skin eruptions and constipation often show a toxic condition of the body or suggest an overactive life. Colon purification and mucus elimination from the Lungs (letting go!) are beneficial now. On the other hand, air is dry in fall and can injure the Lungs since they need a certain amount of lubrication to protect against inhaling dry outer air. If dryness invades the Lungs or Large Intestines, then dry coughs, stuffy nose, sinus infections, constipation or dry stools can result.

Fall Ailments: I find people have more difficulty adjusting to fall than any other season. Although evenings are cool, the warm days entice us into enjoying any remaining good weather. We continue to eat summer's cooling foods (watermelon, salads, ice cream, iced drinks, raw foods and juices), dress lightly (few clothes, exposed necks, arms and midriffs) and live as if summer still exists (continuing at summer's hectic pace, adding in night school while still working eight-hour days and gardening afterward). Thus, people experience colds and flu now more than any other time of year. As well, shortness of breath, chronic sinus infections, stuffy nose, nasal drip, mucousy coughs, asthma and other upper respiratory diseases, chapped lips, dry skin and skin diseases often occur.

Even though days are warm, remember your body's energies are moving inward to store for the coming winter. Support your immunity by stopping all cooling foods and eating only cooked food and warm drinks, adding in spices such as **garlic**, **black pepper** and **ginger**. Also limit intake of sugar as it depletes the immune system by 50%. Layer your clothes so you stay warm or cool as needed. Cover your neck with a scarf, even if it's warm outside, as fall winds are cool (colds and flu invade the body through the back of the neck, the area most vulnerable to Wind). However, when it warms up, take off a few layers so you don't lock summer's heat in, as this leads to coughs with fever.

Begin reigning in your energy - slow down and let go. Do yogic breathing exercises regularly as they strengthen the Lungs (see section Breathing Exercises, in *Home Therapies*), helping protect from respiratory problems. Warm your abdomen and lower back with moxibustion, and on cooler nights, sleep with a hot water bottle over these areas. If you keep windows open at night, make sure they aren't near your bed to prevent waking with stiff neck and shoulders.

Eat more warming foods now. Eliminate juices and raw foods and have salads less frequently as these cooling foods are inappropriate for fall and winter. Excessive intake of cooling and dampening foods (greasy foods, flour products such as breads, muffins, pasta, cookies, pastries and chips, raw foods, juices and frozen foods and drinks, dairy) cause coughs or upper respiratory diseases, especially in fall. Eating all cooked food, root vegetables, winter squash, barley, rice, spices such as **garlic**, **ginger** and **black pepper**, increased protein and roasted foods support Lung functions and alleviate Dampness. Cook seasonal fruit and add **ginger**, cinnamon or cardamom to prevent mucus formation. For dry coughs, cook pears with some whole sugar and eat.

Fall Herbs for Balance: Spicy herbs like **garlic** and **black pepper** clear Lung mucus, as do expectorants such as **elecampane**, **mullein**, **coltsfoot**, **mulberry** root bark, **platycodon**, **wild cherry** bark and **loquat**. Herbs that strengthen immunity, such as **astragalus**, support Lung function and help prepare the body for winter. A good fall immune tonic, called *Jade Screen*, is made of 1 part **astragalus**, $1/2$ part **white atractylodes** and $1/4$ part **sileris** (Formula #4). It helps the Lungs regulate the opening and closing of the pores, keeping Wind from invading and preventing colds and flu, chronic coughs and runny noses.

Other fall herbs moisten the Lungs to protect against Dryness, such as **black sesame seeds**, **marshmallow** and **ophiopogon**, and the Intestines to prevent constipation (**flaxseeds**). **Grapefruit seed extract** is extremely effective for sinus infections so prevalent now. Take 10-15 drops liquid, 3 times daily, internally and use the nasal spray several times a day (both forms may be purchased at health food stores).

WINTER

Whether you live in tropical Hawaii or frosty Minnesota, the energy of winter is the same: storage. At this time, winter's cold drives your life fires deeply inward, collecting itself like a hibernating bear for the coming spring. Winter is the time to retreat and go within to replenish your reserves. The Water Element rules winter, associated with the Kidneys, Adrenals and Bladder. These regulate fluid metabolism, bone health, reproduction and the endocrine system. They also store the deep inherited constitutional energies of the body. Thus, strengthening the Kidneys helps maintain and protect a healthy trust fund.

Winter gives us cues to follow: the sun sets early and rises late. With less sunlight and colder weather, we naturally stay inside more. It's time to stoke you inner furnace, to rest, nourish and replenish your trust fund

energies spent throughout the prior year. Conserve and preserve your resources, essence and energy in winter; it is not a time for extravagance.

Winter provides us with the opportunity for inner reflection, assessing the past year and learning from our experiences. Exhaustion at this time is more harmful than during any other season, even though the consequences may not be felt until later in the year when the energy you expect to have isn't there. When Kidney energy is low, fear (the Kidney's emotion) can become a year-round problem that intensifies in winter. Now is the time to protect your vital constitutional energy and metabolic fires. Doing so helps prevent winter's imbalances and keeps you well throughout the entire year.

The Kidney is a unique organ in Chinese medicine. Although its element is Water, which is cooling, it also has a fiery aspect that's linked to the adrenal, hormonal and reproductive processes. Too much cold can injure the Fire quality, just as too much heat can harm the Water aspect. Those with coldness usually dread winter. Likewise, those who overly expended energy in summer, or who ate inappropriately then and in the fall, also feel cold in winter.

Winter Ailments: People who feel worse when winter arrives often fear the cold. Usually they have chilly hands and feet, sit hunched over, experience lower back pain, urinate frequently, have a groaning and gravely voice and look pale with dark circles under their eyes. They may even experience a sense of insufficiency or fearfulness, and lack the will or determination to follow anything through.

Those who continue eating cold foods in the winter (iced drinks/foods, juices, raw foods, salads, soymilk) not only impair their digestive soup pot and metabolic fires, but also create Coldness in the body. This engages the immune system to maintain body warmth: extra work means a taxed system and, therefore, the body becomes more susceptible to illness. Symptoms then arise, such as feeling cold all the time, fear of the cold, frequent urination, cold and sore lower back, lowered sex drive, nighttime urination, weakness, tiredness, poor immunity, frequent colds and flu, joint aches and pains, digestive problems, cold hands and feet, depression and poor memory.

Pay careful attention to the energy of food and herbs in winter. The outside cold drives the body's heat deep inside and food and herbs should be taken to reinforce and support this. Spicy foods, like salsa and curries, seem warm but are used in hot climates to induce perspiration, which takes heat out of the body.

Instead, now is the time to eat all cooked food to aid digestion, free energy in maintaining vigor and immunity and add heat to the body to keep our inner fires burning strong. Include plenty of protein and foods that warm the body and strengthen the Kidneys, Blood and Energy, such as lamb cooked with **dang gui** and **ginger**, oxtail or bone marrow soups, pork and beef, root and leafy green vegetables, adzuki and black beans, roasted buckwheat, winter squash and walnuts. Instead of juices, eat small amounts of cooked fruits, especially berries, adding spices like **cardamom**, **ginger** and **cinnamon** for digestion, or drink hot apple cider with these spices. Cook food with warming spices such as onions, **garlic**, **ginger**, cumin, **fennel**, basil, **fenugreek** and **parsley**.

Vegetarians especially need to guard against the cold energies of winter, as vegetarian diets tend to create Coldness in the body. Increase your protein intake, eat only cooked foods, liberally use spices in cooking and forego juices, fruit, salads, tofu, soymilk, raw and cooling foods and iced drinks/foods.

Salty is the Water element taste. A little salt and herbs high in mineral salts, such as seaweed and **nettles**, can be added to teas, grains and soups to help Kidney energy. Too much salt, on the other hand, causes water retention. A salt craving often indicates weak Kidneys/Adrenals.

Dress warmly to maintain body heat: wear plenty of clothes, cover your head outdoors and don scarves and warm socks. Be sure to keep your low back warm, too, as the waist is the site of the Kidneys and your life fires. Jackets and clothing should be long enough to cover this area completely (bare midriffs invite sickness and, in women, menstrual problems later in life). Alterna-

tively, use moxibustion over your abdomen and low back and put a hot water bottle in these areas while asleep. Likewise, keeping hot temperatures indoors creates tiredness and sluggishness, and stresses the body when we go outdoors through the temperature extremes. Therefore, keep the heat down indoors to more closely match the temperature outside and dress warmly instead.

On the other hand, excessive use of hot tubs and saunas to get warm in winter actually causes more Internal Coldness because you loose valuable inner heat through sweating. Guard against further heat loss by taking cool showers, going into the cold plunge or rolling in the snow after hot tubs and saunas to push heat back into the body (you'll actually feel more vitalized and warm afterwards).

Those who exploited summer's fast pace and full activity may now experience exhaustion, tiredness, weakness, "burn-out", night sweats, nocturnal dry mouth or restless sleep even though you may rest more now. Whether you work late at night, frequently jog in the icy dark, or get caught in the holiday whirl, you withdraw energy from your constitutional trust fund when you most need replenishment. Drinking coffee to push through tiredness depletes the trust fund reserves even further, as does alcohol. Use grain drinks instead of coffee, and warming teas in place of alcohol.

Early to bed, late to rise is the key to winter: slow down and replenish your energy (make deposits into your trust fund). Use the extra quiet time to reflect, dream, share stories around the fire, stay warm and cozy, reflect, meditate, write in your journal and take naps. Include more protein in your diet (this also helps reduce sugar cravings). Continue at a slower pace throughout the year to follow, including summer, so that your trust fund is stronger next winter and you won't experience the same exhaustion.

It's not unusual to experience depression, irritation, or "cabin fever" in winter. While rest is essential in winter, guard against lethargy as this causes your body's energy to stagnate. You'll then seek stimulation, which usually is interpreted as hunger. Turning to food rather than exercise causes unnecessary weight gain and further stagnation, which then results in spring's symptoms. Instead, exercise regularly and pursue creative outlets.

Winter Herbs for Balance: Herbs that internally warm, strengthen and move Blood circulation are specific now, such as **cinnamon** bark, **deer antler**, **fenugreek**, dried **ginger**, **American ginseng**, **elder** flowers and berries, **prickly ash**, **bayberry**, galangal, celery seeds, **saw palmetto** and spices such as dill, cloves and **cardamom**. Continue any immune tonics started in the fall, such as **astragalus** and **eleuthro**. Cook herbs with soups or in food, an excellent way to increase nutrition and strengthen the body's reserves, or decoct as teas. Tinctures, especially those made with red wine, are most appropriate in winter because alcohol has a Heating energy.

CHAPTER 11

Home Therapies

Quite often it is not enough to just take herbs internally. Rather, various therapies are needed as important supplementary healing approaches. These help correct any internal imbalances causing the illness as well as speed the healing process. Folk people and professionals alike continue to use many of these therapies in China, Korea, Japan, Indonesia, India, Malaysia, Turkey, Iran, Iraq, Greece, France and several countries in South American and Africa. Incredibly valuable and effective, these therapies have been employed around the world and by various cultures for thousands of years. Fortunately, you can learn to use them in your own home.

BREATHING EXERCISES: THE FOUR PURIFICATIONS

In Chinese medicine, the Lungs are considered responsible in part for giving the body strength. Associated with air and its essential and vital life-giving properties, breathing exercises strengthen the Lungs and body. The Four Purifications are a set of four different breathing techniques that quiet the mind, tone the lungs, blood, circulation, brain, internal organs and heart, give strength, calmness and energy to the whole body, and purify the nerve channels, stimulating digestion and strengthening the nervous system. Thus, they alleviate such ailments as nervousness, insomnia, indigestion,

lung and breathing problems, poor circulation, low energy and vitality, fatigue, lethargy and poor memory. As such, they are invaluable for helping recovery from many health problems.

For those who have never done any breathing practices, these four techniques are safe to begin. For those already doing their own form of breathing practices, these are a perfect adjunct and starting exercise. Sit quietly with your back straight, either in a chair with your feet on the floor, or on the floor with your legs crossed. You may also concentrate your attention on the space between the eyebrows while doing these exercises. Do the breathing exercises in the order given. After practicing for a few months, move to the intermediate method described at the end.[1]

Alternate Nostril Breathing (Nadishodhana)

Begin by gently exhaling all air. Then close the right nostril with the thumb of the right hand and inhale slowly and deeply through the left nostril. When finished, close the left nostril with the ring finger of the right hand, releasing the thumb, and exhale slowly and fully through the right nostril. Next, immediately inhale

---

[1] The Four Purifications are thoroughly described and illustrated, along with many other valuable breathing and yogic techniques, in *Ashtanga Yoga Primer*, by Baba Hari Dass, Sri Rama Publishing, 1981 (Box 2550, Santa Cruz, CA 95063).

through the right nostril in a slow and steady manner. Finally, close the right nostril with the right thumb again, releasing the ring finger, and exhale through the left nostril. This completes one round. Begin with ten rounds and gradually increase to forty.

This exercise alone is extremely beneficial to the body. It quiets the mind and strengthens the nervous system, inducing a wonderful calm state, releasing nervous tension, anxiety, agitation, anger and other disruptive emotions and inducing better sleep. It also oxygenates the system, enhancing energy and blood circulation and stimulating the proper functioning of all the internal organs. Continued practice of alternate nostril breathing strengthens the lungs and breath control.

Skull Shining (Kapala Bhati)

Skull shining is a series of forced exhalations with the breath. Begin by inhaling quickly and lightly through both nostrils. Then quickly and fully exhale all the breath through both nostrils. Emphasize the exhale, letting the inhalation come as a natural reflex. Repeat this pattern for thirty exhalations, or one round. After each round, which should last no longer than one minute, rest and breathe naturally. Then repeat the round. Begin with three rounds of thirty exhalations each and gradually increase to ten rounds of sixty exhalations each.

This technique purifies the head area, calming thoughts and enhancing breath and mind. As in alternate nostril breathing, skull shining helps release nervous tension, balances emotions and circulates Qi and Blood. It also strengthens the Lungs and breath control.

Cautions: Persons with high blood pressure or lung disease should not practice skull shining.

Fire Wash (Agnisara Dhauti)

Perform this exercise with all air held out of the body. Begin by taking a normal inhalation and exhalation, expelling all air. While holding the breath out, pull the diaphragm up and toward the backbone, and then release it suddenly. Repeat this in-and-out movement rapidly, as long as the breath can be held out without strain,

about thirty pulls. Then inhale *gently*. This makes one round. Start with three rounds, gradually increasing to ten, beginning with thirty pulls per breath and working up to sixty.

This technique strengthens the "navel lock" (frequently used in breathing exercises), creating heat at the navel center (*manipura chakra*) that purifies nerve channels, stimulates digestion, increases gastric fire, strengthens lungs and alleviates indigestion, abdominal diseases and menstrual disorders.

Horse Mudra (Ashvini Mudra)

This fourth exercise is an internal movement of the anal sphincter muscle. Begin by inhaling a complete and full breath and hold it in. Then contract and release the anal sphincter muscle rapidly and repeatedly. Hold the breath only so long as the following exhalation can be slow and controlled. Do not force your breath or length of holding. Begin with three rounds of thirty pulls each, and increase gradually to ten rounds of sixty contractions each. The horse mudra strengthens *mula bandha*, the anal lock, which increases concentration, strengthens reproductive glands and stimulates gastric fires.

Intermediate Method

When you've done the Four Purifications regularly for two to three months and feel comfortable with them, you may begin the intermediate method. In this the Four Purifications are performed with no "resting breaths" in between, that is, they are done consecutively without a breath or rest in between. To perform, do 10-30 rounds of alternate nostril breathing, then after the last exhalation through the left nostril, inhale partially and immediately begin skull shining. At the end of one series of skull shining exhalations, inhale slowly and completely, then exhale all air, hold the breath out and do the fire wash. After one round of the fire wash, inhale completely, hold the breath and do the horse mudra. This entire series now completes one round.

After the horse mudra, exhale completely and immediately begin again with alternate nostril breathing, thus starting the next round. Do five rounds, gradually increasing the numbers of alternate nostril breathing and the duration of retention in each of the other three techniques.

CUPPING

Cupping is an ancient technique that was (and still is in rural areas) widely used as folk medicine by people throughout Europe, the Middle East, South America, Indonesia and the Far East. I have even seen glyphs of cups on ancient Egyptian healing temple walls. Cupping is shown in the movies *Zorba the Greek* and *Dangerous Liasons,* and can be read about in the book *Every Month Was May,* by Evelyn Eaton.

Cupping is the treatment of disease by suction of the skin surface. This is done by creating a vacuum in small jars and attaching them to the body surface. The vacuum draws the underlying tissues into the cups, pulling inner congestion and Heat out of the body. When effective in its job, the skin may appear reddened, or even bruised, after the cup is removed (with no discomfort). This marking can take several days to disappear, yet, relief is immediate and noticeable.

Cupping is done over areas of swelling, pain or congestion, edema, asthma, bronchitis, dull aches and pains, arthritis, abdominal pain, stomachache, indigestion, headache, low back or menstrual pain and places where bodily movement is limited and painful. I have also seen cupping relieve depression, anger and moodiness.

Technique: To do cupping, you'll need several lightweight jars or cups with even and smooth rims. Good cups to use include small votive cups easily found where candles are purchased. Yet, wineglasses or other lightweight and thin glasses or bamboo cups may also be used. "Modern" plastic cups using a plunger to create suction are commonly used today (see *Resources* for obtaining cups). You'll also need cotton balls, tweezers or forceps, rubbing alcohol and matches (you may also use a candle instead of cotton, tweezers and alcohol).

Make sure the person is comfortable and all tools are in place before starting. Then attach cotton ball to tweezers and dip in alcohol. Hold cup so its mouth opening faces down, or the flame will burn your hand. Ignite cotton and while burning with a low to medium flame, insert into downward mouth of cup for about 2 seconds. Then *moving swiftly,* withdraw cotton and place mouth of cup firmly against skin at desired location (if using a candle, hold cup with flame inside cup, just past its rim, for a short time, then *quickly* place on skin). The flame consumes the oxygen in the cup, causing a vacuum when placed on the skin, and suction holds the cup in place. Check by lightly tugging cup to make sure it doesn't release into your hand.

It's important that you don't leave flaming cotton in the cup too long or it'll heat the cup's rim, possibly burning the skin. Conversely, if flaming cotton isn't left in long enough, a vacuum won't occur and the cup will fall off when tugged gently. Practice yields desired results, and it's actually easier to do than it may sound. How you remove the cup is quite important, too. Rather than rip it off the body, first break suction by holding the cup in one hand while gently sliding a finger from your other hand down and under the cup's rim. This breaks the seal and the cup pops off.

My favorite cupping method, native to India, requires a few pennies and some tissue along with the cups. Put one penny in a tissue and twist to form a wick (cut excess tissue, leaving $1/2$ inch). Place wrapped penny on body surface where desired and light. Immediately place cup over wick. Within a second the consumed oxygen extinguishes the flame and underlying skin sucks into cup.

Cups should be retained in place 5-15 minutes, depending on the strength of suction. Especially in hot weather, or when cupping over shallow flesh, the duration of treatment should be short. Often I have seen the cups pop off for no apparent reason. If suction was good in the first place, this generally indicates that suction wasn't needed, or excessive body hair or wrong body angle doesn't allow the cups to hold. Further, several skin marks may occur that can be used for diagnosis: bruising indicates there's stagnant Blood; redness indicates Heat; water bubbles indicate Dampness; and no mark indicates stagnant Qi. Marks disappear within a few hours to several days.

Cautions: Cupping should not be done during high fever, convulsions or cramps, over allergic skin conditions, ulcerated sores, or on the abdomens or lower backs of pregnant women. Cups won't hold over irregular body angles, excessive body hair, or thin muscles.

DERMAL HAMMER

A dermal hammer is an acupuncture tool with a long handle supporting a head of small individual dull needles clustered together. Several needles striking the skin simultaneously cause less pain and stimulate a wider surface area than does a single needle. They are more suitable for use on small children, the elderly and those sensitive to pain or who desire to treat themselves.

Other names for dermal hammers include seven star needle and plum-blossom needle, referring to their number and arrangement of needles (see *Resources* for purchasing dermal hammers). Alternatively, bundling 20 toothpicks together with a rubber band makes a home dermal hammer (although it isn't as effective as the traditional dermal hammer with a springy handle that provides more leverage).

Dermal hammers are tapped *over* local areas of pain, congestion, numbness, hair loss, aches or spasms and *around* (never on) sites of wounds and skin diseases. If acupuncture meridians are known (acupressure and shiastu books give these diagrams and instructions), tap along each meridian's natural flow to influence its corresponding Internal Organ. With this approach, many internal and chronic diseases can be treated, especially when used on babies and the elderly, since their meridians are closer to the skin surface.

Technique: By its handle, hold dermal hammer 1-2 inches above skin, then lightly and repeatedly tap over desired area with a flexible movement of the wrist. This stimulates local circulation, improving healing to that place. Tap continuously for 5-10 minutes, until skin reddens and moistens. Treatment may be repeated several times daily for many days, or until problem is alleviated. If treating several areas of body, or along acupuncture meridians, then follow this traditional sequence: first tap the center of the body, then sides, beginning at the top of the body then moving toward the feet. Begin this sequence with the back, then move to the front.

Sterilization: You may sterilize your dermal hammer so it can be used on more than one person: cook in a pressure cooker on a rack over a little water at 15 lbs. pressure for 20 minutes before and after each use. However, since they are easy to make or inexpensive to buy, I recommend each person uses his or her own dermal hammer.

Cautions: Do not use on anyone who has a blood-carrying disease, such as hepatitis or AIDS (unless with their own dermal hammer), on ulcerated areas, open wounds, infectious skin regions, traumatic injuries, or during acute infectious disease or acute abdominal disorders. If bleeding occurs (this is often a purposeful part of the technique), wear rubber gloves to cleanse skin with alcohol.

JOURNAL WRITING

When emotions are blocked or hidden, they fester, causing stagnant Liver Qi and a multitude of disease symptoms. Many people do not have an outlet for their feelings, either from lack of a listener, appropriate environment, or ability to express feelings. Writing in a journal provides a safe outlet for expressing these feelings, allowing the release to occur before it builds and adversely affects the body. Doing so is different than diary writing where you record the events of the day. In journal writing, you describe your feelings, ideas or thoughts currently experienced. Since the journal is for your eyes only, write any feeling, thoughts or ideas desired—get them out and expressed.

Writing your feelings is quite different than just thinking or feeling them, a process that only creates an endless mental loop. Instead, writing opens a door of expression, allowing what's occurring inside to come out. As a result, your feelings aren't bottled up, unknown, or unacknowledged. For another, you create an outlet, a doorway or thoroughfare if you will, for thoughts and feelings to freely travel between your conscious, subconscious and superconscious minds. This process not only releases trapped emotions, but also reveals inner connections, new ideas, past experiences, or hidden thoughts and feelings, all of which often form new meanings and awareness of yourself.

You may also use the journal to write about your healing process, asking and answering such questions as: Do I truly want to get well? And am I ready? Am I willing to do what is necessary to make the needed changes? If not, what is blocking this? What do I feel about it and why? Most people are amazed by the outcome of a journal writing session. It is a constantly revealing and nourishing process. Journal writing is incredibly healing, for when emotions are given vent and thoughts provided a channeled pathway, a release occurs on the emotional and mental levels that beneficially affects the entire body-mind-spirit complex.

To help you write more openly, imagine you're talking with a good and trusted friend (you might even record his/her imagined "responses" as well). If focusing on your healing process, it's also helpful to "dialogue" with the body part needing help, writing down your words and recording any imagined response (although this may sound weird, it is actually quite revealing and helpful).

There are a few helpful tips for keeping a journal. First, purchase a blank book so attractive to you, you'll enjoy viewing and holding it frequently. Doing so invites you to open and write in the book more often. Next, keep it in a secure yet easily accessible place—near your bed is usually a good choice so it's available to record your dreams upon awakening, too (since dreams directly reflect hidden thoughts and feelings, they're also valuable to include).

When to write is another important consideration. As in all things, it's best to establish a routine if possible, as this ensures frequent and regular use of your journal. Many find that nighttime is especially good, since it benefits sleep to empty mind and heart, offering emotional issues to your subconscious and superconscious for solutions during sleep. Regardless of any set routine, journal writing is an essential tool during times of stress, mental or emotional upset, creative blocks and so forth, no matter when these occur. For this reason, I suggest carrying your journal with you wherever you go, so it's available when needed.

Lastly, trust the process of journal writing. Even if you think you're fully aware of all that you're feeling and thinking and so have no need to write anything down, go ahead and write anyway. You'll be surprised and amazed at what comes through and seeks expression. Journal writing is an intensely personal, yet very powerful, process that brings enormous emotional, mental, physical and spiritual benefits.

MAGNETS

I first learned about magnets while treating a patient with such a severely torn meniscus, his knee was swollen to twice its normal size. He could only walk with crutches and doctors warned that surgery was the only (and necessary) alternative. Since he didn't like that option, he learned about magnets from a friend and taped four large magnets together of alternating polarity, placing them over his knee for several hours every day. Within many months, his knee was normal again and he could walk without crutches.

Magnets have long been used in Japan to treat pain, eliminate scars, speed healing of broken bones and skin and eliminate tumors and cancer (in fact, almost 50% of the people in Japan sleep on magnetic mattresses). In our clinic, we mainly use magnets to treat pain and inflammation, and have found it extremely effective for this.

Easy to obtain and use, magnets are rated according to their gauss (strength), which has nothing to do with their size, but the materials from which they are made. Some are made of alloys of several metals, while ferrite magnets are quite powerful. Low gauss is around 300-700g, medium around 1000-2500 and high at 7000-12,000g. We find medium gauss to be quite sufficient and they come in tiny rounds, easy to wear under clothing (see *Resources* for suppliers).

Magnets have two poles, negative (north) and positive (south).[2] The negative polarity is dispersing, slowing cellular metabolism. It usually has a small indentation on it. The positive pole is consolidating, augmenting cellular metabolism. It normally has a smooth, unmarked side. If neither side is marked, use a compass: the end of the magnet attracted to north is the negative side and its opposite end is the positive side.

Technique: Place magnet with chosen positive or negative pole directly against skin and tape in place (purchased magnets usually already have tape on them). Keep in place until problem heals or disappears. If problem gets worse, turn magnet over so opposite polarity rests against skin. Problem should then improve (if it doesn't, remove magnet). Periodically, tap magnet for 1 minute to intensify magnetic field.

Negative Pole: Use to disperse (clear, eliminate, detoxify and cool) an area—acute pain (sharp, stabbing or burning quality) or conditions caused by Heat, Excess and inflammation, hypertension, insomnia, nervousness, infections, arthritis, spondylitis, prostitis, lumbago, chronic and acute headaches, bruises, injuries, bacterial infections, dysentery, skin ailments, eczema, psoriasis, ringworm, tumors, cataract, glaucoma, neuralgia and initial stage of hernias. Do not use on Deficiency conditions, coldness, low metabolism, or weakness.

Positive Pole: Use to consolidate (tonify, strengthen, build or heat) an area to treat pains caused by weakness, Coldness and Deficiency (usually more chronic and "achy" in nature with accompanying weak digestion

and immunity, energy and vitality), paralysis, leucoderma, alopecia, chronic hernia, asthma, tingling and numbness, comatose conditions, gastroenteritis, scars, tuberculosis, debilitating illness and to strengthen weak muscles and tissues. Avoid using on inflammatory conditions, bacterial infections, cancer and tumors.

Combined Positive and Negative Poles: Certain conditions or pains respond better to a combination of both positive and negative poles used together. Either alternate the application of these poles every 15 minutes, or apply them simultaneously on the area. This harmonizing approach is commonly used because it strengthens the magnetic field and treats a larger range of complex problems. However, quicker results occur if optimum polarity is used. If pain or the condition worsens, revert to using single polarity. Use on chronic pain, arthritis, rheumatism, speed mending of fractures or breaks and to strengthen organ systems and functions.

Cautions: Do not wear magnets if you're pregnant, wear a pacemaker or have epilepsy; do not place over the heart; use with care on small infants, children and on the eyes or brain. Be cautious with magnets around computer hard drives and discs, credit cards, recording tapes, videos, CDs, battery operated watches or clocks, hearing aids, homeopathic remedies, areas of the body with inserted metallic parts and other magnetically, battery, or energetically charged items.

MOXIBUSTION

Pain usually results from blockage, improper flow of Qi, Blood or Fluids, or stagnation of Cold, Wind, Damp, Heat or food. Moxibustion, a method of burning herbs on or above the skin, alleviates these blockages, stimulates Qi, Blood and Fluid circulation and warms areas of Coldness. It is especially wonderful for sprains, traumas and injuries, although it treats other types of pain, such as arthritis, rheumatism, sciatica, menstrual pain and muscle aches and pains. In addition, it stimulates and supports immunity and eliminates Cold and Damp, thus promoting normal Organ functioning.

---

[2] There's great confusion amongst those using magnets if the south pole is actually south, or south-seeking, and if the north pole is actually north, or north-seeking. This is why I'm using the terms negative and positive, rather than north and south.

Although made from a variety of herbs, moxa (short for moxibustion) is generally made from the **mugwort** plant (*Artemesia vulgaris*). This herb has a mild heat, burns easily and penetrates deeply. It comes in a variety of forms, either as loose wool, in cones or as sticks, often called moxa cigars (see *Resources* for suppliers). Moxa sticks may be made at home by picking and drying mugwort (usually from 7 to 14 years—the older the better—although you may use it within a few months). Next, grind dried herb into a fine powder, sift and filter to remove coarse materials and repeat this entire process until fine, soft, wooly powder results. Then tightly roll in tissue paper to form a 6" long thick "cigar".

There are other uses for moxa. The ashes stop bleeding (put 1 tsp. in water and drink for internal bleeding, or apply topically for external wounds—beware, this can tattoo the spot for several months), and the smoke beneficially treats sinus infections and blockages by closing one nostril and inhaling smoke into open nostril, alternating nostrils and repeating for about 5 minutes.

Technique: If using purchased moxa, remove commercial paper wrapper from stick (not white inner paper) and light one end. Hold about 1 inch from skin surface over chosen area, the distance varying with the person's tolerance and the amount of heat stimulation desired. There are three methods of using moxibustion: 1) either hold stick still and only move when heat tolerance is reached, returning after a few seconds and repeating process; 2) move stick in circular fashion to warm larger areas—especially good for soft tissue injuries, skin disorders and larger areas of pain; 3) rapidly 'peck' moxa at one small area without touching the skin, enabling heat to penetrate deeply, beneficial when strong stimulation is desired. If several areas need treatment, alternate between them. Continue with moxa until area turns red, about 5-15 minutes. In the meantime, it's extremely important to periodically scrap ashes off stick into a container, as else they'll fall on the person's skin (or carpet, clothing, etc.) and burn. (Keep ashes as first aid remedy to stop bleeding).

Extinguishing moxa is just as important as learning to use it, for otherwise it can easily continue smoldering and cause a fire. To do, either gently twist sick into container of uncooked rice, place in jar and screw on lid, or tightly wrap lit end in tin foil. Sometimes the stick fits into a small-holed candleholder and placing the lit end inside effectively puts it out. Whichever you choose, do NOT put moxa in dirt, for it doesn't work but continues smoldering.

Applications: When used over the following areas, moxibustion helps the indicated conditions:

Chest: Lung congestion, cough, cold, flu, allergies, asthma, bronchitis, mucus, difficulty in breathing, other lung complaints.

Upper abdomen: Poor digestion, gas, poor appetite, nausea, vomiting, local spasms and cramps, food congestion. *Caution:* Don't use over person's right upper abdomen near rib cage as this is residence of the liver, an organ already too prone to Heat.

Middle abdomen: Poor digestion, gas, diarrhea, local cramps and spasms, weakness, low energy.

Lower abdomen: Gas, diarrhea, local cramps and spasms, bladder infections (without the appearance of blood), low energy, body coldness, lowered immunity, menstrual cramps, frequent urination, nighttime urination, weakness, leukorrhea and other discharges, poor circulation, prostate difficulty.

Upper back: Treats same conditions as listed under chest, only this area isn't as sensitive or vulnerable to treat on most people.

Middle back (waist level): Kidney and Urinary Bladder disorders, frequent and nighttime urination, low back pain, bone and disc problems, hair loss, knee and other joint pains, sciatica, lowered immunity and resistance, poor circulation, coldness, weakness, low energy. Heating this area increases immunity and energy, relieving any diseases experienced. It is also especially good for vegetarians or those with more Internal Coldness.

Lower back: Low back pain, menstrual difficulties, leukorrhea, bladder infections, diarrhea, sciatica.

Joints: Local pain and swelling, arthritis, aches, soreness, local injuries, coldness, congestion, sciatica.

Other body parts: Use over any area of tension, soreness, ache, arthritis, cramps, spasms, blockage and non-healing places.

Cautions: Do not burn the skin or use over the liver (lower right ribcage region), areas of severe inflammation or infection; over the lower backs or abdomens of pregnant women, during a fever; in the vicinity of sensory organs or mucous membranes and over areas of numbness, little feeling or poor circulation (unless with great caution and awareness, or the person can burn easily). If burning occurs, apply salve or aloe vera immediately to prevent blistering; if blister rises, dress to prevent infection.

Note: While Western medicine advocates an ice application over injuries and inflammations, TCM uses heat. In the short term, ice alleviates pain, yet in the long run, it causes stagnant Blood and Qi, eventually resulting in arthritic pain in that area later in life. As well, it slows the healing process (ice and coldness slow circulation and congeal Blood and Qi, just as cold turns water to ice). Heat, on the other hand, stimulates fresh Blood and Qi circulation, alleviating pain and quickening the healing process, especially over the long run. Although other heat applications exacerbate inflamed conditions, moxa heat is different and doesn't aggravate most of these conditions. The only time moxa should not be used is when the application of moxa doesn't feel good. Alternatively, you may interchange cold and moxa applications, using ice no more than 20 minutes at a time, and ending the session with moxa.

Although this approach sounds doubtful to most Western ears, I can only suggest you give it a try and see for yourself. I've personally seen many cases benefit from moxa where ice aggravated the condition. I've had people with three-week-old knee injuries throw away their crutches after only one moxa session. I've seen

sprains heal faster than most doctors admit possible. And I've watched arthritic conditions and frozen joints (that even surgery didn't improve) disappear after regular moxa treatment. Experiment yourself and see how amazingly effective it is.

Other: If moxibustion is not available and heat is needed, a hot water bottle, hair dryer and stones or bags of sand or salt heated in an oven or on a wood stove are useful alternatives, although they can't be used on inflamed areas like moxa can.

NASAL WASH

Nasal wash is a procedure of rinsing the entire nasal tract with a saltwater solution. Doing this clears sinus congestion and infections, allergies, stuffy nose, difficulty of breathing through the nose, sore throats and especially recurring sinus and throat infections. It may be done on a preventative basis once a day first thing in the morning, or several times a day in the case of an infection.[3]

Techniques: To do a nasal wash, you'll need a water container with a small spout, such as a netipot or small watering can (alternatively, you may use a bulb syringe, squeeze bottle or turkey baster). Fill with saltwater (about 1/2 tsp. salt/2 cups water) and, over a sink or tub, place end of spout in right nostril while tilting head to left. Slowly pour solution into nostril, making sure it runs out left nostril (adjust your head as needed). Now reverse sides, inserting spout into left nostril while tilting head to right, making sure solution comes out right nostril. Continue alternating nostrils until solution is gone. You'll frequently need to blow your nose in between as fluids collect.

---

[3] Called *neti*, nasal wash is traditionally done by yogis in India to clear air passages before performing breathing practices. The yogic methods of neti are described in *Ashtanga Yoga Primer*, by Baba Hari Dass, Sri Rama Publishing, 1981 (Box 2550, Santa Cruz, CA 95063).

While it may seem difficult, if not impossible, for the solution to flow through a blocked nostril, eventually it does since salt dissolves mucus and moves congestion (if this doesn't occur in the first session, it will during the next one or two). In the meantime, continue blowing your nose. A wonderful clearing of your nasal passages occurs and you'll be amazed at how well you can breathe afterwards.

For stubborn, recurring chronic sore throats, sinusitis, tonsillitis and other throat infections, pour saltwater solution alternatively through the right and left nostrils but tilt head *back*, allowing it to run down throat and out mouth (then spit solution out). This method of nasal wash quickly clears such infections since they recur from lingering bacteria breeding in passages between nose and throat. These bacteria cannot be reached with the traditional gargle or throat medication, but a nasal wash running down the throat effectively treats it.

Although warm saltwater solution prevents and clears infections and inflammations (as many people healing their sore throats with warm saltwater gargles can attest to), an herbal tea may be made and used as the wash instead. Good herbs to use include antibiotic, alterative and antiinflammatory herbs, such as **echinacea**, **chaparral**, **red clover**, **dandelion** and **goldenseal** (especially valuable since it tones the mucous membranes) and astringents, such as **raspberry** and **partridgeberry**. A small amount of demulcent may be added, like **marshmallow** or **licorice**, to soothe inflamed and irritated tissues. Make your own customized solutions and experiment to find your favorite ones.

RITUALS

I frequently suggest patients perform rituals to assist and speed their healing process. Because emotional issues are so frequently involved in (and cause) disease, doing a ritual not only clears them, but also releases past issues, makes decisions, confirms your life choices, establishes a deeper relationship with yourself, ends old habits, creates a new beginning and much more. There

are as many functions and benefits of rituals as there are rituals to do.

A ritual for healing differs from daily ritual routines with one important trait—*intention*. Drinking hot tea or reading the paper first thing every morning is a ritual habit. But if you drink your herb tea *intending* all the while that it heal a particular health problem, then you create meaning that gives a different energy and influence to your body-mind-spirit.

As an example, one ceremony I frequently suggest to patients for making "either/or" tough decisions is a feather ritual. Go alone into nature with a feather and when ready, say aloud the choice you can let go. Then release the feather. If that decision reflects your deeper wish, you'll be able to let the feather go and may even feel liberated seeing it fly away. If it doesn't reflect your deeper desires, then you won't be able to release the feather, or may chase after and retrieve it. Either way, it gives valuable insight to your true hidden feelings and desires, making your decision clearer and easier.

Rituals are fun to create and can be simple or quite elaborate and even involve other people. They can include such things as music, singing, dancing, gestures, prayer, statements of belief, offerings and movement. Whatever ritual you create, I suggest you begin with smudging (described later) to "set the stage". Several ritual elements to try are listed in the table Ritual Components. Combine as appropriate for your needs.

Creating *talismans* is a ritual using the subtle healing energies of plants. A talisman is the wearing of herbs imbued with intention for certain effects. Talismans are a known part of folk traditions worldwide and more often than not, there is solid scientific basis behind these "quaint" ways. Wearing plants such as **garlic**, **asafoetida** or camphor to ward off "evil spirits" and contagion actually works because their volatile oils either attract beneficial insects, or repulse harmful pathogens. To make a talisman, choose your desired herbs, make or purchase a little pouch and create a ritual to "empower" it (transmit your intentions into it). Select herbs based upon their properties and traditional uses.

For instance, **valerian root**, an herbal sedative, was traditionally used to restore peace between two people. Dried pansy or periwinkle flowers were carried as talismans of love. **Angelica root**, whose sweet scent was said to resemble the scent of angels, may be carried to prolong life. **Mugwort** in dream pillows evokes dreams when sleeping and opens intuitive knowledge of the future when worn during the day. The familiar rose increases feelings of love and devotion.

You may directly wear an herb around your neck or carry it in your pocket. As well, it may be wrapped in a special leaf, cloth or leather pouch and held in a pocket, pinned on a shirt, or worn around the neck, depending on whether you want a constant visual or tactile reminder, or a less obvious and more intimate connection with your talisman. Whatever is done, I suggest making the carrier personally meaningful, such as using a silk string, an embroidered bag or utilizing something which has been given to you. This makes the talisman that much more special to you, thus increasing its effectiveness.

Ritual, the final step for making the talisman, is one of the most important as this empowers the herbs with your intentions, resulting in a powerful magnet and transmitter of healing properties. Example rituals include lighting a candle, fasting with the plants, meditating, drumming and chanting, reciting of prayers, smudging, blowing the breath on the herbs, sprinkling them with some special water from a sacred stream or river, adding a special stone, or any other single or combination of ceremonies.

Choose what creates a relaxed and focused state of consciousness. After performing the ritual, hold the herb(s) or pouch of herbs in your hands and project your healing intentions into them verbally. This transfers your thoughts to the herbs, empowering them as talismans. Then carry your talisman until your healing intentions are realized. You may desire to periodically renew or reinforce your intentions, or refresh the herbs as needed.

Smudging, another ritual, is a Native American term for using the smoke of burning herbs to cleanse and renew. It's very similar to using incense for purification, but rather than using stick incense, loose dried herbs are burned in a container, such as a bowl or shell. The smoke is then wafted over the area to be cleansed—the body, room, car, objects or whatever you choose.

RITUAL COMPONENTS

ENDINGS	TRANSITION	BEGINNINGS	OTHER
Cutting hair	Symbolic clothing	Hair style change	Smudging
Smashing	Solitude	Clothing style change	Journal writing
Burning	Vigils	Feasting	Dream recall
Cutting	Making vows	Tying knots	Power walks
Tearing	Wearing masks	Mending	Night walks
Burying	Period of silence	Symbol of new status	Purification
Washing	Immersion in water	Weaving	Collages
Veiling	Fasting	Unveiling	Lighting candles
Cleaning out stuff	Celibacy	Exchanging gifts	
Crossing a threshold	Staying in sacred space	Re-crossing threshold	
Stripping away		Joining together	

Smudging centers the body, mind and spirit, helping you focus and concentrate better. It also clears the mind of all previous activities and wholly (holy!) prepares one for the next, creating one-pointed attention to the matter at hand and funneling the mental, emotional and spiritual energies in a focused and attentive manner. Smudging calms the mind and nervous system, evens emotions and purifies the outer physical body. When done in a group, it aligns each individual's energy with the whole. It also serves as a ritual, providing a focus and preparatory rite.

SWEATING

Sweating therapy is used in the early stages of acute colds, flu and fevers to stimulate elimination of toxins through skin pores, cleanse the lymphatic system and eliminate mucus conditions. It also stimulates a sluggish appetite and treats conditions such as chills, stubborn fevers, arthritis and rheumatism. When we "catch" cold, it means our immune system is weakened so Cold, Heat, Wind and/or Dampness penetrate through the skin (see Pernicious Influences in *The Energy of Illness*). This invading energy stimulates the body to close its pores, locking the invading Influence into the muscles below the skin. The body's next recourse is to raise surface temperature, dilate pores and sweat out the invading pathogens if it can.

Immunity is compromised in many ways—poor eating and lifestyle habits, mental, emotional and/or physical stress, inappropriate dress for the weather, or overexposure to the elements are some. However these pathogens intrude, sweating not only opens the pores and releases the invading Influence, it also eliminates through the skin any internally accumulated toxins.

Sweating therapy is well known and highly used throughout the world. The Native American sweat lodge incorporates sweating therapy along with spiritual renewal. Ayurvedic medicine of India performs *swedan* treatments, a method of sweating that consists of lying in an enclosed box (covering all but the head) under which an herbal steam cooks, causing a sweat. Traditional Swedish sweating includes sitting in a wet or dry sauna with periodic rolls in the snow for relief and further stimulation. Sweating therapies used by the European, American folk and naturopathic traditions are useful home methods you can use yourself.

There are two basic kinds of sweating therapy: 1) Sweating with fire, including saunas, hot baths, applications of dry heat with sand, poultices and fomentations (raising the temperature only in a local part of the body) and drinking hot stimulating liquids and; 2) sweating without fire, including being closed in a hot unventilated room, exercise and sun bathing. Of these two, we will learn several variations of sweating with fire: cool sponge, cold sheet and stool methods.

Whichever of these methods you use, drink hot herbal teas at the same time—warming stimulating diaphoretics for those with strong chills and low fever (such as fresh **ginger**, **cinnamon branches**, **garlic**, **mustard**, **horseradish**, **angelica**, **lovage**, scallion bulbs, **ephedra**, osha, sage and hyssop), or cooling stimulating diaphoretics for those with little to no chills and a higher fever (such as **mint**, **lemon balm**, catnip, **elder**, **feverfew**, **chrysanthemum**, **bupleurum**, **yarrow** and **pueraria**).

In undergoing sweating therapy, no heavy or solid foods should be in the stomach, or it will detract from the body's ability and energy to fight the infection. The patient should also keep feet warm, such as dipping a towel in a diluted solution of hot apple cider vinegar with grated **ginger** and/or **garlic**, wrapping around the feet, then apply a heating pad, hot water bottle, or a hot brick against feet to keep warm. This is tremendously effective in helping normalize the circulation during acute fevers.

It's important to remember that as high fevers can be dangerous, they should be reduced as quickly as possible. Be sure the person drinks plenty of liquids to prevent dehydration. After sweating therapy, keep drinking fluids, eat simple nourishing food (if at all) and rest to rebuild strength.

Cool Sponge Method

This method of sweating is a sure-fire treatment for

breaking stubborn fevers, either occurring alone or with colds and flu. I have seen it break a 2-3 day old high fever in a child when nothing else worked. It's equally effective for adults—it saved me once in Mexico from spoiling too much of my vacation.

The cold sponge method simply uses a cloth or sponge, water and lots of blankets. Completely sponge the sick person's skin off, head to toe as quickly as possible, using room to cool temperature water. Then *immediately* dress and put person in bed covered by as many blankets as can be tolerated. The body reacts by sweating, so repeat sponging every 1-2 hours until fever breaks.

It's important to do this process quickly or else a chill could set in, complicating the condition even further. This method isn't always a comfortable one for the patient, as the coolness of the sponge feels rather shocking to a fevered body, but it's so effective there are times its necessary. Be sure to keep the head and male genitals cool by regularly applying a cool damp cloth to those areas. Administer appropriate sweating teas throughout the day.

Cold Sheet Treatment

Here, the person removes all clothes and completely wraps in a large sheet wet with cool water. S/he is then enveloped in plastic (large cut-up garbage bags do) and immediately placed in bed under a pile of blankets. Cover head (and male genitals) with a cool cloth and let person sweat. The cool sheet wrapped by plastic causes sweating, reducing fever and releasing toxins. After sweating for 10-15 minutes, unwrap person, dress in clean dry clothes and return to a clean dry bed, covered adequately, to rest. Be sure to give plenty of fluids and simple nourishing food when appropriate. If necessary, repeat every several hours.

Foot Soak Method

Remove shoes and socks, sit on a stool or chair and stick feet in pot of hot water or herbal tea (such as **ginger** tea). Then drape blankets around person, head to toe, encompassing the pot of hot water and only leaving an air hole

for breathing. Leave in place until sweating is induced; then sweat for 5-10 minutes. The person should then disrobe, be sponged off, dressed in clean dry clothes and put to bed.

Cautions: Keep head and male genitals cool, as too high a fever can destroy nerve cells in the brain or cause sterility in men. Do not sweat if too weak, obese, thin, severely debilitated or alcoholic, if suffering from hepatitis, jaundice or anemia, if pregnant or during menstruation (causes Deficient Blood), or in a state of shock, fright, grief, anger or other extreme emotional state. Extreme sweating and sweating to the point of exhaustion is counterproductive, especially for individuals with weakness or Deficient Blood. Further, it causes salt loss, severely depleting plasma volume and causing hypotension, weakness, fainting, Deficient Blood and lowered immunity. Thus, be sure to drink lots of fluids during and after the sweating process.

OTHER THERAPIES

There are several other techniques worth mentioning here. Various therapies strengthen an Organ system and can powerfully heal the body-mind-spirit complex. They are as follows:

Creative expression is an essential element in freeing **Liver** energy, helping it flow smoothly and evenly. This in turn treats as well as prevents a myriad of problems from chest and rib pain to depression, menstrual, digestive and eliminative irregularities, feelings of unhappiness, irritability, frustration, anger, loss of life direction, PMS symptoms, nausea, acid regurgitation, abdominal pain, abdominal distension and lumps (or masses) in the neck, breast, groin or flank. It doesn't matter what you choose to do, be it rearranging furniture or painting a picture, just so it creatively expresses your energy.

Similarly, *exercise and movement* also free stagnant **Liver** energy, treating these same symptoms. As well, they increase energy, stimulate metabolism, aid sleep, rejuvenate bodily functions, clear Dampness and improve digestion and elimination. Blood type O's especially need abundant and strenuous exercise—aerobics 3 times/weekly is insufficient (your ancestors walked 10-15 miles a day carrying extremely heavy loads!). Blood type A's need less and more relaxed exercise, such as Tai Chi or yoga. Blood type B's need something in between.

Movement may be any activity that physically moves your body. Putting on music and dancing while performing chores, walking, swimming, bicycling, wrestling with kids, any activity that physically moves your body frees stagnant **Liver** energy. An important note here is to make sure the exercise and movement you choose is FUN. Let it express your unique being; otherwise it defeats the purpose.

Thanks to Norman Cousins, *laughter* therapy has been given the recognition it deserves. Not only does laughter substantially boost immunity and improve all bodily functions, but it's also the sound of the **Heart**, thus improving blood circulation, mental functions (memory, articulation), sleep, anxiety, palpitations and uplifting your spirit, treating lack of joy and sadness. Laughter also dispels grief, sadness and anxiety.

Singing is extremely beneficial to the **Spleen**, stimulating metabolism and circulation and treating digestive and eliminative disorders, such as gas, tiredness, lethargy, diarrhea or constipation, weakness, heaviness and anemia. Singing after eating especially helps digestion, but sing any time of day to improve emotions and treat health disorders. It doesn't matter if you sing a specific song; any tune you hum or chant is beneficial.

Many parts of the world incorporate *siesta* (or *napping*) into their daily schedules to rest during midday, often the hottest part of the day. In the West, it's almost inconceivable to do this since our cultural beliefs teach us to go-go-go, get more done, be productive, don't slack off. Coffee breaks are allowed, but they're just enough time to use the bathroom and get a drink, and one that usually stimulates us to keep going. This is unfortunate because resting is the best activity for replenishing the Kidneys, which revitalizes the body and prevents "burn-out".

Resting also improves symptoms of low back pain, poor memory, knee weakness, lowered libido, infertility, ringing in the ears, hair loss, exhaustion, poor sleep, urinary problems, teeth issues, impaired hearing or eyesight and premature aging symptoms among many others.

Interestingly, resting actually allows you to get more done in the long run, since it replenishes the mind and energy and encourages creative ideas and solutions to emerge. If you can't sleep, take the time anyway to rest—listen to music, or daydream. So go ahead, give yourself permission to rest, even nap, during the day! Its innumerous benefits are well worth it.

CHAPTER 12
Herbal Preparations

It's very enriching to make your own healing tools and empowers us to care for others and ourselves. Internal remedies are the first line of defense in treatment, yet external applications often reach the desired area faster, beginning their work before herbs arrive internally since the skin quickly absorbs into the bloodstream anything that is placed, rubbed or massaged into it. Thus, both should be used together for most effective treatment.

Herbal preparations can be made and used by anyone. Usually made out of items already in the home, they put the power of healing back into each of our hands. You can use any of them upon the first signs of a problem, such as a cold or flu, or to prevent further complications or advancement of health issues. The choice of method used depends on a number of factors, but familiarity with different preparations enables you to choose the best suited for each particular ailment, individual and herb used.

In treating conditions, it is often more effective to combine several remedies for greater effect. For example, when treating a lung complaint, you could first apply a liniment or healing salve as a chest rub, then place an herb pack or fomentation on the chest. In treating a wound, you could use an antiseptic wash followed by applying a soothing healing salve. At the same time you use any of these, you can drink an herb tea, or take a tincture, pills or capsules.

When making herbal preparations, use glass or ceramic containers as much as possible, since most metal containers add metallic "salts" to herbal solutions, diluting and altering their properties. Even stainless steel does this, but to a much lesser extent than iron, aluminum or copper. Iron pots are specifically recommended, however, when certain metal "salts" are a desirable part of the medicine. If glass or enamel containers are not available, stainless steel is the next choice.

For long-term storage, use enamel or glass containers, not metal, and ideally of a dark color to exclude sunlight. Sterilize first by boiling for 10 minutes, or washing in a dishwasher. Use cheesecloth for straining (finer grades can be washed and reused), while for very fine straining, use coffee filters. If very small particles still get through, let the formula sit a few days first to settle particles on the bottom. Then strain liquid into a new bottle and discard sediment.

If you purchase herbs for preparations, get them whole-cut because powdered herbs quickly lose their effectiveness. Powder them yourself in a coffee grinder or a blender when a recipe calls for powdered herbs. Fresh herbs are usually the most effective, but should be used as soon as possible after picking (refer to *Herbal Fundamentals*, for further information on collecting fresh herbs). Because fresh herbs contain more water than dried ones, the water needs to be evaporated, or cooked out of them.

BATHS

Herbal baths treat specific parts of the body, such as hands, hips or feet, or the entire body. Because the skin is the largest digestive organ in the body, it readily absorbs herbal properties in a bath. They are especially useful and effective for treating infants and the elderly, as these folks quickly absorb herbs through their thinner skin.

Herbal baths stimulate blood circulation, warm, heal infections and inflammations, ease headaches, lower fevers, calm nerves, relax, relieve chills and eliminate aches, pains, cramps and spasms, depending on the herbs used. In general, the less severe the condition, the less strong and frequent the bath needs to be, and vice versa.

Bath

METHOD 1—YIELDS A STRONGER BATH:

1. Chop or grate desired herbs.
2. Make infusion or decoction as appropriate (refer to the section Teas).
3. Add tea to hot water in tub, basin or bucket, as needed.
4. Soak and enjoy.

METHOD 2—YIELDS A WEAKER BATH:

1. Chop or grate desired herbs.
2. Place in a thin cloth bag and tie up.
3. Tie bag under bath faucet and let hot water pour through bag when filling tub, or simply place bag in tub.
4. Soak and enjoy.

Amounts: If using Method 1, make 2 gallons herb tea. If using Method 2, use 2-6 oz. herbs, depending on strength desired and herbs used. Weaker herbs need larger quantities, while stimulating herbs can be used more sparingly.

Dose: Take baths as needed.

Storage: Baths are made only as needed.

BOLUS

A bolus is a suppository inserted into the rectum to treat hemorrhoids and cysts, or into the vagina to treat infections, cysts, irritations and tumors. The herbs used in a bolus may include astringents, such as **white oak** bark, or **partridgeberry**; demulcents, such as **comfrey** root or **slippery elm**; and antibiotics such as **garlic**, **echinacea**, **chaparral** or **goldenseal**. A binder is also needed, such as ghee or cocoa butter, both of which also heal. Boluses are usually inserted at night before sleep, allowing cocoa butter to melt (from body heat) and release herbs. Take precautions to protect clothing and bedding, and rinse (or douche) any external residue the following morning.

Bolus

1. Powder desired herb(s) in blender or coffee grinder.
2. Mix herbs together in small bowl.
3. Add enough binder (ghee or cocoa butter) to form a thick, firm, pie-dough consistency.
4. Roll mixture into long strips about 3/4" thick.
5. Place in refrigerator or freezer to harden.
6. When ready to use, cut segment of mixture 1" long.
7. Allow to come to room temperature, then insert into rectum or vagina as needed.
8. Wear underwear or pad to protect clothing from possible leakage.

Amounts: Mix 1 oz. powdered herbs to approximately 1 Tbsp. binder (add more herbs or binder as needed). Some herbs powder more coarsely than others and so need more binder.

Dose: Insert 1" segment, 1-2 times/day, especially before going to bed.

Storage: Make and use bolus preparations as needed; don't store beyond 5 days (unless in freezer).

CAPSULES

Capsules are useful to take herbs in small amounts (1/2

to 3 grams—less than ¹/9th of an ounce) and for herbs that taste bitter, strong or high in mucilage. It's best not to use capsules for mild-tasting herbs since you'd have to take 6-8 capsules or more at a time for it to be effective. You may use roots, barks, leaves or flowers in capsules, but they must be powdered first for digestive ease. You can purchase herbs already powdered, but it's best to buy them whole and powder them yourself.

Capsules come in three sizes: the small "0" (best for children), middle "00" (better for adults) and large "000"caps. Take capsules with warm fluids to aid assimilation. Whenever a formula calls for using capsules, you may take pills instead, using twice as many pills as capsules to get about the same dose. Another method is to wrap the powder in rice paper to the appropriate pill size.

Capsules

1. Powder herb(s) in blender or coffee grinder.

2. Place powdered herb(s) in small bowl. If using more than one herb, combine and blend well with spoon.

3. Separate two parts of capsule and press each into powder so it's forced into capsule. Continue until both ends are filled.

4. Carefully close capsule ends together and place in another bowl. Continue until all powder or capsules are gone.

Amounts: 1 ounce of herbs fills about 60 "0" caps or 30 "00" caps. One "00" capsule holds a little more than ¹/4 tsp. dried powdered herb, equivalent to ¹/2 tsp. dried whole herb.

Dose: Take 1 "0" capsule (children), or 2 "00" capsules (adults), with room temperature water, 2-3 times/ day.

Storage: Store in tightly sealed jar in cool, dark place. As stated before, herbs begin to deteriorate shortly after they've been powdered, yet when put into capsules, they'll keep approximately 1 year.

DRY CONCENTRATE EXTRACTS

A dry concentrate is made when a concentrated extract (usually a decoction) is combined with part of the herb, then dried and granulated. This yields a highly potent herbal product with increased potency and biological availability. Because moisture is removed from the herbs, they preserve well, and since they are 2-5 times stronger than powdered herbs, less needs be taken. Expensive to purchase, you may concoct them in your own home. Dry concentrate extracts may be made from a single herb, or an entire formula, as desired. Avoid using herbs high in volatile oils, as these constituents may be lost during the preparation process.

Dry Concentrate Extract

1. Stuff pot full of desired herb(s) or formula. Remove ¹/10th of herb/formula and set aside.

2. Fill pot with water, cover and bring to boil.

3. With lid cracked, reduce heat to lowest setting. Slowly simmer until 1" liquid remains (this may take a full day).

4. Strain liquid and return to pot. Press marc (pulpy herbal mash) through cheesecloth or winepress and catch remaining liquid. Add pressed liquid to that in pot and discard marc.

5. Very finely powder removed ¹/10th herb/formula (set aside at beginning). Add to liquid in pot.

6. Turn on heat to lowest possible setting and, watching carefully, slowly cook until water evaporates, right before mass burns or sticks, about 1-2 hours.

7. Pour mass onto non-stick cookie trays and place in food dehydrator on medium for 4-6 hr., or overnight in oven on lowest setting with door cracked. Turn mass during drying process and when dry enough, break into large pieces.

8. Crumble dried mass into smaller pieces, then grind to small granules in food processor, blender, or coffee grinder.

Amounts: Depending on final amount desired, use any size pot. Large canning pots work well, while a smaller Crock-Pot is also convenient. Exact amounts of herbs needed depend on which are being used—fresh or dried herbs, flowers, roots, barks, seeds and so on. Whatever is used, fill pot full with chosen herb or formula.

Dose: Take 1 tsp.–1 Tbsp. (3-5 gms.), 3 times/day, depending on need and body size. To take, blend with hot water to create tea, put in capsules, or mix with honey and eat.

Storage: Store in tightly sealed jar in cool, dark place. Dry concentrate extracts last up to 5 years.

FOMENTATIONS

A fomentation, sometimes called a compress, is an herbal fluid wrapped on the body and kept warm. Stimulating fresh blood circulation and warming the area where placed, it treats swellings, pains, coldness, sprains, injuries, sore throats, colds and flu, among other things. Herbs that are too strong to be taken internally can be applied externally, allowing the body to slowly absorb them. In helping restore circulation to an area that's been immobilized or weakened, the hot fomentation can be alternated with a shorter application of cold water. Heat serves to relax the body and open the pores, while cold causes contraction, so the alternation of hot and cold can revitalize an area.

A *wash* is similar in that a cloth is soaked in an herbal tea and then used to spread the tea over a desired area.

Fomentation:

1. Make tea out of herbs, either infusion or decoction (see the section Teas)

2. Dip small cloth (like washcloth) into tea and let soak for 5 minutes to absorb tea.

3. Using pair of tongs, lift cloth out of tea. Quickly wring out and put over part of body where fomentation is desired.

4. Immediately cover cloth with towel, hot water bottle or heating pad, and another towel over everything to keep fomentation warm.

5. Leave on at least 20 minutes. Replace with another, if desired.

Amounts: Make about 3 cups tea for fomentation, using 1 oz. herbs.

Dose: You may want to apply fomentation more than once. Leave on for 20 minutes; then with another cloth soaking in tea, place over same area after first is done. Leave second compress on for another 20 minutes.

Castor Oil Compress

Castor oil compress is a fabulous way to treat scarred and weak tissues and organs. The oil is very close to natural oils in the body and so easily penetrates the cells, healing and rejuvenating them and breaking down fibrous tissues. It also detoxifies, reduces cysts, growths, warts, treats epilepsy, paralysis and other nervous system disorders, stimulates the body's deep circulation, detoxifies the liver and treats chronic bladder infections (place over the liver and bladder respectively for these). Repeated applications are necessary over time to heal these conditions. Often a pattern is followed of applying the castor oil compress for 4 days in a row and then leaving off for 3 days. This is repeated for several weeks to months until condition is healed.

Castor oil compress is made a little differently than other compresses. Soak a piece of felt, cloth or cheesecloth, cut to fit the desired area, in pan of castor oil. Heat in oven or on stove until very warm but still touchable. Apply over desired area, cover with plastic first (since it's sticky) then follow rest of fomentation steps. Leave on an hour at a time. If you plan to leave on overnight, protect bed with several towels before lying down.

Storage: Fomentations are not stored, but made as needed.

LINIMENTS

Liniments are herbal extracts rubbed into the skin for treating strained muscles and ligaments, bruises, arthritis and some inflammations. Liniments usually include stimulating herbs, such as **cayenne**, to warm an area and increase the circulation, and antispasmodic herbs, such as **chamomile**, to relax muscles. Essential oils may be added to liniments to act as stimulants, aromatics and carminatives (use caution in working with them, however, since some are vesicants—cause blisters—and others cannot be taken internally). Avoid rubbing near the eyes.

Liniments may be made from alcohol, vinegar or oil. The application of alcohol can be somewhat cooling but evaporates quickly, leaving herbal principles on the skin. You can use a grain alcohol, such as vodka or gin (this yields a tincture—see section Tinctures), or a food-grade (ethyl) alcohol for external use. Rubbing alcohol may be used for externally applied liniments, but is poisonous if accidentally taken internally. Vinegar acts as a natural astringent and preservative. It may be used directly or diluted to 50% strength with water. Oils are useful for extracting herbs with aromatic oils and for massage (see next section Oils).

Liniments

1–2. Same as steps 1 and 2 in making Tinctures

3. Pour alcohol, vinegar or oil over herbs into glass jar.

4–6. Same as steps 4–6 in making Tinctures.

Amounts: Use 4 oz. dried whole, cut or powdered herbs, or 8 oz. fresh, to 1 pint alcohol.

Dose: Because liniments are applied directly onto body, there's no specific dosage for their use. However, they are messy if you overuse.

Storage: If made with alcohol, liniments keep as long as tinctures. If made with oil, they keep about 1 year. Store in a glass jar (dark is best) in a cool, dark place.

OILS

Herbal oils are a method of extracting the active principles of herbs into oil that's then applied externally, like liniments. Good for sore and aching muscles, cuts and stings, they are also wonderful for massage. Spices, mints and other strong smelling herbs (those with essential oils) are especially good to use in oils. Because powdered herbs make oils gritty, only use whole or cut herbs.

There are generally two types of herbal oils: soothing/emollient and warming/stimulating. Soothing oils are usually made with such herbs as **comfrey**, **calendula**, **sage**, **lemon balm**, or **lavender** and applied over the entire body or specific areas needing treatment. Stimulating oils are made with stimulating herbs, like **cayenne**, or by adding a few drops of pure essential oils (such as **cinnamon**, **thyme**, **cajeput**, **camphor**, **eucalyptus**, **peppermint**, **ginger** or **wintergreen**) to a base oil and applied only over the needed area.

Olive or sesame oils are best to use as base oils since they are warming, preserve well, warm the skin and keep longer. A few other oils may be added in small amounts such as apricot, almond and avocado. Experiment until you find your favorite combination. Besides their therapeutic effects, pure essential oils of lemon, mint, orange, rose and so forth can be added to the vegetable base to make an excellent massage oil. When the oil is made, a bit of tincture of benzoin or vitamin E oil needs to be added as preservative.

Oils

METHOD 1

1. Bruise herbs first by rubbing fresh/dried herbs between palms of hands.

2. Place herbs in glass jar.

3. Pour chosen oil(s) over herbs. Cover jar with tight lid.

4–6. Same as steps 4-6 for making alcohol Tinctures.

7. Add tincture of benzoin or vitamin E as preservative.

METHOD 2

1. Same as step 1 for Method 1.

2. Place bruised herbs in oil in pan. Slowly heat and cook herbs gently, covered, until crispy, about $1/2$–1 hour (cook roots first, then add leaves and flowers last).

3–5. Same as steps 4-6 for making alcohol Tinctures.

6. Same as step 7 for Method 1.

METHOD 3—YIELDS A SUPERIOR OIL

The proportions of herbs to oil are different and water is added to extract additional medicinal properties into oil. This is the Ayurvedic method of making herbal oils.

1. Same as step 1 for Method 1.

2. Place 1 part herbs, 4 parts oil and 16 parts water in pan. Gently heat ingredients until water evaporates.

3–5. Same as steps 4-6 for making alcohol Tinctures.

6. Same as step 7 for Method 1.

Amounts: Use 4 oz. dried herbs, or 8 oz., fresh, to 1 pint oil. Add tincture of benzoin ($1/4$ tsp. per cup oil) or vitamin E (400 IU per cup oil) as preservative.

Dose: Oils do not have a dosage limit, but overuse can be messy and stain clothes or furniture.

Storage: Oils last about 1 year. Store in dark glass jars in cool, dark place.

PILLS

Herbal pills are swallowed like gelatin capsules, but have the advantage of being prepared entirely with herbs. They are particularly advantageous for strict vegetarians since most capsules are made from animal gelatin, and if made small, for children. As well, some may be sucked to coat the throat. Powdered herbs are used in pills, but do not need to be as finely ground as those for capsules. Any formula taken in tea or powder form may also be taken as pills. Fun to make, they are also a tasty treat if a sweet herb, like licorice or slippery elm, is

added. Both of these are also good binders, helping to hold the pill together.

Pills

METHOD 1

1. Mix and powder herbs in blender or coffee grinder.

2. Place powders in mixing bowl and add binder.

3. Slowly add water and mix to form dough. Take care as wet dough takes longer to dry. (Alternatively, add honey instead of water to form sweeter pills.)

4. Roll dough into little balls about size of pea and space apart on cookie sheet. Try to make sides smooth.

5. Place cookie sheet in warm air away from open windows (so they don't get dirty), or in oven on low heat for about an hour or two. Leave until dry (overnight or about 10 hours, depending on wetness of balls). If you use an oven, be sure to watch and see they do not get burned.

METHOD 2—YIELDS A SUPERIOR AND MORE EFFECTIVE PILL

1. Make strong herbal tea from chosen herbs.

2. Strain, then cook down strained liquid to thick paste-like consistency. Watch so material doesn't burn, or overcook (this alters, or destroys, its properties).

3. Cool. Scrape mass from bottom of pan.

4–5. Same as above.

Amounts: Use 1 oz. powdered herbs and $1/10$th oz. binder. Makes about 30 pea-sized pills.

Dose: Pea-sized pills equal about half the dose of 1 "00" gelatin capsule. Therefore, for children, use 1 pea-sized pill per "0" capsule, 2-3 times/day, and for adults, use 2 pea-sized pills per "00" capsule, 1-3 times/day.

Storage: Store in tightly covered glass container in cool, dark (but not wet) place for up to 1 year.

PLASTER

A plaster is an herbal mash wrapped in a protective cloth, or combined in a thick base material such as **slippery elm**, oil, or Vaseline, and then placed on the skin. The mash is first placed in the cloth or oil because the herbs used in a plaster are so strong they can burn or irritate the skin if put directly on it. **Mustard** and **garlic** are two common examples.

Plasters are good for muscle spasms, swelling, arthritis, rheumatism, tumors, fevers, mucus congestion in the chest, bronchitis and pneumonia. They also treat enlarged glands and organs (neck, breast, groin, kidney, liver, prostate) and clear various eruptions (boils, abscesses). A plaster should be kept warm, either by replacing it with a fresh hot one, or by placing a hot water bottle or heating pad over it.

Plaster

1. Choose herb(s) and powder in blender or nut and seed/coffee grinder.

2. Add a little bit of hot water, herbal tea, liniment or a tincture to powdered herbs and mix to form a thick paste. If herbs aren't powdered, make into tea first and add to rest of powdered herbs.

3. Spread paste on thin piece of cheesecloth. Wrap until paste is well enclosed in cloth. Place on skin where wanted. Keep warm with hot water bottle or heating pad. Change frequently if needed.

Amounts: This depends largely on area to be covered, and if fresh or powdered herbs are to be used. Experimentation yields the right amount. For a 4" x 4" area, use approximately ¹/₂ ounce powdered herb(s) and 2 Tbsp. liquid.

Dose: Plasters may be applied continuously and left on overnight. Some need be reapplied and kept in place for several days. Usually, however, they are applied from 20 minutes to several hours or longer. Don't re-heat plasters.

Storage: Plasters are made as needed and not stored.

POULTICE

A poultice is an herbal pack applied directly on the skin. Sometimes poultices are kept warm, other times not, depending on its application. Poultices may be made with fresh herbs—bruise and crush the fresh plant to a pulp and heat, then follow steps 2-3 below, or make in the wild by picking herb leaf, washing and chewing. Don't swallow, but spit it out and put directly on desired area. Cover so it doesn't fall off.

Poultice

1. Choose dried herb(s) and powder in blender or coffee grinder.

2. Add a bit of hot water, herbal tea, liniment or tincture to powdered herbs and mix to form a thick paste. If all herbs aren't powdered, make into tea first and add to powdered herbs in small amounts.

3. Put paste on skin where desired. Cover immediately with gauze bandage and tie or tape in place. Or spread paste on gauze first and then apply to skin area. Leave in place several hours or overnight. Replace with another poultice until problem is healed. Keep warm with hot water bottle or heating pad as needed.

Amounts: This depends largely on the area to be covered, and if fresh or powdered herbs are used. Experimentation yields the right amount. For an area 4" x 4", use approximately ¹/₂ ounce powdered herb(s) and 2 Tbsp. liquid.

Dose: Poultices may be worn continuously and overnight as needed. Some, such as a plantain poultice to draw out splinters, need be reapplied and kept in place for several days. Usually, however, they are left from 20 minutes to several hours or longer.

Storage: Poultices are made as needed and not stored.

SALVES

A salve is a thick herbal oil applied to the skin for reducing pain, stopping itch and quickly healing such conditions as bites, stings, cuts, sores, scrapes, burns and other skin problems. Salves can be made with fresh, dried, whole or powdered herbs. To use, place your finger in the salve and spread on the desired area. Salves can be made to address a single condition, such as itching, dryness, cuts and so on, but a general all-purpose salve may also be concocted.

Use oils that are readily absorbed by the skin, such as sesame and olive oil. Non-drying oils are best for dry skin and massage, since they don't absorb as readily as semi-drying ones. Try combining both types, for instance, sesame and olive. Castor oil is a nice addition to salves as it is very thick and an excellent healing oil (but only add in small amounts as it's very sticky). Possible oils include:

Non-drying oils: coconut, avocado, castor, apricot, cocoa butter, olive

Semi-drying oils: wheat germ, sesame, safflower, sunflower

Drying oils: soybean, linseed (flax)

In addition to these ingredients, herbal tinctures may be included to enhance the salve's healing power. For example, **calendula** tincture added to calendula flower salve makes its healing properties stronger. Lastly, some vitamin E oil, or tincture of benzoin (a tree resin), should be included as preservative. Both also heal the skin.

Salve

1. Make herbal oil with desired herbs (see the section Oils).

2. Pour strained herbal oil into pot and gently heat to simmer.

3. Melt beeswax in old pot (because it's messy).

4. When beeswax is melted, pour into herbal oil. Mix well.

5. Add vitamin E oil or tincture of benzoin.

6. Test salve for hardness: blow on 1 tsp. of salve oil until hard, or put 1 tsp. salve oil in refrigerator for a minute. When it looks hard, test with finger. If too hard, you won't be able to spread salve; add more

oil. If too soft, it feels mushy; add more melted beeswax. In either case, test salve oil until desired hardness is achieved.

7. Immediately pour oil into small jar or tin, as it starts hardening right away. Wash out pots with hot water as soon as possible. Put tight lid on salve container.

Amounts: For about 4 oz. salve, use 2 oz. dried or powdered herbs, or 4 oz. fresh herbs to 1 cup oil, and 1/2 oz. beeswax. Add 1/2 tsp. vitamin E oil or benzoin tincture as preservative.

Dose: Since salves are rubbed directly on the skin and not taken internally, there's no dosage limit. However, too much salve can be messy.

Storage: Salves keep up to 5 years or more.

SYRUPS

Syrups are used to treat coughs and sore throats, relieve tickling and irritation of the throat, loosen phlegm, facilitate expectoration and heal and soothe the throat and lungs. Fun and easy to make, use either fresh or dried whole herbs rather than powdered ones, or the syrup tastes gritty.

The sweetener added can affect the syrup's properties somewhat. White sugar depletes immunity and robs the bones and nerves of calcium and other important nutrients. Honey, on the other hand, adds medicinal properties of cutting mucus and soothing sore and inflamed conditions. A little whole, unrefined sugar, or glycerin gives energy.

Syrup

1. Make tea of desired herbs (see the section Teas).

2. Slowly simmer tea until only half remains, about 1 pint.

3. Strain. While still warm, add 2 oz. honey and/or glycerin. Stir until dissolved.

4. After cooling, pour into glass bottle and cap tightly. Keep in refrigerator.

Amounts: Use 1 quart water and 2 oz. herbs. For simple

syrup, use 2 oz. honey and/or glycerin. This syrup lasts about 1 month refrigerated. For a syrup that lasts unrefrigerated 1 year, use 2 pounds sugar to 1 pint herbal tea. When finished, it yields about 1 pint syrup.

Dose: Children: Take 1 tsp. syrup as needed. Adults: Take 1 Tblsp. syrup as needed.

Storage: Always keep syrups refrigerated. They keep about 1 month, if simple; 1 year otherwise.

TEAS

Herbs with a mild flavor are usually made into teas for medicine or as beverage. Because the body easily assimilates herbal teas, they are highly effective and appropriate for serious illnesses. However, it's important to make the tea strong for medicinal effectiveness. Rather than the typical $1/4$ oz. of herbs/1 cup water as in a beverage tea, the medicinal dosage is 1 oz. dried herbs/1 pint water (or $1/2$ oz. herbs/1 cup water). Anywhere from 2-3 oz. herbs should be used, if fresh.

Teas are made from fresh or dried herbs, either cut or whole. If using fresh herbs, rub between palms of hands first, or break up in mortar and pestle (called "bruising") to help release their active ingredients. Powdered herbs can be used in a pinch, but are gritty in tea form. Teas should be made in non-metallic containers such as glass, earthenware or enamel pots. Stainless steel is fine to use if the others aren't available. Whenever possible, spring or purified water, rather than tap water, should be used.

There are two basic methods of preparing teas: infusion and decoction. An infusion is used with delicate plant parts: flowers and soft leaves and with herbs that contain volatile oils, such as **mint**. Decoctions are used with sturdy herb parts that need breaking down—coarse leaves, stems, roots and barks–and without volatile oils.

Infusions

1. Bring water to boil and turn heat off.
2. Put herbs in teapot or container.
3. Pour boiled water over herbs in container.

4. Put tight lid on to keep volatile oils from escaping. Put in warm place.
5. Let sit (steep) for 15 minutes.
6. Strain by pouring tea through strainer into cup. Drink.

Decoctions

1. Place herbs directly in water and stir well.
2. Bring water to boil, then turn heat down to simmer.
3. Simmer herbs for 20-30 minutes (20 minutes for coarse leaves, up to 30 minutes for stems, roots and barks). Usually water decreases by half through evaporation.
4. Strain by pouring tea through strainer into cup. Drink.

Dose: Drink teas warm. To cause sweating, drink hot, or to effect diuresis, drink cool. Normally drink $1/4$–1 cups (children), or 2-4 cups (adults) tea/day. In acute cases (illness comes on strong and suddenly), drink 4-6 cups tea/day. Often frequent small doses of 2-3 Tbsp. every half-hour are more effective than a few large doses, especially for children. In chronic conditions (illness is mild and chronic), use 2-3 cups/day, taking one day per week off from herbs.

Herb teas can be made in larger amounts and stored in the refrigerator for 2 days. Very bitter or stimulating herbs are used in smaller amounts of herb to water, such as $1/4$–$1/2$ oz. herb/1 pint water. Tea can also be poured into dropper bottle and carried throughout the day, taking a few dropperfuls every several hours. This is very effective for administering herbs to children.

Storage: Herbal teas may be made in large batches of 1 quart to 1 gallon and stored 2 days in tightly sealed container in refrigerator.

TINCTURES

Tinctures are concentrated medicines useful for bitter-tasting herbs, those too strong to drink in teas, herbs taken over a long period of time, and those that don't extract well in water but do better in alcohol. Having a long shelf life, they store conveniently in small bottles and travel easily. It's safe for children to take tinctures in lower dosage with adult supervision, although it's best for them and people with alcohol sensitivity to put tincture drops in water and boil 20 minutes uncovered to evaporate most of the alcohol.

In a tincture, the medicinal parts of herbs are extracted by a solvent, a process called maceration, the solvent termed the menstruum and the insoluble, pulpy residue of herbs left after extraction termed the marc. The final result is called the extract, or extractive. The purpose of the menstruum is to pull the medicinal constituents of the plant into the solution and preserve it. Tinctures are often made on the new moon and strained on the full moon so that the drawing power of the waxing moon extracts further herbal properties (similar to the moon's pull on the ocean, creating tides).

Tinctures are made with alcohol, vinegar or glycerin. Alcohol is an excellent extracting agent, drawing out both volatile oils and plant alkaloids, and acts as a preservative. You can use a grain alcohol, such as vodka or gin, or if only external use is intended as in liniments, a rubbing alcohol. Vinegar acts as an astringent and a natural preservative in liniments, or is useful for those intolerant to alcohol. However, vinegar only extracts plant alkaloids and so isn't effective for all herbs. Glycerin is a preservative and extracts the same properties as alcohol and water, but not as strongly. It's also antiseptic, emollient, soothing and acts as a drawing agent. Because it's sweet, it's wonderful for children's medicines.

For alcohol tinctures, vodka is best to use due to its lack of color and taste. Since most dried herbs need about 50% alcohol and 50% water to extract their properties, this is equivalent to 100-proof vodka. Because fresh herbs have water in them, this needs be taken into account and the alcohol-to-water ratio varied per herb. In general, use the same amount of alcohol and decrease the amount of water by what is in the plant. Because this gets confusing and varies per plant, the instructions here are for using alcohol/water ratio for both dried and fresh herbs. This yields a perfectly adequate tincture for home use.[1]

Tinctures

1. Powder dried herb(s) in blender or coffee grinder.

2. Mix powders together and place in glass jar.

3. Pour alcohol/vinegar/glycerin over herbs in jar. Cover tightly.

4. Shake jar daily so herbs and solvent mix together. Repeat this procedure for at least 2 weeks.

5. After 2 weeks, strain tincture by covering kitchen colander with piece of cheesecloth. Place colander in big bowl and pour herbal solution into colander. If there are still herbs in liquid, strain again. Squeeze herbs in cheesecloth to extract any remaining liquid.

6. Pour contents of bowl into clean glass jar and cover tightly. This is your tincture. You can also pour into eyedropper bottles, making it easier to carry and take.

Amounts: Use 4 oz. dried whole, cut or powdered herbs, or 8 oz. fresh, to 1 pint alcohol/vinegar/glycerin.

Dose: For children, give 5 drops tincture, 2 times/day, on average. If milder herbs are used, then give up to 10 drops, twice/day. For adults, take 10-40 drops tincture (or 1 tsp. for higher doses, depending on the herb), 3-4 times/day. The best way to take tinctures is to put drops into $1/2$ cup water and drink. If you don't want the alcohol, put drops in 2 cups water and boil 20 minutes uncovered to evaporate alcohol. Drink tincture water in 3-4 portions throughout day.

Storage: Because of their antibacterial properties, alcohol tinctures last up to 10 years and vinegar and glycerin last up to 3 years. Keep in tightly sealed bottles (brown dropper bottles are best) in a cool, dark place.

---

[1] If you wish to produce professional-grade tinctures you'll need to get exact solvent information on individual herbs from the *King's American Dispensatory* by Harvey Wickes Felter and John Uri Lloyd, 1983 published by the Eclectic Medical Publications, Portland, OR.

PART IV

❧ *Appendices* ❧

APPENDIX A

Weights and Measures

$\mathcal{X}$

1 pound	= 453 grams
1 ounce	= 28.3 grams = 437.5 grains = 8 drachms
16 ounces (dry)	= 1 pound = 16 fluid oz.
1 gallon	= 4 quarts = 8 pints (10 lb.) = 160 fl oz. = 70,000 grains
1 quart	= 2 pints
1 pint	= 2 cups = 567.93 ml.
1 cup	= 8 fluid ounces
1 cup	= 16 Tablespoons
1 teaspoon	= 60 drops
1 Tablespoon	= 3 teaspoons
1 fluid ounce	= 2 tablespoons = 28.4 ml.
1 fluid ounce	= 8 fluid drachms = 60 grains
1 fluid drachm	= 3.55 ml. = 1 large teaspoon
4 fluid drachm	= 15 ml = 1 Tablespoon
1 kilogram	= 2 lb, 3.27 oz.
15.4 grains	= 1 gram
1 gram	= 1000 ml.
contents 1 "00" capsule	= about 650 mg. = 10 grains (well packed)
contents "0" capsule	= about 500 mg. = 8 grains (well packed)
1 ounce powdered herb	= 25-35 "00" well-filled capsules
1 ounce powdered herb	= 35-45 "0" well-filled capsules

Glossary

Blood: though broader in definition, it encompasses physical blood and is a very dense and material form of Qi; Blood moistens tissues, muscles, skin and hair and nourishes cells and Organs.

Deficient Blood: a lack of Blood with signs of anemia, dizziness, scanty menses or amenorrhea, thin emaciated body, spots in the visual field, impaired vision, numb arms or legs, dry skin, hair or eyes, lusterless, pale face and lips, tiredness and poor memory.

Body Fluids: see Fluids.

Cold, Coldness, Cold signs: lowered metabolism with symptoms of aversion to cold and craving for heat, clear to white bodily secretions, chills, body aches, poor circulation, pale complexion, lethargy, no thirst or sweating, frigidity, impotence, infertility, nighttime urination, frequent and copious urination, loose stools or diarrhea, undigested food in the stools, poor digestion, lack of appetite, low fever but severe chills, and hypo-conditions such as hypothyroidism, hypo-adrenalism and hypoglycemic.

Cools Blood: a function of herbs that clears Heat from the Blood; symptoms include rashes, certain skin disorders, nosebleed, vomiting, spitting or coughing of blood, blood in the stool or urine, night fevers, delirium and hemorrhage.

Damp, Dampness: Excess Fluids in the body with symptoms of sluggishness, feelings of heaviness, secretions that are turbid, sluggish, sinking, viscous, copious, slimy, cloudy or sticky, excessive leukorrhea, oozing, purulent skin eruptions, lassitude, edema, abdominal distension, chest fullness, nausea, vomiting, loss of appetite, lack of thirst and achy, heavy, stiff and sore joints.

Damp Heat: a condition of Dampness and Heat with symptoms of thick, greasy yellow secretions and phlegm, jaundice, hepatitis, dysentery, urinary difficulty or pain, furuncles and eczema.

Deficiency: a condition of weakness; lack of either Qi, Blood, Fluids, Yin, Yang or Essence.

Deficient Heat: the same as Deficient Yin.

Deficient Qi: a lack of Qi (energy) with signs of low vitality, lethargy, weakness, shortness of breath, slow metabolism, frequent colds and flu with slow recovery, low soft voice, spontaneous sweating, frequent urination, palpitations.

Deficient Yang: a condition of Coldness due to lack of metabolic heat; symptoms include lethargy, coldness, edema, poor digestion, lower back pain, the type of constipation caused by weak peristaltic motion and lack of libido.

Deficient Yin: when cooling moistening Fluids (Yin) diminish, Heat appears to be greater than it is, resulting in emaciation and weakness with Heat symptoms (sometimes termed "false heat" or Deficient Heat);

symptoms include night sweats, insomnia, a burning sensation in the palms, soles and chest, flushed cheeks, afternoon fever, nervous exhaustion, dry throat (especially at night), dry eyes, blurred vision, dizziness and nervous tension.

Dry, Dryness: a condition of dehydration with symptoms of extreme thirst, dry skin, hair, mouth, lips, nose, throat, dry cough with little phlegm and constipation.

Essence: a highly refined fluid substance comprised of both Yin and Yang that provides the basis of reproduction, development, growth, sexual power, conception, pregnancy and decay.

Excess: a condition of too much of something, either Yin, Yang, Heat, Cold or Fluids.

Excess Cold: a condition of too much Coldness in the body; see Cold, Coldness, Cold Signs.

Excess Heat: a condition of too much Heat in the body; see Heat.

Excess Yang: the same as Excess Heat; see Heat.

Excess Yin: the same as Excess Dampness: see Damp, Dampness.

External, Exterior: designates the location of illness as on the surface of body; includes colds, flu, fevers, skin eruptions, sore throats and headaches.

False Yang: the same as Deficient Yin; see Deficient Yin.

Fluids: all Fluids in the body including Blood, lymph, and intracellular and cerebrospinal fluids.

Fire: a condition of more extreme Excess Heat, usually associated with the Liver, Stomach or Heart.

Heat, Hot, Heat Signs: hyper-metabolism with symptoms of higher fever, little chills, restlessness, constipation, thirst, dark yellow or scanty urine, aversion to heat and craving for cold, burning digestion, infections, inflammations, dryness, red face, sweating, strong appetite, hemorrhaging, blood in vomit, urine, stool, nose or mucus, strong orders, sticky or thick yellow bodily excretions, irritability, swollen, red and painful eyes or gums, red skin eruptions and hyper-conditions such as

hypertension.

Internal, Interior: designates the location of illness as inside the body; includes conditions affecting Qi, Blood, Fluids, Yin, Yang, Essence and Internal Organs.

Jing: see Essence.

Meridians: the pathways along which Qi circulates to supply energy and nourishment to Organs and surface of body.

Moves Blood: see Regulates Blood.

Organs: Organs in TCM are different than in Western medicine for they have energetic, rather than physical, tasks; the Organs function as dynamic interrelated processes that occur throughout every level of the body; Yin Organs include Heart, Lungs, Kidneys, Spleen, Liver and Pericardium; Yang Organs include Small Intestines, Large Intestines, Urinary Bladder, Stomach, Gallbladder and Triple Warmer.

Qi: energy, life force; Qi circulates, protects, holds, transforms and warms.

Regulates Blood: smoothes Blood flow in body; herbs that regulate Blood are used for symptoms of bleeding, hemorrhaging, excessive menstruation, localized stabbing pain, abdominal masses, ulcers, abscesses and painful menstruation.

Regulates Energy: smoothes Qi flow in body; herbs that regulate Qi treat symptoms of dull, aching pain, abdominal distension and pain, belching, gas, acid regurgitation, nausea, vomiting, stifling sensation in chest, pain in the sides, loss of appetite, depression, hernia pain, irregular menstruation, swollen, tender breasts and wheezing.

Seven Emotions: the seven emotions, a major cause of illness, include sadness, fright, fear, grief, anger, joy (overexcitability) and melancholy.

Shen: a person's overall Spirit and mental faculties, including enthusiasm for life, charisma and the capacity to behave appropriately, be responsive, speak coherently, think and form ideas and live a life of joy and spiritual fulfillment.

Spirit: see Shen.

Stagnant, Stagnation: the congestion of Qi, Blood, Fluids, Cold, Heat or food.

TCM: abbreviation for Traditional Chinese Medicine.

Tonify: strengthen, build and improve the condition of Qi, Blood, Yin, Yang, Essence or Organs and their functions.

Wind: a force similar to wind in nature that arises quickly, changes rapidly, moves swiftly and blows intermittently, causing symptoms such as spasms, twitches, stiff or rigid neck and shoulders, dizziness, rigidity of muscles, deviation of eye and mouth, tremors, convulsions, vertigo and sudden onset of colds, chills, fever, stuffy nose, body aches and headache.

Yang: the body's capacity to generate and maintain warmth, circulation and metabolism.

Yin: the body's substance, including Blood and all other Fluids in the body; these nurture and moisten Organs and tissues.

Zang-Fu: the theory of the Organs; the solid Organs (*Zang*, or Yin Organs) transport, while the hollow Organs (*Fu*, or Yang Organs) store.

APPENDIX C
Bibliography

Ballantine, Rudolph, M.D. *Diet and Nutrition.* Honesdale, PA: The Himalayan International Institute, 1978 (includes Ayurvedic nutrition).

Beinfield, Harriet and Korngold, Efrem. *Between Heaven and Earth.* New York, NY: Ballantine Books, 1991.

Bensky and Barolet. *Formulas and Strategies.* Seattle, WA: Eastland Press, 1990.

Bensky and Gamble. *Chinese Herbal Medicine Materia Medica.* Seattle, WA: Eastland Press, 1986.

Brooke, Elizabeth. *Women Healers: Portraits of Herbalists, Physicians, and Midwives.* Rochester, VT: Healing Arts Press, 1995.

Bulletins of the Oriental Healing Arts Institute of U.S.A. Los Angeles, CA: Oriental Healing Arts Institute.

Chang, But, Yao, Wang and Yeung. *Pharmacology and Applications of Chinese Materia Medica.* Philadelphia, PA: World Scientific Publishing Company, 1986.

Cheung, C.S. *Treatment of Traditional Chinese Medicine.* San Francisco, CA: Traditional Chinese Medical Publisher, 1980.

Christopher, Dr. John R. *School of Natural Healing.* Provo, UT: Biworld, 1976.

Colbin, Annemarie. *Book of Whole Meals.* New York, NY: Ballantine Books, 1983.

Colbin, Annemarie. *Food and Healing.* New York, NY: Ballantine Books, 1980.

Connelly, Diane. *Traditional Acupuncture: The Law of the Five Elements.* MD: Center for Traditional Acupuncture, 1979.

Courtenay and Zimmerman, *Wildflowers and Weeds: A Field Guide in Full Color.* NJ: Prentice Hall 1992.

Crawford, Amanda McQuade. *Herbal Remedies for Women.* Rocklin, CA: Prima Publishing, 1997.

Crittenden, Mabel and Dorothy Telfer. *Wildflowers of the West.* Berkeley, CA: Celestial Arts. 1975.

Culpeper, Nicholas. *Culpeper's Complete Herbal.* 8th Edition. London: W. Foulsham and Co., 1995.

Clymer, R. Swinburne, MD. *Nature's Healing Agents.* Quakertown, PA: The Humanitarian Society, 1973.

D'Adamo, Dr. Peter J. *Eat Right for Your Type.* New York, NY: G. P. Putnam's Sons, 1996.

Dharmananda, S. PhD. *Your Nature, Your Health.* Portland, OR: Institute for Traditional Medicine and Preventive Health Care, 1986.

Duke, James A, PhD. *The Green Pharmacy.* Emmaus, PA: Rodale Press, 1997.

Ellingwood, Finley. *American Materia Medica Therapeutics and Pharmacognosy.* Portland, OR: Eclectic Medical Publications, 1983.

Elpel, Thomas, *Botany in a Day.* Hollowtop Outdoor Primitive School, 1996; PO Box 691, Pony, MT 59747: www.hollowtop.com.

Estella, Mary. *Natural Foods Cookbook*. New York, NY: Japan Publications, 1985.

Fallon, Sally. *Nourishing Traditions*. San Diego, CA: Promotion Publishing, 1995.

Felter, Harvey Wickes, MD. *King's American Dispensatory*. Portland, OR: Eclectic Medical Publications, 1983.

Flaws, Bob. *The Secret of Chinese Pulse Diagnosis*. Boulder, CO: Blue Poppy Press, 1995.

Flaws, Bob and Honora Wolfe. *Prince Wen Hui's Cook: Chinese Dietary Therapy*. Brookline, MA: Paradigm Publications, 1985.

Foster, Steven. *East-West Botanicals*. Brisey, MO: Ozark Beneficial Plant Project. (HCR Box 3, Brisey, MO, 65618).

Foster, Steven. *Herbal Bounty*. Salt Lake City, UT: Peregrine Smith Books, 1984.

Foster, Steven and Yue Chongxi. *Herbal Emissaries, Bringing Chinese Herbs to the West*. Rochester, VT: Healing Arts Press, 1992.

Fratkin, Jake Paul. *Chinese Herbal Patent Medicines, The Clinical Desk Reference*. Boulder, CO: Shya Publications, 2001.

Frawley, Dr. David and Dr. Lad Vasant. *The Yoga of Herbs*. Twin Lakes, WI: Lotus Press, 1988.

Gladstar, Rosemary. *Herbal Healing for Women*. New York, NY: Simon and Schuster, 1993.

Graedon, Joe and Teresa Graedon, PhD. *The People's Pharmacy Guide to Home and Herbal Remedies*. New York, NY: St. Martin's Press, 1999.

Green, James, AHG. *The Male Herbal: Health Care for Men and Boys*. Freedom, CA: Crossing Press, 1991.

Green, James. *The Herbal Medicine Makers Handbook*. Freedom, CA: Crossing Press, 2000

Grieve, Mrs. M. *A Modern Herbal*. New York, NY: Dover Publications, 1971.

Griggs, Barbara. *Green Pharmacy*. New York, NY: Viking Press, 1981.

Griggs, Barbara. *The Food Factor*. New York, NY: Viking Press, 1986.

Hickey, Michael and Clive King. *100 Families of Flowering Plants*. New York, NY: Cambridge University Press, 1981.

Hobbs, Christopher, and Stephen Brown. *Saw Palmetto*. Loveland, CO: Interweave Press, 1997.

Hobbs, Christopher. *Chinese Herbs Growing in the Western U.S.* Capitola CA: Botanica Press, 1987.

Hoffmann, David. *The Herbal Handbook*. Rochester, VT: Healing Arts Press, 1987.

Hoffmann, David. *The Herb User's Guide*, Wellingborough, Northamptonshire and Rochester, Vermont: Thorsons Publishing Group, 1987.

Hoffmann, David. *The Holistic Herbal*. Scotland: Findhorn Press, 1983.

Hsu, Hong-Yen. *How to Treat Yourself with Chinese Herbs*. Los Angeles, CA: Oriental Healing Arts Institute, 1980.

Hsu, Hong-Yen and Chau-Shin Hsu. *Commonly Used Chinese Herb Formulas With Illustrations*. Los Angeles, CA: Oriental Healing Arts Institute, 1980.

Hsu, Hong-Yen and Douglas Easer. *Major Chinese Herbal Formulas*. Los Angeles, CA: Oriental Healing Arts Institute, 1980.

Hsu, Hong-Yen and William Preacher. *Chinese Herb Medicine and Therapy*. Los Angeles, CA: Oriental Healing Arts Institute, 1976.

Hsu, Dr. Hong-yen and Dr. William G. Preacher. *Chinese Herb Medicine and Therapy*. Los Angeles, CA: Oriental Healing Arts Institute, 1994.

Hutchens, Alma. *Indian Herbology of North America*. Boston, MA: Shambhala Publications, 1991.

Hyatt, Richard. *Chinese Herbal Medicine*. New York, NY: Schocken Books, 1978.

Kaptchuk, Ted. *The Web That Has No Weaver*. New York, NY: Congdon & Weed, 1983.

Kirschbaum, Barbara. *Atlas of Chinese Tongue Diagnosis.* Seattle, WA: Eastland Press, 2000.

Kushi, Michio. *How to See Your Health: Book of Oriental Diagnosis.* New York, NY: Japan Publications, 1981.

Kushi, Michio. *Macrobiotic Home Remedies.* New York, NY: Japan Publications, 1985.

L'Orange, LAc. and Gary Dolowich, MD. *Ancient Roots, Many Branches.* Twin Lakes, WI: Lotus Press, 2002.

L'Orange, Darlena. *Herbal Healing Secrets of the Orient.* Paramus, NJ: Prentice Hall, 1998.

Lad, Dr. Vasant. *Ayurveda. The Science of Self-Healing.* Santa Fe, NM: Lotus Press, 1984.

Le, Kim, PhD. *The Simple Path to Health.* Portland, OR: Rudra Press, 1996.

Lee, John R. MD. and Jesse Hanley, MD. and Virginia Hopkins. *What Your Doctor May Not Tell You about Pre-menopause.* New York, NY: Warner Books, 1999.

Lee, John R. MD. and Virginia Hopkins. *What Your Doctor May Not Tell You About Menopause.* New York, NY: Warner Books, 1996.

Li, Shih-Chen. *Chinese Medicinal Herbs.* San Francisco, CA: Georgetown Press, 1973.

Lu, Henry C. *Chinese System of Food Cures.* New York, NY: Sterling Publishing Co., 1986.

Lu, Henry C. *Chinese Foods for Longevity.* New York, NY: Sterling Publishing Co, 1990.

Lu, Henry C. *Chinese Natural Cures, Traditional Methods for Remedies and Preventions.* New York, NY: Black Dog & Leventhal Publishers, Inc., 1986 (reprinted 1994).

Lust, John. *The Herb Book.* New York, NY: Benedict Lust Pub., 1974.

Mabey, Richard. *The New Age Herbalist.* New York, NY: Collier Books, 1988.

Maciocia, Giovanni. *Obstetrics and Gynecology in Chinese Medicine.* New York, NY: Churchill Livingstone, 1998.

Maciocia, Giovanni. *The Foundations of Chinese Medicine.* New York, NY: Churchill Livingstone, 1989.

Maciocia, Giovanni. *The Practice of Chinese Medicine.* New York, NY: Churchill Livingstone, 1994.

Maciocia, Giovanni. *Tongue Diagnosis in Chinese Medicine.* Seattle, WA: Eastland Press, 1987.

Moerman, Daniel E. *Medicinal Plants of Native America.* Ann Arbor, MI: University of Michigan Museum of Anthropology, 1986.

Mooney, James. *Swimmer Manuscript: Cherokee Sacred Formulas and Medicinal Prescriptions.* First published by the U.S. Government Bureau of American Ethnology Bulletins, 1932. Reissued by Botanica Press, Capitola, CA.

Moore, Michael. *Medicinal Plants of the Mountain West.* Santa Fe, NM: Museum of New Mexico Press, 1979.

Muramoto, Naboro. *Healing Ourselves.* New York, NY: Avon Press, 1973.

Ni, Maoshing. *Chinese Herbology Made Easy.* Los Angeles, CA: The Shrine of the Eternal Breath of Tao and College of Tao and Traditional Chinese Healing, 1986.

Ni, Maoshing with Cathy McNease. *The Tao of Nutrition.* Santa Monica/Los Angeles, CA: Seven Star Communications Group, Inc., 1993.

Nissim, Rina. *Natural Healing in Gynecology.* New York, NY: Pandora Publishers, 1986.

Parvati, Jeannine. *Hygieia, A Woman's Herbal.* Sevier, Utah: Freestone Press, 1978.

Phillips, Nancy and Michael. *The Village Herbalist.* White River Junction, VT: Chelsea Green Publishing, 2001.

Pipher, Mary. *Reviving Ophelia, Saving the Selves of Adolescent Girls.* New York, NY: Ballantine Books, 1995.

Pitchford, Paul. *Healing with Whole Foods: Oriental Traditions and Modern Nutrition.* Berkeley, CA: North Atlantic Books, 1993.

Pollack, William. *Real Boys, Rescuing Our Sons from the Myths of Boyhood.* New York, NY: Owl Books, 1999.

Priest and Priest. *Herbal Medication.* Essex, England: L.N. Fowler & Co. 1982.

Romm, Aviva and Tracy. *ADHD Alternatives, A Natural Approach to Treating Attention-Deficit Hyperactivity Disorder.* Pownal, VT: Storey Books, 2000.

Romm, Aviva Jill. *Natural Pregnancy Book.* Freedom: CA: Crossing Press, 1997.

Romm, Aviva Jill. *Vaccinations: A Thoughtful Parent's Guide,* Inner Traditions, 2001.

Romm, Aviva Jill and Sears, William, MD. *Naturally Healthy Babies and Children.* Pownal, VT: Storey Books, 2000.

Rose, Jeanne. *Herbs and Things.* 19th Edition. San Francisco, CA: Last Gasp of San Francisco, 2001.

Ross, Julia. *The Diet Cure.* London, England: Penguin Books, 1999.

Schauenber, Paul and Paris, Ferdinand. *Guide to Medicinal Plants.* New Canaan, CT: Keats Publishing, 1977.

Schmid, Ronald F., ND. *Native Nutrition, Eating According to Ancestral Wisdom,* Rochester, VT: Healing Arts Press, 1987.

Sears, Barry. *Mastering the Zone.* New York, NY: HarperCollins Publications, 1997.

Shook, Dr. Edward E. *Beginning and Advanced Treatise in Herbology.* Beaumont, CA: Trinity Center Press, 1978.

Teeguarden, Ron. *Chinese Tonic Herbs.* New York, NY: Japan Publications, 1984.

The Revolutionary Health Committee of Hunan Province. *A Barefoot Doctor's Manual.* Seattle, WA: Cloudburst Press, 1977.

Tierra, Lesley. *A Kid's Herb Book.* San Francisco, CA: RD Reed, 2000.

Tierra, Lesley. *Healing With Chinese Herbs.* Freedom, CA: Crossing Press.

Tierra, Lesley. *The Herbs of Life.* Freedom, CA: Crossing Press, 1992.

Tierra, Michael and Tierra, Lesley. *Chinese Traditional Herbal Medicine, Vol. I & II.* Twin Lakes, WI: Lotus Press, 1998.

Tierra, Michael. *The Way of Herbs.* New York, NY: Pocket Books, 1983.

Tierra, Michael, *Planetary Herbology,* Santa Fe, NM: Lotus Press, 1988.

Tierra, Michael. *Biomagnetic and Herbal Therapy.* Twin Lakes, WI: Lotus Press, 1997.

Tierra, Michael, *Treating Cancer with Herbs,* NM: Lotus Press, 2003.

Tierra, Michael and Candis Cantin. *The Herbal Tarot.* New York, NY: U.S. Games, 1989.

Tierra, Michael and John Lust. *The Natural Remedy Bible,* New York, NY: Pocket Books, 1990 and 2003.

Tilgner, Sharol, ND. *Herbal Medicine From the Heart of the Earth.* Creswell, OR: Wise Acre Publishing, 1999.

Tillotson, Alan Keith, PhD. *The One Earth Herbal Sourcebook.* New York, NY: Kensington Publishing, 2001.

Tompkins, Peter and Christopher Bird. *The Secret Life of Plants.* New York, NY: Harper Colophon Books, 1973.

Tortora, Gerard J. *Principles of Human Anatomy.* New York, NY: Harper and Row, 1980.

Tyler, Brady and Robbers. *Pharmacognosy.* Philadelphia, PA: Lea & Febiger, 1981.

Upton, Roy, AHG. editor. *American Herbal Pharmacopoeia Monographs.* PO Box 5159, Santa Cruz, CA 95063. (831) 461-6335.

Vander, Sherman and Luciano. *Human Physiology.* New York, NY: McGraw Hill, 1980.

Vogel, Virgil H., *American Indian Medicine.* Norman, OK: University of Oklahoma Press, 1973. (revised 1990).

Weed, Susun. *Wise Woman Herbal for the Childbearing Years.* Woodstock, NY: Ash Tree Publishing, 1986.

Weed, Susun S. *Menopausal Years The Wise Woman Way.* Woodstock, NY: Ash Tree Publishing, 1992.

Weiss, Rudolf Fritz. *Herbal Medicine.* New York, NY: Thieme Medical Publications, 2000.

Willard, Terry. *Reishi Mushroom.* Issaquah, WA: Sylvan Press, 1990.

Willard, Terry. *Helping Yourself with Natural Remedies,* Reno, NV: CRCS Publications, 1986.

Willard, Terry. *The Wild Rose Scientific Herbal.* Calgary, Alberta, Canada: Wild Rose College of Natural Healing Ltd., 1991.

Willard, Terry, PhD. *Textbook of Modern Herbology.* Calgary, Alberta, Canada, Progressive Publishers, Inc., 1988.

Willard, Terry, PhD. *Reishi Mushroom: Herb of Spiritual Potency and Medicinal Wonder.* Issaquah, WA: Sylvan Press, 1990.

Wood, Matthew, AHG. *The Book of Herbal Wisdom: Using Plants as Medicine.* Berkeley, CA: North Atlantic Books, 1997.

Wood, Matthew. *The Magical Staff: The Vitalist Tradition in Western Medicine.* Berkeley, CA: North Atlantic Books, 1992.

Winston, David. *Saw Palmetto for Men and Women,* Pownal, VT: Storey Books, 1999.

Wren, F.C. and R.C. *Potter's New Cyclopaedia of Botanical Drugs and Preparations.* Woodstock, NY: Beekman Publications, 1989.

Yance, Donald AHG. *Herbal Medicine, Healing & Cancer,* Los Angeles, CA: Keats, 1999.

Yeung, Him-che LAc., OMD, PhD. *Handbook of Chinese Herbs.* Rosemead, CA: Institute of Chinese Medicine, 1983.

Yeung, Him-che LAc., OMD, PhD. *Handbook of Chinese Herbal Formulas.* Rosemead, CA: Institute of Chinese Medicine, 1983.

Yeung, Him-che. *Handbook of Chinese Herbs and Formulas, Vol. I and II.* Brookline, MA: Redwing Books, 2000.

Zhen, Li Shi. *Pulse Diagnosis.* Brookline, MA: Paradigm Publications, 1981.

APPENDIX D

Resources

Ayurvedic herbs and products: Banyan (800) 953-6424, www.banyantrading.com; Ayush Herbs (800) 925-1371

Beta Glucan cream, capsules: Life Source Basics, 3388 Mike Collins Drive, Eagan, MN 55121, (877) 346-6863

Candida products: Standard Process (800) 321-9807

Chinese patents and other formulas: Mayway (800) 262-9929; www.herbsnet.com; The Herb Room, 1130 Mission Street, Santa Cruz, CA, (831) 429-8108

Coptis Purge Fire: Health Concerns (510) 639-0280

Herbal extracts, singles and formulas: Sun Ten Formulas, Brion Herbs (800) 333-4372

GERD: www.theherbalshoppeonline.com (use Digestive Formula One)

Neem Tree Farms, 601 Southwood Cove, Brandon, FL 33511; (813) 661-8873, www.neemtreefarms.com

Planetary Formulas: 1(800)717-5010; www.planetherbs.com

Skin zinc (active ingredient is zinc pyrithione): www.selfworx.com

Soil-based organisms: Primal Defense by Garden of Life: (800) 622-8986, www.gardenoflifeusa.com; *Nature Earth* by Lifeline (888) 532-7845

Moxa, cupping, etc. supplies: OMS, 1950 Washington St., Braintree, MA 02184, (617) 328-0672

Good Manufacturing Practices (GMP) Companies (for patents): Lanzhou Foci Pharmaceutical Company Ltd.,

Guangzhou Pangaoshou Pharmaceutical Co. Ltd., Guangzhou Qixing Pharmaceutical Co. Ltd.

American Herbalists Guild: 1931 Gladdis Road, Canton, GA 30115. (770) 751-6021, email: ahgoffice@earthlink.net; http://www.americanherbalistsguild.com

United Plant Savers: A grassroots nonprofit educational corporation dedicated to preserving native medicinal plants. A very worthwhile cause and worthy of support. Publish *United Plant Savers Nursery and Bulk Herb Directory.* Specializing in Native Medicinal Plants. PO Box 98, East Barre, VT 05640. (802)496-7053.

Alkaline/Acid Effects of Foods: ELISA/ACT Biotechnologies, Inc. 800-553-5472; clientservices@ elisaact.com

Business of Herbs: www.herb-biz.com; northwind@sulphurcanyon.com

Celtic Sea Salt: The Grain and Salt Society, 273 Fairway Dr., Asheville, NC 28805, (800) 867-7258; www.celtic-seasalt.com

Consultations: Lesley and Michael Tierra www.planetherbs.com; (831)429-8066

Flaxseeds: Dakota Gold Flax, (800) 333-5813; www.flaxgold.com

Herbalgram: www.herbalgram.org, P.O. Box 12602, Austin, TX 78711

Medical Herbalism Journal: www.medherb.com, P.O. Box 20515, Boulder, CO 80308

APPENDIX E

Formulas

While there are many excellent herbal formulas available on the market today that can be located at a local health food or herbal store, the following formulas are included because they're readily available through the internet. See *Resources* for obtaining them.

Formulas #1–113: Planetary Formulas

Formulas #130–202: Plum Flower brand ·

Formulas #230–242: Min Shan brand

Formulas #260–266: other brands

TABLETS: dose is 2 tablets, 3 times/day

LIQUID EXTRACTS: take 1 dropperful, 3 times/day

#1 **Antler Velvet:** tonifies Yang; use for low sex drive, coldness, peri/menopause disorders, fatigue, infertility, impotence, cold extremities, ringing in the ears, weak low back and knees, frequent urination.

#2 **Ashwagandha Liquid Herbal Extract:** tonifies Yang; use for sexual debility, nervous exhaustion, problems of old age, poor memory, rheumatism, fatigue, infertility, insomnia.

#3 **Astragalus Full Spectrum Extract:** tonifies Qi; use for fatigue, frequent colds and flu, poor digestion, exhaustion, poor appetite, diarrhea, non-healing sores, night sweats.

#4 **Astragalus Jade Screen:** astragalus, white atractylodes, sileris; tonifies Qi and releases the surface; use to strengthen protective energy and prevent frequent colds and flu.

#5 **Avena Sativa Oat Complex for Men:** oat extract, saw palmetto, damiana, nettle, epimedium, ginseng, sarsaparilla, rose hips, cinnamon bark, ginkgo; use for low sex drive and sexual debility.

#6 **Avena Sativa Oat Complex for Women:** oat extract, *dang gui*, white peony, ligusticum, curculigo, alfalfa, vitex, ginger, cinnamon bark, jujube, ginger; use for low sex drive and sexual debility.

#7 **Bacopa-Ginkgo Brain Strength:** bacopa extract, ginkgo leaf extract, ashwagandha, guggul, saussurea, cardamom, gotu kola, asparagus root, Chebulic myrobalan, Indian valerian root; use for poor memory and concentration.

#8 **Bilberry Eye Complex:** bilberry extract, eyebright, lycii, prepared rehmannia, chrysanthemum, dioscorea, white peony, tribulus, *fu ling*, alisma, cornus; use to strengthen and improve eyesight, clear red, painful eyes, improve night vision.

#9 **Bilberry Vision**, full spectrum.

#10 **Black Cohosh**, full spectrum.

#11 **Borage Super GLA 300:** borage seed oil.

#12 **Bupleurum Calmative Compound** (Traditional Chinese Formula: *Xiao Yao Wan*): bupleurum, *dang gui*, white atractylodes, white peony, ginger, *fu ling*, licorice, mint; regulates Liver Qi and clears Heat;

use for PMS, irregular menstruation, irritability, anxiety, depression, headache, breast distension, poor appetite, chronic hepatitis, malaria and peri/menopausal disorders with Heat signs.

#13 Bupleurum Liver Cleanse: bupleurum, wild yam, Oregon grape, lycii, milk thistle extract, cyperus, dandelion extract, *dang gui*, white peony, fennel, ginger, dandelion root, *dang gui* extract; clears Liver Heat; use for constipation, headache, irritability, red eyes.

#14 Cat's Claw Tablets

#15 Calm Child: gotu kola extract, chamomile extract, zizyphus, hawthorn berry, catnip, lemon balm, longan pepper, licorice, chamomile flower, amla, anise, magnesium taurinate, calcium carbonate, clove, cinnamon bark; use for ADD, stress, hyperactivity, insomnia (hard to fall asleep), colds and flu.

#16 Calm Child Herbal Syrup: zizyphus, hawthorn, catnip, lemon balm, longan pepper, licorice, chamomile, gotu kola, amla, essential oils of anise, cinnamon bark and clove; use for ADD, stress, hyperactivity, insomnia (hard to fall asleep), colds and flu.

#17 Candida Digest: asafoetida, caraway, cumin, ginger, longan pepper, black pepper, slippery elm, dandelion, white atractylodes, rock salt, cyperus; use for loose stools, vaginal itching, poor digestion with gas, bloatedness, abdominal distension, nausea, vomiting, Candida symptoms, all due to Cold.

#18 CholestGar: garlic, guggul, salvia, *dang gui*, gambir, *he shou wu*, cayenne; use to lower cholesterol.

#19 Comfrey Care Salve: comfrey, calendula, plantain, St John's wort, yarrow, echinacea, barberry, lavender, lavender essential oil, chamomile essential oil, gum benzoin, olive oil, beeswax; use topically on wounds, cuts, sores, insect bites and so on.

#20 Complete Cat's Claw Complex: cat's claw, andrographis, echinacea, isatis, oldenlandia, astragalus, reishi, reishi extract, jujube, cardamom; use for viral conditions.

#21 Cordyceps Power CS-4: cordyceps standardized extract, astragalus, codonopsis, adenophora, eucom-

mia, eleuthro (Siberian ginseng), white atractylodes, ginger; use for chronic coughs with weakness, low-back pain, difficulty inhaling and fatigue.

#22 Cramp Bark Comfort: vitex, cramp bark, *dang gui*, *fu ling*, partridgeberry, cyperus, ginger, *dang gui* extract; use for menstrual cramps.

#23 Cranberry Bladder Defense: cranberry extract, uva ursi extract, *fu ling*, echinacea, coptis, polyporus, marshmallow, alisma; use for bladder infections from Heat with scanty, dark, painful urination.

#24 Damiana Male Potential: ginseng, saw palmetto, epimedium, sarsaparilla, damiana, morinda, schisandra, ophiopogon, cinnamon bark, ginkgo.

#25 Digestive Comfort: *fu ling*, coix, white atractylodes, angelica, kudzu, magnolia bark, agastache, saussurea, leavened wheat, sprouted rice, trichosanthes, chrysanthemum, cyperus, gastrodia, mint; removes food stagnation; use for abdominal bloating, gas and cramps, belching, hiccups, nausea, abdominal distension and pain, hyperacidity, overeating, hangover, motion sickness, morning sickness, stomach flu and food poisoning.

#26 Digestive Grape Bitters: angelica, gentian, artemisia, astragalus, dill, goldenseal, juniper, magnolia, Oregon grape, yerba santa, cardamom, sarsaparilla, white atractylodes, pau d'arco, yarrow, coriander, galangal, ginger, cyperus, essential oils of anise and sweet orange, grape juice; use to promote good digestion and prevent gas, bloatedness, abdominal distension.

#27 Echinacea Glycerite: available in peppermint, lemon and orange flavors, especially suitable for kids.

#28 Echinacea Full Spectrum Extract

#29 Echinacea Root Tablets (pure).

#30 Echinacea-Elderberry Syrup: elderberry, echinacea, isatis, honeysuckle, forsythia, boneset, platycodon, licorice, apricot, gastrodia; antiviral and antibacterial for colds, flu, fever and cough.

#31 Echinacea Defense Force: echinacea root extract, schisandra, ligustrum, astragalus, pau d'arco extract, garlic, reishi, eleuthro (Siberian ginseng), pau d'arco, goldenseal, ginger, echinacea, suma; preventing and treating colds and flu Yin Deficiency.

#32 Echinacea Elderberry Syrup: elderberry, *Echinacea purpurea* root, isatis, honeysuckle, forsythia, boneset, platycodon, licorice, apricot seed, gastrodia; antiviral/antibacterial for colds, flu, fever and cough.

#33 Echinacea-Goldenseal Liquid Extract: *Echinacea purpurea* root, goldenseal root, *Echinacea purpurea* seed; use for infections and inflammations.

#34 Echinacea-Goldenseal with Olive Leaf: echinacea, goldenseal, olive leaf, garlic, andrographis extract, isatis extract, dandelion extract, licorice extract, ginger extract; antiviral for acute and prolonged colds, flu and fever, infections, inflammations.

#35 Elderberry Fluid Extract, full spectrum.

#36 Elderberry Syrup: elder berry, honey.

#37 Feverfew Head Aid: willow bark extract, feverfew extract, schizonepeta leaf and stem, notopterygium root, green tea leaf, licorice root, ligusticum rhizome, angelica root, siler root, cyperus rhizome, ginger root; use for headaches due to Liver Heat with irritability, stress.

#38 Flex-Ability (Tablets or Liquid): *Angelica pubescent* root (*du huo*), chaneomales, gambir, achyranthes, ligusticum, teasel, angelica, tienchi ginseng, lycii, notopterygium, siler, *dang gui*; use for joint and muscle aches and pains.

#39 GarliChol (Enteric-coated, Standardized 650 mg); lowers high cholesterol and blood pressure.

#40 Ginger Tablets, full spectrum and standardized extract.

#41 Ginger Warming Compound: ginger, cinnamon bark, cayenne, white pine bark, cloves, bayberry, marshmallow, licorice; warms the body; use for colds, flu, fever, sore throats, cough or runny nose with white mucus, cold hands and feet, menstrual cramps and pain, all due to Coldness.

#42 Ginkgo Awareness: Indian valerian, dendrobium, polygala, calamus, eclipta, nutmeg, cardamom, gotu kola extract, ginkgo extract; use to improve memory, concentration and eyesight.

#43 Ginseng Classic (Traditional Chinese Formula: *Four Gentlemen*): Asian ginseng, white atractylodes, fu ling, licorice; tonifies Spleen Qi; use for poor appetite, energy and digestion.

#44 Ginseng Elixir (Traditional Chinese Formula: *Bu Zhong Yi Qi Wan*): Asian ginseng, astragalus, licorice, molasses, white atractylodes, bupleurum, cyperus, cimicifuga, jujube, *dang gui* extract and root, ginger; tonifies Spleen and Lung Qi; use for poor appetite, energy and digestion, prolapsed organs.

#45 Ginseng Revitalizer: angelica, white atractylodes, codonopsis, Asian ginseng, polygonum, licorice, astragalus, eleuthro (Siberian ginseng), American ginseng, ginger, tienchi ginseng, *fu ling*, eleuthro extract, Asian ginseng extract; use for poor energy, fatigue, exhaustion and weakness.

#46 Glucosamine-MSM Herbal: d-glucosamine sulfate, MSM, molybdenum aspartate citrate, rehmannia, wild yam, teasel, eucommia, boswellia, drynaria, calcium citrate, myrrh; use for painful joints.

#47 Guggul Cholesterol Compound: guggul, plumbago root, harada (*Terminalia chebula*), behada (*Terminalia belerica*), amla (*Emblica officinalis*), longan pepper, vidanga, cumin, cardamom, deodar cedar bark, tribulus, nut grass rhizome, ginger, cinnamon bark, vetiver grass, barley grain, Himalayan fir bark; use to lower high cholesterol.

#48 Hawthorne Extract, full spectrum.

#49 Hawthorne Extract, glycerin syrup.

#50 Hawthorne Heart: hawthorn berry, hawthorn leaf and flower extract, tienchi ginseng, motherwort, salvia, polygala, *dang gui*, codonopsis, *dang gui* extract, juniper berry, longan; use for palpitations, arrhythmias, irregular heartbeat, chest pain, insomnia due to Deficient Heart Blood.

#51 "Horny Goat Weed": epimedium; use for low sex drive, peri/menopausal disorders, hot flashes, night sweats, dry throat at night, heat in palms and soles, malar flush, thirst, weakness, tiredness, low back pain.

#52 Horse Chestnut Cream: horse chestnut seed and bark extract, butcher's broom extract, witch hazel extract, white oak bark extract, myrrh extract, rosemary oil, purified water, aloe vera gel, glycerol stearate, caprylic/capric triglyceride, glycerin, stearic acid, beeswax, cetyl alcohol, cetearyl alcohol, methyl glucose, lecithin phospholipid, jojoba oil, Vitamin E, xanthan gum, grapefruit seed extract, methylparaben, sorbic acid, proplparaben; use externally for hemorrhoids, bruises and varicose veins.

#53 Horse Chestnut Vein Strength: horse chestnut seed extract, witch hazel, butcher's broom, bitter orange, dang gui, ginkgo extract; use internally for hemorrhoids, bruises and varicose veins.

#54 Jiagulan Full Spectrum Tablets; use to regulate blood sugar.

#55 Kava Concentrate: *full spectrum and standardized* extract–liquid or tabs.

#56 Super Kava 80: standardized to 80% or greater kavalactones in softgel capsules.

#57 Kava Dreams: zizyphus, kava kava extract, *fu ling*, American ginseng, ligusticum, anemarrhena, licorice; use for insomnia, restlessness and night sweats due to Deficient Yin.

#58 Kudzu Recovery: kudzu root and flower, havenia fruit, coptis, *fu ling*, grifola, white atractylodes, codonopsis, saussurea, *shen qu* (*Massa fermentata* extract), cyperus, cardamom, ginger; use for quick recovery from hangovers.

#59 Lower Back Support: loranthes, achyranthes, eucommia, angelica (*du huo*), rehmannia, dioscorea, alisma, *fu ling*, psoralea, moutan peony, cornus; use for low back, hip and knee pain.

#60 Maca Extract, full spectrum and standardized.

#61 Maitake Beta-Factor, Dr. Nanba's.

#62 Maitake Mushroom, full spectrum.

#63 MenoChange (modified Traditional Chinese Formula: *Jia Wei Xiao Yao Wan*): Magnesium citrate, chaste tree berry, *dang gui* extract, wild yam extract, calcium citrate, anemarrhena, white atractylodes, bupleurum, epimidium, gardenia, moutan peony, phellodendron, *fu ling*, black cohosh extract, white peony, ginger, motherwort, licorice; use for PMS and peri/menopause disorders, night sweats, hot flashes, palpitations, headaches, depression, irritability, breast distension and so on.

#64 Mullein Lung Complex: platycodon, ephedra, ophiopogon, elecampane, licorice, mullein, wild cherry, ginger, cinnamon twig, wild ginger; use for cough, asthma, wheezing, bronchitis, etc.

#65 Myelin Sheath Support, Dr. Alan Tillotson's: guggul, elderberry, ginseng, tienchi ginseng, hawthorn berry, shilajit mineral resin, bromelain, amla, boswellia, licorice, ashwagandha, salvia, vitamin B12, pantothenic acid, calcium, kelp, magnesium citrate and malate, zinc picolinate, selenium, copper sebaceae, manganese citrate, chromium picolinate, molybdenum chelate, potassium citrate, turmeric root extract, hericium erinaceus mycelium, astragalus, bacopa plant extract, black pepper, ginger root, longan pepper, boron chelate and black pepper extract; highly effective for MS when taken as prescribed over a long time.

#66 Narayana Muscle Oil (Traditional Ayurvedic formula): sesame seed oil, ashwagandha, bael fruit, Indian nightshade herb, mallow, *Trianthema monogyna* root, Chinese flower plant, asparagus root, saffron, musk, black pepper, valerian, catechu wood, natural fragrance; for sore and aching muscles and joints.

#67 Neck and Shoulders Support: kudzu root, notopterygium, ligusticum, turmeric, *dang gui*, white peony root, kava kava root extract, astragalus root, cinnamon twig, millettiae stem, clematis root and stem extract; effective for stiff and painful neck and shoulders, upper back pain, shoulder joint pain.

#68 Old Indian Herbal Syrup: yerba santa, echinacea, osha, grindelia, wild ginger, elecampane, horehound, hyssop, platycodon, white pine bark, polypodii, wild cherry bark, mullein, Irish moss, marshmallow, nettle, loquat leaf, fritillaria, licorice, bitter almond seed, angelica root; fabulous for all sorts of coughs.

#69 Olive Leaf, full spectrum extract.

#70 Pau d'Arco Deep Cleansing: burdock root, pau d'arco bark, red clover, echinacea, *fu ling*, astragalus, licorice, ginger, American ginseng, kelp, reishi mushroom; for toxic conditions.

#71 Prosta Palmetto Concentrate, full spectrum and standardized.

#72 Pumpkin Seed Oil, full spectrum.

#73 Red Clover Cleanser: honeysuckle, forsythia, red clover, echinacea, sarsaparilla, yellow dock, echinacea extract, ginger, goldenseal, licorice, cinnamon twig, American ginseng; clears Heat and toxins; use to cleanse the blood, and for skin eruptions.

#74 Rehmannia Endurance (modified Traditional Chinese Formula: *Liu Wei Di Huang Wan*): rehmannia, cornus, lycii, alisma, dioscorea, *fu ling*, moutan peony, *he shou wu*, chrysanthemum, ligustrum, saw palmetto; use for dry eyes, mouth, throat or vagina, weak lower back, headache, dizziness, tinnitus, hypertension, insomnia, night sweats, anxiety, fatigue and peri/menopausal disorders, all due to Deficient Kidney Yin.

#75 Rehmannia Vitalizer (modified Traditional Chinese formula: *Ba Wei Di Huang Wan*): morinda, cistanche, cuscuta, rehmannia, psoralea, cornus, dioscorea, moutan peony, alisma, Asian ginseng, *dang gui*, epimedium, *fu ling*, schisandra, saw palmetto, cinnamon bark, lycii; use for low-back pain or weakness, weak knees, frequent urination, impotence, infertility, cold limbs, edema (especially of ankles), chronic nephritis, chronic prostatitis, and as a geriatric tonic; all due to Deficient Kidney Yang.

#76 Reishi Mushroom, full spectrum extract: reishi mushroom body and mycelia biomass.

#77 Reishi Mushroom Supreme: reishi, shiitake, eleuthro (Siberian ginseng), schisandra, astragalus, atractylodes, grifola, ligustrum, poria cocos, reishi extract, polygala, ginger, cyperus; use for poor energy, lowered resistance to colds and flu, weakness, low immunity in general.

#78 Rhodiola Rosea, full spectrum extract and standardized: *Rhodolia rosea* root.

#79 Saw Palmetto Classic: saw palmetto berry extract, pygeum bark extract, pumpkin seed oil extract, echinacea root, gardenia, alisma, salvia, gravel root, codonopsis, cuscuta, ligustrum, plantain seed, *dang gui*; use for prostate issues, including swollen prostate and frequent urination.

#80 Schisandra Adrenal Complex: schisandra, dioscorea, cornus, *fu ling*, alisma, rehmannia, cuscuta, plantain, rubus, lycii; astringes and holds Yin and Fluids and tonifies adrenals.

#81 Shiitake Mushroom, full spectrum extract: mature shiitake fruiting body and mycelia biomass.

#82 Shitake Mushroom Supreme: shiitake, reishi, schisandra, angelica, lycii, salvia, turmeric, milk thistle extract, ligustrum, rehmannia, cyperus, shiitake extract, reishi extract, *Letinus edodes mycelium* extract; use to tonify immunity, particularly of Liver in cirrhosis, and hepatitis.

#83 Silymarin 80, full spectrum extract and standardized: milk thistle seed extract and whole seeds.

#84 Sinus Free: horseradish, thyme, yarrow, eyebright; use for sinus infections.

#85 Soy Genistein Isoflavone 1000: isoflavone-rich soybean powder Soylife.

#86 Stevia Powder, full spectrum.

#87 Stinging Nettles, freeze-dried.

#88 St. John's Wort Junior Syrup: St. John's wort leaf and flower, lemon balm, hawthorn berry, elder, zizyphus, passionflower, chamomile, jujube; use for hyperactivity, insomnia, restlessness and crying.

#89 St. John's Wort, full spectrum and standardized extract: St. John's wort extract and St. John's wort extract prepared from flowering tops.

#90 St. John's Wort–Kava Compound: St John's wort extract, kava kava extract, bupleurum, moutan peony, atractylodes, *dang gui*, *fu ling*, lemon balm, licorice, cyperus, ginger; depression from Liver Heat.

#91 Stone Free: turmeric, gravel root, dandelion extract, ginger, lemon balm, marshmallow, parsley, dandelion root, licorice; effective for gallbladder or kidney stones.

#92 Stress Free: zizyphus, skullcap, valerian, American ginseng, hawthorn, black cohosh, ginger, licorice, valerian extract, wood betony, chamomile, hops, magnesium citrate and oxide, eleuthro (Siberian ginseng), eleuthro extract, calcium carbonate; relieves and helps one handle stress without inducing sleepiness.

#93 Suma: 500 mg suma per tablet.

#94 Three Spices Sinus Complex (Traditional Ayurvedic formula: *Trikatu*): ginger, longan pepper, black pepper, dehydrated honey; sinus infections, cough with white mucus.

#95 Tri-Cleanse Internal Cleanser with Triphala (modified Traditional Ayurvedic Formula): psyllium husk, Triphala, flaxseed (partially defatted to prevent rancidity), guar gum, oat bran, wild yam, anise, stevia, cyperus, ginger, natural licorice flavor; use for constipation and as a bowel tonic.

#96 Triphala-Garcinia Program: spirulina, garcinia berry extract, Triphala compound (amla, behada and harada fruits), kelp, guar gum fiber, atractylodes root, L-tyrosine, cleavers leaf and stem, fennel seed, bladderwrack, astragalus, echinacea, ginger, licorice, watercress leaf and stem, lecithin, apple cider vinegar, vitamin B6, burdock root and zizyphus seed.

#97 Triphala Internal Cleanser (Traditional Ayurvedic formula): harada fruit (*Terminalia chebula*), amla fruit (*Emblica officinalis*) and behada fruit (*Terminalia beterica*); constipation.

#98 Upper Back Support: pueraria (Kudzu), notopterygium, ligusticum, turmeric, *dang gui*, white peony, kava kava, astragalus, cinnamon twigs, milettiae, clematis; pain in upper back, neck and shoulders.

#99 Uva Ursi Diurite: cleavers, *fu ling*, dandelion extract, dandelion root, ginger, marshmallow, parsley, uva ursi extract, uva ursi leaf; use for bladder and kidney infections.

#100 Valerian Easy Sleep: zizyphus, valerian, skullcap, passionflower, chamomile, hops, wood betony, cal-

cium citrate, magnesium taurinate, amber, American ginseng, *dang gui*, ginger, licorice, pinellia, *fu ling*, valerian root extract; use for insomnia when it's difficult to fall asleep.

#101 Valerian, full spectrum and standardized extract: valerian root.

#102 Vitex, full spectrum and standardized extract: vitex extract and vitex whole berry.

#103 Well Child Echinacea Elderberry Herbal Syurp: honeysuckle, elder, lemon balm, chamomile, catnip, echinacea root and leaf, cinnamon twig, licorice root; use for colds, flu and fever.

#104 Wild Yam–Black Cohosh Complex: American ginseng, black cohosh, *dang gui* extract, *dang gui*, licorice, sarsaparilla, wild yam extract, kelp, wild yam root, ginger, saw palmetto extract, saw palmetto berry, goldenseal; use for hormonal imbalances to ease menstrual and peri/menopausal complaints.

#105 Willow Aid: willow bark extract, corydalis, *dang gui*, valerian, guggul, boswellia extract; relieves pain from headaches, painful joints and general pain.

#106 Women's Dong Quai Tonifier: *dang gui* extract, white peony, white atractylodes, codonopsis, rehmannia, *fu ling*, molasses, ligusticum, licorice; tonifies Blood and Qi; use for pale complexion, tiredness, dizziness, vertigo, tinnitus, amenorrhea, threatened miscarriage, postpartum anemia, a pale tongue, and a thready and weak pulse. This is the main formula to tonify Deficient Blood and Qi.

#107 Women's Dong Quai Treasure (modified Traditional Chinese Formula: *Si Wu Tang*): *dang gui* extract, cramp bark, false unicorn root, cooked rehmannia, *dang gui*, white atractylodes, white peony, ligusticum, moutan peony, blue cohosh, ginger, *fu ling*; use for menstrual pain, abdominal masses.

#108 Yellow Dock Skin Cleanse: yellow dock, bupleurum, echinacea extract, echinacea root, gentian, myrrh, Oregon grape, *fu ling*, wild yam, wild yam extract, marshmallow; use for skin problems.

#109 Yin Chiao Classic (Traditional Chinese Formula): forsythia, honeysuckle, mint, phragmities, burdock seed, platycodon, soybean, licorice, schizonepeta, bamboo; use for colds and flu with fever, aversion to heat, thirst, sweating, all due to Wind Heat.

#110 Yin Chiao-Echinacea Complex (modified Traditional Chinese Formula): forsythia, honeysuckle, phragmites, notopterygium, bamboo leaf, burdock root, echinacea, horehound, schizonepeta, boneset, elecampane, isatis root and leaf, platycodon, soybean, licorice, mint; use for colds and flu with fever, sweating, stuffy nose, cough, all due to Wind Heat or Wind Cold.

#111 Full Spectrum Andrographis

#112 Arjuna CardioComfort: hawthorn leaf and flower, tienchi ginseng, guggul extract, salvia, arjuna; use for irregular heartbeat and rate, angina, palpitations, heart weakness.

#113 Saliva, full spectrum.

CHINESE PATENTS: standard dose is 8 pills, 3 times/day.

#130 Abundant Yin Teapills (*Da Bu Yin Wan*): cooked rehmannia, fresh water turtle shell (*gui ban*), anemarrhena, phellodendron; nourishes Kidney Yin, clears Heat and Deficient Heat, stops sweating; use for peri/menopausal hot flashes, nightsweats, palpitations, insomnia, anxiety, feverish palms and soles, spermatorrhea, lower back pain, Deficiency bleeding, hyperthyroidism.

#131 An Mien Pien: zizyphus seeds, polygala (*yuan zhi*), *fu ling*, gardenia, *massa fermentata*, licorice; Clears Heat, settles Heart, calms Shen; use for insomnia, restlessness, anxiety, palpitations, vivid dreams, mental fatigue, anxiety disorders, depression and panic attacks.

#132 An Shui Wan Teapills: polygala, cooked rehmannia, schisandra, biota, zizyphus seed, citrus, *fu ling*, Chinese wild yam, codonopsis, *dang gui*, scrophularia, ophiopogon, platycodon, stephania (*jin bu huan*), white atractylodes, acorus (*shi chang pu*), licorice; use for insomnia, palpitations, restlessness, anxiety, panic attacks, depression, mental fatigue and vivid dreaming from Deficient Heart Blood and Yin.

#133 Autumn Rain (*Sha Shen Mai Men Dong Tang Wan- Glehnia and Ophiopogon Decoction*): ophiopogon, polygonatum, glehnia, mulberry leaf, trichosanthis root, hyacinth bean (*Dolichoris lablab-bai bian dou*), licorice; use for dry throat, cough with scanty sputum, thirst, sore throat, dry nostrils and lips, and smoker's dry cough all due to Deficient Lung and Stomach Yin.

#134 Bai Xing Shi Gan Teapills (modified *Ma Xing Shi Gan Wan*): gypsum, apricot seed, cynanchum (*bai qian*), licorice; use for colds, flu, asthma and cough due to Wind Heat or Wind Cold.

#135 Bi Yan Pian: xanthium (*cang er zi*), magnolia buds, forsythia, siler (ledebouriella), angelica (*bai zhi*), anemarrhena, licorice, schizonepeta, chrysanthemum, schisandra, platycodon; clears pathogenic Wind, eliminates Heat, clears toxins, transforms Phlegm, dispels turbidity, benefits the eyes, opens the nasal passages; for nasal congestion or rhinitis with watery or thick yellow discharge, sneezing, red, itchy eyes, hay fever, common cold and sinus infection.

#136 Bu Nao Pian (*Cerebral Tonic Pills*): schisandra, zizyphus, *dang gui*, cistanche (*rou cong rong*), walnut, lycii, biota (*bai zi ren*), gastrodia, polygala (*yuan zhi*), raw arisaema (jack in the pulpit–*tian nan xing*), acorus (*shi chang pu*), amber (*flu po*), dragon teeth (*long chi*); nourishes the Heart, tonifies Blood, tonifies Kidneys, disperses stagnation, subdues Yang, calms Shen; use for poor memory, concentration and alertness, insomnia, restlessness, palpitation, anxiety or vivid dreaming due to Deficient Blood and Yin.

#137 Calm in the Sea of Life Teapills (*Tong Jing Wan*): peach seed, white peony, salvia, cattail pollen (*pu huang*), lindera (*wu yao*), corydalis, *dang gui*, cyperus, safflower, tien qi, ligusticum; moves and breaks Blood stagnation, regulates menses, relieves pain; use for menstrual cramps due to Cold and stagnant Liver Qi.

#138 Calm Spirit Teapills (*Gan Mai Da Zao Tang-Licorice, Wheat, and Jujube Decoction*): *he shou wu* vine, sprouted wheat (*fu xiao mai*), jujube dates, *fu ling*, lily bulb, licorice, albizzia bark; nourishes the Heart and settles the Spirit; harmonizes the Middle Burner; use for excessive worrying, anxiety, crying spells, inability to control one's self, restless sleep, frequent bouts of yawning, depression, insomnia, anxiety, clouded mind, vivid dreaming, PMS and peri/menopausal disorders.

#139 Central Qi Teapills (*Bu Zhong Yi Qi Wan–Ginseng and Astragalus Combination*): astragalus, licorice, codonopsis, white atractylodes, *dang gui*, Chinese black cohosh, bupleurum, citrus (*chen pi*), jujube dates, fresh ginger; tonifies the Spleen, warms digestion, raises Spleen Yang, harmonizes the stomach, raises prolapsed organs; for Deficient Spleen Qi causing prolapsed organs including the stomach, uterus and intestines; also for poor digestion, tiredness, abdominal distension, loose stools, chronic diarrhea and flatulence.

#140 Chien Chin Chih Tai Wan: *dang gui*, white atractylodes, fennel, corydalis, sausaurea (*mu xiang*), dipsacus (*xu duan*), codonopsis, oyster shell (*mu li*), indigo (*qing dai*); clears Heat and toxins, tonifies Spleen Qi, drains Damp; relieves vaginal itching and discharge, leukorrhea, Trichomonas and Candida.

#141 Ching Fei Yi Huo Pian: scutellaria, gardenia, rhubarb, peucedanum (hogfennel root–*qian hu*), sophora (*ku shen*), trichosanthes (*tian hua fen*), platycodon, anemarrhena; clears Damp Heat in Lungs; use for colds, flu, fever and cough with thick yellow mucus in lungs.

#142 Chuan Xin Lian Pian (*Antiphlogistic Pills*): andrographis, dandelion, isatis root; Clears Heat and toxins, cools Blood, disperses swellings; a great antiviral formula for acute Heat toxin and inflammation of the lymph, Blood or Organs, including hepatitis, tonsillitis, herpes simplex or zoster, common cold, flu, mumps, measles and bacterial or viral infections.

#143 Cinnamon and Poria Teapills (*Gui Zhi Fu Ling Wan–Cinnamon and Hoelen Combination*): cinnamon branches (*gui zhi*), *fu ling*, red peony, moutan peony, peach seeds; moves Blood, breaks Blood stagnation, warms the uterus, dissipates masses, stops bleeding; use for menstrual cramps, uterine masses, endometriosis, irregular periods, ovarian cysts, amenorrhea and prostate swelling due to stagnant Blood.

#144 Clear Mountain Air (*Ding Chuan Wan*): ginkgo nut, mulberry bark, platycodon, perilla, apricot seed, scutellaria, pinellia, licorice, stemona (*bai bu*), aster (*zi wan*); dispels Wind, clears Heat and transforms Phlegm; use for asthma, bronchitis, cough and emphysema due to Deficient Lung Qi.

#145 Coptis Teapills (*Huang Lian Su Wan*): coptis; clears Heat and toxins; use for bacterial dysentery, food poisoning, acute and chronic appendicitis, gastroenteritis, canker sores, strep throat and sinus infections.

#146 Curing Pills (*Kang Ning Wan*): coix, black atractylodes, agastache, magnolia bark, saussurea (*mu xiang*), pueraria, angelica (*bai zhi*), massa fermenta (*shen qu*), rice sprout (*gu ya*), *fu ling*, trichosanthes (*tian hua fen*), chrysanthemum, citrus (red part of tangerine peel--*ju hong*), gastrodia, mint; removes food stagnation, harmonizes the Stomach, subdues rebellious Stomach Qi, transforms Dampness, subdues Yang, relieves pain; use for abdominal bloating, gas and cramps, belching, hiccups, nausea, abdominal distension and pain, hyperacidity, overeating, hangover, motion sickness, morning sickness, stomach flu and food poisoning.

#147 Eight Flavor Rehmannia Teapills (*Zhi Bai Di Huang Wan*): prepared rehmannia, cornus, Chinese wild yam, alisma, moutan peony, *fu ling*, phellodendron, anemarrhena; nourishes Kidney Yin, clears Heat, subdues Deficient Fire flourishing upwards; use for hot flashes, night sweats, feverish palms and soles, peri/menopausal disorders, hypertension, hyperthyroidism, anxiety, chronic urinary tract infection, rheumatoid arthritis due to Deficient Yin.

#148 Eight Righteous Teapills (*Ba Zheng San Wan*):

lysimachia (*jin qian cao*), clematis, plantago seed (*che qian zi*), dianthus (*qu mai*), polygonum (knotweed–*bian xu*), gardenia, licorice, phellodendron, rhubarb; dispels Heat and Damp; use for acute and chronic urinary tract infections, frequency of and pain during urination, lower back pain, prostatitis and kidney stone.

#149 Emperor's Teapills (*Tian Wang Bu Xin Dan Wan–Ginseng and Zizyphus Combination*): raw rehmannia, *dang gui*, schisandra, zizyphus, biota, asparagus root, ophiopogon, scrophularia (*xuan shen*), salvia, codonopsis, *fu ling*, platycodon, polygala (*yuan zhi*); cools Blood Heat, nourishes Heart Blood and Yin, calms Heart and Shen; use for insomnia, palpitations, anxiety, restlessness, restless leg syndrome, poor memory, mental fatigue, tongue or mouth sores, nocturnal emission, constipation, hyperthyroidism and peri/menopausal disorders due to Deficient Heart Yin.

#150 Er Chen Teapills: pinellia, citrus (*chen pi*), *fu ling*, licorice, fresh ginger; transforms and dispels Phlegm, dries Dampness, harmonizes the Stomach; use for cough, bronchitis, emphysema, asthma, postnasal drip, nausea, vomiting, poor appetite, dizziness, morning sickness, hangover and acid regurgitation due to Deficient Spleen Qi and Dampness.

#151 Eucommia Combination (*Du Zhong Pian*): eucommia, gambir, prunella (self heal spikes–*xia ku cao*), scutellaria; tonifies Kidneys and subdues Liver: use for hypertension, dizziness, vertigo, headache, pressure behind the eyes, stiff neck and insomnia or restlessness from Deficient Kidneys and Liver Yang rising.

#152 Five Flavor Teapills (*Wu Wei Xiao Du Wan*): honeysuckle, chrysanthemum, dandelion leaves, Chinese violet (*zi hua di ding*), Chinese begonia (*zi bei tian kui*); clears Heat and toxins, cools Blood; use for boils, carbuncles, infected wounds, mastitis, urinary tract or kidney infections, appendicitis, mumps, measles, chickenpox, tonsillitis, flu, hepatitis and other viral infections.

#153 Free and Easy Wanderer (*Xiao Yao Wan–Hsiao Yao Wan–Bupleurum Sedative Pills–Bupleurum and Dang Gui Combination*): bupleurum, white peony, *dang gui*, white atractylodes, *fu ling*, fresh ginger, licorice, mint; soothes Liver Qi, clears Liver Qi stagnation, harmonizes Liver and Spleen, moves Qi and Blood, tonifies Spleen Qi, regulates menses; use for PMS, irregular menstruation, irritability, anxiety, depression, headache, breast distension, poor appetite, chronic hepatitis, malaria and peri/menopause.

#154 Free and Easy Plus (*Jia Wei Xiao Yao Wan–Bupleurum and Peony Combination*): wine-fried white peony, *fu ling*, white atractylodes, moutan peony, gardenia, bupleurum, *dang gui*, fresh ginger, licorice, mint; regulates Liver Qi and clears Heat; use for PMS, irregular menstruation, irritability, anxiety, depression, headache, breast distension, poor appetite, chronic hepatitis, malaria and peri/menopausal disorders with more pronounced Heat signs.

#155 Ge Gen Wan (*Kudzu Teapills–Pueraia Combination*): pueraria, ephedra, fresh ginger, cinnamon twigs, white peony, licorice, jujube dates; releases the Exterior for Wind-Cold invasion; treats colds, flu, cough, acute bronchitis, emphysema, asthma, upper respiratory allergies, intolerance of wind and cold, lack of sweating and stiffness and pain of neck and shoulders.

#156 Gecko Tonic (*Ge Jie Da Bu Wan*): prepared rehmannia, raw rehmannia, polygonatum (*huang jing*), ligustrum, eucommia, dipsacus (teasel), drynaria (*gu sui bu*), cibotium (*gou ji*), gecko (*ge jie*), *dang gui*, codonopsis, astragalus, *fu ling*, Chinese wild yam, lycii, chaenomeles (*mu gua*), morinda (*ba ji tian*), licorice, white atractylodes; tonifies Yang and Qi, nourishes Blood; use for fatigue, cold limbs, weak low back, poor circulation, lowered sex drive, shortness of breath, frequent urination, ear ringing, palpitation, asthma and insomnia due to Deficient Kidneys and Lungs.

#157 Great Corydalis Teapills (*Yan Hu Suo Wan*): corydalis, angelica (*bai zhi*); invigorates Blood, moves Qi, relieves pain; use for trauma, epigastric pain, menstrual pain, headache, migraine, stomach ulcer, sinus pain, tooth pain, hemorrhoids, arthritic pain, angina, sciatica and insomnia due to pain.

#158 Great Windkeeper Teapills (*Xiao Feng Wan*): siler (ledebouriella), sophora (*ku shen*), gypsum, raw rehmannia, schizonepeta, cicada moultings (*chan tui*), burdock seed, sesame seed, anemarrhena, *dang gui*, black atractylodes, clematis (*mu tong*), licorice; disperses Wind, clears Dampness and Heat from the skin, relieves itching; use for weeping eczema, psoriasis, pruritus, dermatitis, hives, diaper rash, rosacea and certain fungal infections.

#159 Gui Pi Teapills (*Restore Spleen Pill*): white atractylodes, *fu ling*, polygala (*yuan zhi*), longan berries, *dang gui*, codonopsis, astragalus, zizyphus, saussurea (*mu xiang*), jujube dates, licorice; tonifies Spleen and Heart Qi, nourishes Heart Blood, calms Shen; use for insomnia, poor memory, palpitations, anxiety, dizziness, fatigue, poor appetite, amenorrhea, prolonged menses, chronic leukorrhea and purpura due to Deficient Spleen Qi and Heart Blood.

#160 Gui Zhi Tang Teapills (*Cinnamon Combination*): cinnamon twigs, white peony, fresh ginger, jujube dates, baked licorice; eat rice congee, 1/2 bowl, 1/2 hour after perspiring; releases Exterior Wind-Cold; use for colds, flu and fever from Deficiency, chills, headache, intolerance of wind, decreased body resistance, spontaneous sweating that doesn't relieve the fever, postpartum care, morning sickness and skin diseases such as eczema, frostbite, and tinea.

#161 Huang Lian Shang Ching Pian: rhubarb, Chinese vitex, chrysanthemum, coptis, schizonepeta (*jing jie*), *dang gui*, platycodon, scutellaria, siler (ledebouriella), gypsum, ligusticum (*gao ben*), licorice; clears Heat and toxins, drains Fire, releases Exterior Wind-Heat, relieves pain; use for sore throat, strep throat, tonsillitis, conjunctivitis, sty, sinusitis, ear infections, fever, headache, tooth infection, mouth ulcer, infected gums, nosebleed, boil and constipation.

#162 Ji Gu Cao Pill: *Abrus fruticulosus* (*ji gu cao*), *Fel serpentis* (*she dan*), salvia, *Bos taurus domesticus bezoar* (*niu huang*), *dang gui*, lycii, pearl; dispels Damp Heat and moves Blood; use for jaundice, gallstone, acid regurgitation, nausea, chronic/ acute hepatitis and gallbladder inflammation.

#163 Jiang Ya Pian: motherwort, achyranthes, raw rehmannia, donkey skin gelatin (*e jiao*), *dang gui*, gambir vine, aquilaria (*chen xiang*), ligusticum, prunella (self-heal spike–*xia ku cao*), moutan peony, gastrodia, rhubarb, coptis, *Saiga tartarica* horn (*ling yang jiao*), amber resin (*hu po*); nourishes Kidney Yin, tonifies Blood, subdues Liver Yang; use for dizziness, vertigo, headache, pressure behind the eyes, ringing in the ears, irritability and high blood pressure due to Deficient Kidney Yin and Liver Yang Rising.

#164 Joint Inflammation Teapills (*Guan Jie Yan Wan*): coix, stephania (*fang ji*), black atractylodes, erythrina bark (*hai tong pi*), cinnamon branches, *Periphloca sepium* root-bark (*xiang jia pi*), achyranthes, gentian (*qin jiao*), evodia (*wu zhu yu*), scutellaria, angelica (*du huo*), ginger; dispels Wind and Dampness, opens and warms the channels and collaterals, relieves pain; use for lower limb arthritis, sciatica, rheumatism, painful joints with swelling, especially in knees or feet and lower back pain.

#165 Kai Kit Wan: vaccaria (*wang bu liu xing*), patrinia (*bai jiang cao*), red peony, astragalus, moutan peony, clematis, saussurea (*mu tong*), corydalis, licorice; clears Heat and toxins, tonifies Qi and moves Blood; use for chronic swollen prostate with slight infection, dribbling urine, urine retention or difficulty and burning, painful urination.

#166 Left Side Replenishing Teapills (*Zuo Gui Wan*): cooked rehmannia, Chinese wild yam, cornus, lycii, cuscuta (*tu si zi*), achyranthes; nourishes Kidney Yin and Essence, strengthens tendons and bones; use for weak or painful lower back, ear ringing, palpitations, insomnia, fatigue, night sweats, impotence, weak eyesight, dizziness, premature ejaculation, peri/menopausal disorders, hypertension, diabetes and chronic nephritis due to Deficient Kidney Yin and Essence.

#167 Li Dan Pian: scutellaria, saussurea (*mu xiang*), lysimachia (*jin qian cao*), honeysuckle, capillaris, bupleurum, isatis, rhubarb; clears Damp Heat and toxins, relieves pain; use for gallstones, jaundice, gallbladder inflammation, acute or chronic hepatitis and pain in the ribs.

#168 Li Fei Pian: bletilla (*bai ji*), stemona ((*bai bu*) schisandra, oyster shell, loquat, lily bulb, licorice, cordyceps, gecko; clears Lung Heat, tonifies Lung Yin; use for dry cough with possible blood, TB

#169 Linking Decoction (*Yi Guan Jian Wan–Glehnia and Rehmannia Combination*): raw rehmannia, lycii, glehnia (*bei sha shen*), ophiopogon, *dang gui*, chinaberry (*Melia toosendan–chuan lian zi*); tonifies Liver and Kidney Yin, regulates Qi, Deficient Liver and Kidney Yin with Liver Qi stagnation; use for chest fullness and pains, dryness of throat and mouth, bitter taste, peri/menopausal symptoms, insomnia, chronic hepatitis, nervous gastrointestinal tract, gastro and duodenal ulcers.

#170 Long Dan Xie Gan Wan (*Gentianna Combination Pill*): gentian, bupleurum, alisma, raw rehmannia, *dang gui*, scutellaria, gardenia, clematis, plantago seed, licorice; drains Liver and Gallbladder Damp Heat, promotes urination; use for jaundice, liver and gallbladder inflammation, rib pain, scanty, painful and difficult urination, leukorrhea, itching and swelling of vulva, oral or genital herpes simplex, shingles, acute prostatitis, chronic PID, migraines, hypertension and hyperthyroidism due to Liver Fire.

#171 Loquat Extract Natural Herb: loquat; use for coughs due to Heat with copious yellow phlegm.

#172 Ma Huang Tang Wan (*Ephedra Combination*): apricot seed, cinnamon bark, ephedra, baked licorice; dispels Exterior Wind-Cold, descends rebellious Lung Qi; use for fever, colds, flu with intolerance of cold, lack of perspiration, body aches, headache, cough, wheezing, shortness of breath, asthma, and bronchitis.

#173 Major Bupleurum Teapills (*Da Chai Hu Wan*): fresh ginger, bupleurum, pinellia, scutellaria, green citrus, white peony, jujube dates, rhubarb; harmonizes Exterior and Interior; use for alternating fever and chills, prolonged unresolved colds and flu, gastrointestinal flu, nausea, vomiting, constipation, irritability, hepatitis, acute cholecystitis or pancreatitis, red eye, migraines, malarial fever and manic behavior.

#174 Margarite Acne Pills (*Cai Feng Zhen Zhu An Chuang Wan*): honeysuckle, raw rehmannia, *Zostera marina* (*hai dai*), pearl, bubalus bubalis horn (*shui niu jiao*), bos taurus domesticus bezoar–synthetic (*niu huang*); clears Heat and toxins, tonifies Blood and Yin; use for acne, rosacea, furuncle, skin rash, allergic hives, eczema, chicken pox and measles.

#175 Peach Kernel Teapills (*Run Chang Wan–Moisten Intestines Pill*): peach seeds, sesame seeds, rhubarb, notopterygium, *dang gui*; moistens intestines; use for chronic constipation due to Deficient Yin and Blood, including for the elderly, weak, postpartum or during fever.

#176 Ping Chuan Wan (*Calm Wheezing Pill*): codonopsis, apricot seed, mulberry root-bark, ficus (*wu zhi mao tao*), *Elaeagnus glabra* fruit (*man hu tui zi*), licorice, citrus (*chen pi*), cynanchum (*bai qian*), gecko (*ge jie*), cordyceps, *Lapis micae* (*meng shi*); Tonifies Lung Qi, Kidney Qi and Yang; use for wheezing, cough, asthma, emphysema or common cold due to Lung and Kidney weakness (inhalation is more difficult).

#177 Qi Guan Yan Wan: loquat, codonopsis, jujube dates, mulberry leaf, fresh ginger, apricot seed, fritillaria (*chuan bei mu*), peucedanum (*qian hu*), polygala (*yuan zhi*), citrus (*ju hong*), coltsfoot, mulberry branch peel, schisandra; transforms and clears Phlegm, regulates Lung Qi, regulates the nutritive and protective levels, relieves cough; use for cough with profuse clear or white phlegm, difficulty inhaling, chronic bronchitis, pneumonia, pertussis and chronic asthma and emphysema.

#178 Red Vessel Teapills (*Huo Luo Xiao Ling Wan*): *dang gui*, salvia, boswellia, myrrh; moves Blood and breaks Blood stagnation, tonifies Blood, stops bleeding, opens the channels and collaterals, relieves pain; use for trauma, bruising and swelling due to sprain, fracture or dislocation, injury to organs, ulceration, ectopic pregnancy, enlarged liver or spleen, angina and pain in general due to stagnant Blood.

#179 Return to Spring Teapills (*Huan Shao Dan*): jujube dates, cooked rehmannia, lycii berries, *Dioscorea hypoglauca* (*bai xie*), *fu ling*, cistanche (*rou cong rong*), fennel, morinda (*ba ji tian*), eucommia, achyranthes, schisandra, cornus, *Broussonetia papyrifera* fruit (*chu shi zi*); tonifies Kidney Yang; use for weak lower back and knees, urinary incontinence, weakness or dizziness following orgasm, nocturnal emission, aging symptoms, fatigue, shortness of breath, palpitations, insomnia, infertility and chronic leukorrhea due to Deficient Kidneys.

#180 Right Side Replenishing (*You Gui Wan*): prepared rehmannia, Chinese wild yam, cornus, lycii, eucommia, cuscuta (*tu si zi*), *dang gui*, cinnamon bark; tonifies Kidney Yang and Yin; use for lower back pain or weakness, weak knees, impotency, infertility, cold limbs, edema, poor digestion, loose stools due to Deficient Kidney Yang.

#181 Rising Courage Teapills (*Wen Dan Tang Wan–Bamboo and Hoelen Combination*): bamboo shavings (*zhu ru*), green citrus (*zhi shi*), pinellia, citrus (*chen pi*), *fu ling*, licorice, fresh ginger, jujube dates; regulates Qi, transforms Phlegm; use for dizziness, vertigo, headache, nausea, vomiting, poor appetite or digestion, anxiety, insomnia (especially awake 5-7 AM), irritability, depression, palpitations, seizures, hepatitis, gastritis, chronic gallbladder inflammation, and obesity.

#182 Salvia Teapills (*Dan Shen Yin Wan–Bamboo and Hoelen Combination*): salvia, sandlewood shavings (*tan xiang*), cardamom (*sha ren*), licorice; moves Blood, breaks Blood stagnation, clears Heat, calms Shen, resolves chest oppression, opens orifices; use for chest pain due to poor blood circulation or accumulation of blood fats, angina, palpitations, tachycardia, insomnia, restless sleep, arrhythmia and stroke.

#183 Seven Treasures for Beautiful Hair (*Qi Bao Mei Ran Dan*): he shou wu, *dang gui*, lycii berries, achyranthes, *fu ling*, cuscuta, psoralea (*bu gu zhi*), sesame seeds; tonifies Blood and Qi, Kidney and Liver; use for hair loss, alopecia, balding, balding patches, postpartum hair loss, hair loss of eyebrows, beard, armpits and pubic hair all due to Deficiency (signs of fatigue, dizziness, insomnia, poor concentration).

#184 Shen Ling Bai Zhu Pian (*Ginseng, Poria, Atractylodes Pill*): codonopsis, *fu ling*, white atractylodes, Chinese wild yam, coix, hyacinth bean (*dolichoris-bai bian dou*), lotus seed, platycodon, cardamom (*sha ren*), licorice; tonifies Spleen Qi, descends rebellious Stomach Qi, dispels Damp, relieves diarrhea; use for loose stools, diarrhea, poor appetite, weight loss, indigestion, nausea, vomiting and rumbling intestines.

#185 Six Gentlemen Teapills (*Liu Jun Zi Wan–Six Major Herb Combination*): codonopsis, white atractylodes, *fu ling*, citrus (*chen pi*), pinellia, licorice; tonifies Spleen Qi, transforms Phlegm, harmonizes the Stomach, descends rebellious Stomach Qi, transforms Damp, stops vomiting; use for poor digestion, loose stools, gas, bloatedness, drooling, nausea, vomiting, postnasal drip.

#186 Six Gentlemen Plus Teapills (*Xiang Sha Liu Jun Zi Wan–Sausserea and Cardamom Combination*): white atractylodes, *fu ling*, codonopsis, pinellia, citrus (*chen pi*), cardamom (*sha ren*), sausserea (*mu xiang*), licorice, jujube date, fresh ginger; tonifies Spleen Qi, transforms Phlegm, descends rebellious Qi; use for poor appetite, bloatedness, loose stools, nausea, vomiting, belching, morning sickness, Crohn's disease and chronic diarrhea due to Deficient Spleen Qi.

#187 Solitary Hermit (*Du Huo Ji Sheng Wan–Tuhuo and Vaeicum Combination*): pseudostellaria (*tai zi shen*), angelica (*du huo*), loranthus, siler, asarum (*xi xin*), cooked rehmannia, eucommia, achyranthes, cinnamon bark, ligusticum, *dang gui*, white peony, licorice, *fu ling*, gentian (*G. macrophylla–qin jiao*); strengthen tendons and bones, Kidneys and Liver, dispel Wind-Cold Damp, moves Blood; use for arthritis, rheumatism, sciatica, chronic lower back pain, slow gait, stiff knees, numbness in limbs and painful joints and tendons, all due to Deficiency with an aversion to cold.

#188 Sophora Japonica Teapills (*Huai Jiao Wan*): sophora (*huai jiao zi*), sanguisorba (*di yu*), scutellaria, citrus (*zhi ke*), siler (ledebouriella), *dang gui*; dispels Damp Heat, cools Blood, stops bleeding, dissipates masses; use for hemorrhoids with or without bleeding, including its pain, swelling and itchiness, also burning anus, anal fissure, intestinal bleeding and constipation.

#189 Soothe Liver Teapills (*Shu Gan Wan*): cyperus, white peony, bupleurum, citrus (*zhi ke*), green citrus (*qing pi*), citrus (*chen pi*), cardamom, magnolia bark, corydalis, moutan peony, citrus (*xiang yuan*), licorice, saussurea (*mu xiang*), turmeric rhizome, finger citron fruit (*fo shou gan*), aquilaria (*chen xiang*), white cardamom (*bai dou kou*), sandalwood shavings (*tan xiang*); Moves Liver Qi and Blood, clears Liver Heat, descends rebellious Stomach Qi, relieves pain; use for rib or epigastric distension or pain, nausea, belching, hiccups, poor appetite, indigestion, esophageal spasm, ulcer, irritability, gastritis, duodenal ulcer and chronic hepatitis or pancreatitis.

#190 Suan Zao Ren Tang (*Zizyphus Decoction*): zizyphus seeds, ligusticum, *fu ling*, anemarrhena, licorice; calms the Mind, clears Liver Heat, nourishes Liver Blood; use for insomnia, palpitations, nervous anxiety, excessive dreaming, night sweats, restlessness, dizziness, dryness of mouth and throat, all due to Deficient Liver Blood.

#191 The Great Mender (*Jin Gu Die Shang Wan*): dipsacus (*xu duan*), notoginseng (*tienqi–san qi*), red peony, boswellia, myrrh, safflower, daemonorops (*xue jie*), scirpus (*Sarganium simplex–san leng*), white peony, sappan wood (*su mu*), licorice, corydalis, *dang*

gui, *Eupolyphaga sinensis* (*tu bie chong*), moutan peony, *Cucumis melo* seed (*tian gua zi*), peach seed, siler (ledebouriella), clematis, drynaria (*gu sui bu*), citrus (*zhi shi*), *Artemisia anomala* (*liu ji nu*), platycodon, turmeric rhizome; moves and breaks up Blood stagnation, tonifies Blood, stops bleeding, strengthens sinews and bones, opens the channels and collaterals, relieves pain; use for traumatic sprain, fracture or dislocation with bruising and possible swelling.

#192 Tian Ma Gou Teng Yin Teapills (*Gastrodia and Uncaria Decoction*): abalone shell (*Haliotidis concha-shi jue ming*), loranthus, gambir, *he shou wu* vine, *fu ling*, achyranthes (*chuan niu xi*), motherwort, gastrodia, gardenia, scutellaria, eucommia; clears Heat, descends rising Liver Yang, nourishes Yin; use for migraines, headaches, vertigo, blurry vision, dizziness, paralysis, convulsions, mild hypertension, spasms, trembling, insomnia, coma, Bell's palsy, hemiplegia, hypertension, trigeminal neuralgia, following stroke and early stage Parkinson's disease.

#193 Tian Qi Teapills: *Panax notoginseng* root (*san qi*); dispels stagnant Blood and swelling and relieves pain; use for acute trauma with bleeding, bruising or swelling (internal or external), excessive menses, postpartum bleeding, blood in urine or stool, nosebleed, bleeding ulcer.

#194 True Warrior Teapills (*Zhen Wu Tang Wan–Vitality Combination*): *fu ling*, white peony, fresh ginger, prepared aconite, white atractylodes; tonifies Spleen and Kidney Yang and Qi, eliminates Dampness; use for low metabolism including edema of limbs and body, heavy and painful sensation of arms and legs, abdominal pain, intolerance of cold, diarrhea, difficult urination, chronic nephritis, liver cirrhosis, arthritis, congestive heart failure, dizziness and vertigo due to Deficient Yang and Excess Dampness.

#195 Two Immortals (*Er Xian Tang*): curculigo (*xian mao*), epimedium, morinda (*ba ji tian*), phellodendron, anemarrhena, *dang gui*; tonifies Kidney Yang and Essence, tonifies Blood, drains Kidney Fire; use for peri/menopausal disorders, hot flashes, night sweats, anxiety, fatigue, insomnia, palpitations, irritability, high blood pressure and hyperthyroidism.

#196 Universal Benefit Teapills (*Pu Ji Xiao Do Yin Wan*): wine-fried scutellaria, wine-fried coptis, scrophularia (*xuan shen*), platycodon, bupleurum, citrus (*chen pi*), licorice, forsythia, burdock seed, mint, fruiting body of puff-ball (*Lasiosphaera fenslii–ma bo*), isatis, bombyx mori (*jiang can*), Chinese black cohosh; clears Heat and toxins, dispels Wind; use for flu, colds, sore throat, tonsillitis, fever, chills, thirst, aching neck and shoulders, headache, swollen lymph nodes, ear infections, measles, mumps, chicken pox, skin infections with fever, boils and carbuncles.

#197 White Tiger Teapills (*Bai Hu Tang–Gypsum Combination*): gypsum, Chinese wild yam, anemarrhena, baked licorice; clears Lung and Stomach Heat, promotes Fluids; use for high fever, especially in encephalitis, meningitis, pneumonia, heat stroke, thirst with desire for cold drinks, red face, sweating, aversion to heat, toothache, nosebleeds, gum bleeding and conjunctivitis.

#198 Women's Precious (*Nu Ke Ba Zhen Wan*): prepared rehmannia, *dang gui*, white peony, codonopsis, *fu ling*, white atractylodes, ligusticum (*chuan xiong*), licorice; nourishes Blood, tonifies Qi; use for fatigue, dizziness, poor memory, cracked nails, pale complexion, dry skin and hair, amenorrhea, scanty or irregular menses, anemia, dizziness, palpitations and slow healing of wounds.

#199 Xiao Qing Long Wan (*Minor Blue Dragon Combination*): white peony, pinellia, cinnamon branches, schisandra, ephedra, dried ginger, asarum (*xi xin*), licorice; dispels Wind-Cold and Phlegm; use for cough with white phlegm, stuffy/runny nose, cold, flu, bronchitis, emphysema, chronic asthma & pollen allergies.

#200 Xiao Huo Luo Dan Teapills (*Minor Invigorate the Luo Channel Elixir Pills*): prepared aconite (*zhi chuan wu*), prepared aconite (*zhi cao wu*), lubricus (*di long*), *Pulvis arisaemae cum felle bovis* (*dan nan xing*), boswellia, myrrh; warms Interior, moves Qi and Blood, dispels Phlegm, relieves pain; use for arthritis, rheumatism, sciatica, joint pains due to Coldness, muscle spasms, numbness and hemiplegia following stroke.

#201 Yunnan Pai Yao (*Yunnan Paiyao*): tien qi ginseng plus other undisclosed substances; stops bleeding, moves Blood, disperses swelling, clears Heat and toxins, relieves pain; use internally or externally for trauma, injuries, wounds and hemorrhage and for excessive menstrual bleeding, nosebleeds, bleeding ulcer, blood in urine or stool and postpartum hemorrhage.

#202 Gan Mao Ling: Ilex asprella root (*gang mei gen*), evodia (*san cha ku*), chrysanthemum, Chinese vitex, isatis, honeysuckle; dispels Wind-Heat, relieves cough and toxins; use for colds and flu, fever with chills, headache, sore throat, red eyes, stiff neck and shoulders, nasal discharge, general body aches, swollen lymph glands, ear infections, sinus infection and viral pneumonia.

#230 An Shen Bu Xin Wan: Mother-of-pearl (*zhen zhu mu*), *he shou wu*, ligustrum, salvia, eclipta (*han lian cao*), cuscuta (*tu si zi*), albizzia bark, cooked rehmannia, schisandra, sweetflag (*Acorus gramineus-shi chang pu*); calms Yang, Heart and Shen; use for Shen disturbance due to Heart and Kidneys not communicating, causing rising of Yang with insomnia, vivid dreams, nightmares, palpitations, dizziness, or restlessness with anxiety, chest oppression or pain.

#231 Angelica Dang Gui Teapills (*Dang Gui Wan*): *dang gui*, ligusticum, white atractylodes, jujube dates; nourishes Blood, promotes circulation; use for pale complexion, tiredness, dizziness, vertigo, tinnitus, amenorrhea, threatened miscarriage and postpartum anemia.

#232 Bao He Wan: hawthorn berries, pinellia, massa fermentata, *fu ling*, citrus (*chen pi*), forsythia, sprouted barley (*mai ya*), radish seed (*lai fu zi*); clears food stagnation, subdues rebellious Stomach Qi, clears Heat, drains Damp, tonifies Spleen Qi, promotes digestion; use for acute or chronic food stagnation with indigestion, abdominal or epigastric bloating, belching, hiccups, nausea, poor appetite, poorly formed stools, hangover, morning sickness, overeating and motion sickness.

#233 Chen Xiang Hua Qi Wan (*Aquilaria Pills*): codonopsis, white atractylodes, rhubarb, scutellaria, aquilaria (*chen xiang*); tonifies Qi, clears Stomach Heat, harmonizes the Stomach, descends rebellious Stomach Qi, clears and purges the bowel; use for Stomach Heat causing indigestion, poor appetite, abdominal distension, constipation, epigastric pain, canker sores and bad breath.

#234 Chuan Xiong Cha Tiao Wan (*Cnidium and Tea Combination*): mint, ligusticum (*chuan xiong*), schizonepeta (*jing jie*), notopterygium (*qiang huo*), angelica (*bai zhi*), licorice, siler (ledebouriella), Chinese wild ginger (*xi xin*)—take with green tea; releases the Exterior, warms the channels, frees the collaterals, stops pain; use for colds, flu and headaches due to Wind-Cold.

#235 Fu Ke Zhong Zi Wan: prepared rehmannia, eucommia, cyperus, ligusticum (*chuan xiong*), *dang gui*, dipsacus (*xu duan*), mugwort (*ai ye*), scutellaria, donkey skin gelatin (*e jiao*), white peony; nourishes and moves Blood, warms Kidney Yang, warms the uterus, cools and nourishes the Liver; use for infertility from Deficient Blood and Kidney Yang, threatened miscarriage, amenorrhea, scanty or spotty menses, dry hair and skin, poor memory, weak lower back, cold lower limbs, sore knees, postmenstrual Deficient Blood and a general tonic.

#236 Huo Xiang Zheng Qi Wan (*Huo Hsiang Cheng Chi Pien-Agastache Pill*): agastache, white atractylodes, magnolia bark, platycodon, citrus (*chen pi*), licorice, pinellia, betel husk (*Areca catechu–da fu pi*), angelica (*bai zhi*), perilla (*zi su ye*), *fu ling*, jujube dates, dry ginger; disperses pathogenic factors and releases the Exterior, clears Summer Heat and Damp, dispels turbidity, descends rebellious Qi, harmonizes digestion; use for summer colds and flu with diarrhea, general diarrhea, bloatedness, loose stools,

vomiting, nausea, acute food stagnation, motion sickness, overeating and hangover.

#237 Jian Pi Wan (*Ginseng Stomachic Pills*): white atractylodes, citrus (*zhi shi*), codonopsis, citrus (*chen pi*), sprouted barley (*mai ya*), hawthorn berries; dispels food stagnation, harmonizes the Stomach, descends rebellious Qi, tonifies Spleen Qi; use for digestive problems such as poor appetite gas, bloatedness, abdominal discomfort after eating, loose stools, rumbling intestines, nausea and fatigue.

#238 Lilium Teapills (*Bai He Gu Jin Wan–Lily Combination*): prepared rehmannia, raw rehmannia, ophiopogon, lily bulb (*chuan bei mu*), *dang gui*, white peony, licorice, scrophularia (*xuan shen*) platycodon; tonifies Lung Yin, transforms Phlegm; use for dry cough, blood with cough, sore throat, difficulty breathing, low-grade tidal fever and smoker's and whooping cough with little phlegm.

#239 Mu Xiang Shun Qi Wan: *dang gui*, magnolia bark, saussurea (*mu xiang*), grass cardamom (*cao dou kou*), black atractylodes, black cardamom (*yi zhi ren*), alisma, citrus (*qing pi*), evodia (*wu zhu yu*), dried ginger, citrus (*chen pi*), *fu ling*, pinellia, Chinese black cohosh, bupleurum; tonifies Spleen Qi and Yang, dispels Damp; use for indigestion, abdominal distension, poor appetite, rumbling intestines, loose or erratic stools and sensitivity to cold foods.

#240 Xiang Sha Yang Wei Wan (*Xiang Sha Yang Wei Pian*): white atractylodes, *fu ling*, citrus (*chen pi*), pinellia, sausserea (*mu xiang*), agastache, cyperus, white cardamom cluster (*bai dou kou*), magnolia bark, cardamom seeds (*sha ren*), citrus (*zhi shi*), jujube dates, licorice, fresh ginger; clears Damp, transforms Phlegm, harmonizes the Stomach, descends rebellious Stomach Qi, tonifies Spleen Qi, soothes the Liver, stops vomiting; use for poor appetite, abdominal distension, nausea, acid regurgitation, rumbling intestines, loose or erratic stools, duodenal ulcer, morning sickness and gastritis.

#241 Xiao Chai Hu Tang Wan (*Minor Bupleurum Combination*): bupleurum, pinellia, codonopsis, scutellaria, jujube date, licorice, fresh ginger; cools Liver Heat, harmonizes and resolves half Exterior–half Interior syndrome, transforms Phlegm, tonifies Spleen Qi; use for alternating chills and fever, lingering illness, prolonged colds and flu, nausea, poor appetite, low energy, pain in the ribs, menstrual disorders, irregular periods, PMS irritability, all due to stagnant Liver Qi and Liver Heat.

#242 Yu Dai Wan (*Heal Vaginal Discharge Pill*): ailanthus (*chun gen pi*), white peony, prepared rehmannia, *dang gui*, phellodendron, ligusticum (*chuan xiong*), galanga (*gao liang jiang*); clears Heat and toxins, eliminates Dampness, nourishes Yin and Blood, stops bleeding; use for vaginal discharge, itching and bleeding and vaginal and urinary yeast infections, with or without bleeding.

#260 Ching Chuan Bao (*Qing Chun Bao; Recovery of Youth Tablet*): ginseng (*ren shen*), prepared rehmannia, asparagus root; tonifies Kidney Yang, Qi and Blood, moves Blood, benefits relationship between the Kidneys and Heart; a geriatric tonic useful in promoting good memory, sexual function, immunity, restful sleep, heart function and appetite.

#261 Coix Combination: coix, ephedra, *dang gui*, white atractylodes, cinnamon branches, white peony, licorice; use for rheumatism and arthritis, kidney infections, pulmonary edema and pleurisy.

#262 Coptis Purge Fire (see *Resources* to obtain): coptis, lophatherum (*dan zhu ye*), bupleurum, raw rehmannia, *dang gui*, white peony, akebia (*ba yue zha*), anemarrhena, phellodendron, gentian, alisma, plantago, scutellaria, sophora, forsythia, gardenia, licorice; clears Excess and Deficient Heat in Liver and Heart; use for excessive menstruation and peri/menopausal symptoms due to Heat and Yin Deficiency with rising Liver Yang.

#263 Shen Ching Shuai Jao Wan: astragalus, ginseng (*ren shen*), zizyphus, placenta, ophiopogon, clam shell (*hai ge ke*), schisandra, coptis, *he shou wu*, donkey skin gelatin (*e jiao*), *dang gui*, *fu ling*; tonifies Heart Qi, Blood and Yin, cools Blood Heat, subdues Yang, calms Shen; use for insomnia, nightmares, palpitation, anxiety, vivid dreaming, restlessness, poor concentration, mental fatigue, dizziness and tinnitus all due to Deficiency.

#264 Te Xiao Yao Tong Ling (*Specific Lumbaglin*): eucommia, morinda, *dang gui*, carthamus, achyranthes, gentian (*G. macrophylla–qin jiao*), aconite (*cao wu*), angelica (*du huo*), loranthus, angelica (*bai zhi*), clematis, drynaria (*gu sui bu*); tonifies Kidney Yang, tonifies and moves Blood, strengthens tendons and bones, dispels Wind and eliminates Damp, relieves pain; use for lower back and knee pain, sciatica, arthritis and rheumatism of the lower body, especially if there's accompanying Liver Heat.

#265 Yue Qu Tang: equal parts ligusticum, black atractylodes, gardenia, *shen qu* and saussurea (or cyperus); this formula moves all stagnations: Blood, Damp, Heat, food and Qi.

#266 Shao Yao Tang (*Peony Combination*): white peony, coptis, scutellaria, rhubarb, *dang gui*, cinnamon bark, saussurea, areca, licorice; clears Heat and toxins, relieves pain; use for inflammation of intestines caused by Heat, Dampness or bacterial toxin with symptoms of abdominal pain, bloody stool, diarrhea, burning sensation of anus and short, dark urination.

Identification of Herbs

✦

HERBS BY COMMON NAME

COMMON NAME	LATIN NAME	PIN YIN	SANSKRIT
Agastache	Agastache rugosa	huo xiang	
	Pogostemon cablin	huo xiang	
Agrimony	Agrimonia pilosa	xian he cao	
	A. eupatoria		
Albizzia, bark	Albizzia julibrissin	he huan pi	
Albizzia , flowerheads		he huan hua	
Alisma	Alisma orientale	ze xie	
	A. plantago-aquatica	ze xie	
Aloe	Aloe vera, A. chinensis	lu hui	kumari
	A. ferox	lu hui	kumari
	A. barbadensis		kumari
American ginseng	Panax quinquefolium	xi yang shen	
Andographis	Andrographis paniculata	chuan xin lian	
Angelica	Angelica archangelica		
Angelica	A. dahurica	bai zhi	
	A. pubescens	duo huo	
Angelica sinensis: see Dang gui			
Apricot	Prunus armeniaca	xing ren	
Arjuna	Terminalia arjuna		arjuna
Asafoetida	Ferula asafoetida	ai wei	hingu
Ashwagandha	Withania somnifera		ashwagandha
Asparagus	Asparagus cochinchinensis	tian men dong	shatavari
Astragalus	Astragalus membranaceus	huang qi	
Atractylodes, black	Atractylodes lancea	cang zhu	
Atractylodes, white	Atractylodes macrocephala	bai zhu	
Bacopa: see Gotu kola			
Baptisia	Baptisia tinctoria		

COMMON NAME	LATIN NAME	PIN YIN	SANSKRIT
Barberry: see Oregon grape			
Bayberry	Myrica cerifera		katphala
Bilberry	Vaccinium spp.		
Blackberry	Rubus fruticosus		
Black cohosh	Cimicifuga racemosa		
	C. foetida	sheng ma	
Black haw	Viburnum prunifolium		
Black pepper	Piper nigrum	hu jiao	marich
Blue cohosh	Caulophyllium thalictroides		
Blueberry: see Bilberry			
Boneset	Eupatorium perfoliatum		
Boswellia: see Frankincense			
Bugleweed	Lycopus virginicus		
	L. lucidus	ze lan	
Bupleurum	Bupleurum chinense	chai hu	
Burdock	Arctium lappa	niu bang zi (seeds)	
Cactus	Selenicereus grandiflorus		
	Cereus grandiflorus		
	Cactus grandiflorus		
Calendula	Calendula officinalis		
California poppy	Eschscholzia californica		
Cardamom	Elettaria cardamomum		
	Amomum villosum	sha ren	ela
	A. tsao-ko	cao guo	
Carthamus: see Safflower			
Cascara sagrada	Rhamnus purshiana		
Castor	Ricinus communis	bi ma zi	eranda
Cayenne	Capsicum anuum		marichi-phalam
Chamomile	Matricaria recutita		
	Anthemis nobiles		
Chaparral	Larrea tridentata		
	L. mexicana		
Chaste Tree Berry: see Vitex			
Chickweed	Stellaria media		
Chokecherry: see Wild cherry			
Chrysanthemum	Chrysanthemum morifolium	ju hua	
Cinnamon, bark	Cinnamomum cassia	rou gui	twak
Cinnamon, twigs		gui zhi	
Citrus, aged tangerine peel	Citrus reticulata	chen pi	
Citrus, green	Citrus reticulata	qing pi	

COMMON NAME	LATIN NAME	PIN YIN	SANSKRIT
Citrus, immature bitter orange peel	Citrus reticulata	zhi shi or chih-shih	
Citrus, tangerine seed	Citrus reticulata	ju he	
Codonopsis	Codonopsis pilosula	dang shen	
Coix	Coix lachryma jobi	yi yi ren	
Coltsfoot	Tussilago farfara	kuan dong hua	
Comfrey	Symphytum officinale		
Coptis	Coptis chinensis	huang lian	
Cordyceps	Cordyceps sinensis	dong chong xia cao	
Cornus	Cornus officinalis	shan zhu yu	
Corydalis	Corydalis yanhusuo	yan hu suo	
Cramp bark: see Black haw			
Cuscuta	Cuscuta chinensis	tu si zi	
Cyperus	Cyperus rotundus	xiang fu	
Damiana	Turnera diffusa		
Dandelion	Taraxacum mongolicum	pu gong ying	atirasa
Dang gui	Angelica sinensis	dang gui (dong quai, tang keui)	
Deer antler	Cornu cervi parvum	lu rong	
Dipsacus	Dipsacus asper	xu duan	
Echinacea	Echinacea spp.		
Elder	Sambucus nigra		
	S. canadensis		
Elecampane	Inula helenium		pushkaramula
Eleuthro	Eleutherococcus senticosus		
	I. japonica, I chinensis	xuan fu hua	pushkaramula
Ephedra	Ephedra spp.	ma huang	
Epimedium	Epimedium grandiflorum	yin yang huo	
Eucommia	Eucommia ulmoides	du zhong	
Eyebright	Euphrasia officinalis		
Fennel	Foeniculum vulgare	xiao hui xiang	mahdurika
Fenugreek	Trigonella foenum-graecum	hu lu ba	methi
Feverfew	Tanacetum parthenium		atasi
Fleeceflower: see He Shou Wu			
Forsythia	Forsythia suspensa	lian qiao	
Foxglove, Chinese: see Rehmannia			
Frankincense	Boswellia carterii	ru xiang	shallaki
	B. serrata		salai guggul
Fu ling	Poria cocos	fu ling	
Gambir	Uncaria rhynchophylla	gou teng	
Ganoderma: see Reishi			

COMMON NAME	LATIN NAME	PIN YIN	SANSKRIT
Gardenia	Gardenia jasminoides	zhi zi	
Garlic	Allium sativum	da suan	lasunam
Gentian	Gentiana spp.	long dan cao	kirata, katuki, trayamana
Ginger, fresh	Zingiberis officinalis	sheng jiang	ardraka
Ginger, dried	Zingiberis officinalis	gan jiang	sunthi
Ginkgo, nut	Ginkgo biloba	bai guo	
Ginkgo, leaf			
	yin guo ye		
Ginseng	Panax ginseng	ren shen	
Goldenseal	Hydrastis canadensis		
Gotu kola	Centella asiatica	luo de da	brahmi
	Hydrocotyle asiatica	ji xue cao	mandukaparni
Gravel root	Eupatorium purpureum		
Green Citrus: see Citrus			
Hawthorn	Crataegus oxyacantha, C. spp.		
	C.pinnatifida	shan zha	
He shou wu	Polygonum multiflorum	he shou wu	
Hoelen: see Fu ling			
Honeysuckle	Lonicera japonica	jin yin hua	
Horny Goat Wort (Weed): see Epimedium			
Horse chestnut	Aesculus hippocastanum		
Huckleberry: see Bilberry			
Isatis	Isatis tinctoria	ban lan gen	
Jujube, dates	Ziziphus jujuba	da zao	
Jujube, seeds	Z. spinosae	suan zao ren	
Kava kava	Piper methysticum		
Kuzu, Kudzu root: see Pueraria			
Lemon balm	Melissa officinalis		
Licorice, raw	Glycyrrhiza glabra		
Licorice, raw	G. uralensis	gan cao	madhukam
Licorice, honey-fried	G. uralensis	zhi gan cao	yashti madhu
Ligusticum	Ligusticum wallichii	chuan xiong	
Lobelia	Lobelia inflata		
	L. chinensis	ban bian lian	
Longan	Euphoria longan	long yan rou	
Loquat	Eriobotrya japonica	pi pa ye	
Lycii Berries	Lycium barbarum		
	L. chinensis	gou qi zi	

COMMON NAME	LATIN NAME	PIN YIN	SANSKRIT
Lycopus: see Bugleweed			
Magnolia, bark	Magnolia officinalis	hou po	
Magnolia, flower	Magnolia liliflora	xin yi hua	
Marshmallow	Althea officinalis		
Milk thistle	Silybum marianum		
Mimosa tree: see Albizzia			
Mint	Mentha haplocalyx	bo he	
	M. arvensis	bo he	
	M. piperita		putani
Motherwort	Leonurus heterophyllus	yi mu cao	
	L. cardiaca		
Moutan: see Peony			
Mugwort	Artemisia argyi	ai ye	
	A. vulgaris	ai ye	nagadamani
Mulberry, fruit	Morus alba	sang shen	
Mulberry, leaf	Morus alba	sang ye	
Mulberry, twigs	Morus alba	sang zhi	
Mulberry, root bark	Morus alba	sang bai pi	
Mullein	Verbascum thapsus		
Myrobalans: see Triphala			
Myrrh	Commiphora myrrha	mo yao	daindhava, bola
	C. molmol	mo yao	daindhava, bola
	C. mukul	mo yao	guggulu
Neem	Azadirachta indica		nimba
Nettle	Urtica urens and spp.		
Night-blooming Cereus: see Cactus			
Notoginseng: see Tienqi			
Olive leaf	Olea europea		
Ophiopogon	Ophiopogon japonicus	mai men dong	
Oregon grape	Mahonia spp.		
Oyster shell	Ostera gigas	mu li	
Parsley	Petroselinum spp.		
Partridgeberry	Mitchella repens		
Passionflower	Passiflora incarnata		
Patchouli: see Agastache			
Pau d'arco	Tabebuia heptaphylla		
	T. impetiginosa		
Peony, white	Paeonia lactiflora	bai shao	
Peony, red	Paeonia rubrae,	chi shao	
	P. veitehii	chi shao	

COMMON NAME	LATIN NAME	PIN YIN	SANSKRIT
Peony, tree (or moutan)	P. suffruticosa	mu dan pi	
Platycodon	Platycodon grandiflorum	jie geng	
Plantain	Plantago major		
	P. lanceolata		
	P. asiatica	che qian cao	
Pogostemon: see Agastache			
Polygonum multiflorum: see He Shou Wu			
Poppy: see California poppy			
Poria Cocos: see Fu ling			
Prickly ash	Zanthoxylum americanum (Northern)		tumburu
	Z. clava-herculis (Southern)		tumburu
	Z. bungeanum	chuan jiao	tumburu
Pseudoginseng: see Tienqi			
Pueraria	Pueraria lobata	ge gen	bidari kand
Purple Coneflower: see Echinacea			
Raspberry	Rubus idaeus		
	R. chingii	fu pen zi	
Red clover	Trifolium pratense		vana-methika
Red Sage Root: see Salvia			
Rehmannia, prepared	Rehmannia glutinosa	shu di huang	
Rehmannia, raw	Rehmannia glutinosa	sheng di huang	
Reishi	Ganoderma lucidum	ling zhi	
Rhubarb	Rheum palmatum	da huang	amlavetasa
Safflower	Carthamus tinctorius	hong hua	
Salvia	Salvia miltiorrhiza	dan shen	
Sarsaparilla	Smilax medica		
	S. officinalis and other spp.		
	S. glabra	tu fu ling	
Sassafras	Sassafras albidum		
	S. varifolium		
	S. officinale		
Saw palmetto	Serenoa repens		
Schisandra	Schisandra chinensis	wu wei zi	
Scute	Scutellaria baicalensis	huang qin	
Shepherd's purse	Capsella bursa-pastoris	ji cai	
Skullcap	Scutellaria lateriflora		
Slippery elm	Ulmus fulva		
Squawvine: see Partridgeberry			
St. John's wort	Hypericum perforatum		
Tangerine: see Citrus			

COMMON NAME	LATIN NAME	PIN YIN	SANSKRIT
Teasel: see Dipsacus			
Thyme	Thymus vulgaris		
Tien qi (Tian qi, Tienchi)	Panax notoginseng	san qi	
	P. pseudoginseng	san qi	
Triphala: three fruits:			
Indian gooseberry	Emblica officinalis		amla
	Terminalia chebula	he zi	haritaki
	Terminalia belerica		vibhitaki, bhibitaki
Turmeric, tuber	Curcuma longa	yu jin	haridra
Turmeric, rhizome	Curcuma longa	jiang huang	
Uncaria: see Gambir			
Usnea	Usnea barbata		
Uva ursi	Arctostaphylos uva ursi		
Valerian	Valeriana officinalis		tagara
Vitex	Vitex agnus-castus		
	V. rotundifolia, V. trifolia	man jing zi	
Walnut, black	Juglans nigra		
Walnut, nut	J. regia	hu tao ren	
Wild cherry	Prunus serotina		padmaka
	P. virginiana		
Wild indigo: see Baptisia			
Wild yam, Chinese	Dioscorea opposita	shan yao	
Wild yam, Western	Dioscorea villosa		
Yarrow	Achillea millefolium		gandana
Yellow dock	Rumex crispus		amla vetasa

HERBS BY LATIN NAME

LATIN NAME	COMMON NAME	PIN YIN	SANSKRIT
Achillea millefolium	Yarrow		gandana
Aesculus hippocastanum	Horse chestnut		
Agastache rugosa	Agastache	huo xiang	
Agrimonia eupatoria	Agrimony		
Agrimonia pilosa	Agrimony	xian he cao	
Albizzia julibrissin	Albizzia, bark	hu huan pi	
Albizzia, flowerhead		hu huan huas	
Alisma orientale	Alisma		
Alisma plantago-aquatica	Alisma	ze xie	
Allium sativum	Garlic	da suan	lasunam

LATIN NAME	COMMON NAME	PIN YIN	SANSKRIT
Aloe barbadensis	Aloe		
Aloe chinensis	Aloe	lu hui	kumari
Aloe ferox	Aloe	lu hui	kumari
Aloe vera	Aloe	lu hui	kumari
Althea officinalis	Marshmallow		
Amomum tsao-ko	Cardamom	cao guo	
Amomum villosum	Cardamom	sha ren	ela
Andrographis paniculata	Andographis	chuan xin lian	
Angelica archangelica	Angelica		
Angelica dahurica	Angelica	bai zhi	
Angelica pubescens	Angelica	duo huo	
Angelica sinensis	Dang gui	dang gui (dong quai, tang keui)	
Anthemis nobiles	Chamomile, Roman		
Arctium lappa	Burdock	niu bang zi (seeds)	
Arctostaphylos uva ursi	Uva ursi		
Artemisia argyi	Mugwort	ai ye	
Artemisia vulgaris	Mugwort	ai ye	nagadamani
Asarum canadensis	Wild ginger		
Asparagus cochinchinensis	Asparagus	tian men dong	shatavari
Astragalus membranaceus	Astragalus	huang qi	
Atractylodes lancea	Atractylodes, black	cang zhu	
Atractylodes macrocephala	Atractylodes, white	bai zhu	
Azadirachta indica	Neem		nimba
Baptisia tinctoria	Baptisia		
Boswellia carterii	Frankincense	ru xiang	shallaki
Boswellia serrata	Frankincense		salai guggul
Bupleurum chinense	Bupleurum	chai hu	
Cactus grandiflorus	Cactus		
Calendula officinalis	Calendula		
Capsella bursa-pastoris	Shepherd's purse	ji ca	
Capsicum anuum	Cayenne		marichi-phalam
Carthamus tinctorius	Safflower	hong hua	
Caulophyllium thalictroides	Blue cohosh		
Centella asiatica	Gotu kola	luo de da	brahmi
Cereus grandiflorus	Cactus		
Chrysanthemum morifolium	Chrysanthemum	ju hua	
Cimicifuga foetida	Black cohosh	sheng ma	
Cimicifuga racemosa	Black cohosh		
Cinnamomum cassia	Cinnamon, bark	rou gui	twak

LATIN NAME	COMMON NAME	PIN YIN	SANSKRIT
Cinnamomum, twigs		gui zhi	
Citrus reticulata	Citrus, aged tangerine peel	chen pi	
	Citrus, green	qing pi	
	Citrus, immature bitter orange peel	zhi shi or chih-shih	
	Citrus, tangerine seed	ju he	
Codonopsis pilosula	Codonopsis	dang shen	
Coix lachryma jobi	Coix	yi yi ren	
Commiphora molmol	Myrrh	mo yao	daindhava, bola
Commiphora mukul	Myrrh	mo yao	guggulu
Commiphora myrrha	Myrrh	mo yao	daindhava, bola
Coptis chinensis	Coptis	huang lian	
Cordyceps sinensis	Cordyceps	dong chong xia cao	
Cornu cervi parvum	Deer antler	lu rong	
Cornus officinalis	Cornus	shan zhu yu	
Corydalis yanhusuo	Corydalis	yan hu suo	
Crataegus oxyacantha, spp.	Hawthorn		
Crategus pinnatifida	Hawthorn	shan zha	
Curcuma longa	Turmeric, tuber	yu jin	haridra
	Turmeric, rhizome	jiang huang	
Cuscuta chinensis	Cuscuta	tu si zi	
Cyperus rotundus	Cyperus	xiang fu	
Dioscorea opposita	Wild yam	shan yao	
Dioscorea villosa	Wild yam		
Dipsacus asper	Dipsacus	xu duan	
Echinacea spp.	Echinacea		
Elettaria cardamomum	Cardamom		
Eleutherococcus senticosus	Eleuthro (Siberian ginseng)		
Emblica officinalis	Indian gooseberry (a Myrobalan)		amla
Ephedra spp.	Ephedra	ma huang	
Epimedium grandiflorum	Epimedium	yin yang huo	
Eriobotrya japonica	Loquat	pi pa ye	
Eschscholzia californica	California poppy		
Eucommia ulmoides	Eucommia	du zhong	
Eupatorium perfoliatum	Boneset		
Eupatorium purpureum	Gravel root		
Euphoria longan	Longan	long yan rou	
Euphrasia officinalis	Eyebright		
Ferula asafoetida	Asafoetida	ai wei	hingu
Foeniculum vulgare	Fennel	xiao hui xiang	mahdurika
Forsythia suspensa	Forsythia	lian qiao	

LATIN NAME	COMMON NAME	PIN YIN	SANSKRIT
Ganoderma lucidum	Reishi	ling zhi	
Gardenia jasminoides	Gardenia	zhi zi	
Gentiana spp.	Gentian	long dan cao	kirata, katuki, trayamana
Ginkgo biloba	Ginkgo, nut	bai guo	
	Ginkgo, leaf	yin guo ye	
Glycyrrhiza glabra	Licorice, raw		
Glycyrrhiza uralensis	Licorice, raw	gan cao	madhukam
	Licorice, honey-fried	zhi gan cao	yashti madhu
Hydrastis canadensis	Goldenseal		
Hydrocotyle asiatica	Gotu kola	ji xue cao	mandukaparni
Hypericum perforatum	St. John's wort		
Inula helenium	Elecampane		
Inula japonica	Elecampane	xuan fu hua	pushkaramula
Isatis tinctoria	Isatis	ban lan gen	
Juglans nigra	Walnut, black		
Juglans regia	Walnut	hu tao ren (nut)	
Larrea mexicana	Chaparral		
Larrea tridentata	Chaparral		
Leonurus cardiaca	Motherwort		
Leonurus heterophyllus	Motherwort	yi mu cao	
Ligusticum wallichii	Ligusticum	chuan xiong	
Lobelia chinensis	Lobelia	ban bian lian	
Lobelia inflata	Lobelia		
Lonicera japonica	Honeysuckle	jin yin hua	
Lycium chinensis	Lycii berries	gou qi zi	
Lycopus lucidus	Bugleweed	ze lan	
Lycopus virginicus	Bugleweed		
Magnolia liliflora	Magnolia, flower	xin yi hua	
Magnolia officinalis	Magnolia, bark	hou po	
Mahonia spp.	Oregon grape, Barberry		
Matricaria recutita	Chamomile, German		
Melissa officinalis	Lemon balm		
Mentha arvensis	Mint	bo he	
Mentha haplocalyx	Mint	bo he	
Mentha piperita	Mint		putani
Mitchella repens	Partridgeberry		
Morus alba	Mulberry, fruit	sang shen	
	Mulberry, leaf	sang ye	
	Mulberry, twigs	sang zhi	

LATIN NAME	COMMON NAME	PIN YIN	SANSKRIT
	Mulberry, root bark	sang bai pi	
Myrica cerifera	Bayberry		katphala
Olea europea	Olive leaf		
Ophiopogon japonicus	Ophiopogon	mai men dong	
Ostera gigas	Oyster shell	mu li	
Paeonia lactiflora	Peony, white	bai shao	
Paeonia rubrae	Peony, red	chi shao	
Paeonia suffruticosa	Peony, tree (or moutan)	mu dan pi	
Paeonia veitchii	Peony, red	chi shao	
Panax ginseng	Ginseng	ren shen	
Panax notoginseng	Tien qi (Tian qi, tienchi)	san qi	
Panax quinquefolium	American ginseng	xi yang shen	
Panax pseudoginseng	Tien qi (Tian qi, tienchi)	san qi	
Passiflora incarnata	Passionflower		
Petroselinum spp.	Parsley		
Piper methysticum	Kava kava		
Piper nigrum	Black pepper	hu jiao	marich
Plantago asiatica	Plantain	che qian cao	
Plantago lanceolata	Plantain		
Plantago major	Plantain		
Platycodon grandiflorum	Platycodon	jie geng	
Pogostemon cablin	Agastache	huo xiang	
Polygonum multiflorum	He shou wu	he shou wu	
Poria cocos	Fu ling	fu ling	
Prunus armeniaca	Apricot	xing ren	
Prunus serotina	Wild cherry		padmaka
Prunus virginiana	Wild cherry		
Pueraria lobata	Pueraria	ge gen	bidari kand
Ramulus Sangjisheng	Loranthus	sang ji sheng	
Rehmannia glutinosa	Rehmannia, prepared	shu di huang	
	Rehmannia, raw	sheng di huang	
Rhamnus purshiana	Cascara sagrada		
Rheum palmatum	Rhubarb	da huang	amlavetasa
Ricinus communis	Castor	bi ma zi	eranda
Rubus chingii	Raspberry	fu pen zi	
Rubus fruticosus	Blackberry		
Rubus idaeus	Raspberry		
Rumex crispus	Yellow dock		amla vetasa
Salvia miltiorrhiza	Salvia	dan shen	
Sambucus canadensis	Elder		

LATIN NAME	COMMON NAME	PIN YIN	SANSKRIT
Sambucus nigra	Elder		
Sassafras albidum	Sassafras		
Sassafras officinale	Sassafras		
Sassafras varifolium	Sassafras		
Schisandra chinensis	Schisandra	wu wei zi	
Schizonepeta tenufolia	Schizonepeta	jing jie	
Scutellaria baicalensis	Scute	huang qin	
Scutellaria lateriflora	Skullcap		
Selenicereus grandiflorus	Cactus		
Serenoa repens	Saw palmetto		
Silybum marianum	Milk thistle		
Smilax glabra	Sarsaparilla	tu fu ling	
Smilax medica	Sarsaparilla		
Smilax officinalis and other spp.	Sarsaparilla		
Stellaria media	Chickweed		
Symphytum officinale	Comfrey		
Tabebuia heptaphylla	Pau d'arco		
Tabebuia impetiginosa	Pau d'arco		
Tanacetum parthenium	Feverfew		atasi
Taraxacum mongolicum	Dandelion	pu gong ying	atirasa
Terminala arjuna	Arjuna		arjuna
Terminalia belerica	a Myrobalan		vibhitaki, bhibitaki
Terminalia chebula	a Myrobalan	he zi	haritaki
Thymus vulgaris	Thyme		
Trifolium pratense	Red clover		vana-methika
Trigonella foenum-graecum	Fenugreek	hu lu ba	methi
Turnera diffusa	Damiana		
Tussilago farfara	Coltsfoot	kuan dong hua	
Ulmus fulva	Slippery elm		
Uncaria rhynchophylla	Gambir	gou teng	
Urtica urens and spp.	Nettle		
Usnea barbata	Usnea		
Vaccinium spp.	Bilberry		
Valeriana officinalis	Valerian		tagara
Verbascum thapsus	Mullein		
Viburnum prunifolium	Black haw		
Vitex agnus-castus	Vitex		
Vitex rotundifolia	Vitex	man jing zi	
Vitex trifolia	Vitex	man jing zi	
Withania somnifera	Ashwagandha		ashwagandha

LATIN NAME	COMMON NAME	PIN YIN	SANSKRIT
Zanthoxylum americanum (Northern)	Prickly ash		tumburu
Zanthoxylum bungeanum	Prickly ash	chuan jiao	tumburu
Zanthoxylum clava-herculis (Southern)	Prickly ash		tumburu
Zingiberis officinalis	Ginger, fresh	sheng jiang	ardraka
	Ginger, dried	gan jiang	sunthi
Ziziphus jujuba	Jujube, dates	da zao	
Ziziphus spinosae	Jujube, seeds	suan zao ren	

HERBS BY PIN YIN CHINESE NAME

PIN YIN NAME	COMMON NAME	LATIN NAME	SANSKRIT
Ai wei	Asafoetida	Ferula asafoetida	hingu
Ai ye	Mugwort	Artemisia argyi	
		A. vulgaris	nagadamani
Bai guo	Ginkgo nut	Ginkgo biloba	
Bai shao	Peony, white	Paeonia lactiflora	
Bai zhi	Angelica	Angelica dahurica	
Bai zhu	Atractylodes, white	Atractylodes macrocephala	
Ban bian lian	Lobelia, Chinese	Lobelia chinensis	
Ban lan gen	Isatis	Isatis tinctoria	
Bi ma zi	Castor	Ricinus communis	eranda
Bo he	Mint	Mentha haplocalyx, M. arvensis	
Cang zhu	Atractylodes, black	Atractylodes lancea	
Cao guo	Cardamom	A. tsao-ko	
Chai hu	Bupleurum	Bupleurum chinense	
Che qian cao	Plantain	Plantago asiatica	
Chen pi	Citrus, aged tangerine peel	Citrus reticulata	
Chi shao	Peony, red	Paeonia rubrae, P. veichii	
Chih-shih	Citrus, immature bitter orange peel	Citrus reticulata	
Chuan jiao	Prickly ash	Z. bungeanum	tumburu
Chuan xin lian	Andographis	Andrographis paniculata	
Chuan xiong	Ligusticum	Ligusticum wallichii	
Da huang	Rhubarb	Rheum palmatum	amlavetasa
Da suan	Garlic	Allium sativum	lasunam
Da zao	Jujube, dates	Ziziphus jujuba	
Dan shen	Salvia	Salvia miltiorrhiza	
Dang gui	Dang gui (dong quai, tang keui)	Angelica sinensis	
Dang shen	Codonopsis	Codonopsis pilosula	
Dong chong xia cao	Cordyceps	Cordyceps sinensis	

PIN YIN NAME	COMMON NAME	LATIN NAME	SANSKRIT
Dong quai: see Dang gui			
Du zhong	Eucommia	Eucommia ulmoides	
Duo huo	Angelica	Angelica pubescens	
Fang feng	Siler	Ledebouriella divaricata	
Fu pen zi	Raspberry	Rubus chingii	
Gan cao	Licorice, raw	Glycyrrhiza uralensis	madhukam
Gan jiang	Ginger, dried	Zingiberis officinalis	sunthi
Ge gen	Pueraria	Pueraria lobata	bidari kand
Gou qi zi	Lycii Berries	Lycium chinensis	
Gou teng	Gambir	Uncaria rhynchophylla	
Gui zhi	Cinnamon, twigs	Cinnamomum cassia	twak
He huan hua	Albizzia, flowerhead	Albizzia julibrissin	
He huan pi	Albizzia, bark	Albizzia julibrissin	
He shou wu	He shou wu	Polygonum multiflorum	
He zi	a Myobalan	Terminalia chebula	haritaki
Hong hua	Safflower	Carthamus tinctorius	
Hou po	Magnolia bark	Magnolia officinalis	
Hu jiao	Black pepper	Piper nigrum	marich
Hu lu ba	Fenugreek	Trigonella foenum-graecum	methi
Hu tao ren	Walnut, nut	Juglans regia	
Huo xiang	Agastache	Agastache rugosa, Pogostomon cablin	
Huang lian	Coptis	Coptis chinensis	
Huang qi	Astragalus	Astragalus membranaceus	
Huang qin	Scutellaria	Scutellaria baicalensis	
Ji cai	Shepherd's purse	Capsella bursa-pastoris	
Ji xue cao	Gotu kola	Hydrocotyle asiatica	mandukaparni
Jie geng	Platycodon	Platycodon grandiflorum	
Jiang huang	Turmeric, rhizome	Curcuma longa	
Jin yin hua	Honeysuckle	Lonicera japonica	
Ju he	Citrus, tangerine seed	Citrus reticulata	
Ju hua	Chrysanthemum	Chrysanthemum morifolium	
Kuan dong hua	Coltsfoot	Tussilago farfara	
Lian qiao	Forsythia	Forsythia suspensa	
Ling zhi	Reishi	Ganoderma lucidum	
Long dan cao	Gentian	Gentiana spp.	kirata, katuki,
Long yan rou	Longan	Euphoria longan	
Lu hui	Aloe	Aloe vera, A. chinensis, A. ferox	kumari
Lu rong	Deer antler	Cornu cervi parvum	
Luo de da	Gotu kola	Centella asiatica	brahmi
Ma huang	Ephedra	Ephedra spp.	

PIN YIN NAME	COMMON NAME	LATIN NAME	SANSKRIT
Mai men dong	Ophiopogon	Ophiopogon japonicus	
Man jing zi	Vitex	V. rotundifolia, V. trifolia	
Mo yao	Myrrh	Commiphora myrrha	daindhava, bola
		C. molmol	daindhava, bola
		C. mukul	guggulu
Mu dan pi	Peony, tree (or moutan)	Paeonia suffruticosa	
Mu li	Oyster shell	Ostera gigas	
Niu bang zi	Burdock, seeds	Arctium lappa	
Pi pa ye	Loquat	Eriobotrya japonica	
Pu gong ying	Dandelion	Taraxacum mongolicum	tirasa
Qing pi	Citrus, green	Citrus reticulata	
Ren shen	Ginseng	Panax ginseng	
Rou gui	Cinnamon, bark	Cinnamomum cassia	twak
Ru xiang	Frankincense	Boswellia carterii	shallaki
San qi	Tien qi, Tian qi, Tienchi	Panax notoginseng, P. pseudoginseng	
Sang bai pi	Mulberry, root bark	Morus alba	
Sang shen	Mulberry, fruit	Morus alba	
Sang ye	Mulberry, leaf	Morus alba	
Sang zhi	Mulberry, twigs	Morus alba	
Sha ren	Cardamom	Amomum villosum	ela
Shan yao	Wild yam	Dioscorea opposita	
Shan zha	Hawthorn	Crataegus pinnatifida.	
Shan zhu yu	Cornus	Cornus officinalis	
Sheng di huang	Rehmannia, raw	Rehmannia glutinosa	
Sheng jiang	Ginger, fresh	Zingiberis officinalis	ardraka
Sheng ma	Black Cohosh	Cimicifuga foetida	
Shu di huang	Rehmannia, prepared	Rehmannia glutinosa	
Suan zao ren	Jujube, seeds	Zizyphus spinosae	
Tang Kuei: see Dang Gui			
Tian men dong	Asparagus	Asparagus cochinchinensis	shatavari
Tian Qi: see San Qi			
Tien Qi: see San Qi			
Tu fu ling	Sarsaparilla, Chinese	Smilax glabra	
Tu si zi	Cuscuta	Cuscuta chinensis	
Wu wei zi	Schisandra	Schisandra chinensis	
Xi yang shen	American ginseng	Panax quinquefolium	
Xian he cao	Agrimony	Agrimonia pilosa	
Xiang fu	Cyperus	Cyperus rotundus	
Xiao hui xiang	Fennel	Foeniculum vulgare	mahdurika
Xin yi hua	Magnolia flower	Magnolia liliflora	

PIN YIN NAME	COMMON NAME	LATIN NAME	SANSKRIT
Xing ren	Apricot	Prunus armeniaca	
Xu duan	Dipsacus	Dipsacus asper	
Xuan fu hua	Elecampane	Inula japonica	pushkaramula
Yan hu suo	Corydalis	Corydalis yanhusuo	
Yi mu cao	Motherwort	Leonurus heterophyllus	
Yi yi ren	Coix	Coix lachryma jobi	
Yin guo ye	Ginkgo, leaf	Ginkgo biloba	
Yin yang huo	Epimedium	Epimedium grandiflorum	
Yu jin	Turmeric, tuber	Curcuma longa	haridra
Ze lan	Bugleweed	Lycopus lucidus	
Ze xie	Alisma	Alisma orientale	
		A. plantago-aquatica	
Zhi gan cao	Licorice, honey-fried	Blycyrrhiza uralensis	yashti madhu
Zhi shi	Citrus, immature bitter orange peel	Citrus reticulata	
Zhi zi	Gardenia	Gardenia jasminoides	

HERBS BY SANSKRIT NAME

SANSKRIT NAME	COMMON NAME	LATIN NAME	PIN YIN
Amla	Indian gooseberry	Emblica officinalis	
Amla vetasa	Yellow dock	Rumex crispus	
Amlavetasa	Rhubarb	Rheum palmatum	da huang
Ardraka	Ginger, fresh	Zingiberis officinalis	sheng jiang
Arjuna	Arjuna	Terminalia arjuna	
Ashwagandha	Ashwagandha	Withania somnifera	
Atasi	Feverfew	Tanacetum parthenium	
Atirasa	Dandelion	Taraxacum mongolicum	pu gong ying
Bhibitaki	a Myrobalan	Terminalia bellerica	
Bidari kand	Pueraria	Pueraria lobata	ge gen
Bola	Myrrh	Commiphora myrrha, C. molmol	mo yao
Brahmi	Gotu kola	Centella asiatica	luo de da
Daindhava	Myrrh	Commiphora myrrha, C. molmol	mo yao
Ela	Cardamom	Amomum villosum	sha ren
Eranda	Castor	Ricinus communis	bi ma zi
Gandana	Yarrow	Achillea millefolium	
Guggulu	Myrrh	Commiphora mukul	
Haridra	Turmeric, tubor	Curcuma longa	yu jin
Haritaki	a Myrobalan	Terminalia chebula	he zi
Hingu	Asafoetida	Ferula asafoetida	ai wei

SANSKRIT NAME	COMMON NAME	LATIN NAME	PIN YIN
Katphala	Bayberry	Myrica cerifera	
Katuki	Gentian	Gentiana spp.	long dan cao
Kirata	Gentian	Gentiana spp.	long dan cao
Kumari	Aloe	Aloe spps.	lu hui
Lasunam	Garlic	Allium sativum	da suan
Madhukam	Licorice, raw	Glycyrrhiza uralensis	gan cao
Mahdurika	Fennel	Foeniculum vulgare	xiao hui xiang
Mandukaparni	Gotu kola	Hydrocotyle asiatica	ji xue cao
Marich	Black pepper	Piper nigrum	hu jiao
Marichi-phalam	Cayenne	Capsicum anuum	
Methi	Fenugreek	Trigonella foenum-graecum	hu lu ba
Nimba	Neem	Azadirachta indica	
Nagadamani	Mugwort	Artemisia vulgaris	ai ye
Padmaka	Wild cherry	Prunus spp.	
Pushkaramula	Elecampane	Inula spp.	xuan fu hua
Putani	Mint	Mentha piperita	
Salai guggul	Frankincense	Boswellia serrata	
Shallaki	Frankincense	Boswellia carterii	ru xiang
Shatavari	Asparagus	Asparagus cochinchinensis	tian men dong
Sunthi	Ginger, dried	Zingiberis officinalis	gan jiang
Tagara	Valerian	Valeriana officinalis	
Trayamana	Gentian	Gentiana spp	long dan cao
Tumburu	Prickly Ash	Zanthoxylum spp.	chuan jiao
Twak	Cinnamon, bark	Cinnamomum cassia	rou gui
Vana-methika	Red clover	Trifolium pratense	
Vibhitaki	a Myrobalan	Terminalia belerica	
Yashti madhu	Licorice, honey-fried	Glycyrrhiza uralensis	zhi gan cao

Index

❧

About the Author

Lesley Tierra is a California State and nationally certified Acupuncturist and Herbalist, with a practice in Santa Cruz. She is a founding member of the American Herbalists Guild and is the author of *The Herbs of Life* (Crossing Press, 1992), *Healing with Chinese Herbs* (Crossing Press, 1997), *A Kid's Herb Book* (Robert D. Reed Publishers, 2000) and coauthor of *Chinese Traditional Herbal Medicine Volumes I and II* with Michael Tierra (Lotus Press, 1998).

Lesley has taught Traditional Chinese Medicine healing theory and techniques and herbology throughout the United States and England since 1983. She and her husband, Michael Tierra, are available for consultations, via email or phone, and include TCM diagnosis along with dietary, lifestyle and herbal remedies. To contact call: (831)429-8066, or email/website: www. planetherbs.com.

A Kid's Herb Book, by Lesley Tierra, is an engaging and creative presentation for teaching herbs to children. Eighteen herbs are covered along with kitchen medicines, herbal first aid, herbal tea parties, medicinal flowers, kids gardens, plant ecology and much more.

Lesley collaborated with Michael Tierra to produce the **East West Herb Course** and is its Dean. Two home study courses in herbal medicine are available by correspondence:

The Home Study Course in Herbal Medicine includes 12 lessons and presents the essential principles of herbs including diet, energies, tastes and the elements of disease and diagnosis for the application of herbs encompassing the Western, Ayurvedic and Chinese medical systems. Herbal preparations, formulary and therapeutics are included.

The Professional Herbalist Course includes more advanced studies in Traditional Chinese diagnosis, herbal medicine and treatment covering: 1) the first 12 lessons of *The Home Study Course in Herbal Medicine*; 2) an extensive and comprehensive Materia Medica; 3) clinical diagnosis of specific diseases and the maintenance of health. On completion you have the option of taking a final examination which, when successfully completed, awards a certificate of completion for studies with Dr. Michael Tierra, Master Herbalist, C.A., O.M.D.

East West Herb School *website: www.planetherbs.com*

Consultations, Planetary Formulas, Tapes, *East West Herb Course, A Kid's Herb Book*

P.O. Box 275, Ben Lomond, CA 95005; (831)336-5010; (800)717-5010